# DOCUMENTS CONCERNING CENTRAL EUROPE FROM THE HOSPITAL'S RHODIAN ARCHIVES, 1314–1428

*Documents Concerning Central Europe from the Hospital's Rhodian Archives, 1314–1428* brings together over 450 texts concerning the Hospitallers during the fourteenth and fifteenth centuries.

These texts are crucial sources for understanding the history of the Hospitallers between 1314 and 1428. Whilst some Hospitaller charters and letters have been published elsewhere, few scholarly editions contain enough sources to permit close analysis of the language and contents of these documents. Moreover, most previous editions focus on certain geographical areas, such as Cyprus, Rhodes and the Aegean Islands. In contrast, this book is the first of its kind to focus on central Europe. It brings together 460 texts dated between 1314 to 1428, and two from 1461.

This book will appeal to scholars and students of medieval history and the history of Central Europe, as well as those interested in the legal structures and personal networks within the Order of St. John.

**Karl Borchardt** is Research Fellow at the Monumenta Germaniae Historica in Munich, Germany.

# THE MILITARY RELIGIOUS ORDERS: HISTORY, SOURCES AND MEMORY

Edited by Jochen Burgtorf and Nicholas Morton

The military religious orders were initially established in the twelfth century to care for and protect Western pilgrims in the Holy Land. They later helped to defend the crusader states, participated in the Iberian Reconquista and eventually played a significant role in warfare, charity, commerce, colonization and cross-cultural encounters in Europe, the Mediterranean World and even the New World. *The Military Religious Orders: History, Sources and Memory* stimulates research on this fascinating phenomenon.

# DOCUMENTS CONCERNING CENTRAL EUROPE FROM THE HOSPITAL'S RHODIAN ARCHIVES, 1314–1428

*Edited by Karl Borchardt*

Routledge
Taylor & Francis Group
LONDON AND NEW YORK

First published 2021
by Routledge
2 Park Square, Milton Park, Abingdon, Oxon OX14 4RN

and by Routledge
605 Third Avenue, New York, NY 10017

First issued in paperback 2022

*Routledge is an imprint of the Taylor & Francis Group, an informa business*



*British Library Cataloguing-in-Publication Data*
A catalogue record for this book is available from the British Library

*Library of Congress Cataloging-in-Publication Data*
Names: Borchardt, Karl, editor. | Luttrell, Anthony, 1932–
Title: Documents concerning Central Europe from the Hospital's Rhodian Archives : 1314-1428 / edited by Karl Borchardt in collaboration with Anthony Luttrel.
Description: Abingdon, Oxon ; New York, NY : Routledge, 2021. | Series: The military religious orders: history, sources, and memory | Includes bibliographical references and index.
Identifiers: LCCN 2020027912 (print) | LCCN 2020027913 (ebook) | ISBN 9780367139834 (hardback) | ISBN 9780429029523 (ebook)
Subjects: LCSH: Hospitalers. | Europe, Central—History—15th century. | Rhodes (Greece)—History.
Classification: LCC BX2825 .D63 2021 (print) | LCC BX2825 (ebook) | DDC 271/.7912—dc23
LC record available at https://lccn.loc.gov/2020027912
LC ebook record available at https://lccn.loc.gov/2020027913

ISBN: 978-0-367-63372-1 (pbk)
ISBN: 978-0-367-13983-4 (hbk)
ISBN: 978-0-429-02952-3 (ebk)

DOI: 10.4324/9780429029523

Typeset in Bembo
by Apex CoVantage, LLC

# CONTENTS

# PREFACE

The present volume has a long history. The plan originated as a by-product of my PhD on ecclesiastical institutions in Rothenburg ob der Tauber which was published in 1988. This imperial town in Franconia had two commanderies, one of the Teutonic Order and one of the Hospital. Research on the Teutonic Order in Central Europe abounded, whereas scholarly publications on the Hospital in these regions were rare. In 1987/1988 Anthony Luttrell received a Humboldt prize and came to Würzburg. In the seminars of my supervisor, Peter Herde, he started teaching German students Hospitaller history. The Rhodian documents we read were virtually unknown at this time, at least among German scholars. So the idea was born to have an edition that would benefit both historians of the Hospital and regional historians in Central Europe. From then on I profited greatly from Tony's expertise. Several times we met in the National Library of Malta. He introduced me to that place which is central for all Hospitaller studies. A first version of the present volume was produced. The texts concerning the Priory of Bohemia were made accessible to Libor Jan, his colleagues and students at Brno, and they were used by Jiří Mitáček in his 2005 PhD. Together with Anthony Luttrell and Ekhard Schöffler, another student of Peter Herde, I was honoured to publish Rhodian documents concerning Cyprus in 2011. Tony read the Manosque accounts from the 1280s, which Damien Carraz, Alain Venturini and myself published in 2015. I read some difficult Latin texts for the Rhodian countryside, which Anthony Luttrell and Gregory O'Malley published in 2019. Now Tony has read again the present volume. It owes a lot to his expertise. All remaining mistakes and deficiencies remain of course exclusively my own fault. But without Tony's advice many problems of Hospitaller history would have escaped my notice. In sum, one can say that the present volume would be impossible without the initiative and counsel of Anthony Luttrell and without the time and energy he spent on discussing many problems.

Thanks are also due to many others. The list of scholars from whose publications and expertise I have profited greatly could be long. Only pars pro toto I would like to mention Libor Jan in the Czech Republic, in Poland Maria Starnawska and many colleagues from the Ordines Militares at Toruń, and Johannes

A. Mol for the Netherlands. Special thanks are also due to the National Library of Malta and its staff. Time and again they made it possible for me to see the volumes and to obtain copies. Last but not least, thanks are due to the series editors and to Routledge for having the courage to accept an edition of sometimes long and complicated Latin texts. Nevertheless, these texts are basic both for Hospitaller and for regional history. And I hope they will be used as source materials for further research on these two subjects.

Karl Borchardt, Munich

# GLOSSARY

***ancianitas*:** seniority valid for promotion in the Hospital

***auberge*:** the house or room where the brethren of a tongue meet for their assemblies

***baiulia* or bailiwick, *baiulus* or bailiff:** generally any office or officer in the Hospital, then any preceptory and preceptor, in a narrow sense the Conventual bailiwicks or bailiffs of Admiral, Drapier, Turcopolier, etc., finally, in the Empire north of the Alps, regional sub-divisions, especially of the Priories of Alamania and Bohemia, such as Brandenburg, Cologne, Westphalia etc.

***camera* or chamber:** any office or preceptory that owes an annual pension payment to the prior or to the Master; hence *camerarius* or chamberlain: the ruler of a *camera*

***capellanus* or chaplain:** fully professed member and ordained cleric Hospital; some of them were the Master's chaplains

***capitulum* or chapter:** any formal meeting of brethren, in a house, a bailiwick, a priory or in the Convent

***capitulum generale* or chapter general:** assembly of the Master with representatives both of the Convent and of brethren living outside the Convent, supreme legislative institution for the Order; hence capitular bailiffs: appointed on the chapter general

***commendator* or commander and *commendaria* or commandery:** synonyms for preceptor and preceptory

***conventus* or Convent:** the Hospital's central headquarters, at Rhodes from 1309 to 1522, or the corporation of brethren in this headquarters, empowered to act together with the Master in important matters, hence Conventual bailiffs: appointed by the Master and Convent

***esgardia*:** lawsuits between brethren and the case law based on sentences in such lawsuits

***familiaris* or familiar:** person living in the Master's household, or at least having the privileges of such a person

***iocalia* or jewels:** precious objects in the personal possession of a Hospitaller, after his death usually due to the Treasury

***langue* or tongue:** the corporation of the brethren in the Convent who came from the same province

***membrum* or member:** revenues belonging to a preceptory but allotted to the upkeep of a Hospitaller who was not the preceptor; the person in charge of the member paid his responsions to the preceptor, not directly to the prior

***mortuarium*:** revenues for the remainder of the current financial year following an office holder's death, usually due to the Treasury; see *vacantia*

***passagium*:** travelling to the Convent by ship for the first time with horse and armour or the monies paid for this

***pilerius* or *pilier*:** the head or senior member of a tongue

***pitancia*, literally consolation:** Western revenues for mainaining brethren of a tongue in the Convent

***plancta*:** claim, action

***preceptor* or preceptor and *preceptoria* or preceptory:** the basic unit for the administration of the Order's possessions, synonyms for commander and commandery

***prioratus* or priory and *prior* or prior:** some 20 Western administrative divisions; also used for the senior priest or the head of the priests in a Hospitaller house, including the prior of the Conventual church on Rhodes who was the supreme priest of the Hospital

***proceres*:** experienced and respected brethren of the Order

***procrassia*, from *procrassium*, also *procassium*:** here probably death duties

**province:** one of seven, since 1462 eight, Western regions from which brethren went to the Convent, grouping several priories

***rauba*:** valuable objects, moveable assets, household furniture, clothes

***receptor* or receiver:** officer for collecting monies, including the Receiver General of the Treasury and the usually two receivers in any priory

***responsiones* or responsions:** annual payments from preceptories, priories and other possessions of the Hospital to the Treasury

***retentus ad manus*, retention:** a brother, preceptory or priory under the Master's special protection

***socius*:** a familiar of the Master charged with duties in the Master's personal service

***spolia*:** effects, monies and other assets of a deceased Hospitaller, normally due to the Treasury

***stagia*, from *stagium* dwelling-place:** maintenance for a Hospitaller according to his rank, including a room, food and drink, clothing and the obligation to be obedient to the local superior

***status*:** the buildings, animals and other possessions belonging to a preceptory or other office which preceptors or officers were not allowed to diminish

***taille* or tax:** imposition on Hospitaller possessions in order to pay for a special purpose

***thesaurus* or Treasury and *thesaurarius* or Treasurer:** the office and officer responsible for collecting and spending the revenues of the Convent, sometimes also revenues of the Master

***vacantia* (neuter plural):** revenues for one whole financial year usually starting on 24 June after the office holder's death, and usually due to the Treasury; see *mortuarium*

***visitator* or visitor:** an officer commissioned to inspect, control and reform priories and preceptories

# EDITORIAL SYMBOLS AND ABBREVIATIONS

| | |
|---|---|
| AOM | Malta, Archivum Ordinis Melitensis |
| Dig. | Digests (Corpus Iuris Civilis) |
| Extra | Liber Extra (Corpus Iuris Canonici) |
| (. . .) | ambiguous abbreviation |
| [. . .] | editorial addition |
| [!] | strange or unusual spelling |
| [?] | doubtful reading, editorial crux |
| . . . | blank space in the MS |
| <. . .> | passage omitted by the editor as irrelevant to Central Europe |
| add. | addidit |
| ante | corr. ante correctionem |
| del. | delevit |
| dupl. | duplicavit |
| expunct. | expunctio |
| in lin. | in linea |
| lac. | lacuna |
| lin. | linea |
| marg. | marginaliter |
| MS | manuscriptum |
| om. | omisit |
| post | corr. post correctionem |
| praem. | praemisit |
| ras. | rasura |
| recent. | recentior |
| supra lin. | supra lineam |
| tr. | transposuit |

# INTRODUCTION

The purpose of this book is to make accessible texts from Hospitaller Rhodes, which concern Central Europe and which are today preserved on Malta in the Hospital's Rhodian archives. Between 1309 and 1522 the Order of the Hospital of St. John of Jerusalem had its headquarters on Rhodes. This island in the Dodecanese was strategically situated on important crossroads of the Eastern Mediterranean, from Constantinople to Egypt and from Europe to the Holy Land. The military-religious order was in a good position there to fight against Muslims, Turks from Asia Minor and Mamluks in Egypt and Syria. Moreover, on Rhodes it could support Western pilgrims on their way to the Holy Land. After the loss of Acre in 1291, the Hospital and many other refugees had moved to Cyprus, but the Hospitallers faced difficulties with the king of Cyprus, and Rhodes had the great advantage that there was no secular lord who might interfere in the Order. So the Hospital's central Convent was permanently established on Rhodes, with perhaps about 200 to 400 brethren from Europe organised in seven, and after 1462 eight, tongues.[1] The Master lived on Rhodes, although sometimes he was absent on business in the West. Men and monies from the Hospital's Western possessions were indispensable for the defence of the Rhodian headquarters. Master and Convent tried hard to ensure that their Western possessions did in fact contribute to their pious and religiously meritorious Eastern duties. As a consequence, documents from Rhodes provide us with many insights into what happened in the West. For studying Hospitaller properties and activities throughout Latin Europe, those Rhodian sources should not be neglected. In order to better understand and interpret these documents, some introductory remarks may be helpful concerning the sources used, the administrative traditions of

1 These tongues were Provence, Auvergne, *Francia*, *Hispania*, Italy, England, *Alamania*. Only in 1462 *Hispania* was divided into (1) Aragón, comprising Aragón, Catalonia and Navarre, and (2) Castile, comprising Castile-León and Portugal: Stabilimenta (2007), 194. For the provinces see note 5 below.

the Hospital,[2] especially as far as Central Europe was concerned, and what one might call Hospitaller diplomatics, that is the way in which the texts were phrased and used.

## Sources

When the Hospitallers surrendered Rhodes to the Ottomans in 1522, they were permitted to leave the island with some of their moveables, including parchments and papers that were considered to be important for the future in this dramatic moment. These remnants of the Rhodian archives finally reached Malta,[3] where the Master and Convent resided from 1530 until 1798. Most financial accounts from Rhodes are today missing,[4] possibly because account books were held to be dispensable when the survivors left Rhodes on ships early in 1523. Apart from original charters which the Hospitallers had been granted, the bulk of the Rhodian parchments, papers and books consisted of registers of the Master and Convent and the acts of the Master's council. These latter acts now begin only in 1460 and are therefore outside the time frame of this publication. Moreover, it would be difficult to look for entries concerning Central Europe there, because the acts of the council are arranged chronologically.

The annual registers of Master and Convent or *Libri Bullarum*, however, were usually arranged in geographical order, according to the Western priories of the Hospital. There was a correlation between these priories and the *langues* or tongues to which most brethren in the Convent belonged; in the documents the term *capitulum provinciale* refers to prioral chapters; modern historians conveniently speak of seven, after 1468 of eight, provinces, one for each tongue.[5] For the present publication, the sections devoted to *Alamania* and Bohemia in the registers were closely studied. Their headings were *prioratus Alamanie, Boemie et partium aliarum Alamanie*,[6] meaning that the Tongue of *Alamania* was

2 Unfortunately, a critical edition of the medieval Hospitaller laws is still missing; but see Estatutos (2006), Stabilimenta (2007). AOM 64 no. 2 contains statutes in French of 1344; on the back in contemporary hand, readable with lamp, it says: *pro priore Boemie*. Thanks for this are due to Anthony Luttrell.

3 Prutz (1883); Mager (2014), 38–40; Luttrell (2017).

4 On exceptions, cf. Luttrell (1999), article XI.

5 In the *Libri Bullarum* and with reference to the tongues as in note 1 these were (1) Saint-Gilles, Toulouse. (2) Auvergne. (3) *Francia*, Champagne, Aquitaine. (4) Venice, Lombardy, Pisa, Rome, Hungary (early in the fourteenth century and again after the 1370s), Capua, Barletta, Messina. (5) Amposta (for Aragón), Catalonia and Navarre, Castile-León and Portugal, (6) England, Ireland, Scotland (usually omitted), (7) *Alamania*, Bohemia, Hungary (for some time up to the 1370s), *Dacia* (usually omitted in the *Libri Bullarum*). In Italy, there were five capitular preceptories, Santo Stefano di Monopoli, Venosa, Alife, Naples and Sant'Eufemia.

6 Cf. AOM 316 and 317. AOM 318 had *prioratus Boemie* on fol. 146r (138r) without any entries and *prioratus Alamanie et aliarum partium Alamanie* on fol. 150r (142r).

also responsible for Bohemia and other parts such as, for instance, *Dacia* or Hungary. Poland was considered to be part of the Priory of Bohemia; the term *Polonia* usually referred to Silesia, a country ruled by the King of Bohemia. From the register for 1365/6 to 1366/67 (AOM 319) onwards the standard heading was *prioratus Alamanie et Boemie.*

The Priory of Hungary could be seen either as an extension of Central Europe or of Northern Italy. In the *Libri Bullarum* Hungary was listed in the headings together with *Alamania* and Bohemia in AOM 324, 326, 327, 328, 329 and 330; in 327, however, Hungary was crossed out again.[7] Later on, Hungary was always listed in the headings together with the priories of Venice, Lombardy, Pisa and Rome. This had its political background in the quarrels between members of the house of Anjou in Provence, Naples and Hungary. In 1373 a compromise was mediated between the Tongues of Italy and of Provence over the priories and capitular preceptories in Southern Italy. It included a clause that the Prior of Hungary should alternate between the Tongues of Provence and of Italy.[8] There were examples of documents being entered under a wrong heading: AOM 348 fol. 129v (127v), under *prioratus Alamanie, Boemie,* has the appointment of Fr. *Bertonus ex marchionibus Ceue,* the 'marchese di Ceva' on the borders between Piedmont and Liguria, as procurator in the Priory of Lombardy, dated Rhodes, 1428 May 28, and an amicable agreement between two brethren from Catalonia, Fr. Lluís Mur and Fr. Lluís de Gualbes, Rhodes, 1428 August 17; this latter document, but not the former one, was cancelled with strokes. In view of this fact it cannot be excluded that the present edition may have missed a few documents for Central Europe in the *Libri Bullarum* which so far have not been exhaustively calendared.[9]

The registers included copies, abbreviated copies and sometimes just short notes of documents. It is not sure that for all these notes there were originals that left the Hospitaller chancery. Nor is it sure that all originals that left Rhodes were copied into the registers. The fact that documents were not copied in full explains why today they are hardly understandable without some knowledge of the Hospitaller formularies. The extant *Libri Bullarum* start in the middle of the fourteenth century. The first two volumes are AOM 317 for 1347/8 and AOM 318 for 1351/2. In the series they are preceded by AOM 316 that starts with 1346/7 and continues with the two years from 1357/1358 to 1358/1359. The Rhodian chancery started its year on the feast of the Annunciation on 25 March and followed the *calculus Florentinus,* so it always included the days from 1 January to 24 March of the following year. As a rule, each volume

7 AOM 327 fol. 103r (92r).

8 1373 November 22, AOM 347 fol. 51r–v, ed. Bosio (1629), 116; Hunyadi (2020), 321–2 no. 49, a notarial document. Three members of the Tongue of *Alamania* were among the witnesses, Fr. Hesso Schlegelholz, Fr. Helfrich von Rüdigheim and Fr. Franchus Langus. See Sarnowsky, Macht (2001), 94–5, and Hunyadi (2010), 85–91 on the last native Hungarian prior, Fr. Janos Palisznai.

9 Calendar of Records (1964/90). See Sarnowsky, Macht (2001), 307–15.

covered one or sometimes two years.[10] It should be noted that errors occurred: No. 172 reads 23 January 1390 and was 1391, as were the preceding and following documents, and the true date is therefore 23 January 1392. No. 369 clearly says 1418, but from the itinerary of the Master it must be 1419. The extant *Libri Bullarum* have an old numeration,[11] but it is not sure whether the numbers go back to Rhodian times. It is unclear how far the *Libri Bullarum* reached back to the period before 1346/47. At any rate, the series marks a thorough reorganisation of the Hospitaller headquarters from the times when many of the Templars' possessions were absorbed by their major surviving rival.

The *Libri Bullarum* are also incomplete today[12] for the period here under consideration, and this raises the question whether the losses occurred already on Rhodes or after 1523. On 15 August 1365 Fr. Bernhard von Chotek asked the new Master Fr. Raymond Bérenger for a copy of his appointment to the preceptories of Glatz and Ploskovice from the registers (*de cartulario*) of Master Fr. Roger des Pins, who had died on 28 May 1365, no. 77; so clearly there were volumes that are now lost.[13] Today there are gaps for the five years from 1359/60 to 1364/5, then again for the whole period between 1367/8 and 1380/1, that is for 14 years, though there is AOM 320, an exceptional volume that starts in 1374 when Fr. Robert de Juilly was elected Master. At that time he was in France and began to register his documents in chronological order. On Rhodes this was not continued. During the papal schism there were for a time two rival Masters, one supporting the pope in Avignon and one the pope in Rome, but at the same time there was only one functioning Convent on Rhodes where the brethren were anxious not to commit themselves too clearly, because one part was always in danger of losing the support of their relatives and their possessions in the West. For the Urbanist or Roman Master Fr. Riccardo Caracciolo there is only AOM 281, a volume that was not included in the *Libri Bullarum*, probably because its contents were mainly acts of chapter or chapter general of Urbanist Hospitallers. All extant volumes in the *Libri Bullarum* series are from the old, now Clementist or Avignonese Master Fr. Juan Fernández de Heredia, who had few adherents in Central Europe. His successor Fr. Philibert de Naillac took a more neutral position similar to

10 Exceptions are three years AOM 322, 333, 338, 343, eight years AOM 339 and nine years AOM 337.

11 Used for instance by Delaville (1913). In order to check his references, it may be convenient to have the modern numbers here: No. 1 = AOM 316, 2 = 317, 3 = 318, 4 = 319, 5 = 320, 6 = 321, 7 = 322, 8 = 323, 9 = 324, 10 = 325, 11 = 326, 12 = 327, 13 = 328, 14 = 329, 15 = 330, 16 = 331, 17 = 332, 18 = 333, 19 = 334, 20 = 335, 21 = 336, 22 = 337, 23 = 338, 24 = 339, 25 = 339, 25 = 340, 26 = 341, 27 = 342, 28 = 343, 29 = 344, 30 = 345, 31 = 346, 32 = 347, 33 = 348.

12 Luttrell (1978), articel III, 65–7; Luttrell (1999), article XIX, 210, 220–1; Luttrell (2017). No. 293 mentioned a document from 3 December 1412 that so far has not been found in the extant volumes.

13 For a now lost fragment until recently preserved in AOM 348 fol. 140, cf. Luttrell (2007), article XXI. See also Luttrell (2017), 44.

that of the Convent. From 1409 onwards he adhered to the Pisan obedience and attended the Council of Constance between 1414 and 1418. While he was in the West, that is from 1409 to 1420, two sets of registers were kept, one set by Fr. Philibert in the West[14] and one by his Lieutenant and the Convent on Rhodes.[15]

The many scribes whose hands can be seen in the *Libri Bullarum* had to finish their work as soon as possible and to save space. So they abbreviated many standard formulae with *etcetera*, or sometimes with *ut supra*.[16] Often, especially when recording standard licences, they just noted the date and the major contents. No. 151 is a striking example of a very short note. Documents with the same contents that were sent out to, for instance, all priors, all receivers or all visitors were copied once in the *Liber Bullarum* and only mentioned in the other sections.[17] It remains an open question how complete registration was. No attempt is here made to retrieve Rhodian originals, or copies made from such originals, in the recipients' archives. It should also be noted that the documents do not reflect every activity of the Master concerning Central Europe. In 1417 for instance, in a quarrel concerning the cemetery at Neuenburg, the Master Fr. Philibert de Naillac defended Fr. Heinrich Boes of Neuenburg, whose right to bury inhabitants of the local parish on the Hospitaller cemetery was denied by the local parson.[18]

## Geography and prosopography

Hospitaller possessions in Central Europe were organised in houses in which a usually small number of brethren lived; preceptories, which were governed by preceptors who paid responsions; bailiwicks, whose bailiffs oversaw a regional group of preceptories; and finally into the two priories of *Alamania* and Bohemia.[19] In Central Europe many preceptors would be appointed by the prior with the advice of senior brethren in his annual chapter, in principle based on the *ancianitas* or seniority of the possible candidates.[20] It could be the first appointment of a brother, his *cabimentum*, or if he had already served as a successful

14 AOM 334 for two years 1407/8–8/9, AOM 335 for 1409/10, AOM 336 for 1410/11, then AOM 337 for 1408/9–16/17 and AOM 338 for 1413/14–15/16, partially simultaneous. The itinerary of Naillac has been compiled by Delaville (1913), 383–6.

15 AOM 339 for 1409/10–15/16, AOM 340 and 341 for 1416/17–17/18.

16 For example, no. 115.

17 In a few cases the present publication edits both the note concerning *Alamania* or Bohemia and the document that was directed with the same contents to another priory.

18 Two documents dated Constance, 1417 July 1, and Constance, 1417 October 19, *Urkunden Stadt Neuenburg* 2 (2019), 91–2 no. 857, 94–5 no. 859, issued by the papal penitentiary and by the vicar general of the bishop of Constance respectively. Thanks for this reference are due to Philipp Wollmann, Munich.

19 On *Alamania*, Klein (1922); Rödel (1972); Wienand (1988); Luttrell (1999), article XII; on Bohemia, Novotný (1900); Svátek (1970); Jan and Jesenský (1998); Mitáček (2005).

20 Bonneaud (2007), 222–9.

administrator, his *melioramentum*. In reality this legal framework was often overlaid by social and political networks which historians can only rarely detect.

Preceptories could have sub-divisions. Certain houses or other possessions might owe their responsions to a neighbouring preceptory. They would then be called a *membrum* of this preceptory. In 1420 Hagenau was elevated from being a *membrum* of Dorlisheim to the status of an independent preceptory, no. 381. The Treasury on Rhodes kept a list, and in 1428 it was found *ex registris responsionum communis thesauri* that Regensburg was not a *membrum* but an independent preceptory because it paid its responsions independently; so Fr. Anton Knoblauch was to be inducted into its possession as an independent preceptor, no. 459. One consequence was that the *mortuarium* and the *vacantia* would only be paid from an independent preceptory, not from a member, no. 409.

Hospitallers who served in the Convent on Rhodes expected to be rewarded. They might get a preceptory in the West or even a priory. The ways in which priors came into office deserve comparative studies. For *Alamania* and Bohemia there was the problem that so few brethren from Central Europe were present on Rhodes. The Master with the Convent could grant a priory, in principle following the suggestions of the tongue to which the priory belonged. The documents here edited, however, prove that the priories of *Alamania* and Bohemia were often only confirmed to brethren who had already been elected priors in *Alamania* or Bohemia, either for ten years or for their lifetime.[21] But there were few brethren from *Alamania* on Rhodes. After the death of Fr. Konrad von Braunsberg in 1390, *Alamania* was coveted, at that time in Germany, by Fr. Friedrich von Zollern, who secured an appointment as Heredia's lieutenant, no. 172, then, in the Convent, by Fr. Hesso Schlegelholz; the real successor, however, became Fr. Henman zu Rhein. The networks of the Oberland region dominated the Hospital in Germany. So the chapter general at Aix in 1410 followed a statute concerning such cases and agreed that the prior might be elected in future in the priory itself, no. 237. For Bohemia there were even fewer brethren on Rhodes. In 1422, after the death of Fr. Heinrich von Neuhaus, his successor Fr. Duke Rupert of Silesia was confirmed on Rhodes, but the Tongue of *Alamania* protested in order to safeguard its rights for the future.[22] In both *Alamania* and Bohemia secular powers had a long tradition of trying to influence the appointment of priors, for the simple reason that these posts were powerful and influential.[23]

For preceptories, the situation was comparable. On behalf of the brethren in the Convent, the Master tried to assert his right to grant preceptories in the Western priories. The documents here edited include dozens of such grants and of confirmations of preceptories, for ten years or for life. The Prior of *Alamania* could only grant preceptories for ten years; but in 1415 no. 299 permitted him to grant preceptories for life. Naturally, brethren in the West were loath to accept

21 Nos. 109, 116, 129, 241, 291, 301.

22 Nos. 411–2.

23 Borchardt (1999).

long-time absentees as their fellow preceptors, so that quarrels about preceptories were not infrequent. An interesting example was Fr. Peter Mersner. In 1408 he was granted for ten years the Preceptory of Rothenburg, no. 213. At that time he was on Rhodes and received a licence to travel to the West, no. 219. In 1411, on Rhodes, he was granted the Preceptory of Reichardsroth, 10 km north of Rothenburg, and received again a licence to travel to the West, nos. 248–9. For Rothenburg, the Prior of *Alamania* had meanwhile appointed two co-preceptors, Fr. Peter Salzfaß and Fr. Johann Jagstheimer, the latter from a local family. They argued that they had spent monies to improve the *status* of this preceptory and could not be removed without a financial compensation. In Constance, during the years 1417 and 1418, Fr. Peter Mersner quarrelled with them, nos. 338 and 341. In 1419 he secured a licence to travel to the Convent, accompanying the Master Naillac, and to rent out Rothenburg for three years, nos. 362–3. But his quarrels with his two opponents continued, nos. 370–72. In fact, he never actually got Rothenburg. In 1427 he resigned both Rothenburg and Reichardsroth and secured a grant of the two preceptories of Erdlingen and Hemmendorf, nos. 417–18. He may have got Erdlingen, but not Hemmendorf.[24] In 1428 he pursued a claim to Altmühlmünster near Regensburg, no. 459. Such events illustrate typical difficulties in implementing Rhodian decisions in the West.

Some preceptories were *camere* or chambers for which their preceptor owed an annual payment that was called a pension to either the prior or the Master: Each Western prior held the right himself to choose four, and after 1367 five, chambers in his priory by himself. Moreover the Master held the right to choose one chamber in each priory. According to no. 66, Fr. Hugo von Werdenberg, Prior of *Alamania*, did not have a chamber in 1358 and was permitted to use the Preceptory of Dorlisheim as his chamber. Apparently it was not easy and took some time until chambers became standard practice. A few decades after 1358 the situation was clearer. In *Alamania* the *camere priorales* were Bubikon, Cologne, Klingnau, Rheinfelden and Utrecht, in Bohemia Prague, Dub, Manětin, Ploskovice and Uhřiněves. But the places could be changed. When Rheinfelden burnt down, the prior was permitted to replace it with another preceptory in 1410, no. 235.[25] In 1400 Frankfurt and its member Mosbach were declared to be the fifth chamber of the Prior of *Alamania*, no. 188.[26]

24 Stälin (1883), 109; Borchardt (1988), 532–3 nos. 119, 123–4.

25 Fr. Henman zu Rhein, Prior of *Alamania* from 1408 to 1411, had held both Basel and Rheinfelden since 1389. Afterwards Rheinfelden became a *membrum* of Basel: Helvetia Sacra (2006), 419–20; this publication did not know document no. 235 and the fire in Rheinfelden.

26 In 1495 the five prioral chambers were Utrecht, Cologne, Heimbach, Bubikon (with Wädenswil) and Leuggern, and the Grand Bailiff had four chambers, Frankfurt, Mainz, Burg an der Wupper and Duisburg: Helvetia Sacra (2006), 42, 137; Ahn (2006), 34–5, who says Luzern for Leuggern. On account of conflicts with both the bishop of Constance and the town of Klingnau the Prior Fr. Hugo von Montfort left that place in about 1415, when the Swiss conquered it, and went to live in Leuggern: Helvetia Sacra (2006), 341. The distance was only about 5 kilometres, but Klingnau was situated east, Leuggern west of the River Aare.

The *camere magistrales* were Buchsee in *Alamania* and Tinz in Bohemia. In 1383 Buchsee was replaced by Sulz, both by the Master Fr. Juan Fernández de Heredia, no. 107, and in 1385 by his rival Master Fr. Riccardo Caracciolo, no. 151. But this was apparently revoked when Fr. Dietrich von Keppenbach was no longer the preceptor or chamberlain.[27] The preceptors of the *camere* could be called *camerarii* or chamberlains and owed an annual pension from their revenues, the *camere priorales* to the prior and the *camere magistrales* to the Master. For Buchsee this pension was reduced from 300 to 200 florins a year in 1358 during the lifetime of the Preceptor Fr. Dietrich von Keppenbach (nos. 35, 86). For Tinz in 1414: 50 florins were due each year, no. 288. In 1384 an unnamed chamber in *Alamania*, probably Buchsee, owed 300 florins of Germany to the Master, no. 132.[28]

This rather elaborate organisation came into being in the early fourteenth century after the Hospitallers had taken over a large part of the Templar possessions, and it remained basically unchanged until the eighteenth century. Hospitaller documents from Rhodes rarely used Latin translations for the German terms *Komtur* and *Kommende*, as for example no. 449, but preferred *preceptor* and *preceptoria*. The similar terms *baiulus* or bailiff and *baiulia* or bailiwick were frequently used on Rhodes with many different meanings; it seems that they could refer to almost any officer and any office. The two Central European priories were divided into regional bailiwicks with bailiffs, eight for *Alamania* and four for Bohemia.[29] This was not unique. At any rate there were also bailiwicks for Flanders, under the Priory of *Francia*, and for Lorraine, under the Priory of Champagne. In general bailiwicks could be an imperial or Central European peculiarity, perhaps because the Teutonic Order had many *Balleien* ruled by *Landkomturen*.[30] The following Hospitaller places are mentioned in the documents here edited:

*Alamania*: (1) Oberland[31] with Basel,[32] Bruchsal, Bubikon,[33] Buchsee, Colmar, Dätzingen, Dorlisheim, Feldkirch,[34] Freiburg im Breisgau,[35] Freiburg im Üchtland, Hagenau, Heimbach,[36] Heitersheim, Hemmendorf, Hohenrain,

27 After 1407: no. 210. In 1477 Buchsee was again a *camera magistralis*: Helvetia Sacra (2006), 387–8 with note 49.

28 In 1469 and in 1540 Cologne owed 150 florins: Ahn (2006), 36.

29 Borchardt, Soll-Zahlen (2003); Dauber (1998).

30 Militzer (1970) and (2011).

31 For Alsace, Buchheit, *Commanderies* (2014); for the preceptories in the Grand Duchy of Baden, Krieger (1904/05); for the Kingdom of Württemberg, Stälin (1883); for the Breisgau, Maurer (1978); for modern Switzerland, Zeininger de Borja (1946); *Helvetia Sacra* (2006).

32 Wyss (1938).

33 Lehmann (1945/47).

34 Burmeister (1969).

35 Seitz (1910) und (1911).

36 Rödel (1973).

Klingnau, Küsnacht, Mainz,[37] Meisenheim, Mülhausen, Neuenburg, Rexingen, Rheinau, Rheinfelden, Rohrdorf, Rottweil,[38] Schlettstadt, Straßburg (Grünenwörth),[39] Sulz, Sulzbach, Tobel,[40] Überlingen, Villingen, Wädenswil,[41] Weisheim, Weißenburg (in Alsace), Worms.

(2) Franconia with Würzburg[42] plus Boxberg, Erdlingen, Hall, Krautheim, Kühndorf, Mergentheim, Münster, Regensburg, Reichardsroth, Rothenburg.[43]

(3) Thuringia with Weißensee.[44]

(4) Wetterau with Frankfurt plus Mosbach,[45] Rüdigheim and Weisel.[46]

(5) Cologne[47] with Adenau, Breisig and Mecheln[48] near Aachen.

(6) Westphalia with Steinfurt[49] plus Duisburg, Horst,[50] Lage,[51] Münster, Walsum and Wesel. The Frisian houses belonged to this bailiwick[52] but were not mentioned in the Rhodian documents here edited.

(7) Utrecht with Arnheim and Haarlem.[53]

(8) The north-eastern bailiwick was at first called Saxony, the March (of Brandenburg) and *Slavia* (*Wendland* in German). At the turn of the thirteenth to the fourteenth century Pomerania was added. After the Hospital took over many Templar possessions in the Neumark, the bailiwick became known as the *Ballei* of Brandenburg only.[54] The documents here edited mention Mirow and Nemerow in Mecklenburg, Quartschen in the Neumark and Rörchen in Pomerania, close to the borders of the Neumark.

*Bohemia*: (1) Bohemia proper with Prague, the capital of the country, and the castle of Strakonice, plus Dub, Glatz,[55] Manětin, Ploskovice, Uhřiněves and Zittau.

37 Dertsch (1962/67); Hartmann (1981).
38 Hecht (1971).
39 Prier et combattre (2009), 887–8.
40 Bühler (1985).
41 Ziegler (1987).
42 Hoh (1950), Thomas (1990).
43 Borchardt (1988).
44 This bailiwick was so small that eventually it was united with Franconia.
45 Dörr (1983).
46 Dersch (1915) and (1940).
47 Ahn (2006).
48 A village in Limburg, 13 km west of Aachen, not to be confounded with the homonymous town in the Burgundian Netherlands.
49 Regelmeier (1911); Schöningh (1974); Sgonina (2014).
50 Rödel (1972), 391–2, 35 km south of Münster near the river Lippe.
51 Borchardt and Luttrell (2013).
52 Schöningh (1973); Mol (2005) and (2008); Prier et combattre (2009), 371–2.
53 van Winter (1998).
54 Opgenoorth (1963); Hubatsch (1972); Borchardt (1998); Prier et combattre (2009), 172–4; Gahlbeck (2015) and (2016).
55 Sauermann (1909).

(2) Moravia with Brünn, Orlovice and perhaps Rumberg.[56]
(3) Poland, in fact Silesia with its capital Breslau plus Brieg, Löwenberg, Oels, Striegau and Tinz. Only Posen was situated outside Silesia, in Greater Poland.[57]
(4) Austria with the castle of Mailberg[58] and its capital Vienna plus Ebenfurt, Fürstenfeld in Styria and Pulst in Carinthia.

*Dacia* or Denmark was seldom mentioned in the *Libri Bullarum*.[59] Its status remained unclear. In the beginning it may have been regarded as a bailiwick, later on as a separate priory. The documents mention Andvorskov (on Zealand), Norway[60] and Eskilstuna[61] in Sweden, plus the estates at Maschenholz[62] on Rügen, an island that belonged to the Danish Diocese of Roskilde.

The importance of these bailiwicks varied. As a rule, each bailiff would be at the same time preceptor of a house in his bailiwick. In the documents here published bailiwicks in the Bohemian priory were never mentioned. In *Alamania* Oberland had a bailiff, but as the prior usually lived there, this bailiff was a more or less negligible figure. The two Bailiffs for Franconia and the Wetterau were mentioned once, no. 449. Cologne, Utrecht and Westphalia were more important. Their bailiffs were sometimes, though not always, preceptors of the houses of Cologne, Utrecht or Steinfurt respectively.[63] In 1422 no. 406 clearly stated the Fr. Johann von Monreal was both the Bailiff of Cologne and the Preceptor of Cologne, and no. 408 did the same for Fr. Johann Cruze as both Bailiff of Westphalia and Preceptor of Steinfurt. Moreover, both Cologne and Utrecht were prioral chambers. This meant that the preceptor, but not the bailiff, could also be called chamberlain and owed a pension payment to the prior. From the second half of the fourteenth century onwards the large north-eastern bailiwick secured for itself some sort of autonomy. Its Hospitallers formed their own networks, more or less detached from the Priory of *Alamania*.

The Tongue of *Alamania* always had only a limited number of brethren in the Convent. Compared with other tongues, they had little influence and were isolated because most of them could not understand Romance languages;[64] they were poorer than the English who had more estates at home to send

56 There were a castle and a small town called Rumberg, Czech Rumberk (Deštná), in Moravia, some 50 km north of Brünn. It is so far not known that the Hospitallers had possessions there.

57 Szczesniak (1969); Starnawska (1999); Smoliński (2008).

58 Lechner (1976).

59 Hatt Olsen (1962); Reitzel-Nielsen (1984/88); Nyberg (1985).

60 As in Sweden, there was only one Hospitaller house in Norway, Værne in the Østfold, about 60 km south of Oslo.

61 About 115 km west of Stockholm.

62 Today a deserted settlement 6 km west of Bergen: Büttner (2007), 206–7.

63 Ahn (2006), 30–4; Sgonina (2014), 30–2.

64 Stabilimenta (2007), 215 no. 2.29 stated that brethren were not allowed to have procurators in quarrels with other brethren, except the English and the Germans because they could not understand the language.

monies to Rhodes. The "province"[65] of *Alamania* included Bohemia and *Dacia*. There were few brethren from *Alamania*, even fewer from Bohemia and usually none from *Dacia* in the Convent. But some Germans were conspicuous, especially Fr. Albrecht von Schwarzburg (d. 1327), Preceptor of Cyprus, Grand Preceptor and then Visitor General in the West,[66] and much later Fr. Hesso Schlegelholz, Preceptor of Kos and Lieutenant Master,[67] and Fr. Johann von Ow, Preceptor of Cyprus. All other tongues had a Conventual bailiff;[68] *Alamania* secured such an office only in 1428, no. 435, the newly created Grand Bailiff.[69] The first holder of this office was Fr. Johann Schlegelholz, not by chance a relative of the late Fr. Hesso Schlegelholz. As Rhodes was always in need of brethren, they might be summoned to the Convent, or might be licensed to travel to the Convent. When brethren wanted to leave the Convent, for instance in order to govern their preceptory in the West, they needed a special licence that usually included a permission to return to the Convent.

The documents mention retentions, donats, familiars and chaplains. These legal concepts deserve further research. In Central Europe retention by the Master meant basically protection against the prior or other Hospitallers in the West. The usual incipit of such documents was *Dum laudabilia probitatis*. If a preceptor was retained, his retention included his preceptory, its members and the preceptor's harness. The retention would become invalid in the event that the responsions and other dues were not paid, no. 340. Some brethren from Central Europe were even accepted as familiars serving in the Master's household. Some of these were chaplains of the Master's household, some other servants. The chaplains of the Master are not to be confused with the ordinary chaplains of the Order who were clerics, some of them priests, and lived in houses of the Order.[70]

Many other Rhodian documents were licences,[71] among them licences to rent out a Western preceptory when its Preceptor served in the East.[72] Essential were licences to receive brethren into the Order and to assign them *stagia* or maintenance in one of the Western houses or preceptories. Usually Western preceptors wished to secure the upkeep of their servants. Sometimes service on Rhodes was rewarded with such maintenance. The *stagia* consisted of a room,

65 For the "provinces" of the tongues see notes 1 and 5.

66 Europäische Stammtafeln 1/3 (2000), no. 313; Prier et combattre (2009), 57.

67 Prier et combattre (2009), 433–4.

68 Provence: Grand Preceptor; Auvergne: Marshal; *Francia:* Hospitalier; Spain, from 1462 onwards Aragón: Drapier; Italy: Admiral; England: Turcopolier; *Alamania* in 1428: Grand Bailiff. In 1462 the new, eighth tongue, Castile, secured the Chancellor, an office that hitherto had not been held by a capitular bailiff.

69 On his duties, Stabilimenta (2007), 186–8 nos. 3.14–17.

70 On retentions and familiars, Sarnowsky, Macht (2001), 240–2, 264–7.

71 No. 6 to buy two houses on Rhodes; no. 165 to travel via Rhodes to the Holy Sepulchre; no. 122 to receive the parents' inheritance; nos. 134 and 458 to study canon law.

72 Several examples from nos. 362 to 458.

a bed, clothes, food and drink, hay, firewood and similar things, according to statutes of the Order or local customs. No members could be received into the Order without being granted maintenance at the same time.[73] Not only on Rhodes, but also in the West such orders[74] or licences to receive someone into the Order were eagerly coveted. In 1358 the Prior of Bohemia asked for a general licence to receive as many brethren into the Order as he needed. This was rejected; he was only permitted to receive one knight or sergeant if two died, nos. 54–5.

There were three classes of fully professed members of the Hospital, knights, clerics and sergeants. The clerics or chaplains could be priests and serve in parish churches which belonged to the Order. The sergeants could be sergeants-at-arms or sergeants-at-office. Some maintenance was also due for donats and sisters who also reckoned among members of the Order. The documents here edited do not mention any houses of Hospitaller sisters;[75] no. 335, however, confirms a foundation by a Hospitaller sister. It is not clear so far whether in Central Europe all sisters were fully professed. Those not fully professed were donats. According to no. 147, *Quia ex premio*, donats worked for the Order; they did not get maintenance, *stagia*, but only *victum et vestitum*, victuals and clothes, according to the established practice of the Hospitallers. In addition there were *confratres* and *consorores* of the Order. They were lay people who swore to the Holy Gospels that they would protect and defend the Order. In case they found out about any dangers or damages to the Hospital they had to inform the Hospitallers immediately. For their souls such *confratres* and *consorores* were granted participation in all religious merits that members of the Order had accumulated and would accumulate from its foundation to the end of the world. According to the formula with the incipit *Attendentes pie devotionis affectum* they would pay one pound of wax each year on 24 June, the feast of St. John the Baptist, no. 295.

## Monies

What Rhodes needed was not only men but also monies from the West. As a consequence, the Rhodian chancery issued orders to pay and quittances. The monies from Central Europe were usually florins and ducats. The documents mention florins of Germany, which soon became florins of the Rhine, florins of Hungary, then in Italy florins of Florence and ducats of Venice, finally on Rhodes florins of Rhodes. Exceptions were francs of gold in 1413, no. 269, and écus in 1419, no. 369. Transfer to Rhodes was difficult, costly and risky. Exchange rates varied according to the quality of the coins, their contents

73 In the same way no clerics could be granted higher orders: Extra 3.5.2, 3.5.4, 3.5.16.

74 Nos. 158, 163.

75 Houses of sisters existed in Frisia, Mol (2006).

of gold or silver. Occasionally, rates were mentioned, for example in 1382: 3,214.5 florins of Germany = 3,096.5 florins of Rhodes, no. 99; in 1413: 28 florins of the Rhine = 41 florins of Rhodes, no. 268, and 30 florins of the Rhine = 24 ducats of Venice, no. 347; in 1420: 36 ducats 2 aspers of Venice = 64 florins 18 aspers[76] of Rhodes, no. 396.[77] Hospitallers in Central Europe collected those monies they wanted to send to Rhodes in Flanders in 1347, no. 7, from *Dacia*, or at Frankfurt in 1383, no. 123. The transfer involved Italian bankers, from Venice or the Medici from Florence, who also worked for the papal curia. An alternative for Venice could be Lyons.[78]

Some sums were quite considerable. In 1351 Bohemia paid the Treasury 5,100 ducats, of which, however, 3,000 florins had to be deducted for paying debts of the Treasury (nos. 9, 12). In 1412 the Bodrum indulgence from Bohemia amounted to 1,090 florins, no. 261. While serving on Rhodes and holding Kos, in 1382 Fr. Hesso Schlegelholz received 3,214.5 florins of Germany, nos. 97, 99, 103–4. So Fr. Hesso could lend money to the Treasury, in 1383: 3,000 florins of Florence, no. 126, in 1402: 1,700 florins of Rhodes, nos. 193, 195. What Rhodes really wanted was a stable supply of monies from the West. Regular payments due to the brethren of one of the tongues in the Convent were known as *pitancia*. In 1391 one German brother on Rhodes got 20 florins a year (nos. 168–9). In 1402 the Pilier or head of the Tongue of *Alamania* received 166 florins of Germany (nos. 197–8), probably to support the other German brethren. The Tongue of *Alamania* on Rhodes may have been small, but it had its own *auberge*, its house or room where the brethren usually assembled.[79]

Compared with some other parts of the West, however, two points were remarkable: Central Europe did not always pay its dues with great discipline. And Central Europe was comparatively unimportant for the Convent. This can be seen from the taxes Pope John XXII imposed on the Western priories and capitular bailiwicks (here preceptories) in 1317 for repaying the Hospital's debts. These were for Bohemia, Moravia, Poland and Austria 1,000 florins, for *Alamania* 1,000 florins, for *Dacia*, Sweden and Norway together 100 marks.[80]

76 1 florin = 20 aspers.

77 For other rates, Spufford (1986), 125, 293–4, 319.

78 1413: no. 269. On merchants, Sarnowsky, Macht (2001), 333–4.

79 AOM 48 fol. 214v-16v: a document issued by Fr. Pierre de Culant, Lieutenant Master, 1386 January 12 (or 1387?, 8th indiction following the stilus of the Roman curia) that names Fr. *Herocichus de Witinders., pilerius albergie Alamanie*. There are other references to the piliers of the Tongue of *Alamania*, for example Fr. Ulrich, 1366 May 30, AOM 319 fol. 302r-3r.

80 Jean XXII (1904), nos. 4450–72. The other sums were much larger and in different currencies. One livre tournois had 20 sous or 240 deniers; in 1318 one florin of Florence was 15 sous 2 deniers at Avignon, Spufford (1986), 175. For Scandinavia it could be the mark of Lübeck that had 16 schilling or 192 pfennig. In 1317/20 the Roman curia took one florin as 12 schillings, Spufford (1986), 279.

Few accounts are extant from the Hospitallers themselves.[81] They confirm that the two Priories of *Alamania* and Bohemia owed only some 5% of the expected Western revenues, as in no. 89 from the year 1374, or a similar list from the year 1383: of 38,300 florins Bohemia was supposed to pay 1,200 florins;[82] *Alamania* was not mentioned, perhaps because Fr. Hesso Schlegelholz had already made a loan or gift to the Treasury. AOM 48 fol. 33v-4r contains accounts for 1379 and 1380, fol. 88v-89r, 118v and 122r for 1384 and 1385, fol. 147r for 1387, fol. 225v-6v for 1394 and 1395.[83] In 1380 the Prior of *Alamania* Fr. Konrad von Braunsberg paid 1,214 florins of the Rhine = 1,365 florins 9 gros current at Avignon and then 1,266 florins of the Rhine = 1,424 florins 3 gros current at Avignon, that is in sum 2,890 florins,[84] to the Treasurer Fr. Henri de Saint-Trond, through the hands of the Preceptor of Basel Fr. Werner von Eptingen. In the following years it was the Preceptor of Freiburg Fr. Hesso Schlegelholz who paid similar sums from Central Europe to the Treasury, through the hands of a merchant from Freiburg, Konrad Stobeker. Fr. Domenico d'Alamania, a Neapolitan, or Fr. Pierre de Provins received these payments for the Treasury.

The most important regular dues were the annual responsions.[85] They could be a considerable burden. In the 1360s and 1370s Bohemia owed 1,200 florins, several decades later 700 ducats of Venice or 500 florins of Hungary, nos. 82, 287, 312, 359; *Alamania* owed 1,000 florins, several decades later 500 ducats of Venice, no. 293.[86] In pre-Hussite times Bohemia was thought to be richer than *Alamania*. Arrears of responsions were a standard concern. For special purposes the Master and Convent could impose a *taille* or tax on Western possessions as in 1374, no. 89. When a priory or preceptory fell vacant following the death of the prior or preceptor, the Order's Treasury claimed the *mortuarium* and the *vacantia*, that is the revenues of the office from the time of the death to the next 24 June, the *mortuarium*, and for the following year, the *vacantia*.[87] This custom resembled the annates in the secular church claimed by bishops and especially by popes. Moreover, the Order's Treasury claimed the *spolia* or assets of a late brother, especially the goods and harness of a late officer.[88] The moveables of a late brother were his *iocalia* or jewels, as opposed to the *status*, the belongings of a preceptory. The procedures for payment were debatable and often led to

81 Luttrell (1999), article XI. There is a long account in AOM 322 fol. 61r-62r.

82 Valence, 1383 March 12 during the chapter general, AOM 322 fol. 292-v, ed. Hunyadi (2010), 332–4 no. 65.

83 Such accounts can only be understood together with additional materials, especially from papal and other Western archives. Their edition poses a number of special problems and would be a rewarding project for future research.

84 1 florin = 12 gros.

85 Prier et combattre (2009), 785–6.

86 Luttrell (1999), article XI, 8–9, edition 10–21 from AOM 16 no. 52. For the 1360s, see Nisbet (1957).

87 Sarnowsky, Macht (2001), 470–3.

88 No. 50: *de bonis et arnesiis fratrum defunctorum*. Luttrell (1999), article XI, 4–5, 8–9 and passim.

quarrels. Occasionally such dues could be fairly considerable; for example in 1417 560 florins of Hungary were paid as the *mortuarium* of a deceased brother in Bohemia, no. 312.

For collecting these monies due to the Master and the Treasury on Rhodes, receivers (*receptores*) were active in the West, one or two of them in each priory, probably since 1358.[89] For the Priory of *Alamania* there were usually two receivers, one for Upper Germany and one for Lower Germany; in 1428 these were Fr. Johann Lösel for the upper and Fr. Johann von Schwalbach for the lower part of the priory, no. 445.[90]

Not only for collecting monies, but also for many other disciplinary and administrative problems, including the proper conduct of divine services and other religious ceremonies, visitors were sent from Rhodes to the West. Such visitations were also made by the prior every three, or later all four, years, but they could also be initiated by the Master and the Convent.[91] The documents mention Fr. Albrecht von Schwarzburg for Bohemia before 1323, no. 3, Fr. Gérard de Montaigu for *Alamania* before 1358, no. 29, Fr. Guillaume de Munte and Fr. Pierre de Provins for *Alamania* in 1390 by the Master Fernández de Heredia, no. 166, Fr. Leonardo de Buonafede for *Alamania* and Bohemia in 1409, nos. 229–31, Fr. Johann Schweidler for Bohemia in 1412, no. 261, Fr. Johann von Monreal and Fr. Henri de Bye for *Alamania* in 1420, no. 378; Monreal also no. 407, Fr. Jean de Patria and Fr. Johann Söler von Richtenberg in *Alamania* and Bohemia also in 1420, no. 379, Fr. Roberto di Diana for *Alamania* and Bohemia in 1428, no. 427. These officers were expected to visit the priories in person, to make sure that the Master and Convent were paid all responsions and other dues, to audit accounts, to depose delinquent preceptors and receivers, to rent out their offices and to summon them to face trial on Rhodes. They were also empowered as procurators to act in lawsuits among brethren and elsewhere as if the Master and Convent were present.[92]

## Historical developments

The three years 1349, 1378 and 1417 can be seen as marking epochs for the Hospitallers in Central Europe. Until 1349, when Charles IV was more or less universally recognised as King of the Romans in Germany, they were busy with paying for the conquest of Rhodes and absorbing former Templar possessions, and they had to face the political difficulties within the Empire under Louis IV

89 Estatutos (2006), 169, with the date 1358. But see Stabilimenta (2007), 144 nos. 7–8 and especially Sarnowsky, Macht (2001), 330 with note 8. Other editions include von Osterhausen (1650); Vertôt (1726); King (1934); Waldstein-Wartenberg (1969); Lagleder (1983); a truely critical edition of the Hospitaller statutes and related legal texts remains a desideratum.

90 Appointments nos. 302, 344, 394.

91 Sarnowsky (2007), 152–4.

92 No. 427.

(d. 1347) from the house of Bavaria.[93] One result was the strengthening of the north-eastern Bailiwick of Brandenburg.[94] Thereafter Charles IV (d. 1378) from the rival dynasty of Luxembourg took over, and at about the same time the plague that began in 1347 caused huge losses and triggered profound economic, social and political changes. Debts had already been a problem for the Hospitallers earlier on in the fourteenth century when they needed enormous sums to persuade secular rulers to hand over confiscated Templar possessions. Now debts became a chronic illness. To mobilise additional funding, those who redeemed estates for the Hospital were allowed to keep them for their lifetime, regardless of whether they were Hospitallers or not, as in no. 106 of the year 1383. In 1418 Naillac informed the town of Bern that the Hospitallers needed the Master's special permission to borrow monies and to pawn estates, no. 353; however, this may have been a special arrangement for the Master's chamber of Buchsee, because usually a licence of the prior sufficed.

The financial situation fuelled reforms, especially in the attempts of the 1360s to reduce the number of brethren in the houses and preceptories.[95] Stricter obedience and spiritual discipline became popular at least among some Hospitallers in Central Europe. Straßburg, the most prosperous city in Alsace, became known for such initiatives. Rulman Merswin (d. 1382), a pious and rich banker, had bought there a place called Grünenwörth. The community he assembled there needed recognition and protection, whereas the Hospitallers hoped to profit from their legal status and religious prestige.[96] So in 1371 Fr. Konrad von Braunsberg, Prior of *Alamania*, accepted an offer by Rulman Merswin and accepted Grünenwörth as a preceptory of the Order.[97]

Then, in 1378, the great papal schism commenced.[98] Most rulers in Central Europe recognised the Roman popes and, after 1409, the Pisan popes, but there was always notable opposition. Duke Leopold of Austria (d. 1386), who ruled the Habsburg possessions in the Alps and especially in the southern part of the Bailiwick of Oberland, adhered to the popes of Avignon; so did the Dukes of Brabant and Guelders in the Netherlands. When the Hospitaller Master Fr. Juan Fernández de Heredia left Rhodes in the spring of 1382 he went to Avignon. In response the Roman pontiff, Urban VI, appointed his fellow-Neapolitan Fr. Riccardo Caracciolo, Prior of Capua, as "his" Master in

93 vonPflugk-Harttung (1900); Füßlein (1905, reprint 1985).

94 Gahlbeck (2016) und (2015); Brandenburgisches Klosterbuch (2007); Smoliński (2009) primarily for the times before 1300.

95 Engel (1955); Borchardt, Soll-Zahlen (2003).

96 Borchardt, Wirtschaft und Ordensreform (2003); Buchheit, Strasbourg (2014).

97 Ed. Buchheit, Commanderies (2014), 281–4. An early modern copy in AOM 47 fol. 70–5 (96–101) mentions a confirmation made by the Master Fr. Raymond Bérenger, Rhodes, 1371 October 20. This is probably based on the original in Straßburg, not on a register now lost.

98 Luttrell (1978), article XIX, and (1999), article IV; Lascurain Bernstorff (2019).

1383.[99] Caracciolo was recognised in many parts of Italy, in Bohemia and England, whereas the Prior of *Alamania* Fr. Konrad von Braunsberg collaborated with Fernández de Heredia's chapter general at Valence. Duke Ziemovit of Teschen, Prior of Bohemia,[100] was amply rewarded by Caracciolo, nos. 127–9 and 145. In 1383 he was constituted as procurator, visitor and corrector in *Alamania*, Saxony and Brabant. An annual pension payment due to Fr. Hesso Schlegelholz for the resignation of his claims to the Priory of Bohemia was annulled. Fr. Ziemovit was confirmed as Prior of Bohemia for ten years. And in 1385 the preceptories in Brandenburg and Saxony were transferred to the Priory of Bohemia.

Although Eastern Central Europe supported Urban VI, Caracciolo's decisions had few lasting consequences. Fernández de Heredia however confirmed in 1383 an agreement between the Priory of *Alamania* and the Bailiwick of Brandenburg, no. 115, which is today often hailed as the foundation charter for Brandenburg's autonomy within the Hospital. But Brandenburg continued to pay responsions to the prior. On the other hand, the personal connections between Brandenburg and *Alamania* ceased to be important for either of the two entities. At 1382/83 the Prior of *Alamania* had claimed the right to appoint four preceptors in the Bailiwick. But the social networks no longer interacted. When *Alamania* and Brandenburg began to quarrel in the middle of the fifteenth century Rhodes intervened. On behalf of the Convent Brandenburg was supposed to be turned into a capitular bailiwick.[101] This meant that the bailiff would be appointed on Rhodes, nos. 461–2. In the end, it turned out that this was not possible.[102] The brethren's networks were stronger than the Order's constitution. This was, however, a general problem in the two Priories of *Alamania* and Bohemia and perhaps elsewhere in the Hospital.

## Diplomatics

For understanding the documents here edited, some preliminary remarks about Hospitaller diplomatics may be helpful. For its top ranks, the Order of the Hospital had the leaden bull of the Master, announced in the documents as *bulla nostra plumbea*, and the leaden bull, which was called the *bulla communis plumbea* and was used for important documents issued by Master and Convent together. In the *Libri Bullarum* the clause that announced the seals was often abbreviated to *In cuius rei etcetera*, but its existence was not tacitly suppressed. One can only guess from the formulary and the contents which bull or seal

99 Delaville (1913), 215, 249.

100 On him, see Mitáček (1999); Starnawska (2011).

101 Between 1440 and 1515 such bailiwicks were recognised at Eagle (England), Manosque (Saint-Gilles), Lureil (Auvergne), Caspe (Amposta), Cantavieja (Amposta, only transitory), La Bovedo (Castile), Sarnowsky, Macht (2001), 52–5.

102 Sarnowsky, Konvent (2001), 46–9 with note 43.

was used. In 1358 and 1365 there was a difference between documents issued by the Master with the consent of the Convent[103] and documents issued by the Master together with the Convent.[104] Both categories of documents did have a clause announcing their authentication. A fairly large number of documents, however, did not mention any seal at all before the dating clause. In 1358 this was almost standard practice.[105] Later on such documents became exceptions.[106] These documents may in fact have had a waxen seal. Clearly the Master had not only his leaden bull but also a personal seal that was made of wax,[107] sometimes described as black.[108] Sometimes the Master's chancellor might add his personal *signum*.[109] Some documents were actually letters with the addressee probably on the back of the original; in the *Libri Bullarum* his name stands above the copied text and the issuer at the end below the this text.[110] A special case was the time between the death of the Master and the election of his successor; there would be a lieutenant of the vacant Master's office who used his personal seal in wax.[111]

The most high-ranking documents were, of course, those issued by Master and Convent during the chapter general, that is, in the presence and with the consent of important brethren from outside the Convent.[112] Such texts were dated *durante nostro generali capitulo*. There was no separate seal for them; they had the *bulla communis plumbea* of Master and Convent as in 1314: no. 1, 1346: no. 5 and 1358: no. 12, then again 1420: nos. 377–88 and 1428: nos. 423–35. When Fernández de Heredia held a chapter general at Valence in 1383 and Caracciolo at Naples in 1384, the *bulla communis plumbea* was on Rhodes, and the Master used his own bull. Fernández de Heredia could boast the presence of three procurators of the Convent and 12 other brethren, nos. 105–19, here no. 109, whereas Caracciolo's nos. 127–8 just mentioned other brethren. The situation was even more complicated at Aix in 1410. Naillac was absent, but he had constituted three procurators. For no. 234 they used their own seals. For the documents of the chapter general nos. 235–42 they collaborated with three procurators of the Convent, 14 named and other unnamed brethren, and they used the Master's bull.

103 Nos. 30–32, 35, 37, 43, 49, 58, 66, 68–9.

104 Nos. 45–7, 57, 73–6, 85.

105 Nos. 16, 29, 36, 39–42, 54–56, 60–65.

106 1365: 67, 71–2, 80; 1383: 124; 1390: 162; 1394: 184; 1408: 221; 1409: 225, 230; 1411: 251, 265; 1414: 274, 280; 1414: 290; 1415: 294; 1417: 314, 317, 323, 337; 1418: 342, 348, 355; 1419: 366, 370–72; 1420: 383, 389 after the chapter general, 397; 1422: 409; 1428: 449, 458–9.

107 Nos. 82, 86, 95, *sigilli nostri impressione munita;* nos. 347, 353, 460, *fecimus apponi sigillum.*

108 No. 419, *bulla nostra, qua utimur in cera nigra.*

109 No. 281, *sub sigillo nostro et signo manuali cancellarii.*

110 Nos. 243–5, 250, 258.

111 No. 400, *bulla nostra cerea ob defectum bulle communis plumbee vacante magisterio.*

112 From 1314 to 1428, Stabilimenta (2007), 417–19, lists 16 chapters general.

While in 1374 the Master Fr. Robert de Juilly was still at Avignon, on his way to Rhodes, he issued nos. 89 and 90 *cum consilio fratrum et procerum*. Such counsellors had to replace the absent Convent in this situation. When Fernández de Heredia and Caracciolo were in the West, between 1383 and 1393 their nos. 123, 145–6, 149–50, 160–61, 166 mentioned in a similar way the Master's consultation with brethren and, in Fernández de Heredia's case, sometimes the consent of brethren, nos. 170, 177, or even of the procurator of the Convent and other brethren, nos. 141, 144, 172. When Fr. Philibert de Naillac was in the West from 1409, no. 229, to 1420, no. 376, three, later two, procurators of the Convent accompanied him. The joint decisions of the Master and these procurators were sealed with the Master's bull in lieu of the common bull, *bulla nostra in absentia bulle communis plumbee.*[113] During these years there was a Lieutenant Master on Rhodes who issued documents together with the Convent. They were not allowed to use the *bulla communis plumbea* because the Master was absent. Some of their documents did not have a seal at all.[114] In 1411 their documents expressly stated that there was no separate Conventual bull, *ob defectum bulle nostri conventus*, nos. 246 and 252. In most cases, however, documents issued jointly by the Lieutenant Master and Convent had the waxen seal of the officer acting as Lieutenant Master.[115] For the future, these turbulences had lasting and important consequences. It became standard practice that on Rhodes the Lieutenant Master and the Master issued their documents *de voluntate, consilio et assensu* of named brethren *et aliorum domus nostre fratrum nobis assistentium.*[116] From these beginnings in the fifteenth century the Order's council developed. On 4 March 1410 Fr. Hesso Schlegelholz as Preceptor of Kos and Fr. Hermann von Ow as Pilier of the Tongue of *Alamania* were mentioned among those who were present.[117] Formed by representatives of the tongues, the council worked as an instrument to seek compromises between these tongues.[118] Few sources of this period have been edited so far, and it is not possible at present to ascertain a date when the council was officially instituted. It may in fact have been a gradual development during the first half of the fifteenth century. In order to reduce the influence of the three tongues from the kingdom of France, the three other tongues strove to strengthen the Tongue of *Alamania*. That is an important background to the decisions of 1422, no. 415, and 1428, no. 435. The first recognised the Tongue of *Alamania* and awarded it the Captaincy of the castle of St. Peter at Bodrum as its office in the East. The

113 Examples from nos. 235 to 376.

114 Nos. 232, 251.

115 Nos. 246, 257. No. 227, *sub sigillo nostro in absentia bulle plumbee;* no. 233, *bulla nostra cerea;* nos. 259, 260, 262, 298, 304, 309, *bulla nostra cerea, qua utimur ob defectum bulle communis plumbee.*

116 See for example nos. 170, 302 etc. On the council, Sarnowsky, Macht (2001), 48–52.

117 AOM 339 fol. 224v; cf. Roger (2010), 97–8.

118 In 1428 no. 456 was issued by Master and Convent and sealed with the Master's bull only, not with the *bulla communis plumbea*. Was this standard practice by that date, an exception or a scribal error?

second one established the Conventual bailiwick of Grand Bailiff as its office in the Convent.

## Orthography, punctuation and capitals

The practice of orthography, punctuation and grammar was continually changing. Basically, texts should be edited in the form as they were written down. But the scribes themselves would correct mistakes. Moreover, editors have to ensure that their readers can understand the edited texts. For all these reasons some normalisation is inevitable. Variations between double and single consonants or between *ci* and *ti*, as in *disposicio* or *dispositio*, should not cause problems for readers of Medieval Latin. Following established principles, u and v are normalised according to their pronunciation, whereas J, j is always changed to I, i, because the so-called i-longa was merely an allograph or variant of the grapheme or letter i in Gothic scripts.[119] This rule also applies to well-known names such as *Novadomo*; only uncommon names are rendered in the exact form given in the manuscript. To be sure, some documents from Rhodes were full of serious orthographical problems.[120] In this edition obvious errors are reported in the notes;[121] less obvious and doubtful errors were left in the text and suggestions can be found in the notes.

No normalisation was applied for proper names. On Rhodes names from Central Europe were often grossly misinterpreted. Sometimes an explanation was felt to be necessary; for example, nos. 64 and 65 *Wernerus Albus alias Wis* (Weiß for German 'White'). An example of a scribe on Rhodes committing a patent error is no. 82 where Fr. Gallus von Lemberg was called prior of *Alamania* instead of Bohemia.

All abbreviations are tacitly expanded. This includes the name Jerusalem (*hospitalis Iherosolimitani* for *hosp. Irlni.* or the like) and the dioceses, usually an adjective of the third declension (*diocesis Poznaniensis* for *dioc. Poznan.*). In some doubtful cases the letters supplied by the editor are in parentheses. Square brackets are reserved for explanations made by the editor. No editorial normalisation was possible for the dating clauses that sometimes start with *Datum*, referring to the legal act, sometimes with *Data*, referring to the *littera*, and sometimes with just *Dat.* A similar problem is the locative of Avignon, simply *Avenion.* or expanded as *Avenione*, *Avenioni*. One should note the difference between the three dots (. . .) that mark a lacuna and the *gemipunctus* (··) that marks a personal name deliberately not given, because an order was to be

119 This may be somewhat unusual for English eyes, but there are parallel cases. For instance, there is only one letter a, g or s, regardless of whether a has a top hook or not, g has a looptail or not, s is long or round.

120 For example, no. 87.

121 Marked as *MS* in the notes; e.g. *supradicti fratri* for *supradicto fratri*.

executed not only by the present holder of an office but also by any future holder of that office.

The complex grammar of many legal and juridical clauses makes a consistent punctuation indispensable for understanding long documents. Following an established practice, the punctuation of the edited texts is basically grammatical. That means that, contrary to English usage, all subordinate clauses are in commas. Also, following an established practice, present participles such as *mandantes* or *committentes* in the sense of 'we order' or 'we instruct' are treated as if they start a new sentence. Capital letters are avoided in the Latin text except for names and at the beginning of a sentence; in the English summaries English practice is followed with a few additions, most notably for the Hospital, the Master and the Convent, which always refers to the Convent on Rhodes.

# DOCUMENTS

## 1

*The Master Fr. Foulques de Villaret and the Convent, acting in chapter general, constitute Fr. Leonardo dei Tiberti, lieutenant in the priory of Venice and visitor general in the priories of the realms of France, England, Scotland, Ireland, Bohemia, Denmark, Spain, Norway and Sweden and in all Upper and Lower Germany and in all other ultramontane regions [north of the Alps], and his nephew Fr. Francesco dei Tiberti, lieutenant in the Preceptory of Bologna, as their procurators at the Roman curia and everywhere else in the regions on the other side of the sea [in the West] for all business concerning the former possessions of the Templars and all the old possessions of the Hospital. They are empowered to take monies as loans, to change monies, to sell valuables, to act in lawsuits and arbitrations, and to constitute sub-delegates.*

*Rhodes, 1314 November 5*

*AOM 16 no. 11, original parchment, no seal extant; cg. Hatt Olsen (1962), 101 no. 3, with 3 November.*

Noverint universi et singuli presentes litteras inspecturi, quod nos frater Fulco de Vilareto Dei gratia sancte domus hospitalis sancti Iohannis Ierosolimitani magister humilis et pauperum Christi custos et nos conventus domus eiusdem priores et fratres ceteri Rodi ad sonum campane more solito et loco deputato pro celebracione generalis capituli congregati inter ceteras sollicitudines nostras illud novimus esse precipuum et necessario convenire, quod nos propter multiplicitatem plurium et diversorum negociorum, que nobis et domui, quam benigna influentia creatoris clementer prospiciens per universum orbem suos effecit faniculos largiores, in plurimis et diversis locis et partibus tractanda et promovenda incumbunt et necesse habent fieri et etiam expediri, talem personam ex nostro consorcio disquitamus, que potens opere et sermone debeat, possit et valeat tanti officii sarcinam subportandam ea magna et ardua, que in presentiarum multipliciter imminent et imposterum imminere contingent, solerter facere, tractare utiliter et fideliter explicare. Considerantes similiter, quod sancta Romana ecclesia, que auctore Domino cunctorum fidelium mater est, domina et magistra, a qua universi et singuli tanquam membra a capite, rami ab arbore et rivuli a fonte largifluo salutis nutrimentum recipiunt et habent refugium singulare, dignum necessarium et utile nobis et domui fore previdimus, ut in eius sollempni curia pertractandis, promovendis et explicandis nostris et domus negociis per alium sufficientem et ydoneum nostra personalis astancia demonstratur. De fide igitur et discretione, legalitate atque circumspectionis industria religiosi in Christo nobis carissimi fratris Leonardi de Tybertis eiusdem domus locum nostrum tenentis in prioratu Veneciarum et visitatoris generalis in prioratibus nostris regnorum Francie, Anglie, Scocie, Ybernie, Boemie, Dacie, Yspanie, Nouergie et Suecie et in tota Alamannia alta et bassa et generaliter in omnibus ultramontanis partibus gerentes in Domino fiduciam pleniorem, eundem fratrem Leonardum, quem Dominus misericordiarum per sui gratiam nobis et toti religioni nostre plantavit fructuosum et utilem, presentem et infrascriptam procuracionem ac mandatum sponte, humiliter et ex certa scientia recipientem et dilectissimum fratrem Franciscum de Tibertis eiusdem fratris Leonardi nepotem et locum nostrum tenentem in preceptoria nostra Bononie absentem tanquam presentem et quemlibet eorum insolidum, ita tamen, quod non sit melior conditio occupentis, set ubi unus ex voluntate vel quacunque causa seu occasione dimittet, alter possit semel et pluries assumere, assumptum incipere et inceptum mediare et finire, facimus, constituimus, creamus et etiam ordinamus in Romana curia et in cunctis partibus ultramarinis[a] citra nostros et domus veros, legitimos et indubitatos procuratores, sindicos, yconomos, actores, institores, administratores cum libera[1]) generales et nuncios speciales ad petendum, exigendum, recuperandum ad ius et proprietatem domus nostre reducendum atque recipiendum a quibuscunque personis ecclesiasticis vel secularibus nomine nostro et domus universa et singula bona, quecunque sint, ubicunque et in quibuscunque consistant, in omnibus partibus seu regionibus ultramarinis[a] citra, que nobis et domui collata, concessa, tradita et unita existunt tam per sedem apostolicam quam per alios catholicos imperatores, reges et principes et fideles alios et que olim fuerunt domus milicie Templi necnon et in omnibus et singulis questionibus, controversiis et litibus, causis et negociis motis et movendis per nos in Romana curia et alibi in partibus supradictis ratione et occasione locorum et rerum dicti quondam Templi et etiam bonorum dicte domus nostre antiquorum per universas ultramarinas partes citra sistentium contra quascunque personas ecclesiasticas vel seculares, collegia, capitula, conventus, universitates et communia cuiuscunque gradus, dignitatis, auctoritatis, condicionis et status existant aut contra nos et domum nostram a quibuscunque personis ecclesiasticis et secularibus, collegiis, capitulis, conventibus vel universitatibus et communibus cuiuscunque gradus, dignitatis, auctoritatis, condicionis et status existant, coram domino nostro summo pontifice, auditoribus sacri palacii et audiencie ac iudicibus quibuscunque vicariis, officialibus, presidibus, rectoribus,

1) *A special form of public administrator: Cf. Gierke 4 (1913), 39.*

magistratibus, baillivis ecclesiasticis secularibusve ordinariis, extraordinariis, delegatis, subdelegatis, compromissariis, arbitris, arbitratoribus, amicabilibus compositoribus et amicis communibus et in quacunque curia sive foro ecclesiastico vel mundano, et insuper ad promovendum, tractandum, ordinandum et prosequendum in dicta curia Romana et alibi, ubi sibi expedire videbitur, omnia et singula nos vel domum nostram universaliter aut particulariter seu alias communiter et distinctim tangencia vel nobis et domui, ut dictum est, pertinencia quoquomodo. Dantes et concedentes ipsis nostris et domus certis, veris et indubitatis procuratoribus, sindicis, yconomis, actoribus, institoribus et generalibus administratoribus cum libera atque nunciis specialibus plenam, absolutam, generalem, expeditam et liberam potestatem, auctoritatem, parabolam, expressam licenciam et speciale mandatum, quascunque quantitates peccunie nostro et domus nostre nomine semel et pluries mutuo recipiendi et mutuum contrahendi ac susceptum pro predictis et in predictis causis et negociis expendendi a quocunque seu quibuscunque creditore vel creditoribus undecunque et ubicunque et cuiuscunque condicionis fuerint, item cambiandi et permutandi et nomine cambii et permutacionis permutandi, recipiendi et tradendi quascunque res et quascunque peccuniam, monetam, aurum vel argentum monetatum vel non monetatum et in quocunque numero aut pondere et cuiuscunque generis vel condicionis, item tradendi et concedendi in gardiam vel comandigiam seu depositum vel alio quocunque titulo et modo quascunque quantitates peccunie et quascunque monetas et quodcunque aurum vel argentum monetatum vel non monetatum et cuiuscunque generis, numeri et ponderis cuiuscunque, item petendi, exigendi, recuperandi ad ius et proprietatem domus nostre reducendi, recipiendi, habendi, tenendi et administrandi, possessionem corporalem vel quasi per se ipsos et quemlibet eorum aut alium seu alios deputandum seu deputandos ab eis vel ab aliquo ipsorum apprehendendi, nanciscendi et adhipiscendi, agendi, accusandi, denunciandi, defendendi, conveniendi et reconveniendi, proponendi, excipiendi, replicandi et replicationibus respondendi, libellum vel libellos offerendi, oblato vel oblatis respondendi, litem contestandi, iurandi de calumpnia, de malicia et de veritate dicenda in animam nostram et cuiuslibet alterius generis iuramentum subeundi, ponendi et posicionibus respondendi, testes, instrumenta et alia legitima documenta probationum quarumlibet procudendi, producto et productis obiciendi, crimina et defectus opponendi, renunciandi, concludendi vel pro concluso habendi, in causa vel causis de iure et de facto sententiam et sententias diffinitivas, interlocutorias et preceptorias honandi[b] et audiendi, earum executionem petendi, ab eis atque graviminibus illatis et inferendis semel vel pluries appellandi, apostolos petendi et oblatos recipiendi, appellationem et appellationes prosequendi, expensas litis et extra litem ac quodlibet interesse iudicis officio aut libelli tenore requirendi et easdem in suam vel animam nostram iurandi, iudicem vel iudices, arbitrum vel arbitros, compromissarios, amicos, comunes vel compositores amicabiles assumendi et eligendi et eos recusandi, compromittendi, componendi, transigendi, paciscendi, restitutionem in integrum petendi, solucionem et soluciones petendi, recipiendi finem, absolucionem, quitationem et plenam refutationem, pactum etiam et iuramentum de ulterius non petendo dandi et faciendi, supplicandi pro nobis et domo nostra impetrandi litteras gratie et simplicis iustitie, legendas et non legendas et impetratis et impetrandis contra nos et domum nostram ubique in audientia et in quolibet curia ecclesiastica vel mundana contradicendi et obiciendi et demum universa alia et singula faciendi, dicendi, procurandi, tractandi et ordinandi, que veri, certi, legitimi et indubitati procuratores nostri et domus nostre sindici, yconomi, actores, institores et generales administratores cum libera et nuncii speciales in ipsa Romana curia et alibi facere valent, possunt et debent et que nos facere, dicere, tractare et ordinare possemus, si presentes essemus, et que merita, exercitium atque iudiciarius ordo causarum civilium atque criminalium, que per procuratores possunt tractari quorumcunque negociorum et contractuum desiderant et requirunt, et omnia, que sub generali et speciali clausula continentur et possunt modo aliquo contineri, etiam si mandatum exigant speciale. Item in predictis omnibus et singulis causis, questionibus et litibus ordinariis, extraordinariis, civilibus et criminalibus, in quibus de iure procurator potest admitti, unum et plures et quot voluerint seu alter eorum voluerint procuratores substituendi et eos revocandi et removendi, quando et quociens ipsi vel alter eorum voluerint seu voluerit et eis vel ei videbitur expedire. Nichilominus tamen ipsa etiam substitutione facta et in sua firmitate manente semel vel quociens voluerint, possint dicti nostri et domus procuratores vel alter eorum adesse cause vel causis sive negociis et predictum procurationis officium reassumere et libere exercere in omnibus et singulis supradictis in iudicio atque extra nec propterea hoc ipso intelligantur substitutum vel substitutos revocare, nisi aliter clare de revocando suam expresserint voluntatem. Et hoc semper procuratorio firmo durante in personas dictorum fratrum Leonardi et Francisci de Tybertis domus eiusdem et utriusque eorum procur(atorio). Promittentes ratum, gratum, firmum et stabile perpetuo habituros, quicquid per eosdem procuratores nostros et domus sindicos, yconomos, actores, factores, institores et generales administratores cum libera et nuncios speciales aut alterum eorum substituendum vel substituendos ab eis seu ab aliquo de ipsis actum, factum, accusatum, denunciatum, petitum, responsum, oppositum, exceptum, probatum, appellatum, supplicatum, impetratum, receptum, defensum, quitatum, mutuatum, solutum, cambitum, depositum, comendatum, tractatum, procuratumque fuerit vel aliter ordinatum. Volentes quoque nostros et domus procuratores predictos, sindicos, yconomos, actores, factores, institores et generales administratores cum libera et nuncios speciales et quemlibet eorundem relevare ab omni gravamine, labore et onere satisdandi, promittimus et ypotheca et obligatione omnium bonorum domus nostre mobilium et immobilium et se moventium presentium et etiam futurorum rem ratam haberi et iudicatum solvi cum omnibus clausulis, que in condempnacione continebuntur, nisi fuerit appellatum et pro ipsis et eorum quolibet substituendo vel substituendis ab eis vel altero eorum fideiussores constituimus et firmamus. In cuius rei testimonium et certitudinem pleniorem bulla nostra comunis plumbea presentibus est appensa. Actum in nostro generali capitulo Rodi anno Domini millesimo trecentesimo quarto decimo, videlicet tertio nonas Novembris sollempniter celebrato.

*a)* ultramarini *corr.* *b) recte* levandi

## 2

*The Master Fr. Foulques de Villaret orders the Preceptor of Utrecht and Haarlem Fr. Jacobus, Bishop of Zuda, to pay 3,000 florins of Florence for responsions and taxes (here* subventiones*) to Fr. Paolo da Modena, who is also to receive the responsions and other payments made to Fr. Ulrich von Rechberg, Preceptor of Colmar, and others in order to pay Brutio Carucci, merchant of Florence, for valuables given to the Prior of Venice and procurator at the papal curia Fr. Leonardo dei Tiberti.*

*Arles, 1319 April 12*

*AOM 16 no. 10, originale, pergamentum, cum lacunis pro filo unius bulle, scriptura multis in locis extincta.* 1319 April 12 *add. in dorso per manum recentiorem. Ed. van Winter (1998), 29–30 no. 1.*

Venerabili in Christo patri domino fratri Iacobo Dei gratia episcopo Zudensi, preceptori domorum Traiectensis et Hairlemensis[a)] frater Fulco de Vilareto Dei gratia sancte domus hospitalis sancti Iohannis Ierosolimitani magister humilis et pauperum Christi custos salutem et sinceram in Domino caritatem. Quia dilectum in Christo nobis carissimum fratrem Paulum de Mutina domus eiusdem vicepriorem per Saxoniam, Thuringiam, Marchiam et Slauiam, de [cuius] fid[e] et sollicitudine et circumspectione plene confidimus, fecimus et constituimus ac ordinavimus nostrum verum et legitimum procuratorem, sindicum, negociorum gestorem, yconomum, pet[it]orem et nuncium specialem ad recipiendum, petendum et exigendum a vobis et singulis vestrum usque ad summam trium milium florenorum auri de Florencia necnon a fratre Ulrico de Rechberc preceptor[e] Columbarie ac aliis quibuscumque nostris procuratoribus alias ordinatis per nos[b)] in partibus ipsis ad petendum, exigendum et recipiendum a vobis et singulis vestrum nobis debitas [re]sp[on]siones et subvenciones, quos tria milia florenos idem frater Paulus de mandato nostro solvere habet Brutio Carucii, mercatori de Florencia, qui a fratre Leonardo de Tibertis priore Veneciarum et procuratore in Romana curia propterea recepit quedam vasa et iocalia nostra in pignore, volumus et vobis auctoritate presencium permittimus, quatenus responsionem, ad quam nobis tenemini et dicto hospitali, dicto fratri Paulo vel eius speciali nuncio persolvatis, ut de dictis tribus milibus florenis possit satisfacere mercatori supradicto[c)], recipientes ab ipso fratre Paulo de hiis, que ei solveritis, vel eius [in hiis commissario] apodixam vel literas quitancie de hiis quo solutis ad cautelam. In cuius rei testimonium et certitudinem pleniorem b[ulla] nostra [plum]bea presentibus est appensa. Datum Arelate die duodecima mensis Aprilis anno domini millesimo trecentesimo decimo nono.

*a) illegibilis MS  b) add. rasuram.  c)* . . . per *add. ante corr.*

*Fr. Jacob van Denemarken was Preceptor of Utrecht from 1309 to 1331. In 1312 he became Auxiliary Bishop of Utrecht with the see of Zuda on the Greek island of Syros in the Cyclades, in the Duchy of the Archipelago. See Koorn (†) / Mol (2009), 146–74, and (2015), 204–5.*

## 3

*The preceptors Fr. Oliver von Sayn in Arnheim, Fr. Gerhard von Hammerstein in Breisig, Fr. Eberhard von Kestenburg in Frankfurt, Fr. Johann von Grumbach in Würzburg and Fr. Rudolf von Masmünster request the Master Fr. Hélion de Villeneuve to replace Fr. Paolo da Modena as Preceptor of Thuringia, Saxony and the March (of Brandenburg) with Fr. Albrecht von Schwarzburg, recently created Prior of* Alamania *and visitor in Bohemia and* Dacia.

*1323 January 12*

*AOM 16 no. 15, originale, pergamentum, cum locis quinque sigillorum perditorum. Ed.van Winter (1998), 30 no. 2.*

Magno religionis viro domino fratri Eliono de Villa Noua sacre domus hospitalis sancti Iohannis Ierosolimitani magistro summo fratres Oliuerius de Seina in Arnheim,[1]) Gerhardus de Hamerstein in Briseke, frater Eberhardus de Kestenburg in Frankenuort[1], Iohannes de Grunbach de Herbipoli, Rudolfus de Masemunster domorum conmendatores regularem obedienciam in omnibus debitam et devotam. Cum hactenus in commissis honor(abilis) vir frater Albertus de Nigro Castro prior noster et ex parte vestri visitator regionum Bohemie et Dacie se trans mare et citra talem sue probitati exhibuerit, quod de eo et per ipsum factis sacrosancta Romana ecclesia ipsum specialius amplectetur et nostra religio incrementa salubria senciat, ut vos laudabile testimonium perhibetis et rei evidencia denotat et ostendit. Hinc cum eidem domino fratri Alberto sarcinam nostri prioratus pre cunctis aliis prioratibus longe magis gravem de ordinamento domini summi pontificis, ut intelleximus, imponere voluistis et in partem sollicitudinis officii vobis crediti evocare, miramur, quare paterna pensacione non respexeritis, dummodo vobis constiterit, ut preceptoriam Duringie, Saxonie et Marchie, quam frater Paulus de Mutina tenet, eidem

1) *According to Hatt Olsen (1962), 101, Fr. Olivier de Seyn was Prior of Antvorskov from 1310 to 1314, Fr. Eberhard von Kestenburg Prior of* Dacia *by papal provision in 1317.*

domino fratri Alberto non duxeritis committendam, cum infra terminos eiusdem preceptorie idem dominus frater Albertus de clariori sanguine principum, comitum et nobilium traxerit originem, qui hodierno tempore dictas partes dominio regunt et potencia defendunt et ipsa preceptoria, sicut nobis commendatores eiusdem exponere curarunt, per fratrem Paulum predictum, eciam si in bono statu existeret, re se habente ut nunc ad utilitatem religionis nostre regi minime posset, tum[a] quia dictus frater Paulus est in ipsis partibus inpotens et extraneus quoad amicos defensivos, tum quia in eisdem partibus quoad nostram religionem iusticia eidem reddenda quasi extra terminos exulavit. Que inquantum dictam religionem in dicta preceptoria pungant atrociter et sine cognicione legittima invadant, vestra paternitas tam verbaliter quam litteraliter, ut credimus, bene novit. Hec si per personam aliquam sub hospitalis vehiculo degentem reformari possent et deberent, esset premissis inspectis per predictum dominum fratrem Albertum faciendum, nam ipsa preceptoria ex absencia fratris Pauli predicti deperit evidenter, ut nobis ex fratribus parcium predictarum innotuit in tantum, quod longum foret committere scripto. Unde sane consulimus, cum dicte partes ab antiquo nostro prioratui fuerint annexe et sicut divisio segregat unitatem, sic et perdit substancialitatem et per consequens desolacioni inducit, ut dictam preceptoriam sic mere depressam, cum alias eius ruine nostro iudicio subvenire non possit, ex vestro officio effectualiter committatis. In cuius rei testimonium sigilla nostra presentibus sunt appensa. Datum anno Domini M° CCC° XX° III die Mercurii post epiphaniam eiusdem.[2]

*a)* dum *corr.*

## 4

*Excerpts from six chapters general concerning Central Europe. The following edition is limited to the names from Central Europe.*

*(1330–44)*

*AOM 280; cf. Hatt Olsen (1962), 101 no. 4.*

*1330: Appointment of Fr. Rudolf von Masmünster as Prior of* Alamania *and* Bohemia, *of Fr. Helfrich von Rüdigheim as Prior of* Dacia *and Norway. Monies to be paid: 1,360 florins from* Alamania *with Thuringia, 1,400 florins from Bohemia, 640 florins from Saxony, the March and* Slavia, *100 marks from* Dacia *and Norway. Annual responsions 680 florins from* Alamania *with Thuringia, 1,200 florins from Bohemia, 320 florins from Saxony, the March and* Slavia, *100 marks from* Dacia *and Norway.*

*2) The date is not 11 January 1324, because in the autumn of 1323 Fr. Gebhard von Bortfelde was already in charge of Saxony and of the March of Brandenburg: Füßlein (1983), 392–4.*

*Retention by the Master in* Alamania *of the Preceptory of Utrecht. Fol. 2r: Montpellier, 1330 November 2,*[1] *appointments from now to 24 June 1331 and then onwards for ten years, fol. 2v* fratrem Radulfum de Ma[s]muster priorem Alamanie et Boemie, fratrem Elfricum de Rudenken priorem Dacie et Norouegie. *Fol. 4r: for the subsidy and the responsions of the current year to be paid on 24 June 1331, fol. 5v:* De prioratu Alamanie. Item prior Alamanie cum Turingia florenos M III$^{c}$ LX. Item Boemie florenos M IIII$^{c}$. Et preceptoria Saxonie, Marchie et Slauie florenos VI$^{c}$ XL. Prioratus Dacie et Norouegie marcas argenti C. *Fol. 6v: annual responsions to be paid between August 15 and September 8, fol. 8r:* De prioratu Alamanie. Prioratus Alamanie cum Turingia florenos VI$^{c}$ LXXX. Prioratus Boemie cum pertinenciis suis florenos M II$^{c}$. Preceptoria Saxonie, Marchie et Slauie cum pertinenciis florenos III$^{c}$ XX. Prioratus Dacie et Norouegie marchas argenti C. *Fol. 14r retentus by the Master up to three brethren [or items?] in each priory, fol. 16r:* In prioratu Alamanie retinuit baiuliam Traiectensem, *fol. 19r:* In prioratu Dacie et Norouegie – .

*1332: Retention by the Master of the Preceptory of Utrecht, of Fr. Gerhard von Hammerstein, Fr. Eberhard von Kestenberg, Fr. Konrad von Rüdigheim, Fr. Berthold von Henneberg, and in the Convent on Rhodes of Fr. Angelinus von Goomesten, Fr. Ardego. Fol. 22r: [Rhodes], 1332 August 30, fol. 27r: retentions, fol. 28v:* In prioratu Alamanie retinuit baiuliam Traiecti, fratrem Girardum de Hambester, fratrem Abstart de Questenbor, fratrem Colradum de Rudeken, fratrem Brodum de Henembus, *all five items* cum eorum baiuliis et arnesiis. *Fol. 29v: . . . living in the Convent on Rhodes,* <. . .> De lingua Alamanie fratrem Angelinum de Godoͧmesten, fratrem Ardego.

*1335: Confirmation of Fr. Berthold von Henneberg in the Preceptory of Boxberg for his lifetime (10 marks as responsion), for ten years in the Preceptory of Weißenburg (11 marks) and the Preceptory of Kühndorf (4 marks), of Fr. Walter in the Preceptory of Mainz. Retention by the Master of Fr. Ardego, Fr. Walter. Fol. 33r to 37v: Rhodes, 1335 September 15 to 28. Fol. 33v:* De prioratibus vero Alamanie et Boemie vaccantibus non fuit ordinatum, sed idem dominus magister auctoritate dicti capituli retinuit potestatem providendi de ipsis prioratibus supra anneam. *Fol. 34r confirming baiulie ad vitam:* Fratri Bertodo de Hennenerch baiuliam de Pochesperch sub responsione decem marcharum argenti. *Fol. 35r confirming* baiulie *for 10 years:* Fratri Bertodo de Henneberch baiuliam de Bizebruch sub responsione undecim marcharum argenti. Item dicto fratri Bertodo baiuliam de Chundorf sub responsione quatuor marcharum argenti. Fratri Galterio Alamanni baiuliam Maguncie. *Fol. 37r, retaining brethren from the Convent:* De lingua Alamanie fratrem Ardego, fratrem Gauterium. *Fol. 37v:* Subsequenter prefatus dominus magister auctoritate dicti capituli et conventus retinuit sibi potestatem super omnibus infrascriptis, ut cum consilio procerum supra anneam possit

*1) Ed. Tipton (1968), 301–8, with slight variations.*

facere thesaurarium aut locumtenentem et de prioratibus Boemie et Alamanie ut superius exprimitur ordinare, <. . .>

*1337: Retention of Fr. Ardego, Fr. Gottfried, Fr. Walter, Fr. Nicolaus of Bohemia. Order to come to Rhodes for Fr. Engelbert Ruselfaf, Fr. Konrad von Rüdigheim, Preceptor of Frankfurt und Rüdigheim, and two other brethren whom the Prior may choose. Fol. 39r: Rhodes, 1337 October 16. Fol. 40v retentions on this side of the sea [in the East], fol. 41v:* De lingua Alamanie fratrem Ardego, fratrem Godofredum, fratrem Gauterium, fratrem Nicolaum de Boemia. *Fol. 41v brethren called from beyond the sea [the West] to the Convent, fol. 42v:* De Alamannia frater Engelbert Ruselfaf, frater Colrat de Rudenken preceptor de Frankenfor et Rodenkeyn, item alii duo fratres secundum discretionem prioris. De prioratu Boemie duo fratres secundum discretionem prioris.

*1340: Retention of Fr. Ardego, Fr. Gottfried, Fr. Walter, Fr. Nicolaus of Bohemia. Fol. 44r: [Rhodes], 1340 August 6. Fol. 44v:* Item recorde est de toute Alamaine que puisque, que les messages non sont encors. Retienirs est retenue a la main dou maistre et dou convent de provizir et ordener subre annea. *Fol. 45v retentions:* De Alamagnia frere Ardiagues, frere Guodofre, frere Gautier, frere Nicolas de Boemia.

*1344: Retentions in the East of Fr. Walter, Fr. Georgius de Botrono, in the West of Fr. Heinrich von Castell. Fol. 47r: [Rhodes], 1344 December 12. Fol. 50v retentions on this side of the sea [in the East]:* De ling[u]a Alamanie frayre Gautier, frayre Iorgi de Botron. *Fol. 51v on the other side of the sea [in the West]:* De Alamanha freyre Enric de Chastel.

## 5

*The Master Fr. Hélion de Villeneuve and the Convent, acting in chapter general, summon Fr. Heinrich von Suymberch, Preceptor of Mailberg, to Rhodes by 24 June 1346. As the Convent needs brethren the chapter general has decided to summon preceptors from the priories in the West. Fr. Heinrich is one of them.*

*Rhodes, 1344 December 23*

*AOM 16 no. 34, originale, pergamentum, cum loco bulle signoque magistri.* Littera repelli fratris Henrici de Suymberch prioratus Boemie *add. in dorso.*

Frater Elyonus de Villanoua Dei gratia sacre domus hospitalis sancti Iohannis Ierosolimitani magister humilis et pauperum Christi custos et nos conventus domus eiusdem cismarinus generale capitulum celebrantes religioso in Christo nobis carissimo fratri Henrico de Suymberch domus eiusdem preceptori de Moymperch salutem et sinceram in Domino caritatem. Cum propter carentia et deffectum fratrum domus nostre preceptorum signanter, qui se sustinere possint et aliis subvenire, nosque eorum salubri consilio dirigere in agendis, quorum commitiam et personalem nobis astanciam prosecutioni arduorum et expressorum agendorum tam ex continuo armorum exercicio quam alias multipliciter nobis et nostre domui iminentium in hiis partibus cismarinis oportunam ymo neccessariam dignoscimus vehementer in presenti nostro generali capitulo multa sit deliberatione provisum, ut de universi orbis prioratibus domus nostre fratres preceptores in certo munere repellentur, quorum vos de prioratu nostro Boemie unus estis, vos ideo ad nostram presenciam tenore presencium repellantes vobis districte precipiendo mandamus sub virtute sancte obediencie nichilominus firmiter iniungentes, quatenus cum equis et armis decentibus tali congruo tempore de ipsis ultramarinis partibus pro veniendo ad has cismarinas ad nostram presentiam arripiatis iter vestrum et arreptum continuo prosequamini, quod ad tardius in festo nativitatis sancti Iohannis baptiste anni Domini millesimi CCC[i] quadragesimi sexti omni excusatione propulsa nostro vos conspectui personaliter presentetis, sic iussa nostra huiusmodi cuiusvis irreverencie vitata contagine executurus prompta paricione devote, quod ad vestra compendia et honores quamvis voluntarios ex ylari promptitudine vestre obediencie nos voluntariores reddatis. In cuius rei testimonium bulla nostra communis plumbea presentibus est appensa. Dat. Rodi sub signo nostri dicti magistri durante dicto nostro capitulo generali die vicesima tercia mensis Decembris anno incarnationis Domini millesimo CCC° quadragesimo quarto.

## 6

*The Master Fr. Déodat de Gozon licenses Fr. Pere Arnau de Paretstortes, Prior of Catalonia, to buy two houses next to the Treasury in Rhodes, one from Fr. Albrecht von Hohenberg, the other from the same Fr. Albrecht and the other brethren of the Tongue of* Alamania, *Fr. Petrus Alamanus and Fr. Georgius de Botrono; these houses are to be used on his death by brethren from Fr. Pere's family or from Catalonia.*

*Rhodes, [134]7 June 1*

*AOM 317 fol. 100v (88v), under* prioratus Cathalonie. *Ed. Luttrell (2003), 239–40; Roger (2010), 83–5.*

Frater Deodatus de Gosono etcetera religioso in Christo nobis carissimo fratri Petro Arnaudi de Parietibus Tortis domus eiusdem priori Cathalonie salutem etcetera. Supplicacioni vestre continenti, quod, cum religiosus in Christo nobis carissimus frater Albertus de Montemagno[1)] domus eiusdem hospicium suum, in quo habitat, situm intra colatum nostrum prope hospicium thesauri conventus nostri Rodi vendere vobis velit et ultra tam dictus frater Albertinus

1) *Probably Hohenberg. Several members of this family of counts in Swabia were called Albrecht, but none of them is so far known to have been a Hospitaller; cf. Monumenta Hohenbergica (1862) and Schmid (1862). There was, however, a family of ministeriales in Franconia with a Hospitaller Fr. Albrecht von Hohenberg, cf. Cart. Hosp. 3, 710 no. 4367. On the foundation on Rhodes by Fr. Pere Arnau cf. Luttrell (1992), article XV, 113.*

quam fratres alii lingue Alamanie, videlicet fratres Petrus Alamanni et Georgius de Botrono, in dicto conventu comorantes hospicium unum modicum dicte lingue[a] contiguum hospicio fratris Albertini prefati pro ipsorum urgentibus necessitatibus supportandis vendere eciam vobis velint, tam dicto fratri Albertino vendendi vobis suum hospicium prelibatum quam sibi et fratribus aliis prefatis dicte lingue nominatum hospicium dicte lingue Alamanie vendendi vobis eciam quam vobis emendi ab ipsis hospicia memorata impertiri licenciam dignaremur, quia in dicta vestra supplicacione exposicione fratrum Albertini, Petri et Georgii predictorum nobis facta comperimus esse vera favorabiliter annuentes et vobis et fratribus superius nominatis tenore presencium per vos licenciam concedimus postulatam. Rursum cum ex dictis hospiciis habitacionem unam decentem[b] sub forma subscripta facere intendatis, sicut vestra continuit exposicio facta nobis, videlicet quod, quamdiu Deus prestiterit vobis vitam, dicta habitacio debeat esse vestra et post decursum vite vestre debeat generis vestri domus nostre fratrum et ipsis defficientibus ita, quod in nostro ordine citra nec ultra[c] mare nullus sit generis vestri frater, esse debeat fratrum prioratus Cathalonie habitacio prelibata ita tamen, quod, si postea quandocumque vestri generis haberi contingat unum vel plures in ordine nostro fratres, ipsius et ipsorum perpetuo esse debeat habitacio memorata, quod illius fratres prioratus Cathalonie antefati possessionem seu quasi semel aut pluries habuerint in aliquo non obstante quodque dicta habitacio per fratres vestri generis aut per fratres prioratus prefati nullo unquam tempore vendi possit nec pignori, obligari, ut fratres prefati, cum ad Dei servicia Rodum venerint, inveniant, ubi reponant eorum capita et non cogantur hospicia mendicare, sicut vos, cum Rodum venistis, mendicastis. Formam prescriptam tamquam racionabilem nobis visam placidam habentes et gratam eamque de et cum consilio fratrum et procerum conventus nostri Rodi nobis assistencium in hac parte ad vestre supplicacionis instanciam presenti serie de certa scientia confirmantes hiis presentibus formam et ordinacionem pretactam per illos, ad quos pertinet et poterint futuris temporibus quomodolibet pertinere, mandamus sub virtute sante obediencie firmiter et districte inviolabiliter perpetuo observari et non contra facere vel venire aliqua occasione vel causa. In cuius rey testimonium etcetera. Data Rodi die prima mensis Iunii anno septimo.

*a)* nominatum hospicium dicte lingue Alamanie *add. ante corr. (homoiotel.)* *b)* datentem *MS* *c)* vel ultra *praem. ante corr.*

## 7

*The Master Fr. Déodat [de Gozon] orders the Prior or Priors of Denmark,* Dacia, *Norway and Sweden to pay his or their responsions to the Preceptor of Flanders in order to assist in the defence of Rhodes against the Turks as the pope and many kings and princes did with galleys and armed men.*

*Rhodes, [134]7 August 25*

*AOM 317 fol. 152r (140r), under* prioratus Alamannie, Boemie et aliarum partium Alamanie. *Ed. Bosio 2 (1629), 76; Paoli (1737), 90–1; Diplomatarium Danicum III/3 (1963), 346–7; cf. Hatt Olsen (1962), 102 no. 3.*

Frater Deodatus etcetera religiosis in Christo nobis carissimis fratri aut fratribus priori vel prioribus de Dinesmarcha ac Dacie, Noruegie et Suecie et eorum cuilibet,[1] ad quem et ad quos presentes pervenerint, salutem in filio Virginis gloriose. Ad ea paterna solicitudine libenter vestros animos exitamus, per que sub professionis gloria, qua Altissimo militatis, perennis boni bravium possitis assequi sempiternum. Multis igitur refferentibus intellecto, quod inter alios ordinis nostri fratres estis vite laudabilis, obedientes filii et vestro comissa regimini utiliter gubernantes, sumus quadam admiracione comoti, quia a longis citra temporibus terra sancta transmarina nullam de bonis nostri ordinis prioratuum predictorum a vobis responsionem habuit nec subvencionis refrigerium senciit alicuius. Scire[a] nempe, quamquam in ultimis terre finibus habitetis, vos credimus et fama volatili vos audisse, quomodo in insula dicta Rodo cum multitudine fratrum dicte sacre[b] domus et gente alia armigera habitamus ducentes bella continua contra Cristiane fidei inmanissimos inimicos Turchos vulgariter noncupatos, quorum[c] efrena temeritas per ipsorum ingenti potencia adversus Cristiani nominis professores hiis temporibus severius solito exitata sic infremuit et invasit[d] Christicolas cismarinos, quod nisi sanctissimus dominus noster papa et multi alii catolici[e] reges et principes eis de galeis et gente armigera subvenissent, quod amodo fidem catolicam in hiis partibus ad nichilum addussissent, illam profficentibus et deffendere satagentibus necatis nece dira prior cum ad deffensionem dicte fidei et augumentum pre ceteris statibus mundi huius nostra professio nos invitet[f] et bona nostri ordinis sint dedicata specialiter[g] ad hunc usum debemus et possumus non sine ratione mirari, que nobis et nostro cismarino conventui in tante deceritatis articullo constitutis vestras renueritis[h] mitere responsiones, sicud faciunt indifferenter priores et preceptores omnes orbis terre. Et quia talia vobis ad eternam vestrarum cedunt dampnationem animarum et nobis in non parvam veniunt lesionem, utrorumque indempnitati volentes occurere potissime, quia aliam subvensionem nisi responsiones prioratuum orbis terre non habemus, vobis et vestrum cuilibet sub virtute sancte obedientie districte precipimus et mandamus, quatenus omni occasione et contradictione cessante responsiones dictorum prioratuum et parcium anno quolibet preceptori domus nostre in Flandria infalibiliter exsolvatis. Sciturit[i] quod, si vos filios reverentes palpaverimus et devotos, nos patrem experiemini beneficium et ad vestros honores et comoda non remissum. In cuius rei testimonium[j] presentes nostras litteras fecimus bulla nostra plumbea comuniri. Dat. Rodi die XXV Augusti anno septimo.

*a)* Sire *MS* *b)* s *praem. ante corr.* *c)* corum *MS* *d)* innvasit *MS* *e)* catoloci *MS* *f) praem. corr.* *g)* spiritualiter *MS* *h)* rensesitis *MS (corr.?)* *i)* Situri *MS* *j)* presens *praem. ante corr.*

1) *In fact there was only one prior for* Dacia *that included Denmark, Norway and Sweden.*

## 8

*The Master Fr. Déodat [de Gozon] licenses Fr. Johann to leave the Convent, to go to the priory of* Alamania *and to receive his maintenance there.*

*Rhodes, [134]8 January 10*

*AOM 317 fol. 152v (140v), under* prioratus Alamannie, Boemie et aliarum partium Alamanie.

Frater Deodatus etcetera religioso in Christo nobis carissimo fratri Iohanni domus eiusdem salutem etcetera. Recedendi de conventu nostro Rodi et eundi ad partes prioratus nostri Alamanie inhibi sub obediencia prioris dicti prioratus pro stagia moraturus vobis tenore presencium licenciam elargimur. Data Rodi die decima mensis Ianuari anno septimo.

## 9

*The Prior of Venice is ordered to repay to Giovanni Benedetti or his procurator 3,000 florins which Nichola Cathelini had given to the Treasury. The prior is to do this from the monies he has received from the Prior of Bohemia.*

*1351 March 27*

*AOM 318 fol. 244r (235r), under* assignaciones solucionum peccuniarum.

Die vicesima septima Marcii mandatum fuit priori Veneciarum, ut de peccuniis, quas habuit et recepit a priore Boemie, solvat intra dies XV a die presentationis Iohanni Benedicti vel eius procuratori florenos auri tria milia[a)], quos Nichola Cathelini assignavit thesauro, ut in forma.

*a)* florenos *add. ante corr.*

*The Prior of Venice was Fr. Napoleone dei Tiberti; cf. AOM 318 fol. 155r (147r) of 23 July 1351.*

## 10

*The Master Fr. Déodat [de Gozon] orders the priors of Mirow, Nemerow, Quartschen and Rörchen to send Fr. Jacobus de Lippa to Eskilstuna [in Sweden] where the prior of the chapel has to maintain him. Jacobus has disobeyed written orders by the Prior of Andvorskov to live in a house of the Order in Norway and wandered around, but received a pardon at Rhodes.*

*Rhodes, [1351] June 10*

*AOM 318 fol. 150r (142r), under* prioratus Alamanie et aliarum partium Alamanie.

Frater Deodatus etcetera religiosis in Christo nobis carissimis fratribus domus eiusdem prioribus de Mairov, de Nemorov, de Carcane[1] et de Roreke et eorum cuilibet[2] insolidum salutem et sinceram in Domino caritatem. Noticie vestre defferimus per presentes, quod eo, quia frater Iacobus de Lippa absque sui superioris licencia hinc inde per mundum vagabundus et inhobediens discurrit[a] et in nostrum Rodi conventum[b] venit, ipsum tanquam inhobedientem privavimus habitu domus nostre. Successive tamen coram nobis et conventus nostri proceribus exposita culpa sua tenoris infrascripti petendo veniam humiliter de conmissis est a nobis et dicti conventus proceribus misericordiam assequatus. Exposicio dicte culpe dignoscitur esse talis: "Cum ego frater Iacobus de Lippa literas quasdam patentes domini prioris de Anwerdesto, superioris mei, pridem recepissem continentes, quod accedere deberem sub virtute sancte obediencie ad monasterium quoddam situm[c] in regno Norwegie pro stagia moraturus, ad locum ipsum mihi assignatum accedere nolui, ymo inhobedientem per mundum hinc inde per longum tempus discurri et in conventu Rodi pro misericordia obtinenda presencialiter proveni." Ideo, si sit ita, ut habet exposicio supradicta, et alios excessus non comiserit, per quos[d] amitere debeat consorcium domus nostre, de consilio dictorum procerum volumus et vobis et vestrum cuilibet insolidum tenore presencium comittimus et mandamus, quatinus ipsum ad vestrum alterum declinante benigne admitatis et eidem habitum domus nostre salva tamen nostri[e] ordinis disciplina restituatis secundum bonos usus et laudabiles consuetudines domus nostre. Postquam eidem in prioratu seu capella Essceltune stagiam assignetis, in qua sibi in suis necessariis provideri faciatis secundum prefatos dicti nostri ordinis bonos usus. Mandantes harum serie firmiter et districte religioso in Christo nobis carissimo fratri domus eiusdem priori capelle predicte de Essceltune, ut fratrem Iacobum eundem ad ipsum prioratum seu capellam declinantem benigne admitat et caritatis pertractet eidemque in dicta capella provideri faciat secundum bonos usus et laudabiles consuetudines domus nostre. Data Rodi die decima mensis Iunii.

*a)* discurcit *MS* *b)* nostro Rodi conventu *MS* *c)* scitum *MS* *d)* qos *MS* *e)* nr *cum abbreviatione MS*

## 11

*The Master Fr. Déodat [de Gozon] grants to Fr. Junior, Count of Reichenberg, for five years the Preceptory of Dorlisheim (Priory of* Alamania), *which is vacant following the death of an unnamed person.*

*Rhodes, [1351] June 20*

1) *Probably Quartschen, not Kraak.*

2) *These priors were the heads of the priests in the four houses.*

*AOM 318 fol. 150r-v (142r-v). under* prioratus Alamanie et aliarum partium Alamanie.

Frater Deodatus etcetera religioso in Christo nobis carissimo fratri Iuniori comitti de Richenberg domus eiusdem salutem et sinceram in Domino caritatem. Propter susceptum de probitatis vestre meritis testimonium comendandum ac sperantes[a], quod in vobis[b] comissis in nostro ordine effectus administracionis utilis dante Domino vos comendet, igitur baiuliam Dorolsheim prioratus nostri Alamannie per mortem presencialiter [vacantem], sicud continet supplicacio pro parte vestra nobis facta, si sit ita, cum omnibus et singulis suis menbris, grangiis, iuribus et pertinenciis universis ad eam spectantibus et pertinentibus quoquomodo habendam, tenendam, regendam, gubernandam, augmentandam et meliorandam in spiritualibus et temporalibus tam in capite quam in menbris sub annua responsione et aliis oneribus impositis et imponendis racionabiliter secundum cursum aliarum baiuliarum prioratus nostri Alamanie supradicti ad annos quinque a die presencium continuo conputandos de voluntate, consilio et asensu fratrum et procerum conventus nostri Rodi nobis assistensium in hac parte de nostra certa scientia [150v] et speciali gratia vobis tamquam digno et benemerito auctoritate presencium conferimus et donamus benefaciendo in eadem, dum tamen ita sit, sicud in dicta supplicacione continetur, quamque absque dicti prioris et alterius cuiuscumque preiudicio nobis conferre[c] eadem possumus et valiamus. Comitentes etcetera. Quocirca etcetera necnon etcetera. Inhibentes etcetera. Data Rodi die vicessima mensis Iunii.

*a)* sprantes *MS* *b)* nobis *MS* *c)* confere *corr.*

*The younger count here mentioned as preceptor may have been a relative of Countess Katharina von Veringen, wife of Count Hugo von Reichenberg (in Alsace), who on 21 July 1351 sold some estates to the Counts Eberhard and Ulrich von Württemberg: Württembergische Regesten 1/2/2 (1925), 334 no. 8741. Other preceptors of Dorlisheim were Fr. Thomas von Grostein in the 1330s and 1340s, Fr. Eberhard von Landsberg in 1359: Buchheit, Commanderies (2014), 157, 194.*

## 12

*The Master Fr. Déodat de Gozon and the Convent nominate as their procurator Fr. Bartolomeo Benini, Prior of Rome and Pisa, to receive from Fr. Gallus von Lemberg, Prior of Bohemia, 5,100 ducats for his responsions. Fr. Napoleone dei Tiberti, Prior of Venice, has deposited this sum in Venice with the procurators of Saint Mark.*

*Rhodes, 1351 July 20*

*AOM 318 fol. 167r-8r (159r-60r), under* prioratus Alamanie et aliarum partium Alamanie.

Noverint universi et singuli, quod nos frater Deodatus de Gosono Dei gratia sacre domus Hospitalis santi Iohannis Ierosolimitani magister humilis et pauperum Christi custos et nos conventus domus eiusdem, nos videlicet dictus magister de voluntate, consilio et assensu dicti conventus et nos nominatus[a)] conventus de licensia, consilio et assensu dicti domini magistri, superioris nostri, ad sonum campane, ut moris est, in nostra santi Iohannis Colocensi ecclesia propterea congregati, confisi de fidei legalitate et circumspectionis industria religiosi in Christo nobis carissimi fratris Bartholomei Benini, domus eiusdem prioris Urbis et Pisarum, eundem priorem licet absentem tamquam presentem tenore presentium facimus, creamus, constituimus et sollempniter ordinamus nostrum et dicte domus nostre procuratorem, actorem, yconomum et nuntium specialem ac negotiorum gestorem ad petendum, recuperandum[b)], recipiendum et habendum nostro et dicte domus nostre procuratorio nomine atque vice a nobilibus et sapientibus viris dominis procuratoribus santi Marchi[c)] Veneciarum aut eorum altero vel aliis quibuscumque personis illos quinque milia centum ducatos auri, quos religiosus in Christo nobis carissimus frater Napoleonus de Tibertis domus eiusdem prior Veneciarum nuper in custodiam tradidit seu comandam procuratoribus prelibatis et quos auri ducatos dictus prior Veneciarum [167v] nostro nomine atque vice pridem habuerat et receperat a religioso in Christo nobis carissimo fratre Gallo de Lemberch, domus eiusdem priore Boemie, pro responsionibus et arreyragiis responsionum dicti prioratus Boemie nobis debitis[d)], et de receptis sive recipiendis recognitiones et quitaciones faciendum et concedendum et pro predictis et ea tangentibus agendum et deffendendum contra quaslibet personas et bona in quibuscumque locis et curiis ecclesiasticis vel secularibus et coram iudicibus, officialibus et personis aliis quibuscumque. Dantes et concedentes dicto procuratori nostro plenam et liberam potestatem et speciale mandatum predicta omnia et singula nostro et domus nostre prefate nomine explicandi, compendi, agendi, deffendendi, requirendi, protestandi et supplicandi litteras quaslibet tam simplices quam legendas impetrandi et obtinendi et impetratis per partem adversam contradicendi libellum seu libellos et alias peticiones simplices offerendi et offerri petendi, litem seu lites contestandi, de calumpnia et de veritate dicenda in animas nostras iurandi et subeundi cuiuslibet alterius generis licitum iuramentum, testes, instrumenta, litteras et alia[e)] quelibet probationum et scripturarum genera producendi et productos seu producta in contrarium repellendi et impugnandi, iudicium vanandi, sententiam et sententias audiendi et ab eis et a quocumque gravamine semel et pluries appellandi et appellationum causas prosequendi, unum et plures procuratores ad lites et causas tantummodo et non ad alia loco sui substituendi et substitutos revocandi et demum generaliter omnia alia et singula super premissis et ea tangentibus dicendi et faciendi, que ad premissa et eorum quodlibet explicanda necessaria fuerint et eciam opportuna et que nos in predictis et circa predicta dicere et facere possemus, si presentes personaliter adessemus, et relevantes dictum procuratorem nostrum et substituendum ac substituendos ab eo modo tamen[f)] premisso ab omni onere satisdandi, promitimus bona fide rem ratam haberi, iudicio sisti et iudicatum solvi suis clausulis opportunis, quicquid[g] per dictum procuratorem nostrum et substituendum ac substituendos ab eo actum, dictum, gestum, factum, procuratum et quitiatum fuerit in premissis et quolibet premissorum sub ypotheca et obligatione omnium bonorum nostrorum et dicte domus nostre presentium et futurorum non intendentes propter presentis procurationis constitutionem[h] procuratores nostros alios ad quecumque nostra negotia alia constitutos revocare, quinymo ipsos et eorum quemlibet de certa nostra scientia potius confirmare. [168r] In cuius rei testimonium presentes litteras per infrascriptum notarium scribi et publicari mandavimus et bulla nostra plumbea comuniri in appenso. Data Rodi die vicesima mensis Iulii anno incarnationis Domini millesimo CCC° quinquagesimo primo presentibus testibus discretis viris magistro Iohanne de Furno notario, Petro de Plano clerico, et me Martino Henecii auctoritate imperiali notario publico, qui hoc instrumentum procurationis manu mea propria scripsi et in testimonium premissorum signo meo consueto signavi.

*a)* nomiatus *MS* *b)* recieperandum *MS* *c) add. abbreviationem MS* *d) supra lin. post corr. MS* *e)* aliam *corr.* *f) supra lin. post corr.* *g) post corr.* *h)* contitutionem *MS*

## 13

*The Master Fr. Roger des Pins, with authority of the chapter general, retains Fr. Walter von Rechberg, Preceptor of Rottweil and Villingen.*

*Rhodes, [13]58 February 28*

*AOM 316 fol. 277r-v (281r-v), after* prioratus Baroli, Capue et aliarum partium regni.

Frater Rogerius de Pinibus etcetera religioso in Christo nobis carissimo fratri Waltehero de Rechperch domus eiusdem preceptori de Rothwel et Winlingen salutem et sinceram in Domino caritatem. Dum laudabilia vestre probitatis merita in considerationis[a] nostre aciem recensemus, digne agimus, cum vos accollimus prerogativa honoris et gratie specialis. Igitur vestram volentes honorare personam, ut proinde vestre fidei et devotionis zelus ad laudabiliora fervencius inantea animetur,[b] vos cum baiulia et arnesiis vestris solutis annuis responsionibus et aliis vobis et dicte vestre baiulie quibuscumque incombentibus oneribus supportandis auctoritate presencium et nostri presentis [277v] capituli generalis ad manus nostras de speciali gratia retinemus secundum bonos usus et laudabiles consuetudines domus nostre. Mandantes harum serie universis et singulis fratribus domus nostre quacumque auctoritate, dignitate vel officio fulgentibus, presentibus et futuris sub virtute sancte obediencie firmiter et districte, ne contra presentem nostram retentionem et gratiam aliquatenus venire presumant, quinymo illam studeant iuxta eius mentem et seriem inviolabiliter observare. In cuius etcetera. Data Rodi durante nostro predicto capitulo generali die vicesima secunda mensis Februarii anno LVIII.[1)]

*a)* considertione *MS* *b)* aminetur *MS*

## 14

*Licence for Fr. Heinrich von Neuenburg to travel overseas [to the West] and return.*

*[1358] June 17*

*AOM 316 fol. 218r (219r), under* prioratus Alamanie, Boemie et parcium aliarum Alamanie.

Die XVII Iunii data fuit licentia fratri Henrico de Novocastro eundi ad partes transmarinas ac[a)] redeundi, quando voluerit, ut in forma.

*a)* et re *praem. ante corr.*

## 15

*Licence for Fr. Heinrich to travel overseas to the Bailiwick (here* preceptoria) *of the March (of Brandenburg), where he is assigned his maintenance.*

*[1358 June 17]*

*AOM 316 fol. 218r (219r), under* prioratus Alamanie, Boemie et parcium aliarum Alamanie.

Eadem die fuit[a)] data licentia dicto fratri Henrico eundi ad transmarinas partes et accedendi ad preceptoriam Marchie, in qua fuit sibi assignata stagia. Et mandatum fuit dicte preceptorie preceptori, ut ei provideat ut in forma.

*a)* assignata stagia dicto fratri He *add. ante corr.*

## 16

*The Master Fr. Roger des Pins declares that there are not enough brethren in the Convent on Rhodes to defend the Order's islands. So he orders Fr. John of Yuele, Preceptor of Chibburn (Priory of England), to come to Rhodes, with the licence of his superior, and*

*1) The date is given as 1359 new style but according to no. 57 from 12 September 1358 the year must be 1358.*

*on 1 August of the following year with the* passagium *from Venice under the captaincy of Fr. Napoleone dei Tiberti, Prior of Venice, together with a fixed number of brethren from the Tongues of England, Italy and* Alamania.

*Rhodes, 1358 July 10*

*AOM 316 fol. 200v-201r (201v-2r), under* prioratus Anglie, Ibernie et Scocie. *Cf. Delaville (1913), 140 with note 2.*

Frater Rogerius de Pinibus etcetera religioso in Christo nobis carissimo fratri Iohannis de Yuele domus eiusdem preceptori de Chiborna[1] salutem et sinceram in Domino caritatem. Quia ad promocionem fidei hostiumve eius resistenciam nostrarumque insularum tutelam pauci fratres degunt presencialiter in nostro cismarino conventu fieri debere passagium de Veneciis ad Rodum intra annum unum a mense Augusti primo venienti continuo computandum sub capitanatu religiosi in Christo nobis carissimi fratris Neapolionis de Tibertis domus eiusdem prioris Veneciarum de certo fratrum numero domus nostre linguarum Anglie, Ytalie et Alamanie presencialiter consulta deliberacione habita cum nostris proceribus ducxerimus ordinandum, et quod vos de prioratu Anglie in ipso passagio venire cum equis et armis sufficientibus debeatis. Vobis ydeo tenore presencium sub virtute sante obediencie districte precipimus et mandamus, quatenus [201r] in dicto passagio cum equis et armis sufficientibus ad Dei obsequia ad has partes infallibiliter veniatis a vestro superiore prius licencia requisita. Data Rodi die decima mensis Iulii anno LVIII.

## 17

*The Master Fr. Roger [des Pins] grants for ten years to Fr. Nikolaus von Heinriet, Preceptor of Boxberg and Dätzingen, the Preceptory of Krautheim (Priory of* Alamania), *which is vacant following the death of Fr. Berthold von Henneberg.*

*Rhodes, [13]58 August 1*

*AOM 316 fol. 218r (219r), under* prioratus Alamanie, Boemie et parcium aliarum Alamanie.

Frater Rogerius etcetera religioso etcetera fratri Nicholao de Hehenriet domus eiusdem salutem et sinceram in Domino caritatem. Religionis[a] decor, morum honestas et alia virtutum dona multimoda, quibus vos carisimatis[!] gratia decoravit, ad impertiendum vobis favoris nostri gratiam rationabiliter[b] nos moventes ac sperantes, quod in comisso vobis regimine effectus administracionis provide vos utilem faciente Domine exibebit, de baiuliis de Boxberg et Detichingen

1) *Chibburn, north of Newcastle upon Tyne.*

per alias nostras litteras vobis noviter facta gracia non obstante baiuliam sive domum de Curchem prioratus nostri Alamanie per mortem condam fratris Bertoholdi de Heneberg vacantem presencialiter et propterea[c] ad disposicionem nostram devolutam[d] cum omnibus et singulis suis membris[e], iuribus et pertinenciis[f] universis ad eam spectantibus et pertinentibus[g], quoquomodo et cum quibus dictus condam frater Bertholdus, dum vixit[h], eam tenuit et possedit, habendam, tenendam[i], regendam, gubernandam[j], auguementandam[!] et meliorandam in spiritualibus et temporalibus[k] tam in capite quam in membris sub anua responsione[l] et aliis oneribus inpositis et inponendis[m] racionabiliter secundum[n] comunem cursum et aliarum baiuliarum prioratus nostri Alamannie supradicti in capitulo provinciali prioratus eiusdem omnibus[o] et singulis infalibiliter[p] exolvendis[q] et, nisi feceritis, destituendi vos de dicta baiulia et illam ad manus suas ponendi iuxta statutum priori et receptori responsionum dicti prioratus hac serie plenam concedimus potestatem gratia huiusmodi vobis facta aliquatenus non obstante[r], hinc ad instans festum nativitatis sancti Iohannis baptiste et ab eodem festo inantea ad annos decem continuos et completos de consilio et assensu fratrum et procerum conventus nostri Rodi nobis assistencium in hac parte auctoritate presencium de nostra certa scientia et speciali gratia vobis conferimus, concedimus et donamus benefaciendo in eadem vosque preceptorem et comendatorem in dicta constituimus baiulia tenore presencium ac eciam ordinamus. Comitentes etcetera. Quocirca etcetera. Inhibentes etcetera. In cuius etcetera. Data Rodi[s] die prima mensis Agusti anno LVIII.

*a)* Religioso *MS* *b)* ratonabiliter *MS* *c)* proptera *MS* *d)* de volumtam *MS* *e)* memebris *MS* *f)* pertineciis *MS* *g)* pertinetibus *MS* *h)* iuxta *MS* *i)* tenedam *MS* *j)* gubernadam *MS* *k)* teporalibus *MS* *l)* responsionem *MS* *m)* inponedis *MS* *n)* secudum *MS* *o)* anis *MS* *p)* in falibiter *MS* *q)* ex o *praem. ante corr.* *r)* o *supra lin.* *s)* anno LVIII *add. ante corr.*

## 18

*The Master Fr. Roger [des Pins] grants for ten years to Fr. Nikolaus von Heinriet, who recently received the Preceptories of Krautheim and Dätzingen, the Preceptory of Boxberg (Priory of* Alamania), *which is vacant following the death of Fr. Berthold von Henneberg.*

*Rhodes, [13]58 August 1*

*AOM 316 fol. 218v (219v), under* prioratus Alamanie, Boemie et parcium aliarum Alamanie.

Frater Rogerius etcetera fratri Nicolao de Hehenriet domus eiusdem salutem etcetera. Religionis decor, morum honestas et alia virtutum dona multimoda, quibus vos carismatis gratia decoravit, ad impertiendum vobis favoris nostri gratiam rationabiliter nos moventes ac sperantes, quod in comisso vobis regimine[a] effectus administrationis provide vos utilem faciente Domino exhibebit, de baiuliis[b] de Cruchein et de Detichingen per alias nostras litteras vobis noviter facta gratia non obstante baiuliam de Boxberg prioratus nostri Alamanie per mortem condam fratris Bertholdi de Hennenberg vacantem presencialiter et propterea ad disposicionem nostram devolutam cum omnibus et singulis suis membris, iuribus et pertinenciis universis ad eam spectantibus et pertinentibus ac spectare et pertinere debentibus quoquomodo, et cum quibus dictus condam frater Berhtoldus eam, dum vixit, tenuit et possedit[c], habendam, tenendam, regendam, augmentandam et meliorandam in spiritualibus et temporalibus tam in capite quam in membris sub annua responsione et aliis oneribus impositis et imponendis racionabiliter secundum comunem cursum aliarum baiuliarum prioratus nostri Alamannie supradicti in capitulo provinciali prioratus eiusdem annis singulis infallibiliter exolvendis et, nisi feceritis, destituendi vos dicta baiulia et illam ad manus suas ponendi iuxta statutum priori et receptori responsionum dicti prioratus hac serie plenam concedimus potestatem gratia huiusmodi vobis facta[d] non obstante, hinc ad instans festum nativitatis sancti Iohannis baptiste et ab[e] eodem festo inantea ad annos decem continuos et completos de consilio et assensu fratrum et procerum conventus nostri Rodi nobis assistencium in hac parte auctoritate presencium de nostra certa scientia et speciali gratia vobis confirmamus, concedimus et donamus benefaciendo in eadem vosque preceptorem et comendatorem in dicta constituimus baiulia tenore presencium et eciam ordinamus. Comitentes etcetera. Mandantes etcetera ac religioso in Christo nobis carissimo fratri ·· domus eiusdem priori dicti prioratus Alamanie seu eiusdem prioratus regimini quovis titulo nunc vel imposterum presidenti, ut vos vel procuratores vestrum in corporalem possesionem pacificam et quietam dicte baiulie inducat omni contradictione remota et conservet inductum amoto abinde quolibet ilicito detentore, si quis sit, quem nos amovemus per presentes et decernimus amovendum, necnon universis et singulis fratribus domus nostre quacumque auctoritate, dignitate vel officio fulgentibus, presentibus et futuris, ne contra presentem nostram donacionem, concessionem et gratiam aliquathenus venire presumant, quinymo illam iuxta eius mentem et seriem studeant inviolabiliter observare. Inhibentes etcetera. In cuius etcetera. Data Rodi[f] die prima mensis Agusti anno LVIII.

*a)* regiminibus *corr.* *b)* baiulias *corr.* *c)* possidit *MS* *d)* facte *MS* *e)* ad *corr.* *f)* anno LVIII *del.*

## 19

*The Master Fr. Roger [des Pins] grants for ten years to Fr. Nikolaus von Heinriet, who recently received the Preceptories of Krautheim and Boxberg, the Preceptory of Dätzingen (Priory of* Alamania), *which is vacant following its resignation by Fr. Walter von Rechberg.*

*Rhodes, [13]58 August 1*

*AOM 316 fol. 219v-20r (220v-21r), under* prioratus Alamanie, Boemie et parcium aliarum Alamanie.

Frater Rogerius etcetera religioso etcetera fratri Nicolao de Hehenriet domus eiusdem salutem etcetera. Religionis decor, morum honestas et illa virtutum dona multimoda, quibus vos almi neupmatis[1] gratia insignivit, ad impertiendum vobis favoris nostri gratiam rationabiliter nos moventes ac sperantes, quod in comisso vobis regimine effectus administrationis provide vos utilem faciente Domino exhibebit, ad baiulias[a] de Cruchem et de Boxberg per nos noviter vobis facta gratia non obstante baiuliam sive domum [220r] de Tithingen prioratus nostri Alamanie presencialiter vacantem[b] per resignacionem fratris Wlcheri de Bechberg et ad nostram propterea[c] disposicionem devolutam, sicut vestra continuit supplicacio data nobis, si sit ita, cum omnibus et singulis suis membris, iuribus et pertinenciis universis ad eam spectantibus et pertinentibus, quoquomodo et cum quibus eam tenuit et possedit dictus frater Walterus, habendam, tenendam, regendam, gubernandam, augmentandam et meliorandam in spiritualibus et temporalibus tam in capite quam in membris sub annua responsione et aliis oneribus impositis et imponendis racionabiliter secundum comunem cursum aliarum baiuliarum prioratus nostri Alamanie supradicti[d] in capitulo provinciali prioratus eiusdem annis singulis infalibiliter exsolvendis[e] et, nisi feceritis, destituendi vos dicta baiulia et illam ad manus suas ponendi priori et receptori responsionum dicti prioratus hac serie plenam concedimus potestatem gracia huiusmodi vobis facta aliquatenus non obstante, hinc ad instans[f] festum nativitatis sancti Iohannis baptiste et ab eodem festo inantea[g] ad anos decem continuos et complectos de consilio et assensu fratrum et procerum conventus nostri Rodi nobis assistencium in hac parte auctoritate presencium de nostra certa [scientia] et speciali[h] gratia vobis conferimus, concedimus et donamus benefaciendo in eadem vosque preceptorem[i] et commendatorem in dicta constituimus baiulia presencium serie et eciam ordinamus. Comitentes etcetera. Quocirca[j] etcetera ac religioso in Christo nobis carissimo fratri ·· domus eiusdem prioris dicti prioratus Alamanie seu eiusdem prioratus regimini nunc vel[k] in futurum[l] quovis titulo presidenti, ut vos vel procuratorem vestrum in corporalem possessionem pacificam et quietam dicte[m] baiulie inducat omni contradicione[n] remota et conservet inductum amoto abinde quolibet detentore, si quis sit, quem nos amovemus per presentes et decernimus firmiter amovendum, necnon universis et singulis fratribus domus nostre, cuiuscumque status, gradus vel condicionis existant, presentibus et futuris, ne contra presentem nostram donacionem et gratiam aliquatenus venire presumant, quinymo illam iuxta eius mentem et seriem studeant inviolabiliter observare. Inhibentes etcetera. In cuius etcetera. Data Rodi die prima mensis Agusti anno LVIII.

*a)* baiuliis *MS* *b)* vacantes *MS* *c)* popterea *corr.* *d)* superdicti *MS* *e)* exolvendis *corr.* *f)* instas *MS* *g)* inatea *MS* *h)* specialis *MS* *i)* preceptoram *MS* *j)* Quonsirqua *MS* *k)* condicionis *del.* *l)* fratrum *MS* *m)* decem *MS* *n)* contradicionem *MS*

*1) Du Cange 5, 590, cf. ibid. 6, 378–9 s.v. pneuma.*

## 20

*The Master Fr. Roger [des Pins] confirms Fr. Konrad von Braunsberg for ten years in the Bailiwick of Utrecht (Priory of* Alamania).

*Rhodes, [13]58 August 1*

*AOM 316 fol. 219r (220r), under* prioratus Alamanie, Boemie et parcium aliarum Alamanie. *Ed. van Winter (1998), 31 no. 3.*

Frater Rogerius etcetera religioso etcetera fratri Cůnrado de Brunsperg domus eiusdem preceptori seu bailivo Tragetensi salutem etcetera. Propter probitatis vestre merita et administrationem accomodam, quam in comissis vobis regiminibus in nostro ordine, sicut testimonio fidedigno accepimus, habuistis, illa vobis libenter annuimus, que conservationem vestri status concernere dignoscuntur. Igitur preceptoriam seu baiuliam Tragetensem seu in Traiecto prioratus nostri Alamanie cum omnibus et singulis suis membris, iuribus et pertinenciis universis ad eam spectantibus et pertinentibus, quoquomodo et cum quibus eam tenetis et presencialiter possidetis, habendam, tenendam, regendam[a)], gubernandam, augmentandam et meliorandam in spiritualibus et temporalibus tam in capite quam in membris sub annua responsione et aliis oneribus impositis et imponendis rationabiliter secundum communem cursum aliarum baiuliarum prioratus nostri Alamanie supradicti in capitulo provinciali dicti prioratus annis singulis exolvendis et, nisi feceritis, destituendi vos de dicta baiulia et illam ad manus suas ponendi iuxta statutum priori et receptori responsionum dicti prioratus hac serie plenam concedimus potestatem huiusmodi facta vobis gratia in aliquo non obstante, hinc ad instans festum nativitatis sancti Iohannis baptiste et ab eodem festo inantea ad annos decem continuos et completos de nostrorum procerum consilio auctoritate presencium de nostra certa scientia et speciali gratia vobis confirmamus benefaciendo in eadem. Comitentes etcetera. Quocirca etcetera. Inhibentes[b)] etcetera. In cuius etcetera. Data Rodi die prima mensis Agusti anno LVIII.

*a)* s *del.* *b)* inhbentes *corr.*

## 21

*The Master Fr. Roger [des Pins] confirms Fr. Johann von Steinweg for ten years in the Preceptory of Cologne (Priory of* Alamania).

*Rhodes, [13]58 August 1*

*AOM 316 fol. 219r-v (220r-v), under* prioratus Alamanie, Boemie et parcium aliarum Alamanie.

Frater Rogerius etcetera religioso etcetera fratri Iohanni de Via Lapidea domus eiusdem preceptori domus seu preceptorie de Colonia salutem etcetera. Propter probitatis vestre merita et administracionem accomodam, quam in comissis vobis regiminibus in nostro ordine, sicut fidedigno testimonio accepimus, habuistis, illa vobis libenter annuimus, que conservationem vestri status concernere dignoscuntur. Igitur preceptoriam seu baiuliam supradictam de Colonia prioratus nostri Alamanie cum omnibus et singulis suis membris, iuribus et pertinenciis universis ad eam spectantibus et pertinentibus, quoquomodo et cum quibus eam tenetis et presencialiter possidetis, habendam, tenendam, regendam, gubernandam, augmentandam et meliorandam in spiritualibus et temporalibus tam in capite quam in membris sub anua responsione et aliis oneribus impositis et imponendis racionabiliter secundum comunem cursum aliarum baiuliarum prioratus Alamanie supradicti in capitulo provinciali dicti prioratus annis singulis exolvendis et, nisi feceritis, destituendi vos de dicta baiulia et illam ad manus suas ponendi iuxta statutum[a] priori et receptori responsionum dicti prioratus hac serie plenam concedimus potestatem huiusmodi facta vobis gratia in aliquo non obstante, hinc ad instans festum nativitatis sancti Iohannis baptiste et ab eodem festo inantea ad annos decem continuos et completos [219v] de nostrorum procerum[b] consilio auctoritate presencium de nostra certa scientia et speciali gratia vobis confirmamus benefaciendo in eadem. Comitentes etcetera. Quocirca etcetera. Inhibentes etcetera. In cuius etcetera. Data Rodi die[c] prima mensis Agusti anno LVIII.

*a)* statuum *MS* *b)* preceptorum *del.* *c)* dei *MS*

## 22

*The Master Fr. Roger [des Pins] grants for ten years to Fr. Friedrich von Zollern the Preceptory of Rohrdorf (Priory of* Alamania), *which is vacant following the death of Fr. Konrad Waloh.*

*Rhodes, [13]58 August 5*

*AOM 316 fol. 219v (220v), under* prioratus Alamanie, Boemie et parcium aliarum Alamanie.

Frater Rogerius etcetera religioso etcetera fratri Friderico de Zolera domus eiusdem salutem etcetera. Religionis decor, morum honestas et alia virtutum dona multimoda, quibus vos carisimatis[!] gratia decoravit, ad[a] impertiendum[b] vobis favoris nostri gratiam racionabiliter nos moventes ac sperantes, quod in comisso vobis regimine effectus administracionem provide vos utilem faciente[c] Domino exhibebit[d], baiuliam sive domum de Rodrof prioratus nostri Alamanie vacantem presencialiter obitu condam fratris Cůnradi dicti Waloh[e] ultimi eiusdem preceptorie preceptoris, ut continuit exposicio[f] per vos facta nobis, si sit ita[g], cum omnibus et singulis suis membris[h], iuribus[i], et pertinenciis[j] universis ad eam spectantibus et pertinentibus quoquomodo habendam, tenendam, regendam, augementandam[!] et meliorandam in spiritualibus et temporalibus[k] tam in capite quam membris sub annua responsione et aliis oneribus inpositis et inponendis racionabiliter secundum comunem cursum aliarum baiuliarum prioratus nostri Alamanie supradicti in capitulo provinciali prioratus eiusdem annis singulis infallibiliter exolvendis[l] et, nisi feceritis, destituendi vos dicta baiulia et illam ad manus suas ponendi iuxta statutum priori et receptori responsionum dicti prioratus hac serie plenam concedimus potestatem huiusmodi vobis facta gratia non obstante, hinc ad instans festum nativitatis sancti Iohannis baptiste et ab eodem festo[m] inantea ad annos decem continuos et completos de consilio et assensu fratrum et procerum conventus nostri Rodi nobis assistencium in hac parte auctoritate presencium de nostra certa scientia et speciali gratia vobis confirmamus, concedimus et donamus benefaciendo in eadem vosque preceptorem et comendatorem in dicta constituimus baiulia tenore presencium et eciam ordinamus. Comitentes etcetera. Quocirca etcetera. Inhibentes etcetera. In cuius etcetera. Data Rodi die quinta mensis Agusti anno LVIII.

*a)* in *del.* *b)* impendum *MS* *c)* facientem *MS* *d)* exhlicit *MS* *e)* Wloh *corr.* *f)* expocio *MS* *g)* itam *MS* *h)* memebris *MS* *i)* sub anua *del.* *j)* pertineciis *MS* *k)* teporalibus *MS* *l)* *del. et add. ante corr.* racionabiliter secundum comunem cursum aliarum baiuliarum *(homoiotel.)* *m)* inantea *del.*

## 23

*The Master Fr. Roger [des Pins] confirms Fr. Nikolaus Wildungsmauer for ten years in the Preceptories of Mailberg and Vienna (Priory of Bohemia).*

*Rhodes, [13]58 August 5*

*AOM 316 fol. 223v (224v), under* prioratus Alamanie, Boemie et parcium aliarum Alamanie.

Frater Rogerius etcetera religioso etcetera fratri Nicolao Wilugsmaurer domus eiusdem, comendatori in Mewerg et de Wienna, salutem etcetera. Propter probitatis vestre merita et administrationem accomodam, quam in[a] comissis vobis regiminibus in nostro ordine, sicut fidedigno testimonio accepimus, habuistis, illa vobis libenter annuimus, que conservationem vestri status concernere dignoscuntur. Igitur baiulias de Mewerg et de Wienna prioratus nostri Boemie cum omnibus et singulis suis membris, iuribus et pertinenciis universis ad eas spectantibus et pertinentibus, quoquomodo et cum quibus eas tenetis [et] presencialiter possidetis, habendas, tenendas, regendas, gubernandas, augmentandas et meliorandas in spiritualibus et temporalibus tam in capite quam in membris sub annua responsione et aliis oneribus impositis et imponendis rationabiliter secundum comunem cursum aliarum baiuliarum prioratus nostri Boemie supradicti in capitulo provinciali dicti prioratus annis singulis exolvendis et, nisi feceritis, destituendi vos de dictis baiuliis et illam ad manus suas ponendi iuxta statutum priori et receptori responcionum dicti prioratus hac serie plenam concedimus potestatem huiusmodi facta vobis gratia in aliquo non obstante, hinc ad instans festum nativitatis sancti Iohannis baptiste et ab eodem festo inantea ad annos decem continuos et completos de nostrorum procerum consilio auctoritate presencium de nostra certa scientia et speciali gratia vobis confirmamus benefaciendo in eadem. Comitentes etcetera. Quocirca[b)] etcetera. Inhibentes etcetera. In cuius etcetera. Data Rodi die quinta mensis Agusti anno LVIII.

*a) add. supra lin.* *b)* Qorica *MS*

## 24

*The Master Fr. Roger [des Pins] confirms Fr. Peter von Waleczevo for ten years in the Preceptory of Brünn (Priory of Bohemia).*

*Rhodes, [13]58 August 5*

*AOM 316 fol. 224r-v (225r-v), under* prioratus Alamanie, Boemie et parcium aliarum Alamanie.

Frater Rogerius etcetera religioso etcetera fratri Petro de Waleczovo domus eiusdem, comendatori in Cruce, salutem etcetera. Propter probitatis vestre merita et administracionem accomodam, quam in comissis vobis regiminibus in nostro ordine, sicut fidedigno testimonio accepimus, habuistis[a)], illa vobis libenter annuimus, que conservacionem vestri status concernere dignoscuntur. Igitur baiuliam predictam[b)] de Cruce prioratus nostri Boemie cum omnibus et singulis suis membris, iuribus et pertinenciis universis ad eam spectantibus et pertinentibus, quoquomodo et cum quibus eam tenetis et presencialiter possidetis[c)], habendam, tenendam, regendam, gubernandam, augmentandam et meliorandam in spiritualibus et temporalibus tam in capite quam in membris sub annua responsione et aliis oneribus inpositis et imponendis rationabiliter secundum comunem cursum aliarum baiuliarum prioratus nostri Boemie supradicti in capitulo provinciali dicti prioratus annis singulis exolvendis et, nisi feceritis, destituendi vos de dicta baiulia et illam ad manus suas ponendi iuxta statutum priori et receptori responsionum dicti prioratus hac serie plenam concedimus potestatem huiusmodi facta vobis gratia in aliquo [224v] non obstante, hinc ad instans festum nativitatis sancti Iohannis baptiste et ab eodem festo inantea ad annos decem continuos et completos de voluntate[d)], consilio et assensu fratrum et procerum conventus nostri nobis assistensium in hac parte auctoritate presencium de nostra certa scientia et speciali gratia vobis confirmamus benefaciendo in eadem. Comitentes etcetera. Quocirca etcetera necnon etcetera. Inhibentes etcetera. In cuius etcetera. Data Rodi die quinta mensis Agusti anno LVIII.

*a)* habistis *MS* *b)* baiulia predicta *MS* *c)* possitis *MS* *d)* nostra *praem. ante corr.*

## 25

*The Master Fr. Roger [des Pins] and the Convent confirm Fr. Konrad von Randeck for his lifetime in the Preceptory of Weißenburg (Priory of* Alamania).

*Rhodes, [13]58 August 6*

*AOM 316 fol. 220r-v (221r-v), under* prioratus Alamanie, Boemie et parcium aliarum Alamanie.

Frater Rogerius etcetera et nos conventus etcetera religioso etcetera Cůnrado de Randech domus eiusdem, comendatori in Wisenburg, salutem etcetera. Propter probitatis vestre merita et administracionem accomodam, quam in comissis vobis regiminibus in nostro ordine, sicut fidedigno testimonio accepimus, habuistis, illa vobis libenter annuimus, que conservacionem vestri status concernere dignoscuntur. Igitur preceptoriam in Wisenburg supradictam prioratus nostri Alamanie cum omnibus et singulis suis membris, iuribus et pertinenciis universis ad eam spectantibus et pertinentibus, quoquomodo[a] et cum quibus eam tenetis et presencialiter possidetis, habendam, tenendam, regendam, gubernandam, augmentandam et melio[220v]randam in spiritualibus et temporalibus tam in capite quam in menbris sub annua responsione et aliis oneribus impositis et imponendis rationabiliter secundum comunem[b] cursum aliarum baiuliarum prioratus nostri Alamanie supradicti in capitulo provinciali[c] dicti [prioratus] anis singulis exolvendis et, nisi feceritis, destituendi vos de dicta baiulia et illam ad manus suas ponendi iuxta statutum[d] priori et receptori responsionum dicti prioratus hac serie plenam concedimus potestatem huiusmodi facta vobis gratia in aliquo non obstante, invicem deliberato consilio auctoritate presencium de nostra certa sciencia[e] et speciali[f] gratia ad vitam vestram vobis conferimus[g] benefaciendo in eadem. Comitentes etcetera. Quocirca[h] etcetera necnon etcetera. Inibentes etcetera. In cuius etcetera. Data Rodi die[i] sexta mensis Agusti anno LVIII.

*a)* quoquomo *MS* *b)* comucem *MS* *c)* proviciali *MS* *d)* statum *MS* *e)* sencia *MS* *f)* specialis *MS* *g)* conc *del.* *h)* Qonosiqua *MS* *i)* vicesima *del.*

## 26

*The Master Fr. Roger [des Pins] confirms Fr. Zdeněk von Wartenberg for ten years in the Preceptories of Prague and Orlovice (Priory of Bohemia).*

*Rhodes, [13]58 August 6*

*AOM 316 fol. 220v (221v), under* prioratus Alamanie, Boemie et parcium aliarum Alamanie.

Frater Rogerius etcetera religioso etcetera fratri Schercono de Wartebreh domus eiusdem preceptori seu commendatori de Praga et de Orlabicz salutem etcetera. Propter probitatis vestre merita et administracionem accomodam, quam in comissis vobis regiminibus in nostro ordine, sicut fidedigno testimonio accepimus[a)], habuistis[b)], illa vobis libenter anuimus, que conservacionem vestri status concernere dignoscuntur. Igitur preceptorias seu comendatorias supradictas de Praga et de Orlabicz prioratus nostri Boemie cum omnibus et singulis suis membris, iuribus et pertinenciis universis ad eas spectantibus et pertinentibus, quoquomodo et cum quibus eas tenetis et presencialiter possidetis, habendas, tenendas, regendas, gubernandas, augmentandas et meliorandas in spiritualibus et temporalibus tam in capite quam in membris sub annua responsione et aliis oneribus impositis et imponendis racionabiliter secundum communem cursum aliarum baiuliarum prioratus nostri Boemie[c)] supradicti in capitulo provinciali dicti prioratus annis singulis exolvendis et, nisi feceritis, destituendi vos de dictis baiuliis seu comendatoriis et illas ad manus suas ponendi iuxta statutum priori et receptori responsionum dicti prioratus hac serie plenam concedimus potestatem huiusmodi facta vobis gratia in aliquo non obstante, hinc[d)] ad instans festum nativitatis sancti Iohannis baptiste et ab eodem festo inantea ad anos decem continuos et completos cum consilio et assensu fratrum et procerum conventus nostri Rodi nobis assistencium in hac parte auctoritate presencium de nostra certa scientia et speciali gratia vobis confirmamus benefaciendo in eadem. Comitentes etcetera. Quocirca etcetera necnon etcetera. Inhibentes etcetera. In cuius etcetera. Data Rodi[e)] die sexta mensis Agusti anno LVIII.

*a)* accepmus *MS* *b)* habuisti *MS* *c)* Boeme *MS* *d)* hic *MS* *e)* Ro *del.*

## 27

*The Master Fr. Roger [des Pins] confirms Fr. Eberhard von Landsberg for ten years in the Preceptory of Dorlisheim (Priory of* Alamania).

*Rhodes, [13]58 August 6*

*AOM 316 fol. 221r (222r), under* prioratus Alamanie, Boemie et parcium aliarum Alamanie.

Frater Rogerius etcetera religioso etcetera fratri Eberhardo de Lantsperg domus eiusdem, comendatori in Thorolzhen, salutem etcetera. Propter vestre[a)] probitatis merita et administrationem accomodam, quam in comissis vobis regiminibus in nostro ordine, sicut fidedigno testimonio accepimus, habuistis, illa vobis libenter annuimus, que conservationem vestri status concernere dignoscuntur. Igitur baiuliam predictam in Thorolzhen prioratus nostri Alamanie cum[b] ecclesia parrochiali sancti Georgii, membro baiulie supradicte, et[b] cum omnibus et singulis suis membris, iuribus et pertinenciis universis ad eam spectantibus et pertinentibus, quoquomodo et cum quibus eam tenetis et presencialiter possidetis, habendam, tenendam, regendam, gubernandam, augmentandam et meliorandam in spiritualibus et temporalibus tam in [capite quam in membris] sub anua responsione et aliis oneribus inpositis et inponendis[c] racionabiliter secundum comunem cursum aliarum baiuliarum prioratus nostri Alamanie supradicti in capitulo provinciali dicti prioratus annis singulis exolvendis et, nisi feceritis, destituendi vos de dicta baiulia et illam ad manus suas ponendi iuxta statutum[d] priori et receptori responsionum dicti prioratus hac serie plenam concedimus potestatem huiusmodi facta vobis gratia in aliquo non obstante, hinc ad instans[e] festum[f] nativitatis sancti Iohannis baptiste et ab eodem festo inantea ad anos decem continuos et completos de nostrorum procerum consilio auctoritate presencium de nostra certa scientia[g] et speciali[h] gratia vobis conferimus benefaciendo in eadem. Comitentes etcetera. Quocirca[i] etcetera necnon etcetera. Inibentes etcetera. In cuius etcetera. Data Rodi die sexta mensis Agusti anno LVIII.

*a) supra lin.* *b)* cum – et *add. in marg.* *c)* inponedis *MS* *d)* eius *del.* *e)* instas *MS* *f)* sancti *del.* *g)* sencia *MS* *h)* specialis *MS* *i)* Quonsirqua *MS*

## 28

*The Master Fr. Roger [des Pins] confirms Fr. Konrad von Randeck, Preceptor of Weißenburg, and Fr. Anselm von Eltville for their lifetime in the tithe in Wörrstadt that was given them by the former Preceptor of Mainz Fr. Peter von Frankfurt in return for 150 malters of corn as an annual pension payment. The grant was confirmed by the former lieutenant of the Master and the Convent in* Alamania *Fr. Hugo von Werdenberg.*

*Rhodes, [13]58 August 8*

*AOM 316 fol. 221r-v (222r-v), under* prioratus Alamanie, Boemie et parcium aliarum Alamanie.

Frater Rogerius etcetera religiosis[a] etcetera fratribus Cůnrado de Randech domus eiusdem preceptori[b] de Wisembug et Anschelmo de Eltfil eiusdem domus salutem etcetera. Ut exposicione pro parte vestra nobis facta percepimus[c], religiosus in Christo nobis carissimus frater Petrus de Fraliefurt domus eiusdem preceptor olim preceptorie Maguncie prioratus nostri Alamanie, dum ipsius preceptorie regimini preerat, cum consilio fratrum preceptorie[d] eiusdem decimam Werstat[e] vobis ambobus contulit et concessit sub annua responsione seu pensione centum quinquaginta maltrorum siliginis presidenti dicte preceptorie regimini[f] in annis singulis infalibiliter exolvendi et postea religiosus in Christo nobis carissimus[g] frater Hugo de Werdembreg domus eiusdem, tum locumtenens[h)] noster et nostri conventus [221v] in dicto prioratu Alamanie, vobis decimam confirmavit eandem. Et propterea nobis humiliter suplicastis[i)], ut dignaremur vobis ad vitam vestram dictam decimam confirmare. Nosque vestris suplicacionibus, quantum decenter[j)] possumus, vestre probitatis exigentibus[k)] meritis favorabiliter anuentes decimam in Werstat supradictam, si et prout per dictum fratrem Petrum de Franbefurt[l)] vobis collata extitit[m)], et sub eadem responsione seu pensione et per fratrem Hugonem de Wrdembrg locumtenentem supradictum confirmata de consilio et assensu fratrum et procerum conventus nostri Rodi nobis assistencium in hac parte auctoritate presencium de nostra certa scientia et speciali[n)] gratia ad vitam vestram vobis confirmamus. Mandantes sub virtute sante obendiencie firmiter et districte universis et singulis fratribus domus nostre quacumque auctoritate, dignitate vel officio fulgentibus, presentibus et futuris, ne contra presentem nostram confirmationem et gratiam aliquatenus venire presumant, quinymmo illam studeant iuxta eius mentem inviolabiliter observare. Data Rodi die octava mensis Agusti anno LVIII.

*a)* religioso *MS* *b)* perceptori *MS* *c)* precepimus *MS* *d)* perceptorie *MS* *e)* Westat *corr.* *f) del.* *g)* carisimo *MS* *h)* locumtenentes *MS* *i)* suplicasti *MS* *j)* decentur *MS* *k)* exignetibus *MS* *l)* Breg locumtenentem *del.* *m)* exititit *MS* *n)* specialis *MS*

## 29

*The Master Fr. Roger [des Pins] confirms to Fr. Konrad von Randeck, Preceptor of Weißenburg, 80 malters of corn as an annual pension payment from the tithe of the church in Wörrstadt within the Preceptory of Mainz given him by the former visitor in* Alamania *Fr. Gérard de Montaigu, Preceptor of Romans. This was done in compensation for damages suffered by Fr. Helfrich von Rüdigheim, Preceptor of Mainz. This gift had been confirmed by the Master's former lieutenant in* Alamania, *Fr. Hugo von Werdenberg. Fr. Konrad is also confirmed in possession of the* hospitium *or* habitaculum *called Nuremberg in the Preceptory of Mainz and of 35 malters of corn to be paid by Fr. Johann Maxden, Preceptor of Worms, for goods redeemed from laymen while Fr. Konrad was Preceptor of Worms.*

*Rhodes, [13]58 August 8*

*AOM 316 fol. 221v-2r (222v-3r), under* prioratus Alamanie, Boemie et parcium aliarum Alamanie.

Frater Rogerius etcetera religioso etcetera fratri Cůnrado de Bandech domus eiusdem preceptori de Wisenburg salutem etcetera. Ob vestra laudabilia portamenta vestreque merita probitatis, quibus comendabimini[a)] multipliciter testimonio fidedigno, peticiones vestras exaudientes favorabiliter et benigne octuaginta maltra siliginis per religiosum in Christo nobis carissimum fratrem

Girardum de Montagnino domus eiusdem preceptorem de Romania,[1] dum visitator noster et conventus nostri erat in prioratu nostro Alamanie, vobis assignata super decima ecclesie nostre in Werstat[b)] in preceptoria Maguncie prioratus[c)] predicti pro nonnullis dampnis per fratrem Helfricum de Růdiken domus eiusdem preceptorem dicte preceptorie Maguncie vobis in eadem illatis et per religiosum etcetera fratrem Hugonem de Werdemberg tunc locum nostrum tenentem in dicto prioratu Alamanie vobis postea confirmata necnon hospicium unum seu habitaculum appellatum Nůremberg situm infra preceptoria Maguncie per religiosum [etcetera] fratris Iohannis Maxden domus eiusdem preceptoris dicte preceptorie Wormancie pro aliquibus bonis a manibus secularium per vos ereptis et eidem baiulie acquisitis, dum ipsius eratis preceptor, sicut vestra continuit exposicio facta nobis, ad vitam [222r] vestram de consilio et assensu fratrum et procerum conventus nostri Rodi nobis assistencium in hac parte auctoritate presencium de nostra certa scientia et speciali gratia vobis confirmamus, si et prout vobis ut premittitur[d)] premissa omnia et singula fuerunt collata et assignata. Mandantes sub virtute sancte obediencie religionis etcetera fratribus ·· preceptori preceptorie Maguncie supradicte et ·· preceptori preceptorie Wormacie memorate seu quibuscumque aliis earundem preceptoriarum regiminibus nunc vel imposterum[e)] quibusvis titulis presidentibus, ut presidentes[f)] videlicet dicte preceptorie Maguncie prefata octuaginta maltra siliginis et presidentes preceptorie Wormacie supradicte suprascripta triginta quinque maltra siliginis vobis vel procuratori vestro dent et tradant annis singulis contradicione remota necnon universis et singulis fratribus domus nostre quacumque auctoritate, dignitate vel officio fulgentibus, presentibus et futuris, ne contra presentem nostram confirmacionem et gratiam aliquatenus venire presumant, quinymmo illam iuxta eius mentem et seriem studeant inviolabiliter observare. Data Rodi die octava mensis Agusti anno LVIII.

*a)* comendabimi *MS* *b)* Wersat *corr.* *c)* vob *del.* *d)* promititur *MS* *e)* imposterumt *MS* *f)* prosidentes *MS*

## 30

*The Master Fr. Roger [des Pins], with consent of the Convent, constitutes Fr. Dietrich von Keppenbach, Preceptor of Freiburg im Breisgau and Neuenburg and Chamberlain of Buchsee, as lieutenant and visitor in the Priory of* Dacia *with its possessions in the Kingdoms of Denmark, Sweden and Norway. Fr. Dietrich is to go in person to the priory. He may constitute there a lieutenant, prior or viceprior and one of more preceptors; all these officers have to pay their responsions. Fr. Dietrich may convoke one or more*

1) *Fr. Gérard de Montagny, Preceptor of la Romagne, was Marshal of the Order between 1340 and 1345, visitor in Spain 1341: Delaville (1913), 120, 139.*

*assemblies. He may hear complaints and find decisions for quarrels. As his many duties in the Priory of* Alamania *may prevent him from going to* Dacia, *he may constitute one or more Hospitaller brethren as his substitutes. The Hospitallers and vassals of the Hospital in the priory are to be obedient to him.*

*Rhodes, [13]58 August 15*

*AOM 316 fol. 222r-3r (223r-4r), under* prioratus Alamanie, Boemie et parcium aliarum Alamanie. *Ed. Diplomatarium Danicum III/5 (1967), 130–1; cf. Hatt Olsen (1962), 102 no. 6.*

Frater Rogerius etcetera religioso etcetera fratri Dietrico de Lueppenbach domus eiusdem preceptori de Friburgo Briscaudie et de Novo Castro ac camerario nostro in camera nostra de Buhus[a)] salutem etcetera. Nova informacione suscepta[b)], quod prioratus nostre et domus nostre Dacie cum omnibus eius bonis in regno Dacie necnon in regnis Suecie et Noruagie constitutus per nonnullos domus nostre fratres a longis citra temporibus sine predecessorum nostrorum collacione aut titulo iusto alio est detentus[c)] et adhuc in perniciosum[d)] exemplum detinetur[e)] ad presens, cum hoc potius tirannidem sapiat quam decentiam concernat regularem, insolenciam huiusmodi pati sicut nec convenit non volentes, ne de errore[f)] in errorem ulterius[g)] procedatur, vos, de cuius legalitate fidei, circuspectionis industria et utilis administracionis providencia[h)] plenam in Domino fiduciam obtinemus, de et cum voluntate, consilio et assensu fratrum bayliorum et aliorum procerum conventus nostri Rodi nobis assistencium in hac parte locum nostrum tenentem et visitatorem in dicto prioratu Dacie et omnibus et singulis baiuliis, domibus et bonis et aliis quibuscumque nostris et dicte nostre domus in dictis regnis[i)] constitutis auctoritate presencium de nostra certa scientia ordinamus[j)], donec per alias nostras litteras constiterit nos aliud ordinasse. Dantes [222v] et concedentes vobis hac serie licenciam, potestatem et auctoritatem plenariam vos ad dictum prioratum et bona supradicta ut locum nostrum tenentem et visitatorem personaliter conferendi et inhibi[!] in spiritualibus et temporalibus tam in capite quam in membris visitandi, corrigendi ac prioratu et bonis predictis locum nostrum tenentem seu priorem vel vicepriorem vel preceptorem et preceptoris sub congrua annua responsione nobis annis singulis exolvenda auctoritate nostra[k)] ordinandi ad anos quinque vel decem, prout vobis expedicius videbitur, pro directione[l)] utili et bono regimine prioratus et bonorum predictorum quodque capitula[m)] et assembleyas fratrum dicti prioratus semel et quociens oporteat mandandi, celebrandi et tenendi, de dictis prioratus baiuliis et bonis aliis ad nostram et dicte nostre domus disponendi et ordinandi, inter fratres, sorores[n)], donatos, homines et vassalos prioratus iamdicti[o)] iusticiam ministrandi, rebelles et inobendientes puniendi per iusticiam domus nostre et omnia et singula alia exercendi et faciendi, que nos in prioratu ipso, si in eo personaliter adhessemus[!], facere et exercere possemus ad refformacionem accomodam et directionem utilem prioratus prescripti. Ceterum, si propter alia nostra vobis comissa negocia in prioratu Alamanie exequenda aut iusto alio impedimento superveniente vobis ad premissum prioratum[p)] Dacie vos conferre personaliter forsitan non possitis, quod loco vestri unum vel plures domus nostre fratres sufficientes et ydoneos et semel et pluries ad prefatum prioratum[p)] destinare possitis, qui omnia et singula supradicta in prioratu ipso exequantur, faciant, compleant auctoritate nostra pariter atque vestra vobis et illi vel[q)] illis domus nostre fratri seu fratribus, quem vel quos propterea ad dictum prioratum provideritis destinandos, potestatem, licenciam et auctoritatem plenam hac serie indulgemus. Mandantes sub virtute sancte obediencie firmiter et districte universis et singulis fratribus, sororibus et donatis et hominibus et vassalis nostris et domus nostre in dicto prioratu constitutis sub sacramento fidelitatis et homagii, quo nobis et nostre religioni tenentur, ut vobis aut fratri seu fratribus ad dictum prioratum mitendo vel mittendis pro[r)] prescriptis reverenter pareant, obediant et intendant tamquam nobis assistendo vobis vel mitendo seu mitendis predictis per vos consiliis, adiutoriis et favoribus salubribus in concernentibus utilitatem prioratus prescripti. Inhibentes vobis districcius sub virtute sancte obediencie supradicta, ne pretextu locumtenencie et visitacionis nostre huiusmodi aliqua de bonis, rebus aut iuribus prioratus prescripti vendatis, inpigno[223r]retis, obligetis, distrahatis seu quocumque[s)] alio colore quesito extra nostram religionem transferatis sine nostra speciali licencia et mandato. Et si, quod absit, contra inhibicionem nostram huiusmodi aliquid vel aliqua operari[t)] vel facere vos contingat, illud et illa exnunc prout extunc et extunc prout exnunc cassamus, anullamus ac decernimus irritum et inane nulliusque existere penitus efficacie[u)] vel valoris. In cuius rei etcetera. Data Rodi die XV[a] mensis Augusti anno quinquagesimo octavo.

*a)* Bus *del.* *b)* sucepta *MS* *c)* decitus *MS* *d)* preniciosum *MS* *e)* detinentur *MS* *f)* erare *MS* *g)* ultreius *MS* *h)* providicia *MS* *i)* reginis *MS* *j)* ordinad *corr.* *k)* nostri *MS* *l)* direcionem *MS* *m)* capitulo *MS* *n)* sororis *MS* *o)* imadicti *MS* *p)* prioratu *MS* *q)* ullis *del.* *r)* pre *del.* *s)* quoq *praem. ante corr.* *t)* de bonis rebus *praem. ante corr.* *u)* effacie *MS*

## 31

*The Master Fr. Roger [des Pins], with consent of the Convent, confirms Fr. Kenche von Haugwitz for ten years in the Preceptory of Tinz (Priory of Bohemia).*

*Rhodes, [13]58 August 15*

*AOM 316 fol. 223r-v (224r-v), under* prioratus Alamanie, Boemie et parcium aliarum Alamanie

Frater Rogerius etcetera religioso etcetera fratri Kenche de Hugwiez[a)] domus eiusdem comendatori in Tyncia salutem etcetera. Propter probitatis vestre merita et administracionem accomodam, quam in comissis vobis regiminibus in nostro ordine, sicut testimonio fidedigno accepimus, habuistis, illa vobis libenter anuimus, que conservacionem vestri status concernere dignoscuntur. Igitur baiuliam supradictam de Tyncia[b] prioratus nostri Boemie cum omnibus et singulis suis membris, iuribus et pertinenciis[c] universis ad eam spectantibus, quoquomodo et cum quibus eam tenetis et presencialiter possidetis, habendam, tenendam[d], regendam[e], gubernandam[f] et meliorandam in spiritualibus et temporalibus[g] tam in capite quam in membris sub anua responsione et aliis oneribus inpositis et inponendis[h] racionabiliter secundum[i] comunem cursum aliarum baiuliarum prioratus nostri Boemie supradicti in capitulo provinciali dicti[j] prioratus anis singulis exolvendis [et, nisi feceritis, destituendi] vos de dicta baiulia et illam ad manus suas ponendi iuxta statutum priori, receptori[k] responsionum dicti prioratus hac[l] serie plenam [223v] concedimus potestatem huiusmodi facta vobis gratia[m] in aliquo non obstante, hinc ad instans[n] festum nativitatis sancti Iohannis[o] baptiste et ab eodem festo inantea ad anos decem continuos et complectos de voluntate[p], consilio fratrum et procerum conventus nostri Rodi nobis assistencium in hac parte auctoritate presencium de nostra certa scientia et speciali[q] gratia vobis concedimus benefaciendo in eadem. Comitentes etcetera. Quocirca[r] etcetera necnon etcetera. Inibentes etcetera. In cuius etcetera. Data Rodi die quinta decima mensis Agusti anno[s] LVIII.

*a)* Tr *praem. ante corr.* *b)* Teni *praem. ante corr.* *c)* pertineciis *MS* *d)* tenedam *MS* *e)* regedam *MS* *f)* gubernadam *MS* *g)* teporalibus *MS* *h)* inponedis *MS* *i)* sedum *corr.* *j)* dictis *MS* *k)* rep *praem. ante corr.* *l)* annis singulis exolvendis et nisi feceritis destituendi *praem. ante corr. (homoiotel.)* *m)* gratiam *MS* *n)* instas *MS* *o)* Iohanni *MS* *p)* volutate *MS* *q)* specialis *MS* *r)* Qonsirqua *MS* *s)* annon *MS*

## 32

*The Master Fr. Roger [des Pins], with consent of the Convent, confirms Fr. Konrad Hauspeli for ten years in the Preceptory of Laa (Priory of Bohemia).*

*Rhodes, [13]58 August 15*

*AOM 316 fol. 223v-4r (224v-5r), under* prioratus Alamanie, Boemie et parcium aliarum Alamanie.

Frater Rogerius de etcetera religioso etcetera fratri Conrado dicto Hauspeli domus eiusdem[a] preceptori in Lohoc salutem et sinceram in Domino caritatem. Propter[b] vestre merita probitatis et administracionem accomodam, quam in comissis [224r] vobis regiminibus, sicut testimonio fidedigno percipimus[c], habuistis, illa vobis anuimus libenter, que conservacionem vestri status concernere dignoscuntur. Igitur dictam baiuliam sive domum in Loch prioratus nostri Boemie cum omnibus et singulis suis membris, iuribus et pertinenciis universis ad eam spectantibus et pertinentibus[d], quoquomodo et cum quibus eam tenetis et presencialiter possidetis, habendam, tenendam, regendam, augementandam[!] et meliorandam in spiritualibus et temporalibus[e] tam in capite[f] quam in membris sub anua responsione et aliis oneribus inpositis et inponendis racionabiliter secundum comunem cursum aliarum baiuliarum prioratus nostri Boemie supradicti in capitulo provinciali prioratus eiusdem annis singulis exolvendis[g] et, nisi feceritis, destituendi vos [de] dicta baiulia et illam ad manus suas ponendi iuxta statutum[h] priori et receptori responsionum dicti prioratus hac serie plenam concedimus potestatem gracia huiusmodi vobis facta non obstante, hinc ad instans[i] festum nativitatis sancti Iohannis baptiste et ab eodem festo inantea ad anos decem continuos et complectos de consilio[j] et assensu fratrum et procerum conventus nostri Rodi nobis assistencium in hac parte auctoritate presencium de nostra certa scientia et speciali[k] gratia vobis confirmamus benefaciendo in eadem. Comitentes etcetera. Quocirca[l] etcetera necnon etcetera. Inibentes etcetera. In cuius etcetera. Data Rodi die quinta decima mensis Augusti anno LVIII.

*a)* eiusdem *dupl.* *b)* preceptor *MS* *c)* precipimus *MS* *d)* pertinetibus *MS* *e)* teporalibus *MS* *f)* quapite *MS* *g)* exolundu *MS* *h)* statum *MS*, eius *praem. ante corr.* *i)* instas *MS* *j)* de consilio *dupl.* *k)* specialis *MS* *l)* Qonsirqua *MS*

## 33

*The Master Fr. Roger [des Pins] appoints Fr. Jacobus de Praga, Preceptor of Glatz, as a chaplain of the Master and retains him.*

*Rhodes, [13]58 August 15*

*AOM 316 fol. 225r (226r), under* prioratus Alamanie, Boemie et parcium aliarum Alamanie.

Frater Rogerius etcetera religioso etcetera fratri Iacobo de Praga domus eiusdem preceptori domus in[a] Glacz salutem etcetera. Dum laudabilia probitatis vestre merita in consideracionis nostre aciem recensemus, digne agimus, si vos actolimus[!] prerrogativa[!] honoris et gracie specialis. Igitur vestram volentes honorare personam, ut provide vestre fidei et devocionis zelus ad laudabiliora fervencius[b] inantea animetur, vos in capellanum nostrum tenore presencium retinemus et aliorum capellanorum nostrorum consortio[c] agregamus ac[d] ad uberiorem gratiam vos cum dicta domo et arnesiis vestris ac bonis et aliis quibuscumque solutis annuis responsionibus et aliis vobis et dicte vestre baiulie incumbentibus oneribus suportandis auctoritate presencium ad manus nostras de speciali gratia retinemus secundum bonos usus et laudabiles consuetudines[e] domus nostre. Mandantes harum serie universis et singulis fratribus domus nostre quacumque auctoritate, dignitate vel officio fulgentibus, presentibus et futuris sub virtute sancte obediencie firmiter et districte, ne contra presentis retencionis nostre gratiam aliquatenus venire presumant, quinymmo illam iuxta eius mentem et seriem studeant inviolabiliter observare. In cuius etcetera. Data Rodi die quinta decima mensis Agusti anno LVIII.

*a)* in *praem. ante corr.* *b)* frevencius *MS* *c)* constrincio *MS* *d)* ad *praem. ante corr.* *e)* cosuetudines *MS*

## 34

*The Preceptors of Zittau Fr. Nikolaus and of Mailberg and Vienna Fr. Nikolaus Wildungsmauer (both of the Priory of Bohemia) are retained, but not as the Master's chaplains.*

*[Rhodes, 1358 August 15]*

*AOM 316 fol. 225r (226r), under* prioratus Alamanie, Boemie et parcium aliarum Alamanie.

Item frater Nicolaus preceptor in Citauia et frater Nicolaus Willigssmaurer preceptor in Mewberg et in Wienna[a] prioratus Boemie, isti duo in forma predicta et die predicta fuerunt retenti ad manus domini, set non in cappellanos[b].

*a)* W *praem. ante corr.* *b)* Item die II Febroar *add. ante corr.*

*This text is repeated in AOM 316 fol. 227r (229r):* Die quinta decima mensis Augusti anno quinquagesimo octavo frater Nicolaus preceptor in Mewberg et in Vienna et frater Nicolaus preceptor in Citauia fuerunt retenti ad manus domini magistri cum eorum baiuliis in forma consueta.

## 35

*The Master Fr. Roger [des Pins], with consent of the Convent, reduces for Fr. Dietrich Keppenbach, Preceptor of Freiburg im Breisgau and Neuenburg, the annual pension payment due for the Master's chamber of Buchsee from 300 florins to 200 florins for the rest of his lifetime.*

*Rhodes, [13]58 August 15*

*AOM 316 fol. 225r-v (226r-v), under* prioratus Alamanie, Boemie et parcium aliarum Alamanie.

Frater Rogerius etcetera religioso etcetera fratri Dietrico de Keppenbach domus eiusdem preceptori in Friburgo Brisgaudie et in Novo Castro ac camerario nostro in camera nostra de Buhs salutem etcetera. Vestra et aliorum fidedignorum procerum domus nostre relacione informati, quod de pensione annua trecentorum florenorum, sub qua dudum cameram concessimus supradictam vobis, nimium agravamini, ne pressus inportabili onere subcumbatis, vobis, cum in hac parte volentes agere graciose cameram nostram predictam de Buchs prioratus nostri Alamanie cum omnibus et singulis suis membris, pertinenciis et iuribus ad eam spectantibus ac spectare et pertinere debentibus quoquomodo habendam, tenendam, regendam, gubernandam, augmentandam et meliorandam in spiritualibus et temporalibus tam in ca[225v]pite quam in membris de et cum voluntate, consilio et assensu fratrum et procerum conventus nostri Rodi nobis assistensium in hac parte sub annua pensione ducentorum florenorum auri de Florencia et boni ponderis in festo nativitatis sancti Iohannis baptiste nobis aut cui mandaverimus et ubi annis singulis infalibiliter exolvenda ad vitam vestram vobis auctoritate presencium conferimus, concedimus et mandamus de nostra certa scientia et speciali gratia et vos in illa nostrum pariter camerarium ordinamus benefaciendo in eadem sic et taliter, quod de dicta nostra camera nulla alia teneamini suportare onera nec solvere responsionem nisi[a] predictam anuam pensionem tantummodo[b] ducentorum florenorum, cum nostre camere a solucionibus responsionum et supportacione aliorum quorumlibet onerum ubilibet sint[c] inmunes, vosque camerarium nostrum locum nostrum tenentem pariter in tam nostra dicta[d] camera et omnibus et singulis eius membris et iuribus, quamdiu vite comodo potiemini, hac serie ordinamus. Comitentes etcetera. Quocirca etcetera. Inhibentes etcetera. In cuius etcetera. Data Rodi die quinta decima mensis Agusti anno LVIII.

*a)* misi *MS* *b)* tantumodo *MS* *c)* sin *MS* *d)* nostram dictam *MS*

## 36

*The Master Fr. Roger [des Pins] licenses Fr. Konrad von Randeck, Preceptor of Weißenburg, to receive a kinsman previously made knight into the Order and to maintain him in that preceptory.*

*Rhodes, [13]58 August 15*

*AOM 316 fol. 225v (226v), under* prioratus Alamanie, Boemie et parcium aliarum Alamanie.

Frater Rogerius etcetera religioso etcetera fratri Cůnrado de Randeck domus eiusdem preceptori[a] de Wissemburg salutem etcetera. Vestre proceritatis respectum in peticionibus vestris vobis redditi liberales, quod unum ex iunctis vobis linea parentele in fratrem domus nostre recipere valeatis solempniter, ut est moris, si aptus sit sanusque et integer membris suis et prius per vos vel alium milicie[b] cingulo insignito, si ex utroque parente nobili fuerit legittime procreatus[c] eique assignare stagiam in dicta vestra preceptoria[d], in qua sibi in suis necessariis provideri faciatis secundum bonos usus et laudabiles consuetudines domus nostre, vobis tenore presencium licenciam elargimur. Data Rodi die quinta decima mensis Agusti anno LVIII.

*a)* priori *corr.* *b)* milie *corr.* *c)* procretus *MS* *d)* preceptori *MS*

## 37

*The Master Fr. Roger [des Pins], with consent of the Convent, confirms Fr. Johann von Swerzitz for ten years in the Preceptory of Manětin (Priory of Bohemia).*

*Rhodes, [13]58 August 15*

*AOM 316 fol. 224v (225v), under* prioratus Alamanie, Boemie et parcium aliarum Alamanie.

Frater Rogerius etcetera religioso etcetera fratri Iohanni de Swerzccicz comendatori in Menetyn[a] domus eiusdem salutem etcetera. Propter probitatis vestre merita et administracionem accomodam, quam in quomissis[!] vobis regiminibus in nostro ordine, sicut fidedigno testimonio accepimus, habuistis, illa vobis libenter anuimus, que[b] conservacionem vestri[c] status concernere dignoscuntur. Igitur baiuliam predictam de[b] Mentyn prioratus nostri Boemie cum omnibus et singulis suis membris, iuribus et pertinenciis[d] universis[e] ad eam spectantibus et pertinentibus, quoquomodo et cum quibus[f] eam tenetis [et] presencialiter possidetis, habendam, tenendam[g], regendam, gubernandam[h], augementandam[!] et meliorandam in spiritualibus et temporalibus tam in quapite[!] quam in membris sub annua responsione et aliis oneribus inpositis[i] et inponendis[j] racionabiliter secundum comunem cursum[k] aliarum baiuliarum prioratus nostri Boemie supradicti [in capitulo] provinciali[l] dicti prioratus annis singulis exolvendis et, nisi feceritis, destituendi vos de dicta baiulia et illam ad manus suas ponendi iuxta statutum priori[m] et receptori responsionum dicti prioratus hac serie plenam concedimus potestatem huiusmodi facta gratia in aliquo non[n] obstante, hinc ad instans[o] festum nativitatis santi Iohannis baptiste et ab eodem festo inantea ad anos decem continuos et complectos de voluntate[p], consilio et asensu fratrum et procerum conventus nostri Rodi nobis assistencium in hac parte auctoritate presencium de nostra certa [scientia] et speciali[q] gracia vobis conferimus benefaciendo in eadem. Comitentes etcetera. Quocirca[r] etcetera necnon etcetera. Inibentes[s] etcetera. In cuius etcetera. Data Rodi die quinta decima mensis Agusti anno LVIII.

*a)* Mon *praem. ante corr.* *b)* et *MS* *c)* viri *MS* *d)* pertineciis *MS* *e)* univs *praem. ante corr.* *f)* aliquo *praem. ante corr.* *g)* tenedam *MS* *h)* gubernadam *MS* *i)* in *MS* *j)* inponedis *MS* *k) del.* *l)* provinciali *dupl.* *m)* prio *MS* *n) del.* *o)* instas *MS* *p)* volutate *MS* *q)* specialis *MS* *r)* Qonsirqua *MS* *s)* inbentes *MS*

## 38

*The Master Fr. Roger [des Pins] permits Fr. Dietrich von Keppenbach, Preceptor of Freiburg im Breisgau and Neuenburg and Chamberlain of Buchsee, to send two brethren of his kin to the Convent on Rhodes.*

*Rhodes, [13]58 August 15*

*AOM 316 fol. 225v-6r (226v-8r [227 number omitted]), under* prioratus Alamanie, Boemie et parcium aliarum Alamanie.

Frater Rogerius etcetera religioso etcetera fratri Dietrico de Keppenbach domus eiusdem preceptori de Friburgo Brisgaudie et de Novo Castro ac camerario nostro in camera nostra de Buhs salutem etcetera. Vestrorum comendabilium gratia meritorum supplicaciones vestras exaudientes benigne ad vestram supplicacionem, quod [226r] fratres duos domus nostre vobis affinitate coniunctos cum equis et armis[a] sufficientibus ad Dei obsequia ad conventum[b] nostrum Rodi mitere valeatis ab eorum superiore licencia prius requisita, vobis hac serie licenciam[c] elargimur. Data Rodi die XV[a] mensis Agusti anno LVIII.

*a)* arnis *corr. (forsan* arnesiis). *b)* centum *praem. ante corr.* *c)* licencia *MS*

## 39

*The Master Fr. Roger [des Pins] orders [Fr. Dietrich von Keppenbach], Preceptor of Freiburg im Breisgau, to receive one son of the knight Konrad von Keppenbach into the Order and to maintain him in that preceptory.*

*Rhodes, [13]58 August 15*

*AOM 316 fol. 226r (228r), under* prioratus Alamanie, Boemie et parcium aliarum Alamanie.

Frater Rogerius etcetera religioso etcetera fratri domus eiusdem nunc vel in futurum regimini preceptorie de Friburgo Brisgaudie quovis titulo presidenti salutem etcetera. Ad deprecacionis instanciam viri nobilis domini Cůnradi de Keppembach militis nostri et nostre religionis amici volumus et vobis tenore presencium districte precipimus et mandamus sub virtute sancte obendiencie nichilominus firmiter iniungentes, quatenus unum ex eiusdem domini Conrandi[a] filiis aptum[b] et ydoneum ac integrum[c] membris suis ad eius requisicionem recipiatis[d] in domus nostre fratrem solempniter, ut est moris, eo prius per vos vel alium milicie[e] cingulo decorato, si ex utroque parente nobili fuerit legittime procreatus, sibique in predicta baiulia in necessariis suis provideri faciatis secundum bonos usus et laudabiles consuetudines domus nostre. Data Rodi die quinta decima mensis Agusti anno LVIII.

*a)* Conrando *MS* *b)* apir *praem. ante corr.* *c)* inregrum *MS* *d)* recipiates *MS* *e)* nilicie *MS*

## 40

*The Master Fr. Roger [des Pins] orders his lieutenant in the Priory of* Alamania *to send two brethren from Weißenburg, as soon as two other brethren die, to other preceptories, because Fr. Konrad von Randeck, Preceptor of Weißenburg, has complained that he cannot support and maintain them.*

*Rhodes, [13]58 August 15*

*AOM 316 fol. 226r-v (228r-v), under* prioratus Alamanie, Boemie et parcium aliarum Alamanie.

Frater Rogerius etcetera religioso etcetera fratri ·· domus eiusdem locum nostrum [tenenti] in prioratu Alamanie et cuicumque fratri alteri domus nostre quovis titulo dicti prioratus regimini inantea presidenti salutem etcetera. Exposicione[a] religiosi in Christo nobis carissimi fratris Cůradi[!] de Randech domus eiusdem preceptoris in Wissenbrug capelani nostri noviter intellecto, quod sua preceptoria predicta secundum tenues[b] eius redditus et exiles facultates nimia fratrum multitudine agravatur, sue in hac parte oppressioni compassi ad eiusdem nostri capellani suplicacionem[c] volumus et vobis tenore presencium comitimus et expresse mandamus[d] sub virtute sante obendiencie nichilominus firmiter iniungentes, quatinus preceptoriam ipsius nostri cappellani eundem pariter de duobus allevietis[e] et exoneretis fratribus in huc modum videlicet, quod, cum primum duos fratres[f] in prioratu predicto mori contiget, loco defunctorum huiusmodi duos fratres alios de comendatoria eiusdem nostri capellani transportetis. Mandantes auctoritate nostra comendatori seu [226v] comendatoribus comendatorie seu comendatoriarum, ad quam vel quas transportetis[g] dictos duos fratres, sub virtute sante obendiencie, ut eos benigne recipiant et caritative pertractent ipsisque in eorum necessariis provideri secundum bonos usus et laudabiles consuetudines[h] domus nostre. Data Rodi die XV[a] mensis Agusti anno LVIII.

*a)* exposicionem *MS* *b)* teneues *MS* *c)* fal *praem. ante corr.* *d)* compassi *praem. ante corr. (homoiotel.)* *e)* allevietes *MS* *f)* fratribus *MS* *g)* trasportatibus *MS* *h)* consuetudine *MS*

## 41

*The Master Fr. Roger [des Pins] orders [Fr. Dietrich von Keppenbach], Preceptor of Freiburg im Breisgau, to receive Berthold Hcinguer as sergeant brother into the Order and to maintain him in Freiburg.*

*Rhodes, [13]58 August 15*

*AOM 316 fol. 226v (228v), under* prioratus Alamanie, Boemie et parcium aliarum Alamanie.

Frater Rogerius etcetera religioso etcetera fratri ·· domus eiusdem nunc vel [in] futurum regimini preceptorie de Friburgo Brisgaudie quovis titulo presidenti salutem etcetera. Cum Bercholdus dictus de Hcinguer desideret omnipotenti Deo et beate Marie virgini, matri eius, ac sancto Iohanni baptiste, patrono nostro, et Christi pauperibus sub regulari domus nostre habitu[a] perpetuo[b] familiari, nosque eius piis desideriis in hac parte deflexi vobis comitimus et expresse mandamus sub virtute sancte obediencie firmiter iniungentes, quatinus dictum Bertholdum, si aptus sit sanusque et integer membris suis, ad eius requisicionem recipiatis in fratrem servientem domus nostre solempniter, ut est moris, et ei assignetis stagiam in dicta preceptoria, in qua sibi in suis necessariis provideatur secundum bonos usus et laudabiles consuetudines domus nostre. Data Rodi die quinta decima mensis Agusti[c] anno LVIII.

*a)* habitum *MS* *b)* perpetua *MS* *c)* ag *praem. ante corr.*

## 42

*The Master Fr. Roger [des Pins] orders the Preceptor of Weißenburg to receive as a donat Friedrich von Frankfurt and to maintain him in Weißenburg.*

*Rhodes, [13]58 August 15*

*AOM 316 fol. 226v (228v), under* prioratus Alamanie, Boemie et parcium aliarum Alamanie.

Frater Rogerius etcetera religioso etcetera fratri ·· domus eiusdem preceptori in Wissen seu cuicumque[a] nunc vel in futurum regimini eiusdem baiulie quovis titulo presidenti salutem etcetera. Cum Fredericus de Frantoria ferventer desideret omnipotenti[b] Deo et beate Marie virgini, matri eius, et beato Iohani baptiste, patrono nostro, et Christi pauberibus[!] in religione nostra perpetuo familiari, nosque eius piis desideriis in hac parte defflexi[c] vobis tenore presencium comitimus et mandamus sub virtute sante obendiencie nichilominus iniungentes[d] et vestrum cuilibet, quatinus dictum Fredericum, si aptus[e] sit sanusque[f] et integer[g] membris suis, recipiatis[h] in donatum domus nostre solepniter, ut est moris, eique assignetis stagiam in dicta preceptoria, in qua sibi in suis necesariis provideri faciatis secundum bonos usus et laudabiles consuetudines domus nostre. De quam[i] quidem donacionem faciatis fieri duo consimilia publica instrumenta, quorum unum tradatur dicto donato, si eum[j] [h]abere voluerit[k], alterum vero in thesauro domus nostre ad rei memoriam perpetuam[l] reponatur. Data Rodi die quinta decima mensis Agusti anno LVIII.

*a)* quicumque *MS* *b)* omnidotenti *MS* *c)* deb *praem. ante corr.* *d)* innugentes *MS* *e)* apus *MS* *f)* samusque *MS* *g)* integre *MS* *h)* reg *praem. ante corr.* *i)* quia *MS* *j)* eu *MS* *k) volerit MS* *l)* perpetum *MS*

## 43

*The Master Fr. Roger [des Pins], with consent of the Convent, confirms his chaplain Fr. Johannes de Danubio for ten years in the Preceptory of Pulst (Priory of Bohemia).*

*Rhodes, [13]58 August 15*

*AOM 316 fol. 227r (229r), under* prioratus Alamanie, Boemie et parcium aliarum Alamanie.

Frater Rogerius etcetera religioso etcetera fratri Iohanni de Danubio domus [eiusdem] capellano salutem et sinceram in Domino caritatem. Religionis decor, morum honestas et alia virtutum dona multimoda, quibus vos carismatis gratia decoravit, ad inperciendum vobis favoris nostri gratiam[a)] rationabiliter nos moventes ac sperantes, quod in comisso vobis regimine effectus administracionis provide vos utilem faciente[b)] Domino exhibebit, baiuliam dictam de Pulst prioratus nostri Boemie cum omnibus et singulis suis membris, iuribus et pertinenciis universis ad eam spectantibus et pertinentibus ac spectare et pertinere debentibus quoquomodo habendam, tenendam, regendam, augmentandam et meliorandam in spiritualibus et temporalibus tam in capite quam in membris sub annua responsione et aliis oneribus impositis et imponendis rationabiliter secundum comunem cursum aliarum baiuliarum prioratus nostri Boemie supradicti in capitulo provinciali prioratus eiusdem annis singulis infalibiliter exolvendis et, nisi feceritis, destituendi vos dicta baiulia et illam ad manus suas ponendi iuxta statutum priori et receptori responsionum dicti prioratus hac serie plenam concedimus potestatem gratia huiusmodi vobis facta non obstante, hinc ad instans festum nativitatis sancti Iohannis baptiste et ab eodem festo inantea ad annos decem continuos et completos de consilio et assensu fratrum et procerum conventus nostri Rodi nobis assistensium in hac parte auctoritate presencium de nostra certa scientia et speciali gratia vobis confirmamus, concedimus et donamus benefaciendo in eadem vosque preceptorem et comendatorem in dicta constituimus baiulia tenore presencium et eciam ordinamus. Comitentes etcetera. Quocirca etcetera ac religioso in Christo nobis carissimo fratri ·· domus eiusdem priori dicti prioratus Boemie seu eiusdem prioratus regimini quovis titulo nunc vel inposterum presidenti, ut vos vel procuratorem vestrum in corporalem possesionem[!] pacificam[c)] et quietam dicte baiulie inducat omni contradiccione remota et conservet inductum amoto[d)] abinde quolibet illicito detentore, si quis sit, quem nos amovemus per presentes et decernimus amovendum necnon etcetera. Inhibentes etcetera. In cuius etcetera. Data Rodi die quinta decima mensis Agusti anno LVIII.

*a)* gratia *MS* *b)* faciendo *MS* *c)* facidam *MS* *d)* amote *MS*

## 44

*Fr. Nikolaus Wildungsmauer, Preceptor of Mailberg and Vienna, and Fr. Nikolaus of Zittau are retained with their preceptories (here* baiulie).

*1358 August 15*

*AOM 316 fol. 227r (229r), under* prioratus Alamanie, Boemie et parcium aliarum Alamanie.

Die quinta decima mensis Augusti quinquagesimo octavo frater Nicolaus preceptor in Meurberg et in Vienna et frater Nicolaus de Citauia fuerunt retenti ad manus domini magistri cum eorum baiuliis in forma consueta.

## 45

*The Master Fr. Roger [des Pins] and the Convent order Fr. Gallus von Lemberg, Prior of Bohemia, to send each year to the brothers Costantino and Marco Zuccoli in Venice his priory's responsions, the pension payments due to the Master for his chamber and all other payments that are due to the Master and Convent.*

*Rhodes, [13]58 August 20*

*AOM 316 fol. 227v-8r (229v-30r), under* prioratus Alamanie, Boemie et parcium aliarum Alamanie.

Frater Rogerius[a] etcetera et nos conventus etcetera religioso etcetera[b] fratri Gallo de Lemberch domus eiusdem priori Boemie salutem etcetera. Cum ordinaverimus responciones nostri dicti prioratus ac nostre dicti magistri camere pensionem et omnia et singula alia iura et bona nobis comuniter vel divisim expectancia et debencia pervenire[c] ad civitatem Veneciarum discretis viris Constantino et Marco Zucoli fratribus seu alteri annis singulis per vos miti, vobis ideo tenore presencium sub virtute [228r] sancte obediencie districte mandantes precipimus, quatinus responsiones[d] ac pensionem predictas et alia predicta nominatis Costantino et Marco vel eorum alteri anno quolibet ad civitatem prescriptam infallibiliter transmitatis et tradi pariter nostro[e] nomine faciatis super [h]oc vos taliter habiturum, quod vos obediencie transcressio nulla culpet. In cuius etcetera. Data Rodi die vicesima mensis Augusti anno LVIII.

*a)* de P *add. ante corr.* *b)* etcetera *supra lin.* *c)* prevenire *MS* *d)* rersponsiones *MS* *e)* nostre *MS*

*Mattio, not Marco Zuccoli according toLongo (1817), 119–20.*

## 46

*The Master Fr. Roger [des Pins] and the Convent order Fr. Dietrich von Keppenbach, Preceptor of Freiburg im Breisgau and Neuenburg, Chamberlain of Buchsee and receiver of responsions in the Priory of* Alamania, *to send his responsions of this priory, the pension payments due to the Master for his chamber of Buchsee and all other payments due to the Master and Convent to Venice to the brothers Costantino and Marco Zuccoli.*

*Rhodes, [1358] August 20*

*AOM 316 fol. 228r (230r), under* prioratus Alamanie, Boemie et parcium aliarum Alamanie.

Frater Rogerius etcetera et nos conventus etcetera religioso etcetera fratri Dietrico de Keppembach domus eiusdem preceptori de Friburgo Brisgaudie et in Novo Castro ac camerario[a)] nostri dicti magistri in camera nostra de Buhs et responsionum receptori in prioratu nostro Alamanie salutem etcetera. Cum ordinaverimus responsiones dicti prioratus ac camere nostre dicti magistri supradicte pensionem et omnia et singula alia iura et bona nobis[b)] comuniter vel divisim expectancia et debencia pervenire ad civitatem Veneciarum discretis viris Constantino et Marco Zucoli fratribus seu eorum alteri annis singulis per vos miti, vobis ideo tenore presencium sub virtute sancte obediencie districte mandantes precipimus, quatinus responsiones ac pensionem predictas et alia predicta nominatis Constantino et Marco vel eorum alteri anno quolibet ad civitatem prescriptam infallibiliter transmitatis et tradi nostro nomine pariter faciatis super hoc vos taliter habiturum, quod vos obediencie transgressio nulla culpet. In cuius etcetera. Data Rodi die vicesima mensis Agusti anno [LVIII].

*a)* cameracio *MS* *b)* viris *praem. ante corr.*

## 47

*The Master Fr. Roger [des Pins] and the Convent quit Fr. Gallus von Lemberg, Prior of Bohemia, for his responsions and other payments he owed up to 24 June 1358, which they have received from Fr. Nikolaus Wildungsmauer, Preceptor of Mailberg and Vienna.*

*Rhodes, [13]58 August 20*

*AOM 316 fol. 228r-v (230r-v), under* prioratus Alamanie, Boemie et parcium aliarum Alamanie.

Noverint universi et singuli presentem recognicionem et quitanciam visuri et pariter audituri, quod nos frater Rogerius etcetera et nos conventus etcetera tenore presencium confitemur et in verbo recognoscimus veritatis, quod posita racione thesauro nostro seu eius ministris nostro nomine atque vice per religiosum etcetera fratrem Nicolaum Wilugsmaurer domus eiusdem preceptorem in Mewberg et in Wienna, procuratorem et nuncium religiosi etcetera fratris Galli de Lemberch domus eiusdem prioris Boemie de omnibus et singulis responsionibus [et] quarti[s] responsionum prioratus prescripti de toto tempore, quo idem frater Gallus prefuit ut prior dicti regimini prioratus, usque per totum annum finitum in festo nativitatis sancti Iohannis baptiste anni incarnacionis Domini millesimi trecentesimi quinquagesimi octavi proximo lapsi, per dictam racionem fuit compertum premissum priorem de toto dicto tempore et usque ad festum predictum nominato thesauro suas omnes responsiones et quarta responsionum et alia, que racione sui passagii eidem tenebatur thesauro sive nobis, integre exolvisse sic, quod usque ad festum sancti Iohannis prescriptum [228v] in nullo penitus de toto suo tempore nobis tenetur seu nostro prelibato thesauro. Quamobrem de predictis omnibus responsionibus et quartis responsionum et aliis supradictis contenti plenarie eundem priorem eiusve bona et arnesia presencium serie liberamus perpetuo et quitamus. In cuius etcetera. Data Rodi die vicesima mensis Augusti anno LVIII[a].

*a)* LVII *MS*

## 48

*The Preceptor of Heimbach Fr. Johann von Saulenheim is retained with his preceptory and harness.*

*[1358] August 22*

*AOM 316 fol. 227v (229v) under* prioratus Alamanie, Boemie et parcium aliarum Alamanie.

Die vicesima secunda Augusti frater Iohannes de Sŏwelnhen preceptor de Heinbach retentus fuit cum sua preceptoria et arnesiis ad manus domini in forma consueta.

## 49

*The Master Fr. Roger [des Pins], with consent of the Convent, grants for ten years to Fr. Otto von Heßberg the Preceptory of Kühndorf with the parish church in Schleusingen (Priory of* Alamania*), which is vacant following the death of Fr. Berthold von Henneberg.*

*Rhodes, 1358 August 23*

*AOM 316 fol. 227v (229v), under* prioratus Alamanie, Boemie et parcium aliarum Alamanie.

Frater Rogerius etcetera religioso etcetera fratri Ottono de Hesburg salutem etcetera. Religionis decor etcetera baiuliam seu preceptoriam de Kundorf cum ecclesia parrochiali in Slusingue per mortem quondam fratris Bercholdi de Hennenberg vacantem presencialiter, prout vestra continuit supplicacio data nobis, si sit ita, habendam, tenendam, regendam, gubernandam, augmentandam[a] et meliorandam in spiritualibus et temporalibus tam in capite quam in membris sub annua responsione et aliis oneribus impositis et imponendis rationabiliter secundum comunem cursum aliarum baiuliarum prioratus nostri Alamanie in capitulo provinciali prioratus eiusdem annis singulis infallibiliter exolvendis et, nisi feceritis, destituendi vos de dicta baiulia et illam ad manus suas ponendi iuxta statutum priori et receptori responsionum dicti prioratus hac serie plenam concedimus potestatem gratia huiusmodi vobis facta aliquathenus non obstante, hinc ad instans festum nativitatis sancti Iohannis baptiste et ab eodem festo inantea ad anos decem continuos et completos de consilio et assensu fratrum et procerum conventus nostri Rodi nobis assistencium[b] in hac parte auctoritate presencium de nostra certa scientia et speciali gratia vobis confirmamus, concedimus et donamus benefaciendo in eadem vosque preceptorem et comendatorem in dicta baiulia constituimus tenore presencium ac ecciam ordinamus. Comitentes etcetera. Quocirca etcetera ac religioso etcetera fratri ·· domus eiusdem priori dicti prioratus Alamanie seu eiusdem prioratus[c] regimini nunc[d] vel in futurum quovis titulo presidenti, ut vos vel procuratorem vestrum in corporalem possessionem pacificam et quietam dicte baiulie inducat omni contradictione remota et conservet inductum amoto abinde quolibet illicito decentore, si quis sit, quem nos per presentes amovemus firmiter amovendum necnon etcetera. Inhibentes etcetera. In cuius etcetera. Data Rodi die vicesima tercia mensis Agusti anno incarnacionis Domini millesimo CCC$^{mo}$ quinquagesimo octavo.

*a)* agmentandam *corr.* *b)* assistensium *MS* *c)* priortus *corr.* *d)* nuc *MS*

## 50

*The Master Fr. Roger [des Pins] has received 40 florins, as composition for pension payments due from the Master's chamber of Buchsee and for goods of deceased brethren, from Fr. Gallus von Lemberg, Prior of Bohemia, through Fr. Dietrich von Keppenbach, Preceptor of Freiburg im Breisgau and Neuenburg and Chamberlain of Buchsee.*

*Rhodes, [13]58 August 24*

*AOM 316 fol. 228v (230v), under* prioratus Alamanie, Boemie et parcium aliarum Alamanie.

Noverint universi et singuli presentem recognicionem et quitanciam visuri et pariter audituri, quod nos frater Rogerius etcetera tenore presencium confitemur et in verbo recognoscimus[a] veritatis nos habuisse et recepisse per manus fratris Dietrici de Keppembach domus eiusdem preceptoris in Friburgo Brisgaudie et in Novo Castro ac camerarii nostri in Buhs a religioso etcetera fratri[!] Galo de Lemberch domus eiusdem priore Boemie florenos auri quatrigentos, in quibus idem prior ex composicione[b] facta cum dicto fratre Dietrico ad hec procuratore nostro de pensionibus nostre camere et bonis et arnesiis fratrum defunctorum[c] in dicto prioratu ad manus nostras retentorum nobis tenebatur, de quibus quatragintis[d] florenis ut premititur per nos habitis et receptis contenti plenarie premissos priorem et fratrem Dietricum eorumque bona et arnesia liberamus et quitamus. In cuius etcetera. Data Rodi die vicesima quarta[e] mensis Agusti anno LVIII.

*a)* recogocimus *MS* *b)* composcione *MS* *c)* defontorum *MS* *d)* qutragintis *MS* *e)* quara *MS*

## 51

*Licence for Fr. Konrad von Randeck, chaplain of the Master and Preceptor of Weißenburg, to leave the Convent.*

*[Rhodes, 1358] August 27*

*AOM 316 fol. 228v (230v), under* prioratus Alamanie, Boemie et parcium aliarum Alamanie.

Die XXVII Augusti data fuit licentia fratri Conrado de Randech, capellano nostro et preceptori de Wisemburg, recedendi de conventu et redeundi pro suis negociis exequendis.

## 52

*Licence for Fr. Friedrich von Zollern, Preceptor of Rohrdorf, to leave the Convent for his preceptory and return.*

*[Rhodes, 1358] August 28*

*AOM 316 fol. 228v (230v), under* prioratus Alamanie, Boemie et parcium aliarum Alamanie.

Die XXVIII Augusti data fuit licentia fratri Frederico de Zolra preceptori de Rordorf recedendi de conventu ad regendum suam preceptoriam et redeundi cum equis etcetera ut in forma.

## 53

*Licence for Fr. Dietrich von Keppenbach, Preceptor of Freiburg im Breisgau, to leave the Convent on business of the Master.*

*[Rhodes, 1358 August 28]*

*AOM 316 fol. 228v (230v), under* prioratus Alamanie, Boemie et parcium aliarum Alamanie.

Eadem die data fuit licentia fratri Dietrico de Keppembach preceptori in Friburgo Brisgaudie recedendi de conventu et redeundi pro referendis nonnullis negociis per nos vobis comissis ut in forma.

## 54

*The Master Fr. Roger des Pins rejects a petition from Fr. Gallus von Lemberg, Prior of Bohemia, giving him and his successors the right to receive only one knight or sergeant into the Order if two die. The prior had wanted a general licence to receive the necessary brethren into the Order.*

*Rhodes, [13]58 September 6*

*AOM 316 fol. 228v-9r (230v-31r), under* prioratus Alamanie, Boemie et parcium aliarum Alamanie.

Frater Rogerius de Pinibus etcetera religioso in Christo nobis carissimo fratri Gallo de Lemberch domus eiusdem priori Boemie presenti et successive futuris aut quocumque alio titulo dicti prioratus regimini presidenti salutem et sinceram in Domino caritatem. Pro parte vestra nobis suplicato, ut faciendi fratres necessarios [229r] in dicto prioratu vobis generalem licenciam concedere dignaremur, quia licencia huiusmodi adeo generalis non est alicui consueta concedi nec consuetudinem novam introducere in nostra religione, talem videlicet, velut istam expediat, aliasque vota vestra prout decenter possumus, volentes prosequi graciose, quod, quandocumque et quocienscumque duos fratres mori contingat in dicto prioratu et eius aliqua baiulia seu baiuliis, tociens loco duorum fratrum huiusmodi defuntorum fratrem unum militem vel servientem aptum et ydoneum ac integrum membris suis possitis facere solempniter[a)], ut est moris, et ei in baiulia seu baiuliis, in qua seu quibus dictos duos fratres vel ipsorum alterum continget decedere, stagiam assignare, in qua sibi provideri in suis necessariis faciatis secundum bonos usus et laudabiles consuetudines domus nostre, vobis tenore presencium licenciam elargimur. Inhibentes vobis hac serie sub virtute sancte obediencie firmiter et districte[b)], ne aliter quam in forma huiusmodi vobis data fratrem aliquem nostre domus facere presumatis, quod, si secus, quod absit, atemptaveritis facere seu faceritis fratrem vel fratres aliquos, in eum casum vos inobedientem pronunciamus exnunc et tales non esse domus nostre fratres sicut vere non essent, quia factos de facto per non habentem potestatem contra prohibicionem nostram expressam et nostri ordinis statuta. Data Rodi die sexta mensis Septembris anno LVIII.

*a)* solepniter *MS* *b)* discricte *MS*

## 55

*The Master Fr. Roger des Pins announces his decision concerning the reception of brethren (as no. 54) to all present and future preceptors and vice-preceptors in the Priory of Bohemia.*

*Rhodes, [13]58 September 7*

*AOM 316 fol. 229r-v (231r-v), under* prioratus Alamanie, Boemie et parcium aliarum Alamanie.

Frater Rogerius de Pinibus etcetera religiosis[a] in Christo nobis carissimis universis et singulis fratribus preceptoribus[b] seu vicepreceptoribus prioratus[c] nostri Boemie presentibus et sucessive futuris salutem et sinceram in Domino caritatem. Scribimus ecce per alias nostras patentes[d] litteras religioso in Christo nobis carissimo fratri Gallo de Lembrech domus eiusdem priori Boemie in hec verba:

> Frater Rogerius de Pinibus Dei gratia sacre domus hospitalis sancti Iohannis Ierosolimitani magister humilis et pauperum Christi custos religioso in Christo nobis carissimo fratri Gallo de Lembrech domus eiusdem priori Boemie presenti et successive futuris aut quocumque alio titulo dicti prioratus regimini presidenti salutem et sinceram in Domino caritatem. Pro parte vestra nobis[e] suplicato, ut faciendi fratres necessarios in dicto prioratu vobis generalem[f] licenciam concedere dignaremur[g], quia licencia huiusmodi adeo generalis non est alicui consueta concedi nec consuetudinem[h] novam introducere in nostra religione talem videlicet velut istam expediat aliasque [229v] vota vestra, prout decenter possumus, volentes prosequi graciosse[!], quod, quandocumque et quocienscumque duos fratres mori contingat in dicto prioratu et eius aliqua baiulia seu baiuliis, tociens loco duorum fratrum huiusmodi defunctorum fratrem unum militem vel servientem aptum et ydoneum ac integrum membris suis possitis facere solemniter, ut est[i] moris, et ei in baiulia seu baiuliis, in qua seu quibus dictos duos fratres vel ipsorum alterum continget decedere, stagiam assignare, in qua sibi provideri in suis necessariis faciatis secundum bonos usus et laudabiles consuetudines domus nostre, vobis tenore presencium licenciam elargimur. Inibentes vobis hac serie sub virtute sante obendiencie firmiter et districte, ne aliter quam in forma huiusmodi vobis data fratrem aliquem nostre domus facere presumatis[j], quod, si secus, quod absit, atemptaveritis facere seu feceritis fratrem vel fratres aliquos, in eum casum vos inobedientem pronunciamus exnunc et tales non esse domus nostre fratres, sicut vere non essent, quia factos de facto per non habentem potestatem contra prohibitionem nostram expressam et nostri ordinis statuta. Data Rodi die sexta mensis Septembris anno incarnacionis Domini millesimo trecentesimo quinquagesimo octavo.

Sane contenta in huiusmodi nostris litteris volentes absque illorum transgressione per dictum priorem et successores illius efficaciter observari vobis et vestrum cuilibet sub virtute sante obediencie districte[k] mandantes precipimus, quatinus, si, quod absit, premissum priorem aut successores eius contingat contra in aliis nostris prescriptis litteris traditam sibi formam fratrem seu fratres facere per vestrum nuncium vel litteras nostre noticie defferatis dilacione recisa, ut culpa transgresse[l] obediencie penam seu iusticiam meritam senciat[m] indilate. Preterea vobis et vestrum cuilibet sub dicta virtute sante obediencie expresse precipimus per presentes, ne vestrum aliquis fratrem faciat aliquem domus nostre sine nostra licencia speciali. Et ne de predictis omnibus causam ignorancie allegare possitis, presentes nostras litteras in primo vestro provinciali capitulo in presencia omnium ad ipsum conveniencium capitulum precipimus publicari. Data Rodi die septima mensis Septembris anno LVIII.

*a)* religioso *MS* *b)* proceptoribus *MS* *c)* seu *praem. ante corr.* *d)* pantentes *MS* *e)* bo *praem. ante corr.* *f)* generale *MS* *g)* dignaretur *MS* *h)* consuetudines *corr.* *i)* st *corr.* *j)* presumans *MS* *k)* discricte *corr.* *l)* trangresse *MS* *m)* stenciat *MS*

## 56

*The Master Fr. Roger des Pins was informed that in Bohemia not only the seal of the priory but also seals of preceptories had been used to corroborate documents that mortgaged or pledged goods of the Order. After consultation with brethren of the Convent, the Master now orders the destruction of all authentic seals in the Priory of Bohemia except the seal of the priory that is to be kept in a purse by the prior and three or four preceptors of the [prioral] chapter.*

*Rhodes, [13]58 September 10*

*AOM 316 fol. 229v-30r (231v-2r), under* prioratus Alamanie, Boemie et parcium aliarum Alamanie.

Frater Rogerius de Pinibus etcetera religiosis in Christo nobis carissimis[a] universis et singulis fratribus ·· domus eiusdem priori Boemie et preceptoribus prioratus ipsius presentibus et futuris salutem et sinceram in Domino caritatem. Vigilis cura solicitudinis[b] nobis incumbens ex officio magistratus continuo animum nostrum pulsat[c], ut competens illis accelerimus remedium[d], que periculosa et nociva nostre religioni sentimus. Sane non absque grandi admiracione noviter intellecto, quod preter sigilum comunem dicti prioratus, quod per priorem custoditur, sunt in prioratu ipso [230r] comendatorie seu preceptorie alique sigilla adeo habentes autentica[e],[1] quod sigilata per illa per totam ipsam vestram regionem sic obtinent plenum robur, acsi essent comunis sigilli dicti prioratus sigillata sigillo, ex quo per aliquos ex huiusmodi preceptoriam preceptores in districtionem bonorum preceptoriarum ipsarum et impignoracionibus[f] dictorum efficacia sigilorum preceptoriis eisdem plura dispendia

1) *Ordinary seals were held to be credible for affairs of their owner only, authentic seals also for affairs of other people or for public affairs in general: Extra 2.22.2.*

sunt illata et sperantur inferri[g] propter varias fratrum condicionis et regimina[h] indiscreta[i], nisi acceleretur remedium competens et salubre. Nosque super hoc cum baylivis et proceribus aliis nostri[j] conventus consulta deliberacione habita hac invicem attendentes, quod sigilla huiusmodi grandia et irreparabilia possent[k] afferre discrimina et dampna[l] plurima[m] nostre ipsis partibus religioni ac quod in aliis mundi regionibus seu prioratibus nisi sigillum unum autenticum, prioratus videlicet, non habentur, discriminibus[n] et dampnis hiis occurrere cupientes deliberato consilio cum baylivis et aliis nostri conventus proceribus supradictis de nostra certa scientia sigilla omnia supradicta sigillos prioratus dumtaxat[o] excepto tenore presencium cassamus ac ecciam anullamus et pariter ordinamus, ut deinceps nisi sigillum prioratus, quod[p] per priorem hucusque dicitur custodiri, non sit nec habeatur in prioratu prefato, cum quo[q] gratie et alia occurrecia[r] negocia in capitulis sigiletur[s], et quod sigillum istiusmodi in aliqua bursa sigillata sigillis prioris et trium vel quatuor notabiliorum[t] dicti prioratus preceptorum usque ad capitulum servetur diligenter[u] et tunc[v] de consilio et assensu fratrum preceptorum capituli sigilentur sigilanda et sigillatis sigillandis incontinenti sigillum ipsum reponatur in bursa, que ut predicitur sigilletur sigillis prioris et trium vel quatuor notabiliorum preceptorum sic, quod nisi in capitulis in presencia preceptorum capituli dicto[w] non sigilletur[x] sigillo. Quamobrem[y] omnibus et[z] singulis preceptoribus dictarum preceptoriarum premissa sigilla habencium sub virtute sante obendiencie districte mandantes precipimus, quatinus decetero sigillis ipsis aliquatenus non utantur, quinymo ad primum celebraturum capitullum in dicto prioratu illa portent et in presencia capituli[aa] cominuantur et destruantur omnino reficienda temporibus unquam nullius ius predictis[bb] vos taliter habituros, quod de vera obendiencia digne valeatis in Domino comendari. Data Rodi die decima mensis Septe[m]bris anno LVIII.

*a)* carissimos *corr.* *b)* solitutidinis *MS* *c)* pulstat *MS* *d)* remendium *MS* *e)* autencica *MS* *f)* impignoracinibus *MS* *g)* inferre *corr.* *h)* regima *MS; add. ante corr.* *i) praem. corr.* *j)* nostris *MS* *k)* posent *MS* *l)* dapna *MS* *m) dupl.* *n)* discrimibus *MS* *o)* dumtaxta *MS* *p)* qud *corr.* *q)* quod *MS* *r)* occurecia *corr.* *s)* sigiliter *ante corr.*, sigiliteor *post corr.* *t)* notabliorum *corr.* *u)* diligentur *MS* *v)* tuc *MS* *w)* de *praem. ante corr.* *x)* silgilletur *MS* *y)* Quoabrem *MS* *z)* et *praem. ante corr.* *aa)* capl *praem. ante corr.* *bb)* cuius re *praem. ante corr.*

## 57

*The Master Fr. Roger des Pins and the Convent, acting in accordance with the authority awarded to them by the chapter general at Rhodes the previous February, grant for ten years to Fr. Hugo von Werdenberg the vacant Priory of* Alamania *with 1,000 florins of Florence as responsions to be paid to the receiver in the priory. The responsions are due from Fr. Hugo's prioral chambers and from the preceptories of the Priory of* Alamania. *His ten years start on*

*24 June 1358. He is to rule the priory, to grant vacant preceptories, offices, castellanies and houses to new officers, following a statute recently edited by the chapter general. The Hospitallers and the Hospital's subjects in the priory are to be obedient to him.*

*Rhodes, [13]58 September 12*

*AOM 316 fol. 230v-31r (232v-3r), under* prioratus Alamanie, Boemie et parcium aliarum Alamanie.

Frater Rogerius de Pinibus et nos conventus domus eiusdem religioso in Christo nobis carissimo fratri Hugoni de Werdenbercg[a] domus eiusdem salutem et sinceram in Domino caritatem. Digne credimus agere et racionabiliter operari, si naturali fultos industria et provida discrecione dotatos vitaque et moribus multipliciter comendatos ad celsiores gradus nostri ordinis evocamus, cum, dum bene meritorum fructuum graciarum dulcedine se refectos conspiciunt et senciunt honoratos, ad queque religionis acomoda industrie eorum studia iugiter fervenciora[b] convertunt. Attendentes itaque prioratum nostrum Alamannie ad presens prioris solacio destitutum quodque sub vestro fructuoso regimine, vestra industri solicitudine operante prioratus ipse non solum restaurabitur, quinymo divina gracia vobis assistente prosperitatis[c] multiplicis suscipiet incrementa, horum consideracione inducti prioratum predictum Alamannie cum omnibus et singulis suis membris, iuribus et pertinenciis universis ad eundem prioratum Alamannie spectantibus et pertinentibus ac spectare et pertinere debentibus quoquomodo, et cum omni onere, emolumentis et honore habendum, tenendum, administrandum, regendum, gubernandum, augmentandum et meliorandum in spiritualibus et temporalibus tam in capite quam in membris vobis tamquam digno et benemerito invicem deliberato consilio auctoritate presencium et auctoritate nobis retenta et specialiter reservata in nostro generali capitulo apud Rodum de mense Febroarii preterito proxime celebrato,[1] ut de prioratu predicto intra anneam[2] providere possemus auctoritate dicti capituli ea efficacia et valore[d], acsi de illo provisum fuisset in capitulo supradicto, sub responsione annua mille florenorum auri de Florencia et boni ponderis per vos pro rata vestrarum camerarum et per preceptores prescripti prioratus, prout ad quemlibet eorum pertinebit, receptori responsionum in dicto prioratu in capitulo per nos ordinato vel inantea ordinando[e] infalibiliter annis singulis exolvendis et quibuscumque aliis oneribus dicto prioratu qualitercumque et quomodocumque incumbentibus et incumbendis seu inpositis et imponendis per vos ex pacto eciam suportandis de nostra certa scientia et speciali gratia conferimus, concedimus et donamus benefaciendo in eadem ad [annos] decem in festo nativitatis sancti Iohanes baptiste preterito proxime inchoandas[f] et

1) *1358 February: Delaville (1913), 136.*

2) *Priories were granted on chapters general, and this phrase refers to the time between two chapters general; cf. Countryside (2019), 38 with note 11.*

extunc continuo secutores. Dantes et concedentes vobis auctoritatem et potestatem plenariam regendi, gubernandi et administrandi[g] prioratum prefatum tam in capite quam in membris, in spiritualibus et temporalibus et quecumque alia agendi, celebrandi et exercendi, que ad prioris spectant officium et que pro utili regimine prioratus ipsius necesarias fuerint[h] ac eciam oportuna, et insuper dandi et conferendi cum consilio et assensu fratrum et procerum dicti prioratus preceptorias, baiulias, castelanias acque domos vacaturas dicti prioratus Allamanie fratribus ydoneis et benemeritis domus nostre predictum tempus decem [231r] anorum, prout melius et utilius[i] vobis videbitur expedire, secundum continenciam statuti noviter editi in nostro predicto capitulo generali. Comitentes vobis fiducialiter circa curam, regimen[j] et administracionem ac gubernacionem accomodas dicti prioratus Alamanie ac bonorum et iurium eiusdem defensionem[k] et recuperacionem tam in agendo quam defendendo[l] hac serie vices nostras. Quocirca[m] universis et singulis fratribus preceptoribus, balivis et aliis fratribus, confratribus, sororibus et donatis sub virtute sante obendiencie, hominibus[n] et vassalis et quibus aliis nobis et nostre prefate[o] domui subditis in dicto prioratu constitutis, presentibus et futuris sub sacramento fidelitatis et homagii, quo nobis et nostre domui sunt astricti, precipimus et mandamus harum serie districte, quatinus[p] vobis tanquam eorum superiori et maiori reverenter pareant, obendiant et intenda[n]t vobisque suum prebeant auxilium, consilium et favorem in omnibus, que ad curam, regimen[j] et administracionem ac gubernacionem utilem prioratus prescripti pertinere noscuntur, quocie[n]s opus fuerit et eos duxeritis requirendos. Inibentes vobis districtius sub dicta virtute sancte obediencie, ne pretextu concesionis et gratie nostre huiusmodi aliqua de bonis, rebus et iuribus memorati prioratus vendatis, detis, obligetis, impignoretis, distrahatis, alienetis, permutetis seu in emphiteosim perpetuam concedatis vel quocumque alio colore quesito extra nostram religionem[q] transferatis sine nostra speciali licencia et mandato. Et si, quod absit, contra inhibicionem nostram huiusmodi aliquid vel aliqua operari vel facere vos contingat[r], illud et illa exnunc prout extunc et extunc prout exnunc cassamus, anullamus et decernimus irritum et inane nulliusque existere penitus efficacie vel valoris. In cuius etcetera. Data Rodi die duodecima mensis Septembris anno LVIII.

*a)* Werdenbecg *corr.* *b)* fervencora *MS* *c)* posperitatis *corr.* *d)* valoris *corr.* *e)* ordinado *MS* *f)* inchonadas *MS* *g)* administracionem *MS* *h)* fuerit et *corr. MS* *i)* utilis *corr.* *j)* regimine *MS* *k)* desensionem *MS* *l)* defedendo *MS* *m)* Qoncirca *MS* *n)* hacuminibus *MS* *o)* prfate *MS* *p)* quatinus *dupl. ante corr.* *q)* religonem *MS* *r)* constingat *MS*

## 58

*The Master Fr. Roger des Pins, with consent of the Convent, confirms Fr. Friedrich Gremlich for ten years in the Preceptory of Feldkirch (Priory of* Alamania).

*Rhodes, [13]58 September 15*

*AOM 316 fol. 231r-v (233r-v), under* prioratus Alamanie, Boemie et parcium aliarum Alamanie.

Frater Rogerius de Pinibus etcetera religioso in Christo nobis carissimo[a] fratri Friderico Gremlich domus eiusdem preceptori in Veltkilche salutem et sinceram in Domino caritatem. Propter vestre merita[b] probitatis et administracionem acomodam, quam in comissis vobis regiminibus in nostro ordine, sicut testimonio fidedigno accepimus, hactenus habuistis, illa vobis annuimus libenter, que conservacionem vestri status concernere dignoscuntur. Igitur domum seu baiuliam in Veltkilche supradictam prioratus nostri Alamanie cum omnibus et singulis membris, iuribus et pertinenciis universis ad eam spectantibus et pertinentibus, quoquomodo et cum quibus eam tenetis et presencialiter possidetis, habendam, tenendam, regendam, augmentandam et meliorandam in spiritualibus et temporalibus tam in capite quam in membris sub annua [231v] responsione et aliis oneribus impositis et imponendis racionabiliter secundum comunem cursum aliarum baiuliarum prioratus nostri Alamanie supradicti in capitulo provinciali prioratus eiusdem annis singulis exsolvendis et, nisi feceritis, destituendi vos dicta baiulia et illam ad manus suas ponendi iuxta statutum priori et receptori responsionum[c] dicti prioratus hac serie plenam concedimus potestatem huiusmodi vobis facta gratia non obstante, hinc ad instans festum nativitatis sancti Iohannis baptiste et ab eodem festo inantea ad annos decem continuos et completos de consilio et assensu fratrum et procerum conventus nostri Rodi nobis assistencium in hac parte auctoritate presencium de nostra certa scientia et speciali gratia vobis confirmamus benefaciendo in eadem[d]. Comittentes etcetera. Quocirca[e] etcetera necnon etcetera. Inhibentes etcetera. In cuius etcetera. Data Rodi die quinta decima mensis Septembris anno LVIII.

*a)* caririssimo *MS* *b)* meriata *corr.* *c)* resposionum *MS* *d)* ea *corr.* *e)* Quocirqua *MS*

## 59

*The Master Fr. Roger des Pins allows Fr. Hugo von Werdenberg, Prior of* Alamania, *who has no prioral chambers, to keep the next two vacant preceptories he chooses as chambers.*

*Rhodes, [13]58 September 15*

*AOM 316 fol. 231v (233v), under* prioratus Alamanie, Boemie et parcium aliarum Alamanie.

Frater Rogerius de Pinibus etcetera religioso in Christo nobis carissimo[a] fratri Hugoni de Werdemberg domus eiusdem priori Alamanie salutem et sinceram in Domino caritatem. Tam litterarum vestrarum serie quam nunciorum vestrorum relacione instructi, quod cameras per priores Alamanie teneri et haberi solitas non habetis et quod sine eis vel aliis vestrum sustinere statum[b)] condecentem priori non possetis, pro parte vestra per dictos vestros nuncios nobis extitit supplicatum, ut super hoc vobis dignaremur de oportuno remedio providere. Nosque debita meditacione pensantes, quod sine cameris vestrum tenere statum nec prioratus negocia prosequi[c)] comode non possetis, super hoc remedium, quod pro nunc habilius possumus adhibentes, quod primas duas vacaturas baiulias in prioratu nostro Alamanie, quas volueritis et duxeritis acceptandas, cum omnibus et singulis suis membris, iuribus et pertinenciis ad eas spectantibus et pertinentibus, quoquomodo vobis possitis, in cameris retinere, quamdiu preeritis dicti regimini prioratus, solvendo ex illis responciones impositas et imponendas secundum cursum aliarum baiuliarum dicti prioratus per nos ordinato receptori responsionum de et cum voluntate, consilio et assensu fratrum et procerum conventus nostri Rodi nobis assistencium in hac parte vobis auctoritate presencium impertimur licenciam et plenam concedimus potestatem. Mandantes hac serie sub virtute sancte obediencie firmiter et districte universis et singulis fratribus domus nostre presentibus et futuris, cuiuscumque status, gradus vel condicionis existant, ne contra presentem nostram licenciam et potestatem aliquatenus venire presumant, quinymo eam iuxta eius mentem et continenciam studeant inviolabiliter observare. In cuius etcetera. Data Rodi die quinta decima mensis Septembris anno LVIII.

*a)* caris *add. ante corr.* *b)* statutum *MS* *c)* prossequi *MS*

## 60

*The Master Fr. Roger [des Pins] assigns Fr. Johann von Grostein his maintenance for his lifetime in the Preceptory of Dorlisheim.*

*Rhodes, [1358] September 15*

*AOM 316 fol. 277v-8r (281v-2r), after* prioratus Baroli, Capue et aliarum partium regni.

Frater Rogerius etcetera religioso in Christo nobis carissimo[a)] fratri Iohanni de Grostein domus eiusdem salutem et sinceram in Domino caritatem. Vestrorum exhigencia comendabilium meritorum favorabiliter vestre supplicacioni in hac parte deflexi continenti, ut vobis ad vitam vestram in domo de Toroltzhein assignare stagiam dignaremur, in domo ipsa tenore presencium, quamdiu vixeritis, vobis de speciali gratia stagiam assignamus. Mandantes sub virtute sancte obedientie firmiter et districte fratribus ·· domus eiusdem domus administracioni presidenti nunc vel in futurum, ut vos ad dictam stagiam benigne admitat et caritative pertractet vobisque in vestris necessariis provideat, prout aliis domus nostre fratribus providetur ibidem secundum bonos usus et laudabiles consuetudines domus nostre necnon universis et singulis fratribus domus nostre presentibus et futuris, cuiuscumque status, gradus vel condicionis existant, sub virtute sancte obediencie supradicta, ne contra presentem assignacionem[b)] stagie aliquatenus contra facere vel venire presumant, quinymo efficaciter illa servent. Data Rodi die XV[a] mensis Septembris anno quo supra.

*a)* cas *praem. ante corr.* *b)* nr *praem. ante corr.*

## 61

*The Master Fr. Roger [des Pins] empowers Fr. Hugo von Werdenberg, Prior of* Alamania, *to decide how Fr. Johann von Grostein should be maintained in the Preceptory of Dorlisheim; Fr. Johann had asked for hay and oats for one horse and a room to live in.*
*Rhodes, [1358] September 15*

*AOM 316 fol. 278r (282r), after* prioratus Baroli, Capue et aliarum partium regni.

Frater Rogerius etcetera religioso in Christo sibi carissimo fratri Hugoni de Werdenberg domus eiusdem priori Alamanie salutem etcetera. Supplicacionem nobis factam per religiosum in Christo nobis carissimum fratrem Iohannem de Grostein domus eiusdem, ut, cum sibi in domo de Toroltzhein ad eius vitam stagiam assignaverimus, in domo ipsa provisionem pro uno equo feni et aveni ac stabuli cum una camera, in que resideret, dignaremur facere sibi dari toto tempore vite sue, vobis remitentes vobis hac serie comitimus et[a)] concedimus potestatem super hiis disponendi et ordinandi, prout vobis videbitur disponendum. Erit nobis namque acceptum et placidum, quod in predictis duxeritis disponendum. Data Rodi die XV[a] Septembris anno quo supra.

*a)* et *supra lin.*

## 62

*The Master Fr. Roger [des Pins] assigns Fr. Friedrich Gremlich his maintenance for his lifetime in the Preceptory of Überlingen, if he resigns his Preceptory of Feldkirch.*
*Rhodes, [13]58 September 15*

*AOM 316 fol. 278r-v (282r-v), after* prioratus Baroli, Capue et aliarum partium regni.

Frater Rogerius etcetera fratri Friderico Gremlich domus eiusdem preceptori seu comendatori domus in Veltkilch salutem etcetera. Vestrorum exhigencia comendabilium meritorum favorabiliter vestre in hac parte supplicacioni deflexi continenti, ut in casum, quo vestre predicte comendatorie cederetis et administracionis cuiuslibet onus recusaretis subire, in domo seu comendatoria Vberlingen vobis ad vitam vestram assignare stagiam dignaremur, in casum predictum vobis in comendatoria predicta tenore presencium, quamdiu vixeritis, de speciali gratia stagiam assignamus. Mandantes sub virtute sancte obedientie firmiter et districte fratri ·· domus eiusdem quovis titulo eiusdem comendatorie administracioni presidenti nunc vel in futurum, ut in casum predictum vos ad dictam stagiam benigne admitat et caritative pertractet vobisque in vestris[a] necessariis provideat, prout aliis domus nostre fratribus providetur ibidem secundum bonos usus et laudabiles consuetudines domus nostre, necnon universis et singulis fratribus domus nostre presentibus et futuris, cuiuscumque status, gradus vel condicionis existant, sub virtute sancte obedientie [278v] supradicta, ne contra presentem assignacionem stagie aliquatenus contra facere vel venire presumant, quinymo efficaciter illam servent. Data Rodi die XV$^{a}$ Septembris anno LVIII.

*a)* s *praem. ante corr.*

## 63

*The Master Fr. Roger [des Pins] orders Fr. Hugo von Werdenberg, Prior of* Alamania, *to assign Fr. Friedrich Gremlich, if he resigns the Preceptory of Feldkirch, his maintenance with hay and oats and a stable for a horse and a room to live in in the Preceptory of Überlingen.*

*Rhodes, [1358] September 15*

*AOM 316 fol. 278v (282v), after* prioratus Baroli, Capue et aliarum partium regni.

Frater Rogerius etcetera fratri Hugoni de Werdemberg domus eiusdem priori Alamanie salutem etcetera. Supplicacionem nobis factam per religiosum in Christo nobis carissimum fratrem[a] Fredericum Gremlich, comendatorem domus in Weltkilche, ut, cum sibi in domo de Vberlingen ad vitam eius stagiam assignaverimus in casum, quo sue predicte cederet baiulie vel administracionis cuiuslibet subire onus recusaret[b], in eum casum in domo predicta de Vberlingen provisionem pro uno equo feni et avene et stabuli[c] cum una camera, in qua resideret, dignaremur facere sibi dari toto tempore vite sue, vobis remitentes vobis hac serie comitimus et concedimus potestatem super hiis disponendi et ordinandi, prout vobis videbitur disponendum. Erit nobis namque acceptum et placidum, quod in predictis duxeritis disponendum. Data Rodi die XV$^{a}$ mensis Septembris anno quo supra.

*a)* fratri *corr.* *b)* recusare *MS* *c)* stapuli *corr.*

## 64

*The Master Fr. Roger [des Pins] orders [Fr. Hugo von Werdenberg], Prior of* Alamania, *to receive a son of Werner Weiß into the Order as donat, sergeant or chaplain and to maintain him in the Preceptories of Freiburg or Sulz. This had already been ordered by the Master Fr. Pierre Corneillan but had not been executed due to the death of the lieutenant in the priory Fr. Hermann von Hachberg.*

*Rhodes, [13]58 September 18*

*AOM 316 fol. 277r (281r), after* prioratus Baroli, Capue et aliarum partium regni.

Frater Rogerius etcetera religioso in Christo nobis carissimo fratri ·· domus eiusdem priori Alamanie vel quovis alio titulo nunc vel in futurum dicti prioratus regimini presidenti salutem etcetera. Comperto per cartularia bone memorie fratris Petri Cornilhani predecessoris nostri, quod ad suplicationem Werneri[a] Albi alias Wis idem predecessor condam fratri Hermanno[b] de Hachsperg[c] domus eiusdem, locumtenenti in prioratu predicto,[1] comissit et mandavit, ut unum ex filiis suis in[d] donatum reciperet domus nostre et ei in altera baiuliarum de Friborigh aut Sulz stagiam assignaret, in qua ei provideri in suis faceret necessariis, nosque successive ad[e] dicti Werneri supplicationem premissam gratiam renovantes eidem concedimus dicto[f] condam fratri Hermanno precipiendo, ut unum de[d] dicti Werneri filiis in donatum vel fratrem reciperet domus nostre. Cumque, ut eiusdem Werneri suplicatoria denotatione percipimus[g] per mortem dicti condam fratris Hermanni premissa gratia non fuit executa, propter quod premissus Wernerius Albi nobis suplicavit, ut[d] sibi renovare gratiam huiusmodi dignaremur. Nosque propter ipsius antiqua servicia nostre per eum religioni inpenssa suplicationem ipsius exaudientes benigne volumus et vobis tenore presencium comittimus et mandamus, quatinus unum ex filiis dicti Werneri apti[!] et ydonei[!] et integri[!] membris suis recipiatis ad eius requisitionem in donatum vel[h] fratrem servientem vel capellanum domus nostre sollemniter, ut est moris, sibique in baiulia de Friborg aut Sulz stagiam assignetis, in qua ei provideri in suis necessariis faciatis secundum bonos usus et laudabiles consuetudines domus nostre. Data Rodi die decima octava mensis Septembris anno LVIII°.

*a) praem. corr.* *b)* Her *praem. ante corr.* *c)* Hacsperg *corr.* *d)* et *MS* *e)* a *MS* *f)* diecimus dicti *MS* *g)* precipimus *MS* *h)* de *praem. ante corr.*

1) *Fr. Hermann von Hachberg was a priest, lieutenant of the Master and Convent in* Alamania *and died on 25 April 1356: Ruppert (1889), 294.*

## 65

*The Master Fr. Roger [des Pins] confirms the assignation of his prebend and necessities to Fr. Werner Weiß in the Preceptory of Boxberg by the late Prior of* Alamania *Fr. Rudolf von Masmünster and the late Preceptor of Würzburg and Boxberg Fr. Berthold von Henneberg.*

*Rhodes, [13]58 September 18*

*AOM 316 fol. 277v (281v), after* prioratus Baroli, Capue et aliarum partium regni.

Noverint universi et singuli, quod nos frater Rogerius etcetera ad antiqua servicia nostre prestita religioni per Wernerium Albi alias Wis consideracionem habentes eorundem serviciorum respectu prebendam et necessaria unius fratris Wernerio predicto per condam fratres Roudolfum de Masemunster[a] priorem Alamanie et Bertholdum de Hennenberg preceptorem in Herbipoli et in Bogsperg in altera dictarum baiuliarum assignatam recipiendam ibidem provisionem et necessaria ipsa dari et exhiberi eidem Wernerio in hospicio suo per preceptorem de Bogsperg presentem et successive futuros de cetero ordinamus. Mandantes sub virtute sante obediencie firmiter et districte preceptori dicte preceptorie de Bogsperg presenti et futuris, ut eidem Wernerio de dictis prebenda et necessariis in hospicio suo inantea provideat contradicione remota necnon universis et singulis fratribus domus nostre quacumque auctoritate, dignitate vel officio [fulgentibus], presentibus et futuris, ne contra presentem nostram ordinacionem aliquatenus venire presumant, quinymo illam tenaciter servent. Data Rodi die XVIII mensis Septembris anno LVIII°.

*a)* Masm *praem. ante corr.*

## 66

*The Master Fr. Roger [des Pins], with consent of the Convent, revokes the concession of the Preceptory of Dorlisheim to Fr. Eberhard von Landsberg, who is not fit to be a member of the Order, and grants this preceptory for ten years to Fr. Hugo von Werdenberg, Prior of* Alamania, *because Fr. Hugo's predecessor Fr. Herdegen von Rechberg held this preceptory as a chamber and Fr. Hugo has no other chambers.*

*Rhodes, [13]58 September 20*

*AOM 316 fol. 232r-v (234r-v), under* prioratus Alamanie, Boemie et parcium aliarum Alamanie.

Frater Rogerius etcetera religioso in Christo nobis carissimo fratri Hugoni de Werdenberg domus eiusdem priori Alamanie salutem etcetera. Pro parte vestra noviter informati, quod cameras per priores Alamanie haberi et teneri solitas non habetis et quod fratri Heberhardo de Landesberg baiulia in Torolzen[a], quam condam frater Herdegus de Rechberg prior[b] Alamanie habuit pro camera et possedit, in preiudicium prioris Alamanie fuit collata, vice vestra fuit nobis suplicatum, ut predictam baiuliam vobis assignare et concedere in camera dignaremur. Nosque nolentes sicut numquam intendimus nec etiam aliqui in preiudicium alterius gratiam facere vel fecisse, si sit ita, quod predicta baiulia in Torolzen dicti condam fratris Ardegui fuit camera, omnem gratie concessionem et confirmationem de illa per nos aut quemvis alium[c] facta dicto fratri Eberhardo tanquam suprepticie impetratam, cum, si nobis intelligi datum esset, quod dicti condam fratris Ardegui fuisset camera, numquam eam alteri nec specialiter nominato[d] fratri Eberhardo dedicemus, cum quia tacita veritate surrepta[e], cum quia alia nobis per fidedignos relata, que suscitemus ex causa propter nostre religionis honorem ad dictam baiuliam et statum quemvis alium ipsum in nostro ordine reddunt merito inhabilem et indignum, de et cum voluntate, consilio et assensu fratrum et procerum conventus nostri Rodi nobis assistencium hac parte de certa scientia revocantes baiuliam ipsam in Torolzhem cum omnibus et singulis suis membris, ecclesiis, iuribus et pertinenciis universis ad eam spectantibus et pertinentibus ac spectare et pertinere debentibus quoquomodo habendam, tenendam, regendam, gubernandam, augmentandam et meliorandam in spiritualibus et temporalibus tam in capite quam in[f] menbris sub annua responsione[g] et aliis oneribus inpositis et imponendis rationabiliter secundum comunem cursum aliarum baiuliarum prioratus nostri Alamanie supradicti in capitulo provinciali prioratus eiusdem responsionum receptori in eodem prioratu annis singulis infallibiliter exsolvendo ad annos decem in festo nativitatis sancti Iohannis baptiste lapso proxime incohandos et extunc continuo secuturos auctoritate presencium de nostra certa scientia et speciali gratia vobis tanquam digno et benemerito in cameram assignamus ac confermius, concedimus et donamus benefaciendo in eadem quavis gratia de ea dicto fratri Heberardo facta in aliquo non obstante. Comitentes vobis fiducialiter circa curam, regimen et administrationem accomodam prefate baiulie ac membrorum et iurium eius deffenssionem[h] et recuperationem tam in agendo quam deffendendo hac serie vices[i] nostras. Quocirca universis et singulis fratribus, sororibus et donatis sub virtute sancte obedientie ac hominibus et vassalis et quibusvis aliis nobis subdictis in dicta preceptoria constitutis, presentibus et futuris sub sacramento fidelitatis et homagii, quo nobis et nostre domui sunt astricti, precipimus et mandamus, ut vobis tanquam eorum superiori et maiori reverenter [232v] pareant, obediant et intendant vobisque suum prebeant auxilium, consilium et favorem in omnibus concernentibus utilitatem dicte baiulie sive preceptorie, quociens opus fuerit et eos duxeritis requirendos, necnon universis et singulis fratribus domus nostre quacumque auctoritate, dignitate vel officio fulgentibus, presentibus et futuris[j], ne contra presentem nostram donationem, assignationem et gratiam aliquatenus venire presumant, quinymo illam iuxta eius mentem et seriem studeant inviolabiliter observare ac dicto fratri Eberhardo sub dicta[k)] virtute sancte obediencie districte precipimus, ut prefatam baiuliam in Torolzen vobis admittat libere et ei cedat[l)] omni contradictione et dilatione remotis. Inhibentes vobis districtius sub dicta virtute sancte obedientie, ne pretextu assignationis, concessionis et gratie nostre huiusmodi aliqua de bonis, rebus aut iuribus memorate baiulie vendatis[m)], detis, obligetis, impignoretis, alienetis, distrahatis[n)] seu in emphiteosim perpetuam concedatis vel quocumque alio colore quesito extra nostram religionem transferatis sine nostra speciali licencia et mandato. Et si, quod absit, contra inhibitionem nostram huiusmodi aliquid vel aliqua operari vel facere vos contingat, illas et illa exnunc prout extunc et extunc prout exnunc cassamus, anullamus et decernimus irritum et inane nulliusque existere penitus efficacie vel valoris. In cuius rei etcetera. Data Rodi die vicesima mensis Se[p]tembris anno LVIII°.

*a)* Tolo *praem. ante corr.* *b)* priori *MS* *c)* alio *MS* *d) praem. corr.* *e)* surreptam *MS* *f)* inb *praem. ante corr.* *g)* ref *corr. in lin.* *h)* dessenssionem *MS* *i)* vicis *MS* *j)* futurs *MS* *k) corr.* *l)* sedat *MS* *m)* vendate *MS* *n)* distratis *corr.*

*Note on the lower margin:* Ceteras litteras istius capituli anni huius require ante in folio CCLXXXI.

## 67

*The Master Fr. Roger [des Pins] licenses Fr. Hugo von Werdenberg, Prior of* Alamania, *to receive three men as knights or sergeants into the Order.*

*Rhodes, [13]58 September 20*

*AOM 316 fol. 278r (282r), after* prioratus Baroli, Capue et aliarum partium regni.

Frater Rogerius etcetera religioso in Christo sibi carissimo fratri Hugoni de Werdenberg domus eiusdem priori Alamanie salutem etcetera[a)]. Peticiones pro parte vestra nobis factas, prout decenter possimus, exaudientes favorabiliter recipiendi viros tres aptos et ydoneos ac integros membris suis in fratres domus nostre milites vel servientes, prout volueritis, sollempniter, ut est moris, eisque assignandi stagias in baiuliis dicti prioratus, in quibus ipsis[b)] in eorum necessariis provideri faciatis[c)] secundum bonos usus et laudabiles consuetudines domus nostre, vobis licenciam tenore presencium elargimur. Data Rodi die XX Septembris anno LVIII°.

*a)* sinceram *del. post* et. *b)* ipsos *praem. ante corr.* *c)* facietis *corr.*

## 68

*The Master Fr. Roger [des Pins], with consent of the Convent, confirms Fr. Johann Rinderschink, Preceptor of Fürstenfeld, for ten years in the Preceptory of Laa (Priory of Bohemia), which has been granted him by the Prior of Bohemia.*

*Rhodes, [136]5 May 26*

*AOM 319 fol. 190v-91r (184v-5r), under* prioratus Alamanie et Boemie.

Frater Rogerius etcetera religioso etcetera fratri Iohanni dicto Rinderschinch domus eiusdem preceptori in Furstenueld et in Lach salutem etcetera. Propter probitatis vestre merita[a] et administrationem accomodam, quam in comissis vobis regiminibus in nostro ordine, sicut testimonio fidedigno accepimus, [h]actenus habuistis, illa vobis libenter annuimus[b], que conservationem vestri status concernere dignoscuntur. Igitur preceptoriam[c] seu baiuliam predictam de Lach per religiosum in Christo nobis carissimum fratrem ·· domus eiusdem priorem Boemie vobis datam, ut vestra literalis insinuatio facta nobis continuit, cum omnibus et singulis suis membris, iuribus et pertinenciis universis ad eam spectantibus et pertinentibus ac spectare et pertinere debentibus quoquomodo, [191r] et cum quibus eam tenetis et presencialiter possidetis, habendam, tenendam, regendam, gubernandam, augmentandam et meliorandam in spiritualibus et temporalibus tam in capite quam in membris sub annua responsione et aliis oneribus impositis et imponendis rationabiliter secundum communem cursum aliarum baiuliarum prioratus nostri Boemie in capitulo provinciali prioratus eiusdem annis singulis exsolvendis et, nisi feceritis, destituendi vos de dicta baiulia et illam ad manus suas ponendi iuxta statutum priori et receptori responsionum dicti prioratus tenore presencium plenam concedimus potestatem huiusmodi facta vobis gratia in aliquo non obstante, hinc ad instans festum nativitatis sancti Iohannis[d] baptiste[1] et ab eodem festo inantea ad annos decem continuos et completos de et cum voluntate, consilio et assensu fratrum et[e] procerum conventus nostri Rodi nobis assistencium in hac parte de nostra certa scientia et speciali gratia[f] vobis confirmamus ac de novo conferimus, concedimus et donamus benefaciendo in eadem vosque preceptorem et comendatorem in dicta constituimus baiulia tenore presencium et eciam ordinamus. Commitentes etcetera. Quocirca etcetera necnon etcetera. Inhibentes etcetera. In cuius rei etcetera. Data Rodi die vicesima sexta mensis Maii anno quinto.

*a)* re *praem. ante corr.* *b)* anymus *MS* *c)* predictam *add. ante corr.* *d)* Ioh *add. ante corr.* *e)* f *add. ante corr.* *f)* gr *praem. ante corr.*

1) 24 June.

## 69

*The Master Fr. Roger [des Pins], with consent of the Convent, grants for ten years to Fr. Johann Rinderschink, Preceptor of Fürstenfeld and Laa, the Preceptory of Ebenfurt, which is vacant because of its mismanagement by an unnamed person. Like Fürstenfeld and Laa, it is situated in the Priory of Bohemia.*

*Rhodes, 1365 May 27*

*AOM 319 fol. 190v (184v), under* prioratus Alamanie et Boemie.

Frater Rogerius etcetera religioso in Christo nobis carissimo fratri Iohanni dicto Rinderschinch domus eiusdem preceptori in Furstenueld et in Lach salutem etcetera. Vestrorum comendabilium gratia meritorum et quia de administratione provida nobis testimonium laudabile[a] pro[h]ibetur, vobis ad gratiam redditi liberales non obstante, quod predictas baiulias in Furstenueld et in Lach ad presens in prioratu Boemie noscamini obtinere, preceptoriam seu baiuliam de Ebenfurt per inutile regimen administrationi ipsius deputato vacantem presencialiter in prioratu prefato, prout continuit vestra literalis informatio facta nobis, et ad dispositionem nostram propterea devolutam, si[b] sit ita, cum omnibus et singulis suis membris, pertinenciis et iuribus universis ad eam spectantibus et pertinentibus ac spectare et pertinere debentibus quoquomodo habendam, tenendam, regendam, gubernandam, augmentandam et meliorandam in spiritualibus et temporalibus tam in capite quam in membris sub annua responsione[c] et aliis oneribus inpositis et imponendis rationabiliter secundum communem cursum aliarum[d] baiuliarum prioratus nostri supradicti in capitulo provinciali annis singulis exsolvendis et, nisi feceritis, vos de dicta[e] baiulia et illam ad manus suas ponendi iuxta statutum priori seu alias dicti prioratus regimini presidenti et receptoribus responsionum prioratus eiusdem hac[f] serie plenam concedimus potestatem huiusmodi facta vobis gratia in aliquo non obstante, hinc ad instans festum nativitatis sancti Iohannis baptiste[1] et ab eodem festo inantea ad annos decem continuos et completos de voluntate, consilio[g] et asenssu fratrum et procerum conventus nostri Rodi nobis assistencium in hac parte de nostra[h] certa scientia et speciali gratia vobis[i] conferimus, concedimus et donamus benefaciendo in eadem vosque preceptorem et comendatorem in dicta baiulia de[j] Ebenfurd constituimus hac serie et eciam ordinamus[k]. Comittentes etcetera. Quocirca etcetera [l]necnon etcetera[l] ac religioso etcetera. Inhibentes etcetera. Im[!] cuius rey etcetera. Data Rodi die vicesima septima mensis Maii anno incarnationis Domini millesimo CCC° sexagesimo quinto.

*a)* p *praem. ante corr.* *b)* et ex *praem. ante corr.* *c)* responsionem *MS* *d)* aaliarum *MS* *e)* dictos *MS* *f)* anos *praem. ante corr.* *g)* consiljo *corr.* *h)* nostro *MS* *i)* co *praem. ante corr.* *j)* constituimus *praem. ante corr.* *k)* ortine *praem. ante corr.* *l-l) supra lin.*

*1) 24 June. Roger des Pins died apparently on 28 May 1365: Luttrell (2003), 13.*

## 70

*The Master Fr. Raymond [Bérenger] retains Fr. Johann Rinderschink, Preceptor of Fürstenfeld, Laa and Ebenfurt, and his preceptories.*

*Rhodes, 1365 May 30*

*AOM 319 fol. 190r (184r), under* prioratus Alamanie et Boemie.

Frater Raymundus etcetera religioso in Christo nobis carissimo fratri Iohanni dicto Rinderschinch domus eiusdem preceptori in Furstenueld, in Lach et in Ebenfurd salutem et sinceram in Domino caritatem. Dum laudabilia probitatis vestre merita in consideracionis nostre aciem recensemus, digne agimus, cum vos attollimus prerogativa honoris et gratie specialis. Igitur vestram volentes honorare personam, ut proinde vestre fidei et devocionis zelus ad laudabiliora inantea[a)] fervencius animetur, vos cum dictis vestris baiuliis et arnesiis vestris solutis annuis responsionibus et aliis vobis et vestris dictis baiuliis quibuscunque incumbentibus oneribus supportandis auctoritate presencium ad manus nostras de speciali gratia retinemus secundum bonos usus et laudabiles consuetudines domus nostre. Mandantes harum serie universis et singulis fratribus domus nostre quacunque auctoritate, dignitate vel officio fulgentibus, presentibus et futuris sub virtute sancte obediencie firmiter et districte, ne contra presentis retencionis nostre gratiam aliquatenus venire presumant, quinymo illam studeant iuxta eius mentem et seriem inviolabiliter observare. In cuius[b)] rei testimonium bulla nostra plumbea presentibus est appensa. Data Rodi die penultima mensis Maii anno incarnacionis Domini millesimo CCC° sexagesimo quinto.

*a)* inte *corr.* *b)* cius *MS*

## 71

*The Master Fr. Raymond Bérenger permits Fr. Johann Rinderschink, Preceptor of Fürstenfeld and Laa, to receive two noble men as knights into the Order and to maintain them in these preceptories.*

*Rhodes, [136]5 June 1*

*AOM 319 fol. 190r (184r), under* prioratus Alamanie et Boemie.

Frater Raymundus Berengarii Dei gratia etcetera fratri Iohanni dicto Rinderschinch domus eiusdem preceptori in Furstenueld, in Lach salutem etcetera. Meritorum consideratione vestrorum peticiones vestras exaudientes benigne recipiendi viros duos aptos et ydoneos ac integros membris suis in fratres domus nostre solempniter, ut est moris, eis prius per vos vel alium milicie cingulo insignitis, si[a)] ex utroque parente nobili uterque fuerit de legitimo toro natus, ipsisque in predictis vestris baiuliis stagias assignandi, in quibus illis[b)] provideri in eorum necessariis faciatis, secundum[c] bonos usus et laudabiles consuetudines domus nostre tenore presencium licenciam vobis damus. Data Rod. die prima mensis Iunii anno quinto.

*a)* se *MS* *b)* et lis *corr.* *c)* sciendum *corr.*

## 72

*The Master Fr. Raymond Bérenger licenses Fr. Johann Rinderschink, Preceptor of Fürstenfeld, Laa and Ebenfurt, to travel to the Convent on Rhodes with two brethren, horses and arms.*
*Rhodes, [136]5 June 15*

*AOM 319 fol. 190r (184r), under* prioratus Alamanie et Boemie.

Frater Raymundus Berengarii etcetera fratri Iohanni dicto Rinderschinch domus eiusdem preceptori in Furstenueld, in Lach et in Ebenfurd salutem etcetera. Sperantes vestra servicia nobis et nostre domui in citramarinis partibus existere fructuosa veniendi, quando volueritis, ad conventum nostrum Rodi cum duobus fratribus cum equis et armis sufficientibus et per vos et eos a vestro superiore prius licencia requisita presencium serie licenciam vobis damus. Data Rodi die XV mensis Iunii anno quinto.

## 73

*The Master Fr. Raymond Bérenger and the Convent grant for ten years to Fr. Konrad von Heßberg the Preceptory of Rothenburg with its member Reichardsroth (Priory of* Alamania*); this preceptory is vacant following the death of Fr. Dietrich von Zellingen.*
*Rhodes, [136]5 June 19*

*AOM 319 fol. 191v-2r (185v-6r), under* prioratus Alamanie et Boemie.

Frater Raymundus Berengarii etcetera et nos conventus domus eiusdem religioso in Christo nobis carissimo fratri Conrado de Hespurg domus eiusdem salutem etcetera. Ad illos libenter gratiosum nostrum favorem extendimus, quos illo benemeritos[a] reputamus, ut refecti ex gratia et exhilerati ex honore suscepto ad promovenda religionis nostre comoda libencius invigilent et ad virtutum studia fervencius animentur. Grata igitur fidedigna relatione percepto, quod gratiarum largitor Dominus vos morum compositione, vite mundicia[b] et naturali discretiva virtute dotavit, sperantes, quod in comisso vobis regimine favente Domino vos fructus uberes alaturum, preceptoriam seu baiuliam de Retemburg prioratus nostri Alamanie vacantem presencialiter per obitum condam fratris Theodrici de Zellingen, sicut vestra nobis exhibita supplicatio continuit, cum membro suo Rot et cum omnibus et singulis aliis suis membris, pertinenciis et iuribus universis ad dictam baiuliam spectantibus et pertinentibus ac spectare et pertinere debentibus quoquomodo habendam, tenendam, regendam, gubernandam, augmentandam et meliorandam in spiritualibus et temporalibus tam in capite quam in membris sub annua [192r] responsione et aliis oneribus impositis et imponendis rationabiliter secundum comunem cursum aliarum baiuliarum prioratus nostri supradicti in capitulo provinciali eiusdem prioratus annis singulis exsolvendis et, nisi feceritis, destituendi vos de dicta baiulia et illam ad manus suas ponendi iuxta statutum priori seu alias dicti prioratus regimini presidenti et receptoribus responsionum prioratus eiusdem hac serie plenam concedimus potestatem huiusmodi vobis facta gratia in aliquo non obstante, hinc ad instans festum nativitatis sancti Iohannis baptiste et ab eodem festo inantea ad annos decem continuos et completos[c] invicem deliberato consilio de nostra certa scientia et speciali gratia vobis conferimus, concedimus et donamus benefaciendo in eadem et cuiusque alterius iuri propterea minime derogando vosque preceptorem et comendatorem in dicta baiulia constituimus ac eciam ordinamus. Comittentes etcetera. Quocirca etcetera necnon etcetera ac religioso etcetera. Inhibentes etcetera. Et si, quod absit, etcetera. Ceterum si, quod absit, predictam baiuliam sive domum ·· non administraveritis utiliter et vestro priori aut alias vestro superiori in dicto prioratu eius preceptis non obedieritis reverenter, premissam vobis factam gratiam decernimus esse nullam et eam exnunc in eum casum revocamus de certa scientia per presentes. In cuius rey etcetera. Data Rodi die decima nona mensis Iunii anno quinto.

*a)* benemerito *corr.* *b)* mundia *MS* *c)* competos *MS*

## 74

*The Master Fr. Raymond Bérenger and the Convent grant for ten years to Fr. Karl von Lichtenstein the Preceptory of Boxberg with its member of Krautheim (Priory of* Alamania), *which is vacant following the death of Fr. Nikolaus von Heinriet.*

*Rhodes, [136]5 June 19*

*AOM 319 fol. 192r (186r), under* prioratus Alamanie et Boemie.

Frater Raymundus Berengarii etcetera et nos conventus etcetera religioso in Christo nobis carissimo fratri Karulo de Lyechensten domus eiusdem salutem etcetera. Ad illos libenter gratiosum nostrum favorem extendimus, quos illo benemeritos reputamus, ut refecti ex gratia et exhilerati ex honore suscepto ad promovenda religionis nostre comoda libencius invigilent et ad virtutum studia fervencius animentur. Grata igitur fidedigna relatione percepto, quod gratiarum largitor Dominus vos morum compositione, vite mundicia et naturali discretiva virtute dotavit, sperantes, quod in comisso vobis regimine favente Domino vos fructus uberes alaturum, preceptoriam seu baiuliam[a] sancti Iohannis de Bexsp(er)g vacantem presencialiter per obitum condam fratris Nicolai de Hehric, sicut vestra nobis exhibita supplicacio continuit, cum membro suo de Krauchem et cum omnibus et singulis aliis suis membris, pertinenciis et iuribus universis ad dictam baiuliam spectantibus et pertinentibus ac spectare et pertinere debentibus quoquomodo habendam, tenendam, regendam, gubernandam, augmentandam et meliorandam in spiritualibus et temporalibus tam in capite quam in membris sub annua responsione et aliis oneribus impositis et imponendis rationabiliter secundum comunem cursum aliarum baiuliarum prioratus nostri supradicti in capitulo provinciali[b)] eiusdem prioratus annis singulis exsolvendis et, nisi feceritis, destituendi vos de dicta baiulia et illam ad manus suas ponendi iuxta statutum priori[c)] seu alias dicti prioratus regimini presidenti et receptoribus responsionum prioratus eiusdem hac serie plenam concedimus potestatem huiusmodi facta vobis gratia in aliquo non obstante, hinc ad instans festum nativitatis sancti Iohannis baptiste et ab eodem festo inantea ad annos decem continuos et completos invicem deliberato consilio de nostra certa scientia et speciali gratia vobis conferimus, concedimus et donamus benefaciendo in eadem et cuiusque alterius iuri propterea minime derogando vosque preceptorem et comendatorem in dicta baiulia constituimus ac eciam ordinamus. Comittentes etcetera. Quocirca[d)] etcetera necnon etcetera ac religioso etcetera. Inhibentes etcetera. Et[e)] si, quod absit, etcetera. Ceterum si, quod absit, predictam baiuliam sive domum non administraveritis utiliter et vestro priori aut alias vestro superiori in dicto prioratu et eius preceptis non obedieritis reverenter, premissam vobis factam gratiam decernimus esse nullam et eam exnunc in eum casum revocamus de certa scientia per presentes. In cuius rey etcetera. Data Rodi die decima nona mensis Iunii anno quinto.

*a)* baiulia *MS* *b)* provincia *corr.* *c)* priori et receptori responsionum *praem. ante corr.* *d)* Quocica *MS* *e)* Ets *praem. ante corr.*

## 75

*The Master Fr. Raymond Bérenger and the Convent grant for ten years to Fr. Heinrich von Schwarzburg the Preceptory of Striegau (Priory of Bohemia), which is vacant following its resignation of Fr. Johann Rinderschink.*

*Rhodes, [136]5 August 6*

*AOM 319 fol. 191v (185v), under* prioratus Alamanie et Boemie.

Frater Raymundus Berengarii etcetera et nos conventus domus eiusdem religioso in Christo nobis carissimo fratri Henrico de Nigro[a)] Castro[1)] domus

1) *Europäische Stammtafeln 1/3 (2000), no. 314, a great nephew of Fr. Albrecht von Schwarzburg.*

eiusdem salutem etcetera. Ad illos libenter gratiosum nostrum favorem extendimus, quos illo benemeritos reputamus, ut refecti ex gratia et exhilerati ex honore[b)] suscepto ad promovenda religionis nostre comoda libencius invigilent et ad virtutum studia fervencius animentur. Grata igitur fidedigna relacione percepto, quod gratiarum largitor Dominus vos morum compositione, vite mundicia et naturali discretiva virtute dotavit, sperantes, quod in comisso vobis regimine favente Domino vos fructus uberes alaturum, preceptoriam seu baiuliam de Strigen prioratus nostri Boemie vacantem presencialiter per resignationem de ea factam per religiosum[c)] in Christo nobis carissimum fratrem Iohannem de Rinderschenkel domus eiusdem, ultimum preceptorem, ipsius sua spontanea voluntate in manibus religiosi in Christo nobis carissimi fratris ·· domus eiusdem prioris dicti prioratus, ut pro parte vestra continuit expositio facta nobis, de[d)] qua preceptoria dictus[e)] prior nondum providit alicui, ut asserit expositio predicta, sed eam regendam idem prior cuidam fratri nostre dicte domus comisit, si sit ita, cum omnibus et singulis suis membris, iuribus et pertinenciis universis ad dictam baiuliam spectantibus et pertinentibus ac spectare[f)] et pertinere debentibus quoquomodo habendam, tenendam, regendam, gubernandam, augmentandam[g)], et meliorandam in spiritualibus et temporalibus tam in capite quam in membris sub annua responsione et aliis oneribus inpositis et imponendis rationabiliter secundum comunem cursum aliarum[h)] baiuliarum prioratus nostri supradicti in capitulo provinciali eiusdem prioratus annis singulis exsolvendis et, nisi feceritis, destituendi vos de dicta baiulia et illam ad manus suas ponendi iuxta statutum priori[i)] seu alias dicti prioratus regimini presidenti et receptoribus responsionum prioratus eiusdem hac serie plenam concedimus potestatem huiusmodi facta vobis gratia in aliquo non obstante, hinc ad instans festum nativitatis sancti Iohannis baptiste et ab eodem festo inantea ad annos decem continuos et completos invicem deliberato consilio de nostra certa scientia et speciali gratia vobis conferimus, concedimus et donamus benefaciendo in eadem vosque preceptorem et comendatorem in dicta[j)] baiulia constituimus ac eciam ordinamus. Comittentes etcetera. Quocirca etcetera necnon etcetera ac religioso etcetera. Inhibentes etcetera. Et si, quod absit, etcetera. Ceterum si, quod absit, predictam baiuliam sive domum . . . non administraveritis utiliter et vestro priori aut alias vestro superiori in dicto prioratu et eius preceptis non obedieritis reverenter, premissam vobis factam gratiam decernimus esse nullam et eam exnunc in eum casum revocamus de certa scientia per presentes. In cuius rey etcetera. Data Rodi die sexta[k)] mensis Augusti anno quinto.

*a)* Nigcco *praem. ante corr.* *b)* ex honore *supra lin.* *c)* l *praem. ante corr.* *d)* de *supra lin.* *e)* facta *praem. ante corr.* *f)* ac spectare *dupl.* *g)* ag *praem. ante corr.* *h)* aliarum *add. ante corr.* *i)* et receptori responsionum *add. ante corr.* *j)* in dicta *dupl. ante corr.* *k)* sex *praem. ante corr.*

## 76

*The Master Fr. Raymond Bérenger and the Convent confirm the chaplain and Preceptor Fr. Peter Warnsdorfer for his lifetime in the Preceptory of Löwenberg (Priory of Bohemia).*
*Rhodes, [136]5 August 12*

*AOM 319 fol. 191r (185r), under* prioratus Alamanie et Boemie.

Frater Raymundus Berengarii Dei gratia etcetera et nos conventus domus eiusdem religioso in Christo nobis carissimo fratri Petro Warnsdorfe domus eiusdem, capellano ac preceptori de Lemberg, salutem et sinceram in Domino caritatem. Propter probitatis vestre merita et administracionem accomodam, quam in comisso vobis regimine in nostro ordine, sicut testimonio fidedigno accepimus, actenus habuistis, illa vobis libenter annuymus, que conservacionem vestri status concernere[a] dignoscuntur. Igitur preceptoriam seu baiuliam predictam de Lemberg prioratus nostri Boemie cum omnibus et singulis suis[b] membris, iuribus et pertinenciis universis ad eam spectantibus et pertinentibus ac spectare et pertinere debentibus quoquomodo, et cum quibus eam tenetis et presencialiter possidetis, habendam, tenendam, regendam, gubernandam, augmentandam et meliorandam in spiritualibus et temporalibus tam in capite quam in membris sub annua responsione et aliis oneribus impositis et imponendis rationabiliter secundum communem cursum aliarum baiuliarum prioratus nostri supradicti in capitulo provinciali prioratus eiusdem annis singulis exsolvendis et, nisi feceritis, destituendi vos de dicta baiulia et illam ad manus suas ponendi iuxta statutum priori et receptori responsionum prioratus eiusdem tenore presencium plenam concedimus potestatem huiusmodi facta vobis gratia in aliquo non obstante, ad vitam vestram invicem deliberato consilio auctoritate presencium vobis confirmamus de certa nostra scientia et gratia speciali ac de novo conferimus et donamus benefaciendo in eadem vosque preceptorem et comendatorem in dicta constituimus baiulia tenore presencium et eciam ordinamus. Comittentes vobis etcetera. Quocirca etcetera necnon etcetera. Inhibentes etcetera. Ceterum siquidem[c] baiuliam sive domum non administraveritis utiliter, ut vestro priori aut alias vestro superiori in dicto prioratu et eius preceptis non hobedieritis reverenter, premissam vobis factam gratiam decernimus esse nullam et eam in eum casum revocamus de certa nostra scientia per presentes. In cuius rei etcetera. Data Rodi die duodecima mensis Augusti anno quinto.

*a)* consernere *MS* *b)* sui *corr.* *c)* si quod pridem *corr.*

## 77

*The Master Fr. Raymond Bérenger provides Fr. Bernhard von Chotek, Preceptor of Glatz and Ploskovice, at his request with a copy from the registers of his appointment to his preceptory by the former Master Fr. Roger des Pins.*
*Rhodes, [136]5 August 15*

*AOM 319 fol. 192v (186v), under* prioratus Alamanie et Boemie.

Frater Raymundus Berengarii etcetera religioso in Christo nobis carissimo fratri Bernardo de Chontetz domus eiusdem preceptori de Glocz et de Phaschowytz salutem etcetera. Continuit vestra expositio facta nobis, quod bone memorie[a)] frater Rogerius de Pinibus, inmediatus predecessor noster, vobis gratiose contulit prefatas baiulias. Sed quia in dubium vertitis, an littera dicte gratie, quam ad prioratum Boemie misistis, perdita sit vel non, cum nulla nova de illa post missionem illius habueritis, supplicastis nobis humiliter[b)], ut litteram prefatam de cartulario[c)] dicti predecessoris[d)] nostri extrahi et vobis dari sub bulla nostra plumbea mandaremus. Nosque vestre supplicationi velut rationi consone favorabiliter annuentes[e)] litteram memoratam de dicto cartulario sumi et presentibus inseri iubsimus, cuius tenor sequitur et est talis: "Frater Rogerius etcetera." In cuius rey etcetera. Data Rodi die quinta decima mensis Augusti[f)] anno quinto.

*a)* fratris Rogeriis *add. ante corr.* *b)* habuiliter *MS* *c)* cart *praem. ante corr.* *d)* preced *praem. ante corr.* *e)* an *praem. ante corr.* *f)* Augustis *corr.*

## 78

*The Master Fr. Raymond Bérenger retains*, secundum continentiam statuti, *the following brethren, according to priories. From* Alamania *Fr. Gottfried von Rüdigheim, Preceptor of Mainz and Frankfurt; Fr. Dietrich von Keppenbach, Preceptor of Freiburg (im Breisgau) and Chamberlain of Buchsee; Fr. Walter of Rechberg, Preceptor of Villingen; Fr. Hesso Schlegelholz, Preceptor of Klingnau and Schlettstadt. From Bohemia Fr. Nikolaus Wildungsmaurer, Preceptor of Mailberg; Fr. Nikolaus; Fr. Johann Rinderschink, Preceptor of Fürstenfeld.*

*Rhodes, [1365 October 24]*

*AOM 319 fol. 322v-35v (no old foliation), after* Assignationes pecuniarum.

*Fol. 324r:* In prioratu Alamanie. Fratrem Gaufirdum de Růdenken preceptorem de Maguncia et Frangwortya. Fratrem Dietricum de Kepenbach preceptorem in Friburgo [a)]et camerario[b)] domini in Buhs[a)]. Fratrem Gualterium de Reyperch preceptorem in Vilyngen. Fratrem Hessonem [a)]Slegelholz preceptori[b)] in Klingnaue et in Sletzstat[a)]. In prioratu Boemia. Fratrem Nicolaum Wyldungsmaurer preceptorem in Morperg. Fratrem Nicolaum. Fratrem Iohannem Rindersenk preceptorem in Furstenfelden.

*a-a) add. manus posterior.* *b) The accusative would be correct. The dative was used for the address of the letter when the chancery wrote to the brother.*

## 79

*The Master Fr. Raymond Bérenger grants for ten years to Fr. Protiva von Scheckem the Preceptory of Strakonice (Priory of Bohemia) because its present chaplain and Preceptor Fr. Hermann is too old to govern it.*

*Rhodes, 1365 November 8*

*AOM 319 fol. 192v-3r (185v-6r), under* prioratus Alamanie et Boemie.

Frater Raymundus Berengarii etcetera religioso in Christo nobis carissimo fratri Protiwa de Schekem domus eiusdem salutem etcetera. Sicut pro parte vestra nobis exhibita supplicacio continuit, frater Hermannus cappellanus domus eiusdem preceptor de Strakonnicz longa senectute confractus dictam suam preceptoriam regere et gubernare non potest, propter quod ob ipsius inbecillem inpotencia[m] preceptoria predicta dispendiis multis subicitur, ut de die in diem subicietur pocioribus detrimentis, si nostre provisionis remedium celeriter non ocurrat, subiungentes, ut, si vobis de preceptoria seu baiulia supradicta providere dignaremur, eam restauraretis a noxiis, quibus subiacet, et divina vobis assistente gratia regeretis utiliter ad honorem et comodum domus nostre. Nosque vestre huiusmodi supplicacioni faventes propter atributa vobis de vita, moribus et administratione utili testimonia laudedigna, si contenta in vestra supplicatione prefata contineant veritatem, preceptoriam seu baiuliam supradictam de Strakonitz prioratus nostri Boemie, ne ob fragile senium prelibati fratris Hermanni ad destruccionem deveniat, cum omnibus et singulis suis membris, iuribus et pertinenciis universis ad dictam baiuliam spectantibus et pertinentibus ac spectare et pertinere debentibus quoquomodo habendam, tenendam, regendam, gubernandam, augmentandam et meliorandam in spiritualibus et temporalibus tam in capite quam in membris sub annua responsione et aliis oneribus impositis et imponendis rationabiliter secundum comunem cursum aliarum baiuliarum prioratus nostri supradicti in capitulo provinciali eiusdem prioratus annis singulis exolvendis [193r] et, nisi feceritis, destituendi vos de dicta baiulia et illam ad manus suas ponendi iuxta statutum priori seu alias dicti prioratus regimini presidenti et receptoribus responsionum prioratus eiusdem hac serie plenam concedimus potestatem huiusmodi facta vobis gratia in aliquo non obstante, hinc ad instans festum nativitatis sancti Iohannis baptiste et ab eodem[a)] festo inantea ad annos decem continuos et completos invicem deliberato consilio de nostra certa scientia et speciali gratia vobis conferimus, concedimus et donamus benefaciendo in eadem vosque preceptorem et comendatorem in dicta baiulia co[n]stituimus ac eciam ordinamus. Comitentes etcetera. Quocirca etcetera necnon etcetera ac religioso etcetera. Ceterum si, quod absit, predictam baiuliam sive domum de Strakonnicz non administraveritis utiliter et vestro priori aut alias vestro superiori in dicto prioratu et eius preceptis non obedieritis reverenter, premissam vobis factam gratiam decernimus esse nullam et eam exnunc in eum casum revocamus de certa scientia per presentes. Inhibentes etcetera. In cuius rey etcetera. Data Rodi die VIII mensis Novembris anno incarnationis Domini millesimo trecentesimo sexagesimo quinto.

*a)* eadem *MS*

## 80

*The Master Fr. Raymond Bérenger orders Fr. Konrad von Braunsberg, Prior of* Alamania, *to receive at the request of the Lord of Rieneck Dietrich zu Rhein one man of his family as a knight brother into the Order and to maintain this person in a preceptory of his priory.*

*Rhodes, [13]65 November 22*

*AOM 319 fol. 192v (186v), under* prioratus Alamanie et Boemie.

Frater Raymundus Berengarii etcetera religioso in Christo nobis carissimo fratri Conrado de Bruynberg[a] domus eiusdem priori Alamannie salutem etcetera. Ad deprecativam instanciam viri nobilis domini Dyetrici de Rin, militis, domini de Rineckh, volumus et vobis tenore presencium precipiendo mandamus sub virtute sancte obediencie nichilominus firmiter iniungentes, quatinus alterum ex afinibus premissi[b] domini Dyetrici, si aptus sit sanusque et integer membris suis, ad ipsius requisicionem recipiatis in domus nostre fratrem sollempniter, ut est moris, eo prius per vos vel alium milicie cingulo insignito, si ex utroque parente nobili fuerit de legitimo thoro natus, sibique in altera baiuliarum dicti prioratus stagiam assignetis, in qua ei provideri in suis necessariis faciatis secundum bonos usus et laudabiles consuetudines domus nostre. Data Rodi die vicesima secunda mensis Novembris anno sexagesimo quinto.

*a)* Bir *praem. ante corr.* *b)* premisi *MS*

## 81

*Licence for Fr. Protiva von Scheckem, Preceptor of Strakonice [in Bohemia], to travel to* Alamania *and to return to the Convent.*

*[Rhodes, 1366] January 20*

*AOM 319 fol. 193r (187r), under* prioratus Alamanie et Boemie.

Die vicesima mensis Ianuarii data fuit licencia fratri Protiwa de Sczekem domus eiusdem preceptori de Strakonits recedendi de conventu et eundi[a] ad partes Alamannie ac[b] redeundi ad dictum conventum cum equis et armis suficientibus a suo superiore prius licencia requisita.

*a)* r *praem. ante corr.* *b)* et *praem. ante corr.*

## 82

*The Master Fr. Raymond Bérenger quits Fr. Gallus von Lemberg, Prior of Bohemia, about 1,200 florins for his responsions for the year ending on 24 June 1365 which were paid through Fr. Frank [von Hertwitz].*

*Rhodes, [13]66 January 20*

*AOM 319 fol. 193r (187r), under* prioratus Alamanie et Boemie.

Noverint universi et singuli presentem recognicionem et quitanciam visuri et audituri, quod nos frater Raymundus Berengarii etcetera tenore presentis quitancie confitemur et in verbo recogno[s]cimus veritatis thesaurum nostri conventus habuis[s]e et recepisse per manus fratris Franconis a religioso in Christo nobis carissimo ffratre Gallo de Lamberch domus eiusdem priore Alamanie[1)] florenos auri mille ducentos pro responsione prioratus Boemie anni finiti in festo nativitatis sancti Iohannis baptiste anni Domini millesimi trecentesimi sexagesimi quinti[a)] proximo preteriti. De quibusquidem mille ducentis florenis per dictum thesaurum et eius ministros, ut premit[t]itur, habitis et receptis contenti plenarie premissum priorem Boemie ac eius bona et arnesia liberamus hac serie perpetuo et quitamus. In cuius rey testimonium presentem recognicionem et quitanciam iamdicto priori exinde fieri fecimus[b)] sigilli nostri inpresione munitam. Data Rodi die vicesima mensis Ianuarii anni sexagesimi quinti.

*a)* quinto *corr.* *b)* fecicimus *MS*

## 83

*Licence for Fr. Bernard von Chotek, Preceptor of Glatz and Ploskovice, to travel to his preceptories.*

*[Rhodes, 1366] February 18*

*AOM 319 fol. 193r (187r), under* prioratus Alamanie et Boemie.

Die XVIII Febroarii data fuit licencia fratri Bernardo Cotetz preceptori in Glocz et in Ploskowytz eundi ad regendam suas preceptorias prefatas.

## 84

*Note that a council of prud'hommes from the Convent ordered a general clause to be added to letters of appointment for* Alamania *or Bohemia that preceptories, in this example, the Preceptory of Regensburg, are lost in case of mismanagement or disobedience.*

*[Rhodes, 1365–66]*

*1)* Boemie *recte.*

*AOM 319 fol. 193r (187r), under* prioratus Alamanie et Boemie.

Ordinatum fuit per consilium procerum conventus Rodi, ut in litteris preceptoriarum prioratuum Alamanie et Boemie ponatur in fine ante "In cuius rei testimonium" quequidem talis est: "Ceterum si, quod absit, predictam baiuliam sive domum de Regensburg non administraveritis utiliter et vestro priori aut alias vestro superiori in dicto prioratu et eius preceptis non obediveritis reverenter, premissam vobis factam gratiam decernimus esse nullam et eam exnunc in eum casum[a] revocamus de certa scientia per presentes. In cuius rey etcetera."

*a)* cassum *MS*

## 85

*The Master Fr. Raymond Bérenger and the Convent grant to Fr. Ulrich von Weitersdorf the Preceptory of Regensburg with its member of Münster (Priory of* Alamania), *which is vacant following the death of Fr. Wilbrand.*

*Rhodes, 1366 June 1*

*AOM 319 fol. 312r (309r), under* Terrarum.

Frater Raymundus etcetera et nos conventus etcetera fratri Vlrico de Witsdorf domus eiusdem salutem etcetera. Ad illos libenter gratiosum nostrum favorem extendimus, quos illo benemeritis reputamus etcetera. Preceptoriam seu baiuliam de Regemspurg cum membro eius Ministro[1] vacantem per obitum condam fratris Wiltprandi domus eiusdem ultimi preceptoris illius et ad dispositionem et ordinationem nostram propterea devolutam cum omnibus et singulis suis membris, iuribus et pertinentiis universis ad dictam baiuliam spectantibus et pertinentibus ac spectare et pertinere debentibus quoquomodo et habendam, tenendam, regendam, gubernandam, augmentandam et meliorandam in spiritualibus et temporalibus tam in capite quam in membris sub annuis responsibus et aliis oneribus impositis et imponendis rationabiliter secundum communem cursum aliarum baiuliarum prioratus nostri Alamanie, in quo dicta baiulia sita et posita in capitulo provinciali eiusdem prioratus annis singulis exolvendas. Et nisi feceritis etcetera commitentes etcetera. Quocirca etcetera necnon etcetera. Inhibentes etcetera. Ceterum et si, quod absit, predictam baiuliam sive domum de Regenspurg cum administraveritis utiliter ut vestro priori aut alias vestro superiori in dicto prioratu et eius preceptis non obedieritis reverenter, premissam vobis factam[a] gratiam decernimus esse nullam et eam exnunc etiam eum casum revocamus de certa scientia per presentes. In cuius rei etcetera. Data Rodi die prima mensis Iunii anno sexagesimo sexto.

*a)* fam praem. *corr.*

1) *Altmühlmünster.*

## 86

*The Master Fr. Raymond Bérenger quits Fr. Dietrich von Keppenbach, Preceptor of Freiburg im Breisgau and Neuenburg, for 200 florins due to the Master from the Master's chamber of Buchsee, which were due for all past years until 24 June 1366.*

*Rhodes, 1366 June 3*

*AOM 319 fol. 193v (187v), under* prioratus Alamanie et Boemie.

Noverint universsi et singuli presentem quietanciam et appodiciam inspecturi[a)], quod nos ffrater Raimundus Berengarii Dei gratia ssacre domus hospitalis ssancti Iohanis Ierosolimitani magisster humilis et pauperum Christi cusstos tenore presencium de annua penssione camere nostre de Buhs prioratus Alamanie ducentorum fflorenorum[b)] auri, quos nobis annuatim tenetur exssolvere religiosus in Christo nobis carisimus ffrater Dietricus de Keppembach, premis[s]e domus nostre preceptor in Ffriburgo Brisgaudie et in Nouo Castro, recognoscentes in verbo veritatis contentamur de annis preteritis et pressenti ffiniendo[c)] in festo ssancti Iohanis baptiste anni Domini millesimi trecentesimi sexagessimi sexti. Et idem finem facimus pro tempore dicto. De qua pensione ducentorum florenorum usque ad[d)] premissum tempus cotidie plenarie eundem ffratrem Dietricum ac eius bona et arnecia hac serie liberamus[e)] et perpetuo quitatis[f)] ffacimus ipsi ffinem[g)]. In cuius rei testimonium pressentem quietanciam et appodicia[m] iamdicto ffratri Dietrico exinde ffieri[h)] ffecimus et nostri ssigilli impressione muniri. [i)]Data Rodi die tertia mensis Iunii anno millesimo CCC sexagesimo sexto.

*a)* inespecturi *MS* *b)* fflorenarum *MS* *c)* ffinienido *MS* *d)* ac *MS* *e)* libramus *MS* *f)* cqetatis *MS* *g)* ffinen *MS* *h) supra lin.* *i) From here onwards written by another scribe.*

## 87

*The Master Fr. Raymond Bérenger and the Convent order the Preceptor of Freiburg im Breisgau and Neuenburg and Chamberlain of Buchsee Fr. Dietrich von Keppenbach, receiver of responsions in the Priory of* Alamania, *to send the responsions of the priory and the pension payments due to the Master and all other dues to Fr. Giovanni de Rivara, Prior of Venice, and Fr. Pietro Benatti, Preceptor of Verona and receiver in (here Preceptor of) Hungary, in Venice.*

*[1366–67]*

*AOM 319 fol. 193v-4r (187v-8r), under* prioratus Alamanie et Boemie.

Frater Raymundus Berengarii Dei gratia[a)] et nos conventus[a)] religiosso in Christo nobis[b)] carissimo Dietrico de Keppembach domus eiusdem[c)] preceptori in Friburgo Brisgaudie et in Nouocastro ac camerario nostri dicti magistri in camera nostra de Buhs et responsionum receptori in prioratu nostro Alamanie salutem et ssinceram in Domino caritatem. Cum ordinavimus responssiones dicti prioratus ac camera nostra dicti magistri ssupradicte pensionem[d)] et omnia singula alia iura et bona nobis communiter vel divissim expectancia et debencia prevenire[e)] ad civitatem Veneciarum religiossis in Christo nobis carisimis fratribus Iohani de Riparia priori Veneciarum et [194r] Petro Benatto preceptori Veronensis et Vngre[1)] sive[f)] eorum alteri annis singulis per vos miti, vobis ideo tenore pressencium ssub virtute ssancte obidiencie districte mandantes precipimus[g)], quatinus ressponssiones ac penssionem predictas et alia predicta nominatis ffratribus Ioanni de Riparia et Petro Benatto vel eorum alteri anno colibet ad[h)] civitatem Prieestinpto[?] infallibiliter tra[n]smit[t]i[i)] caveatis et tradi nostro nomine pariter ffaciatis ssuper hoc vos taliter habiturum, quod vos hobidiencie tra[n]sgresio nula culpet[j)]. In cuius[k)] rei testimonium bulla nostra comunis plunbea presentibus est appenssa.

*Note the many oddities of spelling in this text.* *a) add. lac.* *b)* humilis et pauperum Christi custos et nos conventus *add. ante corr.* *c)* eisdem *MS* *d)* pensione *MS* *e)* preveniere *MS* *f)* sue *MS* *g)* precimus *MS* *h)* ac *MS* *i)* trasim *MS* *j)* cupet *MS* *k)* cui *MS*

## 88

*The Master Fr. Robert [de Juilly] answers a complaint made on behalf of Fr. Wilhelm Holste, Preceptor of Rörchen. Three brothers, Hasso, Wedego, knights, and Dietz, squire, von Wedel and others from the castle of Uchtenhagen and the town of Königsberg burnt down the buildings of Rörchen, took away all cattle, horses, pigs, sheep, other animals and moveable goods, destroyed the mills, cut down and took away trees in the forests, imprisoned peasants, extorted ransoms from them and robbed large quantities of money in the villages. What is worse, they broke into parish churches which belonged to the preceptory, stole the boxes containing the consecrated host and toppled baptismal fonts. The damages were so enormous that the preceptor obtained his superior's licence and appealed to the Apostolic See. In vain, the preceptor asked princes of the region for their help. When travelling to the Roman curia, the preceptor was taken prisoner by the above-mentioned wrongdoers and paraded in handcuffs on his own horse through towns and villages of three dioceses. Some brethren from Rörchen who accompanied him were deprived of their belongings. Together these Hospitallers were taken to Königsberg. There the preceptor was put in irons together with other thieves and robbers in a dungeon with*

1) *On 1 June 1365 Fr. Giovanni de Rivara and Fr. Pietro Benatti had been appointed receivers in the Priory of Hungary: AOM 319 fol. 323v; Luttrell (2007), article XXI, 294–5, 300.*

*toads and serpents for 98 days until he escaped miraculously. When he reached the Roman curia, a chapter of the Order was being celebrated there. The Grand Preceptor and the Hospitaller heard his case and licensed him to pursue his lawsuit at the Roman curia. Following the preceptor's petition, the Master now confirms the licence to pursue his case in the Roman curia and elsewhere. The preceptor may use all his revenues to rebuild Rörchen, and he may keep Rörchen for ten years onwards, when all lawsuits have come to an end.*

*Avignon, 1374 September 12*

*AOM 320 fol. 28r-v (19r-v).*

Frater Robertus etcetera religioso in Christo nobis carissimo fratri Guillelmo Holste presbitero domus eiusdem preceptori in Roreke Caminensis diocesis salutem et sinceram in Domino caritatem. Supplicatione nobis pro parte vestra porrecta recepimus, quod, cum Hasso, Wedego milites, Tytzo armi[g]er fratres condicti de Wedel morantes in castro Vcchenhaghen[1)] et multi alii castrenses eorum complices necnon proconsules et consules ac tota universitas opidi Conigesberch[a)] dicte diocesis propinqui vicini[2)] domus predicte ipsam domum seu preceptoriam cum omnibus suis bonis et edificiis per incendium destruxerunt, omnibus bobus, equis, porcis et ceteris pecoribus et animalibus, rebus, utensilibus et aliis rebus mobilibus spoliarunt, molendina devastarunt, lignaque de nemoribus et silvis ipsius domus serari et deportari fecerunt, rusticos seu villanos captivatos in vinculis tenuerunt pecunias extorquentes ab eisdem, et omnes villas et possessiones dicte domus in maximis pecuniarum quantitatibus depaccarunt[3)] et, quod deterius est, quasdam ecclesias parrochiales ad ipsam preceptoriam spectantes fregerunt, pixides cum eucharistie sacramentis et sacra unctione deportarunt, baptisteria subverterunt[b)] et alias omnino Dei timore postposita tot et tanta irrecuperabilia dampna dicte preceptorie vestre intulerunt et fecerunt, quod ipsa preceptoria vestra penitus est destructa, nisi cum iuvamine sedis apostolice de remedio provideremus oportuno. Verum cum vos apud diversos principes terrarum de predictis iniuriis preceptorie, ordini et vobis predictis illatis conquesti fuerunt sepe et incessanter, nullum tamen coram eis potuistis consequi iusticie complementum. Cumque dicti iniuriatores vos iter versus curiam Romanam arripuisse perciperent, quamvis id feceritis de consilio et licentia vestri superioris speciali ad prosequendum dictas iniuriarum causas, dicti emuli et adversarii vos insequentes captivarunt, captivumque

1) *Uchtenhagen near Freienwalde. The castle was inhabited by two families with similar coats-of-arms, von Wedel in gold a black cartwheel with eight spokes, von Uchtenhagen in silver a red cartwheel with eight spokes. So the Hospitallers were apparently involved in a feud with a family.*

2) *6 km south-west of Rörchen.*

3) depactare *to extort a ransom.*

pedibus vestris equo proprio colligatum tamquam furem per campos et carrerias opidorum et villarum trium diocesum[4] duxerunt in dispectum tocius ordinis et ecclesiastice libertatis, et quosdam fratres vestros conventuales vobis cum vos sic ligatum omnibus bonis vestris spoliantes duxerunt usque ad predictum opidum Conigesbergh,[5] ubi vos inter malefactores, fures et latrones et alios maleficos supplicio suspendii tradendos, ubi bufones et serpentes sunt, posuerunt et ibidem vos in vinculis ferreis per spacium nonaginta et octo dierum captivum detinuerunt. Tandem divina gratia vobis mirabiliter suffragante evasistis. Venientes ad curiam Romanam contra memoratos iniuriatores causam iniuriarum [28v] predictarum incepistis. Cumque vos ad dictam curiam venientes, capitulum predicti ordinis fieret generale, magnus preceptor et hospitalarius sacre domus hospitalis sancti Iohannis Ierosolimitani factum causarum vestrarum per modum consilii intelligerunt, catholica pietate moti et vobis compacientes quasdam litteras vobis in subsidium vestri et preceptorie predicte gratiose concesserunt, in quibusquidem litteris licentia agendi et defendendi contra dictos iniuriatores et alios quoscumque in curia Romana et extra usque ad finem cause[c] cuiuslibet litis annuerunt, ut dicitur, quare nobis humiliter supplicastis, ut vobis providere dignaremur de remedio gratioso. Nos igitur supplicationibus vestris tamquam dignis favorabiliter inclinati vobis licentiam digendi et defendendi contra prefatos iniuriatores et adversarios vestros et preceptorie vestre predicte et alios quoscumque in curia Romana et extra usque ad finem cuiuslibet litis, prout predicti visitatores in capitulo generali annuerunt, et de uberiori gratia[d] vobis concessimus, ut omnes fructus, proventus et obventiones, si qui fuerint seu reperiri vel recuperari poterunt in dicta vestra preceptoria Roreke, recipere et habere possitis ad defendendum et prosequendum dictas iniuriarum causas et alias quascumque vos et dictam vestram preceptoriam tangentes in curia Romana et extra cum omnibus suis emergentibus, dependentibus et connexis vobis, quicquid pro emenda dampni spoliis et rapinis dicte vestre preceptorie illatis derivaverit, in usum et utilitatem et reformacionem ac recuperacionem structurarum dicte domus convertere debeatis et profectum necnon gubernationem et regimen possessionis dicte preceptorie vobis de speciali gratia ad decennium concedentes, postquam dicta causa sive lis et alia, quecumque contra quoscumque mota seu movenda fuerit, omnino sopita, preceptorie vestra antedicte recuperacionem faciendo vobis auctoritate et tenore presentium licentiam et auctoritatem concedimus et donamus. Quocirca universis et singulis prioribus, baiuliis, preceptoribus et fratribus dicte domus dicta nostra auctoritate et tenore districte in virtute sancte obedientie precipiendo mandantes, quatenus predictum fratrem Guillelmum Holste preceptorem contra

4) *Probably Cammin, Lebus and Posen.*

5) *The parish church at Königsberg belonged to the Hospitallers: Lindenhayn-Fiedorowicz (2014), 255 with note 21. Rörchen was not rebuilt and the preceptor moved from the Neumark to Wildenbruch in Pomerania.*

formam presentium nostrarum litterarum nullatenus inquietent seu molestent nec ipsis litteris et contentis in eisdem audeant seu presumant quovismodo scienter seu ignoranter ausu temerario contraire, quinymo eas iuxta earum continenciam et tenorem studeant inviolabiliter observari. In cuius rei testimonium bulla nostra plumbea presentibus est appensa. Dat. Avinion. die XII mensis Septembris anno Domini millesimo trecentesimo septuagesimo IIII.

*a)* Conesb *praem. ante corr.* *b)* perverter *praem. ante corr.* *c)* ce *cum abbreviatione praem. ante corr.* *d)* gratie *MS*

## 89

*The Master Fr. Robert [de Juilly] orders the Prior of* Francia *to collect 1,000 florins from the preceptories of that priory as a special tax for the Master's* passagium *to Rhodes. This is the priory's share of 10,000 florins agreed upon by a meeting at Avignon with the Castellan of Amposta and Prior of Catalonia, with the Priors of Auvergne, Saint-Gilles and Toulouse and other brethren. Following a special papal licence, the tax is to be regarded as if it had been decided upon jointly by the Master and the Convent. – Further taxes in florins: Champagne 200, Aquitaine 350, Auvergne 700, Saint-Gilles 1,200, Toulouse 700, Castile 600, Amposta 200, Navarre 100, Portugal 300, Spain [Catalonia] 300, England, Scotland and Ireland 1,250,* Alamania *150, Lombardy 150, Bohemia 250, Pisa 150, Rome 150, Venice 150, Hungary 150, Capua 150, Naples 150, Santo Stefano [di Monopoli] 100, Barletta 300, Venosa 50, Sant'Eufemia 50, Messina 100, Alife 150.*

*Avignon, 1374 September 25*

*AOM 320 fol. 41r-v (32r-v).*

Frater Robertus etcetera religioso in Christo nobis carissimo fratri domus eiusdem priori nostri Francie prioratus salutem et sinceram in Domino caritatem. Cum in assembleia seu congregacione virtute bullarum apostolicarum, per quas nobis conceditur, quod quidquid per nos hic fieri continget, habeat eamdem roboris firmitatem, acsi per conventum nostrum Rodio ipso conventu presente facta forent, Avinioni facte de consilio religiosorum in Christo nobis carissimorum fratrum domus eiusdem Emposte castellani ac Cathallonie prioris,[1] Aluernie, Sancti Egidii et Tholose priorum necnon et quam plurium[a] preceptorum et domus nostre fratrum nobis assistentium pariter et assensu[2] vobis ad hoc consencientium fuerit ordinatum, quod summa decem

1) *Fr. Juan Fernández de Heredia.*

2) *Delaville (1913), 184 mentions the assembly and the tax of 9,800 florins. The sums in the document add up to only 9,000 florins. Hunyadi (2010), 196, says 9,1000 florins.*

millium florenorum super prioratibus, castellaniis, preceptoriis et aliis nostre religionis domibus pro passagio nostro de hiis partibus ad conventum nostrum Rodi fiendo levabitur et percipietur vobis in virtute sancte obedientie districte precipiendo mandamus, quatenus mille florenorum summam vobis et vestro prioratui impositam assideatis et imponatis rationabiliter et iuste super preceptores dicti nostri Francie prioratus, ipsam nobis seu thesauro aut procuratori et receptori nostro generali sine deffectu deliberetis, solvatis et tradatis una cum responsionibus prioratus ipsius, sic in premissis taliter vos habentes, quod nota contemptus seu negligentie vobis nullatenus ascribatur, sed de completo mandato possitis in Domino merito commendari. In cuius rei testimonium bulla nostra plumbea presentibus est appensa. Datum Avinion. XXV die mensis Septembris anno predicto. – Item simili modo mandatur priori Campanie de summa $II^{C}$ florenorum et eiusdem date. Item priori Acquitanie de summa $III^{C}$ L florenorum. Item priori Aluernie de summa $VII^{C}$ florenorum. Item priori Sancti Egidii de summa MCC. Item priori Tholose de summa $VII^{C}$. Item priori Castallanie de summa $VI^{C}$. Item castellano Emposte $II^{C}$. Item priori Nauarre de summa C. Item priori Portugallie de summa $III^{C}$. Item priori Ispanie[3] de summa $III^{C}$. Item prioribus Anglie, Scocie[4] et Yllandie de summa M $II^{C}$ L. [41v] Item priori Alamanie de summa C L. Item priori Lombardie de summa C L. Item priori Bohemie de summa $II^{C}$ L[b]. Item priori Pise de summa C L. Item priori Rome de summa C L. Item priori Veneciarum de summe C L. Item regenti[c] prioratus[d] Vngarie de summa C L. Item priori Capue de summa C L. Item preceptori Neapolis C L. Item preceptori sancti Stephani de summa centum. Item priori Baroli de summa $III^{C}$. Item preceptori Venose de summa L[e]. Item preceptori Sancte Eufemie [de] summa florenorum L. Item priori Messane de summa C. Item preceptori cambii comitatus[f] Alicii[5] centum L.

*a)* plurimorum *MS* *b)* C L *ante corr.* *c) supra lin.* *d)* priori *ante corr.* *e)* C L *ante corr.* *f)* comttatus *MS*

## 90

*The Master Fr. Robert [de Juilly] grants, after consultation with brethren, to Fr. Peter Weghener and Fr. Johann Weghener, of the Bailiwick of Saxony, the March,* Slavia *and Pomerania, priests of the Diocese of Cammin, their maintenance for their lifetime in a small house near the main street at Arnswalde. This small house belongs to the endowment of the parish church there (Diocese of Cammin). The person in charge of the parish*

3) *Castile and Amposta = Aragón are already mentioned; so this is Catalonia.*

4) *There was no Prior of Scotland.*

5) *For* Alifi.

*church is to provide the maintenance either according to the established customs of the Order or in the same way as is usual in this place to other brethren.*

*Avignon, 1374 October 3*

*AOM 320 fol. 40r (31r).*

Frater Robertus etcetera religiosis in Christo nobis carissimis fratribus Petro Weghener et Iohanni Weghener presbiteris eiusdem domus baiulie Sancxonie, Marchie, Sclauie et Pomeranie Camminenis[a)] diocesis salutem etcetera. Ob conversacionem honestam per vos, ut accepimus, hactenus observatam ac vestra laudabilia portamenta vos favorabiliter prosequentes in dote seu domo parrochialis ecclesie Arnsweld domus nostre prefate diocesis de et cum consilio fratrum et procerum domus nostre nobis assistentium in hac parte de nostra certa scientia et speciali gratia vobis et cuilibet vestrum, quamdiu vitam duxeritis in humanis, tenore presentium domunculam prope carreriam [et] stagiam assignamus vitam religiosam in illa laudabili et reverenti obedientia testimonio commendatam. Mandantes harum serie districte in virtute sancte obedientie rectori seu maiori in dicta dote seu domo parrochialis ecclesie predicte vel quovis alio titulo nunc vel in futurum in eodem regimine presidenti, quod vos et vestrum quemlibet ad prenominatam domunculam et stagiam[b)] benigne admittant et caritative pertractent vobisque et unicuique vestrum toto tempore vite vestre iuxta nostre domus bonos usus provideant in cunctis necessariis, aut prout in ipsa aliis fratribus est consuetum provideri, ac universis et singulis fratribus domus nostre nobis subditis cuiuscumque status, gradus aut condicionis fuerint, presentibus et futuris, ne contra presentem stagii assignationem aliquatenus venire presumant, quinymo illam iuxta presencium tenorem studeant inviolabiliter observare. In cuius etcetera. Dat. Avinion. die III mensis Ottobris anno incarnationis M° CCC LXXIIII°.

*a)* B *praem. ante corr.* *b)* stagium *MS*

*Arnswalde in the Neumark, 85 km north-west of Rörchen. The parish church belonged to the Hospitallers: Lindenhayn-Fiedorowicz (2014), 255.*

## 91

*Licence for Fr. Hesso [Schlegelholz] and Fr. Pierre de Hauterive to receive Giacomo di Bartolomeo dei Alismari of Florence as a knight into the Order.*

*Avignon, 1374 October 13*

*AOM 320 fol. 54v (45v).*

Commissum fuit per dominum fratribus Hessoni de Alamania et Petro de Alta Rippa, ut Iacobum filium Bartholomei de Alismari de Florencia reciperent in fratrem militem etcetera ad transmittendum ad conventum Rodi etcetera. Actum die XIII[a] Octobris anno predicto Avinioni.

## 92

*Order to Fr. Duke Ziemovit von Teschen, Prior of Bohemia, to induct Fr. Frank von Hertwitz into possession of the Preceptories of Vienna, Rumberg and Brünn, which are at present detained by Fr. Johann Rüdeshausen, Fr. Petrus Bratislavia and Fr. Johannes. Fr. Petrus Bratislavia is also ordered to return a mill he has sold; otherwise he is to come to the Convent within two months and explain his refusal.*

*[Rhodes, 1381] July 20*

*AOM 321 fol. 157r (148r), under* prioratus Alamanie et Boemie.

Die XX mensis Iullii fratri Symouicu duci Tessinensi priori Boemie, ut fratrem Francum de Hoicznicz preceptorem baiuliarum de Branna,[1] de Runperc[2] et de Bruna seu aliquem eius nomine inducat in possessionem pacificam[a] et quietam. Alias contra eum tamquam in rebellem et inobedientem procedetur secundum statuta, bonos usus et consuetudines. Necnon fratribus Iohanni Rudorsheusze, Petro[b] Bratislavia et Iohanni ‥[3] occupantibus et detinentibus[c] dictas domos absque causa rationabili et contra statuta, bonos etcetera in preiudicium dicti fratris Franci, [ut] dimittant dictas domos et restituant fructus et reddictus perceptos a tempore collationis dictarum baiuliarum fratri Franco predicto facte, nisi habeant causam seu rationem, ad quem protendum iter arripiant veniendi presentialiter commodum rationem allegaturi, cur occupant, et hec infra duos menses a tempore presentationis presencium seu notificationis eis et eorum cuilibet facte. Ac eciam dicto fratri Petro, ut molendinum quoddam vendittum et distractum a iure et proprietate religionis redducat ad ius et proprietatem domus celeriter usque infra duos menses. Alias veniat ad conventum avisurum rationem et mandatum, per que seu vigore quorum predictam molendini alienationem presumpsit attemptare sub pena habitus religionis[d], que fratribus talia presumentibus infligitur. Et predicta fuerunt iniuncta[e] mandata et precepta sub virtute sancte obedientie, prout alias per priorem Francie, fratrem Girardum de Lusura, locumtenentem magistri et conventus,[4] predictis et eorum cuilibet extitant adicta.

*a)* preacificam *MS* *b)* lati *del.* *c)* detien. *MS* *d)* nostre *del.* *e)* iniucta *MS*

1) *Dauber 2 (1998), 586, does not mention any preceptor of Vienna between 1373 and 1287. So Mitáček (2005), 132, may be right to identify* Branna *with Vienna.*

2) *Perhaps Rumberg, Czech Rumberk Deštná, north of Brünn.*

3) *Fr. Peter and Johann Fleming from Breslau, Wratislavia, cf. Mitáček (2005), 132 with note 582, 167–8 with note 742.*

4) *Fr. Gérard de Vienne, Prior of* Francia *and lieutenant in the Priories of* Francia, Alamania *and England on 16 September 1379, AOM 48 fol. 164v.*

## 93

*Licence for Fr. Helfrich [von Rüdigheim], Preceptor of Frankfurt, to receive two sergeants and two donats into the Order, whom he needs to administer his preceptory (here* baiulia) *and who shall be maintained there.*

*[Rhodes, 13]81 September 4*

*AOM 321 fol. 157r (148r), under* prioratus Alamanie et Boemie.

Die quarto mensis Septembris anni octuagesimi primi data fuit licentia fratri Hilfrico[1] preceptori de Frangfort recipiendi viros quatuor, ut moris est, duos in fratres servientes et duos in donatos religionis, quibus pro regimine sue baiulie assertum fuit ipsum indigere, casu tamen non haberentur[a] numerum fratrum et donatorum, quem tenetur habere in ipsa baiulia, et data potestas assignandi ipsis stagias in ipsa baiulia.

Non processa isto modo, set infrascripto *marg. (no. 94).* *a)* haberet *forsan recte.*

## 94

*Licence for Fr. Helfrich von Rüdigheim, Preceptor of Frankfurt, to receive two sergeants and two donats into the Order and to maintain them in his preceptory (as no. 93).*

*[Rhodes, 13]81 October 2*

*AOM 321 fol. 157r (148r), under* prioratus Alamanie et Boemie.

Die secundo mensis Octobris anno octuagesimo primo data fuit licentia fratri Hilfrico de Rudenkym preceptori de Frangfort recipiendi viros quatuor sanos et suis membris integros, duos videlicet in fratres servientes et duos in donatos nostre religionis, quibus pro regimine sue baiulie assertum fuit ipsum indigere quibuscumque ordinationibus et constitutionibus non obstantibus et ipsis receptis assignare stagias etcetera.

## 95

*The Master Fr. Juan [Fernández de Heredia] orders Fr. Konrad von Braunsberg, Prior of* Alamania, *no longer to exclude Fr. Berthold von Ura from the Preceptory of Tobel granted him by the former Master Fr. Raymond Bérenger and the Convent on Rhodes on 1 November 1371.*

*Rhodes, [13]81 October 2*

*AOM 321 fol. 157r-v (148r-v), under* prioratus Alamanie et Boemie.

*1) Helfrich von Rüdigheim (no. 94); on him see Hartmann (1981), 106; Dörr (1983), 34–5.*

Frater Iohannes etcetera religioso etcetera fratri Conrado de Brinsperg domus eiusdem priori prioratus nostri Alamanie seu ipsius prioratus regimini presidenti salutem etcetera. Exponente religioso etcetera fratre Bertoldo de Vra[1] domus eiusdem preceptore de Tobel inteleximus, quod eidem possessionem dicte baiulie eius meritis concessam dare et consignare renuistis, licet in capitulo vestro sepe requisitus et hoc vigore quarundam litterarum a predecessore nostro mediato fratre Raymondo Berengarii et conventu nostro concessarum sub data Rodi die prima mensis Novembris anno incarnationis Domini M° CCC$^{mo}$ LXXI. Quarum sumptum seu copiam manu Appollonii dicti Boyen, clerici Monasteriensis dyocesis, publici apostolica auctoritate notarii,[2] excerptum[a] de originalibus nobis exibuit et presentavit etiam[b] per regestra cancellarie nostre videri et inspici fecimus, que continent in effectum vos domos et baiulias vacantes vestre tantummodo [157v] donationi spectantes fratribus domus nostre ad annos decem seu eorum vitam ex causa in dictis litteris scripta posse concedere. Quarum inspecto tenore non sano usus consilio distullistis demandare executioni gratiam predicto fratri Bertoldo factam in eius preiudicium non modicum attentis viarum distancia et periculis iminentibus, que hodiernis temporibus consideranda sunt. Quapropter vobis sub virtute sancte obedientie districte precipimus et mandamus, quatenus dictum fratrem Bertoldum seu eius procuratorem vel procuratores in possessionem pacificam et quietam dicte baiulie omni prorsus excusatione posposita inducatis amoto abinde quolibet alio detentore, si quis sit, faciatisque sibi seu suo procuratori nomine ipsius de fructibus dicte baiulie, redditibus et proventibus ipsius a die gratie sibi facte de eadem integraliter responderi iuribus nostris et nostri communis thesauri ratione et ex causa prime vacantie reservatis. In executione huiusmodi mandati nostri vos sic habiturum[c], quod de vera obedientia mereamini merito comendari. Datum Rodi sub impressione sigilli nostri die secundo mensis Octubris anno octuagesimo primo.

*a)* excertum *MS* *b)* et nos etiam *recte.* *c)* habituri *recte.*

## 96

*Licence and order with consent of the Conventual Bailiffs for Fr. Berthold von Ura to leave the Convent on Rhodes and to travel to his Preceptory of Tobel.*

*[Rhodes, 1382] February 22*

*AOM 321 fol. 157v (148v), under* prioratus Alamanie et Boemie.

1) *Ura was the name of a knightly family from (Alt-)Urach near Lenzkirch in Baden that was mentioned from 1239 to 1385: Krieger 2 (1905), col. 1255–6. According to Helvetia Sacra (2006), 495 Fr. Ulrich von Tettingen was Preceptor of Tobel from 1378 to 1404.*

2) *Appollonius [= Albrecht] von Boyen, clerk of the Diocese of Münster, notary public by papal commission.*

Die XXII Februarii per dominum magistrum fratri Bertoldo de Vra preceptori de Tobel de consilio bailivorum data fuit licentia recedendi de conventu et eundi ad dictam baiuliam regendam et mandatum sub virtute sancte obedientie, ut super primo navigio de portu Rodi discessuro ad prefatam baiuliam regendam se conferat personaliter ut in forma.

## 97

*Mandate to the Receiver General or his deputy to pay to Fr. Hesso Schlegelholz, Preceptor of Freiburg, 3,214.5 florins of Germany within two months of the presentation of the present letter.*

*[Rhodes, 1382 March 15]*

*AOM 321 fol. 242r (234r), under* assignationes pecuniarum.

Anno, mense et die quibus immediate suprascriptis dicto receptori generali[1)] seu officio receptoris fungenti,[2)] ut solvat, det et assignet et solvat fratri Hessoni Sleghiloz preceptori de Filiburgo florenos de Alamania tria millia ducentos quatuordecim cum dimidio unius floreni, mandatum fuit et preceptum infra duos menses computandos a presentacione litterarum inde confectorum eidem facta, quos florenos tria millia ducentos quatuordecim cum dimidio[a)] frater Hesso predictus comuni thesauro consignavit.

*a)* et dimidio *corr.*

## 98

*Mandate to the Receiver General or his deputy to pay 86.5 florins of Florence to the Preceptor Fr. Frank von Hertwitz within one month of the presentation of this letter.*

*[Rhodes, 1382 March 17]*

*AOM 321 fol. 242r (234r), under* assignationes pecuniarum.

Anno, mense et die quibus suprascriptis predicto receptori generali[1)] seu fungenti receptoris officio[2)] scriptum fuit et mandatum, ut solvat Fratri Franco de Hertuicz domus ·· preceptori florenos de Florencia octuaginta sex cum dimidio, quibus comunis thesaurus eidem tenetur ex finali computo. Et hoc expediat et exequatur infra unius mensis spacium.

1) *Fr. Pierre de Provins, Receiver General in Avignon: Sarnowsky, Macht (2001), 332 with note 17.*
2) *Fr. Nicolinus de Lippo, scribe of the Treasury.*

1) *Fr. Pierre de Provins.*
2) *Fr. Nicolinus de Lippo, scribe of the Treasury.*

## 99

*Mandate to the Priors of* Alamania *and Bohemia and to their receivers to pay within a month after receiving this letter to Fr. Hesso Schlegelholz, Preceptor of Freiburg, or to his procurator 3,214.5 florins of Germany or their equivalent value. This amounts to 3,096.5 florins of Rhodes. A receipt is to be secured.*

*[Rhodes], 1382 March 21*

*AOM 321 fol. 241r (233r), under* assignationes pecuniarum.

Dictis die et anno per dominum magistrum et conventum scriptum fuit et mandatum sub virtute sancte obediencie fratribus ·· Alamanie et Boemie prioribus ac in dictis prioratibus receptoribus responsionum et cuilibet eorum, quatenus infra duorum mensium spacium a die presentacionis presencium eis facte computandum fratri Hessoni Slegiloz preceptori de Filiburgo seu eius procuratori de quibuscunque pecuniis responsionum, mortuariorum, areragiorum quam aliarum comuni thesauro pertinentibus per ipsos seu alium ipsorum receptis et recipiendis florenos de Alamania tria millia ducentos quatuordecim cum dimidio seu eorum valorem, qui valent florenos currentes in Rodo tria millia nonaginta sex cum dimidio traditos per ipsum fratrem Hessonem reali remuneratione comuni thesauro, et recipiant cauthelam, quibus solutis pro habitis reputantur ut in forma.

*The whole entry is crossed out. In the margin:* Processit, ut infra continetur, quia dirigitur receptori generali. *See no. 103.*

## 100

*Licence for Fr. Frank von Hertwitz to leave the Convent and travel to the West.*

*[Rhodes, 13]82 April 6*

*AOM 321 fol. 157v (148v), under* prioratus Alamanie et Boemie.

Die sexto Aprilis anno LXXXII per dominum magistrum data fuit licentia fratri Franco de Hertuicz, ·· baiulie preceptori, recedendi de conventu et eundi ad partes ultramarinos ut in forma.

## 101

*Licence for Fr. Frank [von Hertwitz] to travel to the Convent.*

*[Rhodes, 1382 April 6]*

*AOM 321 fol. 157v (148v), under* prioratus Alamanie et Boemie.

Dicta die per dominum magistrum predicto fratri Franco preceptori data fuit licentia veniendi ad conventum etcetera.

*In other cases, nos. 100 and 101 would be merged into one licence to leave the Convent and return.*

## 102

*Order to the Priors of Bohemia Fr. Ziemovit von Teschen and of* Alamania *Fr. Konrad von Braunsberg to attend the chapter general at Valence on 1 March 1383, each with four preceptors and the receiver of his priory. – The Master Fr. Juan Fernández de Heredia has come to the West with three named procurators of the Convent. As the Order needs reforms, and with the consent of unnamed brethren, he summons a chapter general. Each prior is to come with four preceptors and the receiver of the responsions, with familiars and horses but without unseemly expenditures. They are to take with them responsions, arrears of responsions, taxes, subsidies,* passagia, *also* mortuaria *and* vacantia *and all other dues to the Master and Convent. They are also to take with them a list of chambers, offices and other graces to be made by the Master. They are to inform the Master about the date when they receive the present letter. Furthermore, they are to take with them a description of the chambers, offices, houses, granges and members and list with the numbers and names of all brethren in their priories.*

*[Avignon, 1382] August 2*

*AOM 322 fol. 203r (195r), under* prioratus Alamanie et Boemie.

Sub eisdem anno, tenore et data die secundo mensis Agusti[a)] registratis in prioratu Ungarie foliis CCXL et CCXLI, quibus mandatur dicti prioratus priori, ut veniat ad capitulum, cum clausulis ibidem appositis scribitur et mandatur fratribus Semouito[b)] Thesschinensi Boemie et Conrado de Brinsperg Alamanie prioribus et cuilibet per se.

*a)* quibus *del.* *b)* Semonito *propter abbreviationem.*

*Letter to the Prior of Hungary, Avignon, 1382 July 17, AOM 322 fol. 251v-2r (240v-41r), ed. Dobronić (1984), 172–4; Hunyadi (2010), 327–9 no. 58, under* prioratus Vungarie.

Frater Iohannes etcetera religioso etcetera fratri Iohanni de Palisna domus eiusdem priori prioratus nostri Vngarie salutem etcetera. Cum Domino permittente, a quo procedunt gratiarum munera, quamvis immeriti fuerimus promoti[a)] ad domus nostre magistratus regimen, ad ingens pondus eius administrationis suscepte convertentes, tocius nostre consideracionis aciem excitati, eciam assiduis validis clamoribus fratrum bailivorum, priorum, procerum omnium et singulorum residentium ad Dei servicia in nostro Rodi conventu occasionibus et causis pluribus expositorum perplexis, angustiis paupertatis iminentibus amissionis periculis asserentione inspectis, inspiciendis festino expedientes eisdem neccessario remedio per alium quam nos ac nostre solicitudinis industriam calamitatibus ipsorum subveniri non posse neque nostram religionem dirrectionis, correctionis, reformationis et restaurationis incrementum suscipere salutiferum ad has occidentales partes nullo ad antiquitatem nostram respectu habito omnibus postpositis periculis pii patris motum pro filiis capientes consilium et ferentes moleste filiorum incomoda cum religiosis etcetera fratribus Petro Bussoni priore ecclesie conventualis Rodi, Hessone Slegiligloz de Filiburgo et Guillelmo de Fontanay de Spaliaco[1)] preceptoribus solempniter procuratoribus [252r] ellectis per prenominatum conventum cum plena potestate relictis et dimissis nostris insulis bellicis acquisitis sudoribus sub nostri locumtenentis generalis fideli custodia de consilio premissi conventus ordinati non sine gravi periculo, quod Deus avertere[b)] dignetur, non absque immenso labore et onere expensarum dirreximus gressus nostros provisuri in hiis partibus nobis subditis de salubri reformatione et laudabili consolidatione, cum qua nobis possibili diligentia ferventi opere circa premissa et alia concernentia honorem et[c)] utilitatem religionis nostre de premissorum procuratorum consilio, voluntate et assensu fratrum aliorum priorum et procerum nobis assistencium in hac parte in civitate Valentie supra Rodanum dominica prima instante mensis Martii nostrum generale capitulum in Christi nomine celebrandum ordinaverimus. In quo nostrum et nostri conventus principale propositum prosequentes disponere, decernere et ordinare intendimus, ut dicte religionis nostre reducantur abiecta, consolidentur confracta, corrigantur corrigenda et reformentur in melius reformanda divina favente gratia tali modo, ut propter executionis actionem prefati fratres ·· et conventus subleventur et respirent a miserabili statu, quo degent, religio liberata a pondere debitorum in augmentum Christiani fidei et Christicolarum protectionem favores salubres pociores senciant et nos ab altissimo eius [d)]et domino nostro papa Clemente septimo[d)], etiam, regibus, principibus et tocius orbis Christifidelibus valeamus de nostra cura regiminis salutifera commendari. Quapropter fraternitatem vestram in Domino exortamur ac vobis et per vos deputandis, eligendis et ordinandis districte precipiendo mandamus in virtute sancte obedientie districtius iniungentes, quatenus apud civitatem predictam die suprascripta assignata, in qua tunc adesse disponimus Domino favente, cum quatuor fratribus preceptoribus et responsionum receptori predicti prioratus fervore proceritatis et industria comprobatis, quos duxeritis eligendos, et cum familiaribus et equitaturis decentibus veniatis iuxta statutum pro sumptibus evitandis necnon cum responsionibus, arreragiis responsionum, talearum, subsidiorum[e)], passagiorum et cum aliis bonis, rebus, deneriis tam ratione mortuariorum quam baiuliarum vacacionibus et quorumlibet aliorum bonorum, que habetis et habere poteritis, nobis et dicto nostro conventui pertinentium et spectantium communiter vel divisim ac etiam cum litteris vestris prioratus camerarum baiuliarum[f)] et aliarum gratiarum magistralium, prout ad vos et vobiscum conferendum dignoscitur pertinere, nobiscum personaliter excusatione quacunque remota intersitis. Attencius precaventes, ne in premissis adimplendis commictatis negligentiam, sed tamquam veri filii obedientie valeatis a Domino premiari. Alias contra vos et ipsos premissa recusantes adimplere destituendo vos et eos prioratu et baiuliis rigide procedemus, prout nostre religionis regula et statuta continent. Nichilominus rescribatis per vestras litteras diem receptionis presentium, nam aliter presentes ad vestram noticiam pervenisse

*1) Épailly.*

credimus. Ceterum volumus et vobis harum serie precipiendo mandamus sub dicta virtute sancte obedientie, quatenus particulariter et distincte ad eandem civitatem die prescripta vobiscum apportetis statum camerarum, baiuliarum, domorum, grangiarum, membrorum et eorum nomina, que et quanta sit cuiuslibet responsio et in quanta quantitate restat unusquisque teneri, ac nomina et cognomina singulorum fratrum, sororum et donatorum, quot et quanti sint in dicto prioratu, veniatis instructis et plene informatis de omnibus negociis prioratus eiusdem, ut suffragante Domino vestro et aliorum fratrum procerum domus nostre auxilio[g] super hiis providere salubriter valeamus. In cuius etcetera. Datum Avinione die decimoseptimo Iulii anno incarnationis Domini octuagesimo secundo.

*a) supra lin.* *b)* advertere *MS* *c) om. MS* *d-d) marg. manu recent.* *e)* subscidiorum *MS* *f)* gr *add. ante corr.* *g)* auxilium MS

*The document mentioned one receiver in each priory. Later on, there were usually two receivers in* Alamania.

## 103

*Order to the priors of* Alamania *and Bohemia and to the receivers in these priories to pay 3,214.5 gold florins of Germany to Fr. Hesso Schlegelholz, Preceptor of Freiburg, who had lent that sum to the Treasury (see no. 99).*

*[Avignon, 13]82 September 10*

*AOM 322 fol. 203r (195r), under* prioratus Alamanie et Boemie.

Die decima mensis Septembris mandatum fuit fratribus ·· prioribus Alamanie et Boemie et eorum locumtenentibus ac responsionum nostrarum[a] receptoribus in eisdem, ut fratri Hessoni de Slegelholz preceptori de Friburgo seu eius procuratori legitimo solvant[b], dent et assignent florenos auri Alamanie tria millia ducenti quattuordecim cum dimidio unius floreni, quos mutuavit communi thesauro, ut continetur quadam littera super hec confecta bullata bulla communi domini magistri et conventus. Quorum solutione facta retineant presens mandatum et alias prescriptas penes se incisas recipiantque recognicionem, que sufficiat. Anno incarnationis etcetera octagesimo secundo.

*a)* responsionum nostrarum] mensarum *MS* *b)* salvant *MS*

## 104

*Order for paying and giving a receipt as above (no. 103).*

*[Avignon, 13]82 [September 11]*

*AOM 322 fol. 203r (195r), under* prioratus Alamanie et Boemie.

Die decima una mensis prescripti anno octagesimo secundo mandatum fuit prenominatorum prioratuum priorum locumtenentibus, receptoribus mensarum prioratuum eorum, ut predicto fratri Hessoni aut ab eo procurationem sufficientem[a)] habenti solvant summam florenorum predictorum. Casu, qua per dictas litteras non fuerit satisfactum, et presentes et prescripta retinent in testimonium facte solucionis recipiantque recognicionem, que sufficiat.

*a)* sufficiens *MS*

## 105

*Payment of a tax and subsidy of 1,000 florins on the Priory of* Alamania *and a tax and subsidy of 1,200 florins on the Priory of Bohemia. – As the Convent on Rhodes needs monies to fight the Turks and other enemies of the faith, the Master has deliberated at Valence in the house where he lives with three named procurators of the Convent, two capitular preceptors, five lieutenants of priors, other preceptors and brethren. They have imposed a tolerable tax or subsidy on each priory. It is to be paid on 24 June 1383. Each prior is to calculate it for the* fratres commensales *in the priory, with the help of four senior preceptors. Brethren who cannot pay it may pawn goods of their offices; but this is not to impede the payment of responsions. As the Convent on Rhodes has many debts, one fourth of all revenues of each priory is to be paid to the Treasury for four years from 24 June 1383 to 24 June 1387; but this is not to impede the payment of responsions. The prior is to punish those who fail to pay; they may lose their offices and can be jailed.*

*Valence, 1383 March 12*

*AOM 322 fol. 203r (195r), under* prioratus Alamanie et Boemie.

Pro summa seu quantitate mille florenorum impositorum pro talia priori et prioratui Alamanie, preceptoribus et aliis et pro summa mille ducentorum florenorum impositorum priori et prioratui Boemie, preceptoribus et aliis ipsius pro talliis et subsidio, ut exolvantur, scriptum fuit et mandatum cuilibet dictorum priorum modis et formis regestratis in prioratu Aluernie foliis CXL et XLI et sub eadem data.

*Letter to the Prior of Auvergne Fr. Robert de Châteauneuf AOM 322 fol. 145v-6r (140v-41r), under* prioratus Aluernie.

Frater Iohannes Ferdinandi etcetera [a)]generale capitulum celebrantes[a)] religiosis in Christo nobis carissimis fratribus Roberto de Castronouo priori prioratus nostri Aluernie seu eius locumtenenti, preceptoribus et fratribus aliis omnibus et singulis prioratus eiusdem domus preffate salutem et sinceram in Domino caritatem. Considerantes merito curis assiduis et diligenti opere, quibus modis, viis et formis noster Rodi conventus respiret et sublevetur religio nostra ab onerosis noxiis, dispendiosis periculis et pressuris, quibus, quod dolentes referimus, supponuntur, sustentari et propulsari ad Christi laudem, Christicolarum deffencionem, fidei augmentum, etiam ordinis honorem, ad que religionis bona dedicantur specialiter, valeant insultus perfidorum Turcorum, inimicorum fidei catholice, ex nostra impotencia ferentes contra Christicolas plus solito erigencium audatia resumpta deliberacione discussa pensantes circa salubrem et celerem expedicionem premissorum nos magister prefatus cum predicte domus fratribus Petro Bussoni priore ecclesie conventualis Rodi, Hessone Slegiligloz, Guillelmo de Fonteneyo procuratoribus conventus nostri Rodi ac fratribus ·· Campanie, Francie, Aluernie, Sancti Egidii, Tholose, Pisarum prioratuum prioribus et Neapolis, Venuse preceptoribus capitularibus ac etiam fratribus Aquitanie, Alamanie, Boemie, Lombardie et Venetiarum [a]prioratuum priorum[a] locatenentibus nonnullis aliis fratribus preceptoribus proceribusque prioratuum predictorum et aliorum ad sonum campane convenientibus in civitate Valentie [146r] supra Rodanum in domo habitationis nostre eletta ad hec congregatis de voluntate et assensu expressis predictorum vice et nomine tocius religionis nostre priorum prioratuum, preceptorum preceptoriarum suorum et aliorum absencium nominibus tenore presencium et auctoritate presentis nostri generalis capituli statuimus, ordinamus et taxamus pro tailhia et subsidio dicti conventus tollerabili vobis et dicti prioratus preceptoribus ac talhiam imponimus trium milium florenorum auri solvendorum per vos in proximo festo nativitatis[b] sancti[c] Iohannis baptiste, ad quorum solutionem faciendam fratres commensales prioratus predicti considerata uniuscuiusque facultate taxatione facta per vos et quatuor preceptores proceres compelli volumus per omnem cohercicionis modum. Quam tailhiam trium milium florenorum auri distribuendi et recipiendi vobis et receptori harum serie potestate attributa et fratribus non habentibus alias unde solvere, si qui sint, quorum animas in hoc oneramus, impignorandi ad certum tempus emolumenta et iura certa baiuliarum camerarum absque preiudicio responsionis concedimus licenciam. Ceterum ut prefatus conventus oppressus pondere debitorum sub usurarum voragine ab huiusmodi liberetur pressuris, statuimus et ordinamus, quod de quatuor annis incohandis in proximo festo[d] nativitatis beati Iohannis babtiste continuis de omnibus et singulis fructibus, bonis, iuribus et emolumentis ac omni valore prioratus, camerarum, preceptoriarum, domorum et beneficiorum quorumlibet prefati nostri prioratus Aluernie, prout et aliorum cis- et ultramarinorum statutum est, durante ditto quadriennali tempore annuo quarta pars sit communis thesauri et ad ipsum perveniat ex causa solutionis suorum debitorum soluta prius et deducta responsione annua et aliis neccessariis supportatis extimacione facta per vos et eos, quos eligendos duxeritis, prestito prius sacramento per vos et ipsos, quod legitima extimatio fiet, de quibus receptis peccuniis de prescripta quarta parte debita fratribus ·· annuo dicti quadriennii exsolventur pro quarta parte quotta vobis Roberto priori prioratus iamdicti seu ipsius presidenti regimini fratribus ·· preceptoribus et aliis sub virtute sancte obediencie precipimus districte iniungentes sub pena prioratus et preceptoriarum privationis et penis aliis vobis infligendis, quatenus predicta statuta et ordinationes omnia et singula in ipsis[e] contenta inviolabiliter observetis. Dantes et concedentes vobis prefato priori tailhiam impositam prescriptam trium milium florenorum auri et alia quecunque debita communi thesauro religionis nostre solvere recusantes dicti prioratus fratres auctoritatem, potestatem et licenciam compellendi per captionem bonorum, destitucionem et privacionem baiuliarum et facta de talibus plantta habituum domus nostre exhigente eorum inobendiencia [a)]privationem[a)], captionem personarum, incarceracionem et quemcunque alium dicte domus cohercionis modum. Non obstantibus retentione aliqua de ipsis facta ad manus nostras, oppositione, contradictione et appellatione quibuscunque, implorato eciam ad premissa, si opus fuerit, auxilio brachii secularis. [f)]In cuius rei testimonium bulla nostra plumbea presentibus est appensa. Datum Valencie supra Rodanum durante generali capitulo die duodecima mensis Martii anno incarnationis Domini millesimo trecentesimo octuagesimo secundo.

*a-a) supra lin.* *b)* nati *praem. ante corr.* *c)* santi *MS* *d)* beati *add. ante corr.* *e)* ip *praem. ante corr.* *f) From here onwards written by another hand.*

## 106

*The Master Fr. Juan Fernández [de Heredia] and the chapter general permit the brethren and donats of the Preceptory of Freiburg (Priory of* Alamania*) to redeem possessions of their preceptory and to receive the incomes of these possessions for their lifetime, unless they leave the Order; the same permission to redeem possessions is granted to laymen and clerics who may then receive the incomes for their lifetime.*

*Valence, 1383 March 12*

*AOM 322 fol. 207v (197v), under* prioratus Alamanie et Boemie.

Universis et singulis presentes litteras inspecturis nos frater Iohannes Ferdinandi etcetera notum facimus, quoniam inter sollicitudines alias nostris curis assiduis inherentes illa nos instanter evigilat, ut religio nostra et ipsius membra ab onerosis et noxiis, quibus subsunt, dispendiis subleventur, nempe veris assertionibus informati, quod baiulie nostre in Friburgo prioratus nostri Alamannie plurima bona, possessiones et loca, emolumenta et iura alia personis secularibus in pluribus et diversis peccuniarum quantitatibus obligata[a)] et alienata fuerunt et sunt quousque, recepta et habita inde peccunia restituta et soluta fuerit, cum eciam ipse baiulia agravatur[b)] aliarum obligationum multitudine in grave preiudicium religionis nostre, detrimentum dicte baiulie subcumbentis propter hec precipicio, ruine et statui miserrimo, discussa deliberacione pensantes, quod retardata remedia ampliora parerent incomoda, nos oneris et dispendiis huiusmodi providere cupientes, ut ipsa baiulia ad statum optatum deveniat, ad quem modo et via subscriptis fidedigna relatione poterit reduci, tenore presencium de voluntate, consilio et assensu[c)] fratrum suprascriptorum[d)] auctoritate presentis nostri generalis capituli pro expedienti remedio ordinandum et statuendum duximus, consentimus, volumus et ordinamus, quod fratres omnes et singuli, eciam donati, presentes et futuri dicti prioratus, qui bona, possessiones, loca, iura et pertinentie[e)] dicte baiulie impigunorata[f)] modo prescripto seu quocumque alio personis secularibus et eciam ecclesiasticis et ab ipsis detenta redimerent et reduxerint ad ipsam baiuliam et ad[g] ius religionis nostre, ipsa bona sic redempta et reducta habeant, teneant et possideant libere, quamdiu vitam duxerint in humanis, nec de ipsis bonis sic reductis, receptis et liberatis a dictorum manibus per aliquam planctam de quarantona nec alia[s] amittere possunt nec[h] amittant excepto casu, quem Deus avertat, perdicionis habitus, quo casu et eventu[i] mortis talium fratrum et donatorum dicta bona reducta sint, pertineant et reducantur dicte baiulie. Insuper modo consimili quoscumque clericos et laicos bona dicte [baiulie] impignorata[j] et alienata, ut prefertur, redimentes ordinamus et volumus eosdem talia bona ad eorum vitam libere tenere et ipsis peremptis ad ipsam baiuliam de Friburgo pervenire, a qua deppendent manddantes omnibus universis etcetera. In cuius etcetera. Data Valencie supra Rodanum durante dicto generali capitulo die duodecimo mensis Martii anno incarnacionis etcetera millesimo CCC° LXXXII°.

*a)* obi *del.* *b)* agrxavatur *ante corr.* *c)* p *del.* *d)* se *del.* *e)* ptinent *del.* *f)* sic *MS* *g)* ad *del.* *h)* valeant *del.* *i)* mu *del.* *j)* ipignorata *MS*

## 107

*The Master Fr. Juan [Fernández de Heredia] and the chapter general confirm the subjugation of the Preceptory of Buchsee as a member to the Preceptory of Freiburg; 200 florins hitherto paid to the Master by Buchsee are in future to be paid by the Preceptory of Sulz.*

*[Valence, 13]83 March 12*

*AOM 322 fol. 207v (197v), under* prioratus Alamanie et Boemie.

Frater Iohannes etcetera generale capitulum[a] celebrantes considerantes rationi fore consonum ordinata et constituta per predecessores nostros fructuosa presertim et utilia rata et firma habere, intelecto fidedigna relacione domum sive baiuliam in Buchs propter attenuationem fructuum et reddittuum baiulie de Friburgo oneratam multis debitis in sublevationem ipsorum fuisse unitam causis predictis et aliis quampluribus predicte baiulie de Friburgo, prefatam unionem ratam et gratam habentes dictam domum de Buchs ut membrum dicte baiulie de Friburgo per preceptorem ipsius et successores[b] habendi etcetera cum omnibus et singulis suis membris, iuribus et pertinentiis et sub responsione annua ex dicto membro solvi consueta et aliis oneribus impositis et imponendis de consilio etcetera confirmamus et de novo concedimus benefaciendo in eadem ac ut membrum dicte baiulie de cetero haberi volumus et teneri, sic tamen, quod florenorum auri ducentorum super dicta domo in Buchs consuetorum solvi pro camera nostra annuam quantitatem super domo in Sulcz ex ipsis redditibus nobis et cui mandaverimus per rectores ipsius percipere habeamus. Mandantes etcetera. In cuius etcetera. Datum ut supra die XII Martii anno LXXXII.

*a)* capitulo *MS* *b)* preceptorem *del.*

## 108

*The Master Fr. Juan Fernández [de Heredia] and the chapter general confirm a foundation by Fr. Konrad von Braunsberg, Prior of* Alamania, *for the maintenance of priests in certain preceptories of his priory; in case of default these possessions are to be used for existing priests in other preceptories of the priory.*

*Valence, [13]83 March 12*

*AOM 322 fol. 208r (198r), under* prioratus Alamanie et Boemie.

Frater Iohannes Ferdinandi etcetera generale capitulum celebrantes religioso etcetera fratri Conrado de Brunsperg priori prioratus nostri Alamanie domus eiusdem salutem etcetera. Cultum divinum adaugeri et non minui, ut tenemur, cupientes vestrumque pium et laudabile propositum prosequi et deduci ad effectum assignationem et dispositionem de bonis per vos acquisitis et deputatis in augmentum divini cultus pro vita et substentacione presbiterorum certis baiuliis et domibus prioratus nostri predicti commorantium pro celebrando divino officio sub et cum eo modo sive pacto, quod in divinis decenter deserviant altissimo, ut debetur, – aliter dicta bona deputata, ut prefertur, ex causa officii divini celebrandi devolvantur et deveniant propinquioribus domibus nostre domus seu baiuliis prioratus predicti pro vita et substentacione presbiterorum residentium in eis et deservientium in divinis, prout in eisdem litteris continetur – , ratam et gratam habentes ordinacionem et voluntatem vestram de bonis predictis sic dispositis vestro et successorum vestrorum nomine tenore presentium de certa nostra scientia et auctoritate presentis generalis capituli, si et prout in litteris super huiusmodi assignationem et dispositionem confectis continetur, de consilio et assensu religiosorum etcetera ut supra confirmamus, ratificamus et approbamus. Mandantes universis et singulis etcetera. In cuius etcetera. Datum Valencie supra Rodanum durante generali capitulo die XII Martii anno LXXXII.

## 109

*The Master Fr. Juan [Fernández de Heredia], three procurators of the Convent and 12 other brethren, acting in chapter general, confirm Fr. Konrad von Braunsberg for ten years in the Priory of* Alamania, *naming his powers and duties. Among other things he is to pay his responsions each year on 24 June. Furthermore, he is to pay all other dues the Master and Convent have imposed or may impose on the priory. He is to rule the priory according to the statutes of the late Master Fr. Raymond Bérenger.*

*Valence, 1383 March 13*

*AOM 322 fol. 203r-v (195r-v), under* prioratus Alamanie et Boemie.

Frater Iohannes etcetera generale capitulum celebrantes religioso etcetera fratri Conrado de Brunsperg priori prioratus nostri Alamanie domus eiusdem salutem etcetera. Dum ad proceritatis vestre famam gubernacionemque utilem et fructuosam per vos habitam in commissis vobis in nostro ordine regiminibus aciem mentis nostre dirrigimus, illa vobis libenter anuymus, que conservationem vestri status[a] concernere dignoscuntur. Igitur prioratum nostrum Alamanie supradictum cum omnibus et singulis etcetera et prout ipsum habetis et presentialiter possidetis habendi etcetera vobis tamquam digno et benemerito de consilio et assensu religiosorum in Christo nobis carissimorum fratrum Petri Bussonis prioris ecclesie conventualis Rodi, Hessonis Slegiligloz, Guillelmi de Fontanay procuratorum conventus nostri Rodi necnon fratrum ·· Campanie, Francie, Alvernie, Sancti Egidii, Tholose, Pisarum priorum, Dominici de Alamania Neap. et Iohannis Flotte de Venusa preceptorum capitularium necnon prioratuum Aquitanie, Alamanie, Venetiarum et Lombardie locatenentium et aliorum fratrum nobis in hac parte[b] assistentium[1] sub annuam responsionem per vos nobis aut cui et ubi mandaverimus et ordinaverimus [203v] in festo nativitatis sancti Iohannis baptiste annis singulis ex pacto expresso exolvenda et quibuscumque aliis oneribus dicto prioratui qualitercumque et quomodocumque incumbentibus et incumbendis ac impositis et imponendis ex pacto etiam ultra responsionem predictam supportandis de certa nostra scientia et speciali gratia benefaciendo in eadem confirmamus et de novo vobis ad annos decem continuos et completos conferimus, concedimus et donamus, retento[c] nobis, quod de una vel pluribus etcetera, ac etiam retentis et reservatis nobis omnibus ordinationibus per bone memorie fratrem Raymondum Berengarium[2] etcetera, nichilominus retento et nobis reservato, ut, si, quod absit, in solutione etcetera de premisso prioratu etcetera. Dantes vobis et concedentes auctoritatem et potestatem etcetera regendi etcetera, insuper dandi et conferendi baiulias etcetera. Committentes vobis etcetera. Quocirca universis et singulis fratribus preceptoribus, bailivis et aliis etcetera. Inhybentes vobis etceterea insuper tenore presentium quoscumque procuratores et receptores per nos seu conventum nostrum Rodi in dicto prioratu constitutos ad responsiones, arreragia responsionum, mortuaria, talias, subsidias[d], iochalia[!], baiuliarum vacationes exigendum et petendum revocamus vobis premissa omnia et singula et alia queque nostre religioni pertinentes quovis modo, ratione seu causa exigendo, petendi ac habendi nomine nostro[e] et religionis nostre ac communis thesauri Rodi conventus omnimodam potestatem concendentes[!] et de receptis quitandi. In cuius etcetera. Datum Valencie supra Rodanum durante generali capitulo die XIII Martii anno incarnationis Domini millesimo trecentesimo octuagesimo secundo.

1) *Fr. Pierre Boysson, Prior of the Conventual church at Rhodes, Fr. Hesso Schlegelholz and Fr. Guillaume de Fontenoy as the three procurators of the Convent at Rhodes, the Priors of Champagne*, Francia, *Auvergne, Saint-Gilles, Toulouse, and Pisa as well as two Capitular preceptors, Fr. Domenico d'Alamania of Naples and Fr. Jean Flote of Venosa, the lieutenants in the Priories of Aquitaine*, Alamania, *Venice and Lombardy.*

2) *Master Fr. Raymond Bérenger.*

*a)* statutus *MS* *b)* partes *ante corr.* *c)* benefaciendo *del.* *d)* subsidias *post corr.* *e)* nostra *MS*

## 110

*The Prior of* Alamania *Fr. Konrad von Braunsberg is retained with his priory [by the Master Fr. Juan Fernández de Heredia].*

*[Valence, 1383 March 13]*

*AOM 322 fol. 203v (195v), under* prioratus Alamanie et Boemie.

Dictis die et anno prescriptis proximis immediate dictus frater Conradus de Brunsperg prior Alamanie retentus fuit ad manus domini magistri cum dicto prioratu ut in forma.

## 111

*The Master Fr. Juan [Fernández de Heredia] and the chapter general confirm Fr. Helfrich and Fr. Rudolf von Rüdigheim, joint Preceptors of Meisenheim and its members, for their lifetime in the Preceptory of Frankfurt with its member Mosbach, which these two brethren have recovered from laymen.*

*Valence, [13]83 March 13*

*AOM 322 fol. 203v-4r (195v-6r), under* prioratus Alamanie et Boemie.

Frater Iohannes etcetera generale capitulum celebrantes religiosis etcetera fratribus Hilfrico et Rudulfo de Rudekeym baiuliarum in Franchfort cum membro Mospach et de Meysenkeyn cum suis membris preceptoribus domus eiusdem salutem etcetera. Supplicationi vestre nobis exposite continente, ut vobis baiuliam de Franchfort cum membro Maspach sumptibus vestris a secularium manibus extractam ad ius et proprietatem [204r] nostre religionis redagtam[!] et predecessorum nostrorum de ea obtenta confirmatione ad vitam vestram vobis confirmare dignaremur, vestrorum consideracione meritorum favorabilem prebentes assensum supradictam baiuliam de Franchfort cum membro de Mospach prioratus nostri Alamanie cum omnibus et singulis etcetera habendam etcetera sub annua responsione et aliis etcetera – alias secundum continentiam etcetera – de premissa baiulia etcetera de consilio etcetera de certa nostra scientia etcetera ad vitam vestram confirmamus et pro uberiori cautela de novo conferimus etcetera. Committentes etcetera. Quocirca etcetera necnon etcetera. Inhybentes vobis districtius etcetera. Et si, quod absit, etcetera. In cuius etcetera. Datum Valencie supra Rodanum die XIII mensis Martii anno LXXXII.

## 112

*The Master Fr. Juan [Fernández de Heredia] and the chapter general grant for ten years to Fr. Rudolf von Rüdigheim the Preceptory of Meisenheim with its members of Weisheim, Sobernheim and Sulzbach (Priory of* Alamania), *which is vacant following its resignation by Fr. Richard Lauder.*

*Valence, [13]83 March 13*

*AOM 322 fol. 204r (196r), under* prioratus Alamanie et Boemie.

Frater Iohannes etcetera generale capitulum celebrantes religioso etcetera fratri Ridulfo de Rudekeyn domus eiusdem salutem etcetera. Vestre perspicuitatis meritis commendabilis titulus attributus nos inducit, ut vos dono specialis gratie et honoris prosequamur. Hinc est, quod preceptoriam seu baiuliam in Meysekeyn cum suis grangiis et membris Voissen, Sobernheyn, Sulczbach prioratus nostri Alamanie per resignationem religiosi etcetera fratris Richardi Lauder factam in manibus religiosi etcetera fratris ·· dicti prioratus prioris et per ipsum acceptam ipsa ressignatione, ut nobis licuit relatibus religiosorum etcetera fratrum Hessonis Slegiligloz, ·· et Hylfrici domus in Frank[furt] preceptorum et procuratorum eiusdem prioris[1] presentialiter vacantem et ob hoc ad nostram dispositionem rationabiliter devolutam et cum omnibus et singulis aliis suis membris, iuribus etcetera habendum etcetera sub annua responsione etcetera – alias secundum continentiam etcetera – de consilio etcetera de certa nostra scientia etcetera hinc ad instans festum nativitatis sancti Iohannis baptiste et ab eodem festo inantea ad annos decem continuos et completos conferimus etcetera vosque preceptorem etcetera. Comittentes vobis fiducialiter etcetera. Quocirca universis et singulis etcetera necnon etcetera inhybentes vobis districtius etcetera. Et si, quod absit, etcetera ac fratri ·· etcetera. In cuius etcetera. Datum Valencie supra Rodanum durante generali capitulo die XIII Martii anno LXXXII.

## 113

*The Master Fr. Juan [Fernández de Heredia] and the chapter general order Fr. Konrad von Braunsberg, Prior of* Alamania, *to make preceptors pay their responsions, notwithstanding the excuse that they want to resign their offices, and to make donats carry out their duties in his priory in the same way as they did before they became donats.*

*Valence, [13]83 March 13*

*AOM 322 fol. 204r-v (196r-v), under* prioratus Alamanie et Boemie.

1) *Fr. Hesso Schlegelholz and the joint Preceptors of Frankfurt Fr. Rudolf and Fr. Helfrich von Rüdigheim as procurators of the Prior.*

Frater Iohannes etcetera generale capitulum celebrantes religioso etcetera fratri Conrado de Brunsperg priori prioratus nostri Alamanie domus eiusdem salutem etcetera. Aliquorum domus nostre fratrum fidedignorum relatibus percepto certos dicte domus fratres preceptores eiusdem prioratus, [204v] quod dolenter referimur, suarum baiuliarum responsiones et alia communi thesauro debita ob ipsorum ineptum regimen solvere recusare exponentes se baiulias ipsorum renuntiaturos et ipsa facta renuntiatione ad solutionem predictorum minime teneri necnon certos donatos domus nostre ipsius prioratus renuere et recusare illa officia seu ministeria exercere et facere, que, antequam essent in donati[a] nostre religionis suscepti, faciebantur et exercebantur, contra statuta et ordines dicte nostre religionis, voti sancte obedientie contentum et dicti prioratus ac dicte nostre religionis non modicum detrimentum, de consilio et assensu ut supra de certa nostra scientia etcetera vobis committimus et mandamus, quatenus omnes et singulos fratres preceptores et alios ipsius prioratus responsiones et alia communi thesauro debita tam de preteritis temporibus quam presenti solvere et tradere compellatis per captionem bonorum, baiuliarum privationem et facta plenta habituum domus nostre destitucionem et quemcumque alium dicte nostre domus choercitionis modum, quamquam suas vellent baiulias renuntiare ac donatis[a] predictos et alios compellatis officia exercere, que primitus faciebant et exercebant, qua in donati[a] forent suscepti, et recusantes facere priveri[!] beneficio donacie et aliis officiis quibuscumque ad premissa omnia et singula hiis presentibus potestate vobis attributa. In cuius etcetera. Datum Valencie ut supra etcetera die XIII Martii anno LXXXII.

*a)* donatos *recte.*

## 114

*The Master Fr. Juan [Fernández de Heredia] and the chapter general constitute Fr. Johann Melkheim as their procurator for the defence of their Order's privileges in* Alamania. *Noble and ignoble, secular and ecclesiastical persons invade estates of the Priory of* Alamania. *So Fr. Johann is instructed to defend the Hospital's rights, inside and outside law courts, with the help of the* conservatores *of the Hospital's privileges in this region and to conclude arbitration contracts. What Fr. Johann does is valid as if the Master himself were present and the Master will abide by it.*

*Valence, [13]83 March 13*

*AOM 322 fol. 204r and 207r (196v-7r), under* prioratus Alamanie et Boemie.

Noverint universi et singuli presens procuratorium visuri et pariter audituri, quod nos frater Iohannes etcetera generale celebrantes capitulum cordis displicencia intellecto, quod nonnulli nobiles et ignobiles seculares et ecclesiastici et alii Deum pre oculis non habentes seu salutis immemores, non querentes, que sua sunt, set aliena, religionis nostre bona prioratus nostri Alamanie invadunt, usurpant, capiunt et hiis non contenti domus nostre fratribus, hominibus, vassallis et subditis iniurias, minas et verbera inferunt et nonnulla alia, que sub scilentio[!] obmittimur, que redundant in maximum vituperium, offensam et dispendium religionis nostre et que non decet nec possemus sub dissimulatione ullatenus tollerare, quinymo de predictis satisfactionem condignam fieri cupimus et impendi, quorum consideracione privilegiis, immunitatibus et libertatibus a sancta sede apostolica, Romanorum imperatoribus contra tales nostre religioni concessis uti volentes ad reprimendos temerarios conatus predictorum talia committentium ac satisfactionem habendam religiosum in Christo nobis carissimum fratrem Iohannem Melkeym domus nostre confisi de eius industria procuratorem, actorem, factorem, sindicum, yconomum et nuntium specialem negotiorumque gestorem nostrum et dicte nostre religionis de consilio etcetera facimus, creamus, constituimus et solempniter ordinamus ad compellendum conveniendi premissa committentes et compelli faciendum per conservatores[1] privilegiorum papalium, imperialium et aliorum quorumcumque et brachium aliud ecclesiasticum et temporale ad petendum exigendi pro[a] peccatoribus talibus iniuriarum et bonorum satisfactionem et satisfactione facta ipsos liberandum, ad agendum et deffendendum, tractandum et conveniendum de premissis in iudicio et extra coram iudicibus omnibus ecclesiasticis et secularibus dante et concedente dicto procuratori nostro auctoritatem, potestatem et licentiam cum plena, libera et generali administracione in premissis et quolibet premissorum emergentium connexorum et ipsis neccessariorum agendi, deffendendi, faciendi, exercendi, petendi, requirendi, componendi, omnia alia et singula faciendi, que nos facere possemus, si presentes essemus, et cum potestate substituendi unum et plures procuratores et substitutos revocandi. Promittentes bona fide ratum, gratum et firmum habere et tenere quidquid per dictum procuratorem nostrum, substitutum seu substitutos ab eo in premissis, circa premissa et quolibet premissorum ac dependentium emergentibus ex eisdem et ipsis connexis seu neccessariis actum, factum, procuratum, conventum, pactum, generatum gestumve fuerit relevantes dictum nostrum procuratorem, substitutum et substitutos ab ipso ab omni onere satisdandi et a quocumque alio gravamine iudicio sisti et iudicatum solvi cum omnibus suis clausulis opportunis sub ypotheca et obligatione omnium nostrorum de dicte nostre religionis bonorum presentium et pariter futurorum. In cuius etcetera. Datum Valencie ut supra die XIII Martii anno LXXXII.

*a)* a *praem. ante corr.*

## 115

*The Master Fr. Juan [Fernández de Heredia] and the chapter general, having listened to Fr. Hesso Schlegelholz, Fr. Helfrich von Rüdigheim and Fr. Johann Melkheim, confirm*

*1) Bishops and other prelates whom the Pope had constituted as defenders of the Hospital's privileges.*

*the treaty between the Priory of* Alamania *and the Bailiwick of Brandenburg. This amicable composition concerns especially the free election of the Bailiff: When the bailiff dies the brethren of the Bailiwick are to elect a suitable brother and present him to the prior, and the prior is to invest him in his office with a written charter.*

*Valence, [13]83 March 13*

*AOM 322 fol. 207r-v (197r-v), under* prioratus Alamanie et Boemie. *Antea copia expeditionis ex registro per vice-cancellarium de dato 1 February 1633.*

Frater Iohannes etcetera religiosis fratribus ·· priori prioratus nostri Alamanie, bailivo, preceptoribus omnibus et singulis aliis sororibus et donatis domus eiusdem salutem etcetera. Percepimus fidedigna relatione, quoniam ad sedandam et sopitandam suscitatam et agitatam iamdiu discordiam inter vos dicti prioratus priorem et preceptores fratres ex parte una et fratres bailivum et preceptores baiulie marchie Brandenburgensis ex parte alia, que discordia nostre religioni plurima intullit[!] dispendia et inter vos gravia pericula generavit, amicabilis intervenit compositio utilis et proficua[1] inter alia continens, quod dicte baiulie marchie baiulo persolvente carnis[a] tributum quocienscumque fratres preceptores baiulie ipsius debent et possunt communi concordia unum ex ipsis fratrem ydoneum et fructuosi regiminis baiulie ipsius in fratrem baiulum eligere, prout ipsis videbitur expediens pro statu et conservacione bonorum nostre religionis, quem baiulum ellectum priori Alamanie et suis successoribus in prioratu presentandum ipsum presentatum prefati prioratus prior et ipsius successores omni posposita excusatione absque tergiversatione aliqua admittere debeant[b] et teneantur confirmare, quo ellecto, presentato, admisso et confirmato predicti prioratus prior et sui successores prefatam baiuliam marchie regendam, gubernandam et administrandam eidem fratri baiulo cum omnibus et singulis iuribus et pertinentiis ad eam spectantem committere, dare et assignare teneantur per suas litteras. De qua quidem amicabili compositione et pluribus aliis interventis publica scripta confecta fuerunt. Quamquam quidem compositionem amicabilem et omnia et singula in ipsis contenta vice et nomine vestro et successorum nobis supplicatum extitit ratas habere, ut et ea omnia et singula in ipsis contenta dignaremur confirmare, nosque informatione diligenti habita cum dicte domus fratribus Hessoni Slegiligloz et Hilfrico de Rudekun ac Iohanne Melken, quorum relatibus exposita agnoscimus fore vera, volentes dicte disceptacioni finem imponere et provideri paci et tranquillitati vestre et successorum vestrorum prefatam amicabilem compositionem, tractatum et concordiam, si et prout modo, forma, pactis et conventionibus inter vos habitis nomine vestro[c] et successorum vestrorum in dictis prioratu et bailiviatu ac omnia et singula in instrumentis [207v] inde confectis contenta, tenore presentium etcetera de consilio ut supra etcetera de certa nostra scientia confirmamus et ea omnia et

1) *Heimbach, 1382 June 11, ed. von Winterfeld (1859), 675–80.*

singula perpetuam roborem, firmitatem volumus obtinere. Mandantes etcetera, ne contraveniant etcetera. In cuius etcetera. Datum Valencie ut supra die XIII Martii anno LXXXIII[d].

Bulla confirmationis concordiae super baiulivatu Brandenburgensi *marg. (saec. XVI);* Vide bullam de anno 1461 fol. 133 *[AOM 371 fol. 133r-v (135r-v) ut infra no. 461]* marg. (saec. XVI). *a)* quotannis *copia.* *b)* debeat *MS* *c)* et vice *del.* *d)* secundo *copia.*

## 116

*The Master Fr. Juan [Fernández de Heredia] and the chapter general confirm Fr. Duke Ziemovit von Teschen for ten years in the priory of Bohemia with named powers and duties.*

*[Valence,] 1383 March 13*

*AOM 322 fol. 203v (195v), under* prioratus Alamanie et Boemie.

Frater Iohannes etcetera generale capitulum celebrantes religioso etcetera fratri Symouito duci Teschennatensi priori prioratus nostri Boemie domus eiusdem salutem etcetera. Morem laudabilem nostre religionis sequentem, secundum quem nedum ipsa religio antiquos promovere, verum eos in suis conservare statibus consuevit, sperantes, quod in premissi nostri prioratus commisso vobis regimine eritis facientes Domino comendabiliter, fructuosus et tamquam oliva fructifera in eo vos fructus uberes allecturi, prioratum ipsum Boemie cum omnibus et singulis suis membris etcetera, ut superius de verbo ad verbum in confirmatione prioratus Alamanie continetur,[1] sic scribatur hec et registretur et sub eadem data.

Collatio prioratus Bohemię *marg.*

## 117

*Fr. Ziemovit [von Teschen], Prior of Bohemia, and his priory are retained by the Master [Fr. Juan Fernández de Heredia].*

*[Valence,] 1383 March 13*

*AOM 322 fol. 203v (195v), under* prioratus Alamanie et Boemie.

Dictis die, mense et anno frater Symouitus predictus prior Boemie fuit retentus ad manus domini magistri cum prioratu ut in forma.

*1) No. 109.*

## 118

*The Master Fr. Juan [Fernández de Heredia] and the chapter general confirm Fr. Franciscus de Plaga for his lifetime in the Preceptory of Glatz (Priory of Bohemia).*

*Valence, [13]83 March 13*

*AOM 322 fol. 204r (196r), under* prioratus Alamanie et Boemie.

Frater Iohannes etcetera generale capitulum celebrantes religioso etcetera fratri Francisco de Plaga domus eiusdem de Glacz preceptori salutem etcetera. Probitate vestra et aliis virtutum donis, quibus apud nos commendamini, illa vobis libenter annuimus, que conservacionem[a)] vestri status concernere dignoscuntur. Igitur preceptoriam supradictam de Glacz prioratus nostri Boemie cum omnibus et singulis etcetera habendam etcetera sub annua responsione etcetera – alias secundum continentiam etcetera – de consilio etcetera confirmamus et de novo ad vitam vestram conferimus etcetera. Committentes etcetera. Quocirca etcetera inhybentes etcetera. Et si, quod absit, etcetera. In cuius etcetera. Datum Valencie ut supra die XIII Martii anno LXXXII.

*a)* conservacionen *MS*

*Franciscus without family name: Novotny (1900), 67 with note 46.*

## 119

*The Master Fr. Juan [Fernández de Heredia] and the chapter general revoke a statute issued by the former Master Fr. Raymond Bérenger in the chapter general at Avignon in 1367 and renew a statute of the former Master Fr. Hélion de Villeneuve, that henceforth the prior, the preceptors and other brethren, sisters and donats of the Priory of* Alamania *are not to pay their responsions to receivers appointed in their respective priories (as other priories do) but directly to the Receiver General.*

*Valence, 1383 March 14*

*AOM 322 fol. 208r (198r), under* prioratus Alamanie et Boemie.

Frater Iohannes etcetera generale capitulum celebrantes religiosis[a)] etcetera fratribus ·· priori prioratus nostri Alamanie et eius successoribus in eodem prioratu, preceptoribus et aliis fratribus, sororibus et donatis prioratus predicti domus eiusdem salutem etcetera. Que pia consideracione et utilitate nostre dicte domus statuta et ordinata sunt, dum tendunt ad noxam, convenit revocare et expedit reducere et commutari in melius, ne mirrum cum secundum temporum varietatem varientur et statuta. Revocato igitur in nostro generali capitulo loco et die subscriptis celebrato statuto edito per bone memorie mediatum predecessorem nostrum fratrum Raymondum Berengarium in eius capitulo generali in Avinione anno sexagesimo sexto celebrato[1] de dicte domus fratribus receptoribus responsionum in quolibet prioratu deputandis revocationis statuti bone memorie magistri Elyonis de Villanova predecessoris nostri[2] continentis ipsas responsiones per priores quoslibet in ipsorum prioratibus recipiendas sub certis penis, statutum illud dicti magistri Elyonis renovantes vos latere nolumus nec ignorancia posse excusari vos prefatum priorem, successores vestros et quorumlibet aliorum domus nostre prioratuum priores ad solutionem annue responsionis dicti prioratus et eorundem[b] prioratuum aliorum teneri per vos et ipsos exolvendam generali nostro receptori et sub penis in dicto magistri Elyonis statuto contentis. Quapropter ortamur vos ac vobis dicto priori et prioratus eiusdem in posterum presidenti regimini sub virtute sancte obedientie iniungimus et mandamus, quatenus circa exactionem annue responsionis dicti prioratus ac solutionem integraliter faciendam, ad quam tenemini, ut prefertur, sic vos habere contingat maxime necessitate conventus nostri Rodi et imminentibus ipsi periculis consideratis, quibus vos certioratum credimus, ne negligentia reprehendi et penis dicto statuto expressis puniri possitis, quod nobis displiceret, necnon dicti prioratus fratres preceptores presentes et futuros suarum baiuliarum responsiones et alia communi thesauro debita solvere recusantes iuxta dicti statuti tenorem et litterarum seriem de dictarum baiuliarum gratiis factis et faciendis per privacionem et destitutionem suarum baiuliarum et penas alias contentis ipsis statutis solvere compellatis, potestate, auctoritate et licentia ad premissa omnia et singula vobis de consilio ut supra etcetera tenore presentium et auctoritate presentis generalis capituli attributa. In cuius etcetera. Datum Valencie ut supra die XIIII Martii anno LXXXII.

*a)* in *del.* *b)* eosdem *MS*

## 120

*Fr. Helfrich von Rüdigheim, Preceptor of Frankfurt with its member Mosbach, is retained by the Master [Fr. Juan Fernández de Heredia].*

*[Valence, 1383 March 14]*

*AOM 322 fol. 208r (198r), under* prioratus Alamanie et Boemie.

Dictis die et anno per dominum magistrum frater Hylfricus de Rudecheyn preceptor de Franchfort cum membro de Mospach fuit retentus ad manus domini magistri solutis etcetera ut in forma.

1) *1367 March 5: Delaville (1913), 161–2.*
2) *Master from 1319 to 1346: ibid. 53.*

## 121

*Fr. Johann Melkheim is assigned his maintenance in the Preceptory of Rottweil or Weißensee (Priory of* Alamania) *for his lifetime.*

*[Valence, 13]83 March 16*

*AOM 322 fol. 208r (198r), under* prioratus Alamanie et Boemie.

Die XVI Martii anno LXXXII assignata fuit stagia ad vitam fratri Iohanni Melkeyn in preceptoria de Rotvoiler Wyssensee prioratus Alamanie et mandantes preceptori ut in forma.

## 122

*Licence to keep his parents' inheritance for Fr. Johann [Melkheim].*

*[Valence, 1383 March 16]*

*AOM 322 fol. 208r (198r), under* prioratus Alamanie et Boemie.

Dicta die data fuit licencia dicto fratri Iohanni, quod ipse possit tenere et possidere in vita sua bona parentum, que tenet, ut in forma.

## 123

*The Master Fr. Juan [Fernández de Heredia] authorises, after consultation with brethren [of the Convent], Fr. Hesso Schlegelholz, Preceptor of Rottweil and Castellan of Rhodes, to receive the monies due from the Priory of Bohemia in Frankfurt.*

*Avignon, [13]83 April 7*

*AOM 322 fol. 208v (198v), under* prioratus Alamanie et Boemie.

Noverint universi et singuli presentes litteras visuri et pariter audituri, quod nos frater Iohannes etcetera consideratis discriminibus viarum, pluribus causis aliis nos moventibus pro secutiori et tuciori nobis viso modo percipiende responsionis et habende pro tempore futuro et preterito arreragiis ipsarum responsionum et aliorum debitorum in prioratu nostro Boemie nobis et communi thesauro loco tuto et securo deputandum censemus fratrem unum providum et discretum. Quapropter confisi de fidei legalitate et circumspectionis industria religiosi etcetera fratris Hessonis Slegelholcz preceptoris de Rutuiller et castellani Rodi eundem fratrem Hessonem meliori modo et forma, quibus possumus, facimus, creamus etcetera nostrum et dicte domus nostre procuratorem etcetera de voluntate, consilio et assensu religiosorum etcetera ad petendum, percipiendum et habendum a preterito tempore responsionum arreragia, mortuaria, subsidia, tallias, pecunias, res et bona nobis et nostro communi thesauro spectantes a quibuscumque domus[a)] nostre fratribus, personis aliis ecclesiasticis et secularibus, cuiuscumque status et condicionis existant, ac etiam ad petendum, exigendum et habendum pro tempore presenti et futuro a religioso etcetera fratre ·· priore prioratus nostri Boemie seu ipsius regimini presidenti annuas responsiones prioratus eiusdem, quas exolvi, dari et consignari dicto fratri Hessoni seu specialiter deputato ab eodem predicti prioratus priore seu ipsius presidenti regimini ex[b)] causis predictis de consilio et assensu predictorum in domo nostra hospitale in Frankefort decernimus, ordinamus et volumus necnon ad audiendum computa et rationes de premissis et recipiendum habendum, quodquod per dictas rationes et computa compertum fuerit deberi, et ad dandum de receptis litteras quitantes perpetuo valiture. Dantes et concedentes dicto fratri Hessoni procuratori nostro pro premissis et quolibet premissorum ac dependentis ex eisdem potestatem et auctoritatem cum plena, libera et generali administracione in iudicio et extra comparendi, agendi et deffendendi, petendi, exigendi, percipiendi, habendi, audiendi, quitandi, unum et plures procuratores loco sui substitutendi et substitutos revocandi omniaque alia et singula faciendi, que nos ipse facere et exercere possemus, si presentes essemus, etiamsi talia forent, que mandatum exigerent magistri speciale[c)]. Promittentes etcetera et relevare etcetera sub ypotheca etcetera. Mandantes harum serie sub virtute sancte obedientie fratri ·· domus eiusdem dicti prioratus priori seu ipsius prioratus regimini presidenti, ut dicto procuratori nostro seu deputando ab eo dicti prioratus responsiones et ipsarum arreragia, si ad que teneant, dat, solvat, tradat et consignet in villa de Franchfort in domo nostra[d)] omni excusatione posposita. In cuius etcetera. Datum Avinione die septimo Aprilis anno LXXXIII.

*a)* personis *del.* *b)* annuas responsiones *del.* *c)* speciales *MS* *d)* nostri *ante corr.*

## 124

*The Master Fr. Juan [Fernández de Heredia], following a decision of the chapter general at Valence, orders Fr. Duke Ziemovit von Teschen, Prior of Bohemia, to send to Rhodes with horses and armour Fr. Borscho von Riesenburg and Fr. Johann von Oels, and two knights and a chaplain he may choose. The four brethren are to be present on Rhodes on 20 August 1383.*

*Avignon, [13]83 April 10*

*AOM 322 fol. 208v (198v), under* prioratus Alamanie et Boemie.

Frater Iohannes etcetera religioso etcetera fratri Symouito duci Teschennatensi priori prioratus nostri Boemie seu ipsius prioratus regimini presidenti domus eiusdem salutem etcetera. Sequentes ordinationem dudum in nostro generali capitulo in civitate Valencia supra Rodanum celebrato factam per nos et dicte domus fratres ·· procuratorem conventus nostri Rodi ac fratres ·· prioratus etcetera, secundum quam dicte domus certos fratres priores, preceptores et conventuales ad nostrum conventum Rodi transfretare expedit ad tuicionem terrarum nostrarum, Christicolarum deffensionem, ad que nos domus nostre fratres dedicamus et deputantur specialiter, ordinationis cuius pretextu de dicto prioratu fratres eligendum ducimur fratres Borscho de Risemburg[1)] et Iohannem de Olsen[2)] ac duos alios fratres milites et unum capellanum, eligendos quos duxeritis, vobis tenore presentium sub virtute sancte obedientie precipimus et mandamus, quatenus dictos fratres et alios ac capellanum eligendos, ut prefertur, accessuros ad dictum nostrum conventum, ut prefertur, moneatis, compellatis et iniungatis eisdem sub dicta virtute sancte obedientie, sub qua virtute ipsis et cuilibet ipsorum precipimus, ut in XX die mensis Agusti instante proximo cum equis et armis sufficientibus et solitis transfretare sint parati et per totum dictum mensem vel saltim ad plus per mensem Septembris instante iter eundi ad conventum Rodi cum equis et armis arripiant et arreptum prosequantur indesinenter penitus et absque deffectu aliquo orituro pro certo quod, si in executione presentium pro parte vestri intervenerit deffectus seu ipsis negligentibus vel remissis esse contingat, vos et eos ut inobedientes et rebelles, quod minime existere credimus, puniemur et ducemus per iustitiam nostre domus. Datum Avinione die X Aprilis anno LXXXIII.

## 125

*The Master Fr. Juan [Fernández de Heredia] orders (as no. 124) Fr. Konrad von Braunsberg, Prior of* Alamania, *to send four knight brethren to Rhodes selected by himself and by Fr. Hesso [Schlegelholz].*

*[Avignon, 1383 April 10]*

*AOM 322 fol. 209r (199r), under* prioratus Alamanie et Boemie. *Ed. van Winter (1998), 31 no. 4.*

Sub eisdem dato, modo et forma prescriptis scriptum fuit fratri Conradi de Brunsperg priori Alamanie seu ipsius prioratus regimini presidenti et mandatum ut supra, ut quatuor fratres milites eligendos per ipsum et fratrem Hessonem mictat ad conventum termino prescripto, et ipsis, ut accedant cum equis et armis ut in forma prescripta.

## 126

*Fr. Hesso Schlegelholz is ordered to pay to Nicolino de Lippo or his procurator 3,000 florins of Florence or their equivalent within eight days of the presentation of the present*

1) *Boress, Borsso and Borscho are variants of the same first name, diminutives of Borziwoj.*

2) *Johann von Oels was perhaps son to Duke Conrad I, who died in 1366, and his second wife Euphemia von Kosel.*

*letter. The Master and the Convent owe this sum to Nicolino who had granted them a loan on monies due to them from the Priory of* Alamania. *Nicolino is to issue a receipt and to keep the present letter as a proof of payment.*

*1383 April 15*

*AOM 322 fol. 321r (311r), under* assignaciones pecuniarum.

Die XV mensis Aprilis mandatum fuit fratri Hessoni Slegelhocz, ut solvat Nicolino de Lippo seu eius procuratori legitimo florenos de Florencia tria milia seu eorum valorem, in quibus dictus magister et conventus obligantur eidem ratione et ex causa mutui de quibuscunque pecuniis receptis et recpiendi[s] per eum de prioratu Alamanie pertinentibus ipso domino magistro et conventui communiter vel divisim, infra dies octo computandos a presentacione litterarum[a]. Et solucione facta de dicta quantitate[b] recipiat quitanciam, que sufficiat et retineat presentes litteras incisas in signum facte solucionis.

*a)* et facta *add. MS* *b) q(ua)ictit. MS*

## 127

*The Master Fr. Riccardo Caracciolo and brethren, acting in chapter general, constitute Fr. Duke Ziemovit von Teschen, Prior of Bohemia and Poland[!], as their lieutenant, procurator, visitor and corrector in the Priories of* Alamania, *Saxony and Brabant[!]. He is to collect responsions and arrears of responsions, the* procrassia, mortuaria, iocalia *and other dues from Hospitaller brethren according to the statute of 1367, the pension payments of the Master's chamber in each of these priories and all other dues to the Master and Convent. He is to audit accounts. He is to recover all castles and estates alienated from the Hospital in violation of constitutions issued by the late Pope Gregory XI and the modern Pope Urban VI. He is also to issue receipts. Furthermore, he has full powers for legal acts inside and outside law courts. He may constitute and depose one or more Hospitaller brethren as his substitutes. What he does and what they do is valid as if the Master himself were present and the Master will abide by it. All Hospitallers and subjects of the Hospital are ordered to be obedient to Fr. Johann's orders and to pay all past, present and future responsions, arrears of responsions,* mortuaria, spolia *and other dues.*

*Naples, 1384 April 3*

*AOM 281 fol. 26r-7v. Cf. van Winter (1998), 32 no. 5.*

Noverint universi et singuli presentem constitucionem procuracionis visuri et audituri, quod nos frater Ricardus Caraczolus etcetera et nos fratres cum eo in capitulo nostro generali congregati domus eiusdem in nostra sancti Iohannis Neapolis ecclesia pro ordinandis subscriptis ad sonum campane, ut moris est, capitulariter convenientes in unum, [26v] nos, videlicet dictus magister, de voluntate, consilio et assensu fratrum predictorum et nos, fratres predicti, de licencia, consilio et assensu dicti magistri superioris nostri, confisi de fidei legalitate et circumspeccionis industria venerabilis religiosi in Christo nobis carissimi fratris Symouiti ducis Tassinensis ac prioris prioratus nostri Boemie et Polonie eundem priorem absentem tamquam presentem tenore presencium de nostra certa sciencia facimus, creamus, constituimus et sollempniter ordinamus nostrum et nostre dicte domus locumtenentem, visitatorem, correctorem et privatorem secundum statutum nostre religionis in prioratibus Alamannie, Saxonie et Brabanczie procuratorem, actorem, syndicum, yconomum, responsionum petitorem et certum nuncium specialem ad omnia alia et singula infrascripta dependencia et emergencia ab eisdem vel altero eorundem et ipsis et eorum cuilibet quomodolibet connexis, videlicet ad petendum, habendum, recipiendum et recuperandum nostro et dicte domus nostre procuratorio nomine atque vice omnes et singulas responsiones et arreragia responsionum omnium et singulorum preceptoriarum, baiuliarum et domorum prioratuum nostrorum predictorum ac preceptoriarum et baiuliarum ipsarum nobis debitas et debita de preterito tempore presenti et futuro debitas ac debenda tam singularum preceptoriarum et domorum dictorum prioratuum quam camerarum nostrarum dicti magistri. Item ad petendum, recipiendum, recuperandum et habendum nomine quo supra tam de[a] preterito tempore quam presenti et futuro omnia procrassia et mortuaria ac iocalia, res et bona, qualiacumque sint et quovis nomine nuncupata et in quibuscumque consistant, omnium et singulorum fratrum domus nostre preceptorum seu quorumvis aliorum mortuorum iam et inantea moriendorum in predictis nostris prioratibus et in aliis locis superius nominatis ad nos pertinentibus et debentibus pervenire secundum statutum promulgatum et factum super hoc in generali capitulo apud Avinionem de mense Marcii anno sexagesimo sexto celebrato[1] seu quovis alio nomine. Item ad petendum seu recuperandum nomine quo supra pensiones debitas et debendas camere nostre, prelibati magistri, quam habemus in dictis prioratibus. Item ad petendum et recipiendum nomine quo supra omnes[b] et singulas pecuniarum summas ac bona, res et iura alia, quecumque fuerint et quovis nomine nuncupantur, nobis communiter vel divisim debitas et debita, debendas et debenda et nobis pertinencia et debencia pervenire quovis tytulo, ratione vel causa tam per domus nostre fratres quam personas alias quaslibet aliarum religionum religiosas seu ecclesiasticas et mundanas. Item ad petendum et audiendum rationes et computa quo supra nomine et de predictis et altero predictorum prout sibi videbitur expedire et que nobis per dicta computa deberi et perveniri debere compererit petendi, recipiendi et habendi. Item ad petendum[c] seu recuperandum circa castra et bona religionis nostre alienata per certos nostros fratres contra statutum nostre religionis ac contra constitutiones bone memorie Gregorii pape XI et domini nostri Urbani pape VI moderni. Item ad faciendum nomine quo supra de receptis quitancias perpetuo valituras. Dantes et concedentes predicto

1) *1367 March 5: Delaville (1913), 161–2.*

nostro locumtenenti, responsionum receptori et procuratori licenciam, potestatem et auctoritatem cum plena, libera et generali administracione pro omnibus et singulis supradictis et infrascriptis ac dependentibus et emergentibus ex eisdem et altero eorundem aut ipsis et eorum cuilibet qualitercumque connexis coram quibuscumque iudicibus, curiis ecclesiasticis et mundanis semel et quociens fuerit oportunum et eidem videbitur expedire que supra procuratorio nomine et nostrarum dictarum domorum comparendi, agendi et defendendi, libellum seu libellos et quascumque alias summarias peticiones dandi, litem seu lites contestandi, de calumpnia vitanda et veritate dicenda in animas nostras iurandi et subeundi cuiuslibet alterius generis licitum iuramentum, ponendi, proponendi et articulandi positionibus et articulis alterius partis respondendi et datis per eum responderi, petendi, exceptiones dandi, replicandi, duplicandi, triplicandi, testes, instrumenta et quecumque alia probacionum genera producendi et productis per partem adversam obiciendi, testes iurare videndi et in eos et eorumque dicta dicendi, crimina et defectus opponendi, beneficium absolucionis a quacumque excommunicationis sententia lata vel ferenda et restitucionis in integrum semel et pluries simpliciter et ad cautelam petendi et obtinendi, sententiam et sententias tam interlocutorias quam diffinitivas ferri, petendi et audiendi et, si oporteat, eas variandi et ab ea vel ab eis et a quocumque alio gravamine illato vel inferendo appellandi, apostolos petendi, appellationum causas prosequendi, expensas et interesse petendi, procuratores unum vel plures domus nostre fratres ad predicta et subscripta et eorum quemlibet loco sui semel et pluries substituendi et eciam seculares personas ad lites et causas terminendi et eum seu eos recovandi et in se procuracionis officium reassumendi et generaliter ad omnia alia et singula faciendi, dicendi, procurandi et exercendi, que in premissis et premissorum quolibet necessaria fuerint seu eciam oportuna et que quilibet verus et legitimus locumtenens, procurator, negociorum gestor, petitor et receptor facere posset et debet et nos ipsi facere possemus, si personaliter interessemus, eciam si talia sint, in quibus requiratur speciale mandatum. Et relevantes[d)] dictum nostrum locumtenentem, procuratorem et receptorem ac substituendum et substituendos ab eo ab omni onere satisdandi, promittimus bona fide gratum, ratum et firmum habere perpetuo et tenere, quidquid per dictum nostrum locumtenentem, procuratorem et receptorem ac substituendum et substituendos ab eo vel eis actum, gestum, dictum, petitum, habitum, quitatum et procuratum legitime fuerit in premissis et quolibet premissorum, ac iudicio sisti et iudicatum solvi cum omnibus et singulis clausulis oportunis sub ypoteca et obligacione omnium bonorum nostrorum et nostre dicte domus presencium pariter et futurorum. Mandantes per presens procuratorium sub virtute sancte obediencie firmiter et districte universis et singulis fratribus domorum nostrarum prioratuum predictorum et aliorum locorum sibi[e)] decretorum cuiuscumque status et condicionis existant ac aliis quibuscumque quibus predicta seu eorum quolibet pertinebunt et poterunt quomodolibet pertinere, ut premisso nostro locumtenenti, receptori et procuratori ac deputando vel deputandis ab eo suarumque domorum et baiuliarum responsiones, arreragia, mortuaria atque spolia quecumque tam preteriti temporis quam presentis et futuri et omnia alia et singula nobis communiter et divisim spectancia et debencia racionabiliter pervenire tradant et exhibeant ac eidem in omnibus pareant et obediant contradictione qualibet non obstante. In cuius rei testimonium bulla nostra plumbea presentibus est appensa. Datum Neap(oli) durante nostro predicto capitulo generali die tertia mensis Aprilis anno incarnacionis Domini millesimo trecentesimo octuagesimo quarto.

In capitulo generali procuratorium prioratus Alamanie et Boemie *marg.* *a)* p *praem. ante corr.* *b) del.* *c)* et recipiendum *add. ante corr.* *d)* revelantes *ante corr.* *e)* st *add. ante corr.*

## 128

*The Master Fr. Riccardo [Caracciolo] and [brethren, acting in] chapter general, exempt Fr. Duke Ziemovit von Teschen, Prior of Bohemia and Poland[!] and lieutenant in these countries, from an annual payment of 300 florins owed to Fr. Hesso S[chlegelholz] from the Priory of Bohemia; Fr. Hesso had been granted this annual sum when he renounced the priory.*

*Naples, 1384 April 3*

*AOM 281 fol. 29v. Cf. Delaville (1913), 219, 251.*

Frater Ricardus etcetera venerabili religioso in Christo nobis carissimo fratri Symouito duci Tassinensi ac priori prioratus nostri Boemie et Polonie necnon nostro locumtenenti in partibus ipsis salutem etcetera. Cum hoc sit, quod in quadam sembleia seu capitulo generali celebrato apud Avinionem per olim magistrum et fratres predecessorem nostrum vos obligastis dare et solvere fratri Ausoni de Alamannia florenos trecentos singulis annis ex quadam sententia lata per compromissarios ad hoc electos, ut dicitur plenius contineri quodam publico instrumento super hoc confecto manu notarii Martini tunc secretarii fratris Danielis de Carretto, in qua quidem sententia continebatur, quod frater Ausonus predictus deberet renunciare prioratui Boemie et Polonie sibi per conventum Rodi concesso et eidem fratri A. vos Semiuitus dare tunc[a] deberetis florenos tria mille auri et singulis annis trecentos florenos, donec prioratum predictum teneretis.[1] Nos vero considerantes, quod a dicta obligacione trecentorum florenorum estis ipso iure absolutus ex eo, quod dictus frater A. inobediens est et scismaticus domino nostro Urbano pape sexto et nobis, tamen ad cautelam eciam per presentes omni via, modo, iure et forma, quibus magis

1) *In 1372 Fr. Hesso Schlegelholz had resigned the priory Bohemia and Poland in favour of Fr. Ziemovit: Delaville (1913), 172–3.*

et melius possumus, declaramus vos a dicta obligacione absolutum et nullatenus amplius obligatum. Et ideo vobis, fratri Symovito predicto, in virtute sancte obediencie districte precipiendo mandamus, quatenus eidem fratri A. nullatenus de predicto debito seu obligacione trecentorum florenorum predictorum respondere seu solvere debeatis. In quorum testimonium premissorum bulla nostra plumbea presentibus est appensa. Datum Neap. durante nostro predicto capitulo generali die tercia mensis Aprilis anno incarnacionis Domini millesimo CCC$^{mo}$ octuagesimo quarto.

In capitulo generali absolucio cuiusdam debiti *marg.* *a)* tuc *MS*

## 129

*The Master Fr. Riccardo Caracciolo and [brethren, acting in] chapter general, confirm Fr. Duke Ziemovit von Teschen for ten years in the Priory of Bohemia and Poland. He is to pay the responsions each year in August. Furthermore, he is to pay all other levies the Master and Convent have imposed or may impose on the priory. His ten years start on 24 June 1384. The Master reserves his right to make appointments for vacant offices according to a statute of 1367. In case of default the Master reserves his right to depose Fr. Duke Ziemovit with the counsel of brethren and following another statute of 1367. Fr. Ziemovit is to rule his priory and to appoint officers in the way as prescribed by the statutes of the Hospital.*

*Naples, 1384 April 3*

*AOM 281 fol. 33v-4r.*

Frater Riccardus Caraczolus etcetera unacum fratribus etcetera venerabili religioso in Christo nobis carissimo fratri Simovito duci Tassinensi priori prioratus nostri Bohemie et Polonie salutem et sinceram in Domino caritatem. Extimamus digne agere etcetera. Attendentes itaque, quod[a)] in administracione dicti prioratus estis fructuosus, utiliter, comprobatus, igitur prioratum ipsum actenus vobis concessum per predecessores nostros cum omnibus suis menbris, iuribus et pertinenciis universis ad prioratum ipsum spectantibus et pertinentibus ac spectare et pertinere debentibus quoquomodo et cum omni onere, emolumentis et honore unacum suis cameris consuetis et cum omnibus earum menbris, iuribus et pertinenciis universis habendum, tenendum, regendum, gubernandum, augmentandum et meliorandum in spiritualibus et temporalibus tam in capite quam in membris vobis tamquam digno et benemerito invicem deliberato et communicato consilio auctoritate presencium et nostri generalis capituli sub annua responsione per vos, prout pro cameris vestris vos continget, et per preceptores dicti prioratus, prout pro preceptoriis suis pro rata eis pertinebit, receptoribus deputatis vel deputandis per nos ad recipiendum responsiones in prioratu prefato alii vel aliis, quibus et ubi ordinaverimus et mandaverimus, de mense Augusti ex pacto expresso infallibiliter annis singulis exsolvendis et quibuscumque aliis oneribus dicto prioratui qualitercumque et quocumque incumbentibus et incumbendis, impositis et imponendis per vos et dictos preceptores, ut predicitur, ex pacto etiam ultra responsionem predictam supportandis de nostra certa sciencia et speciali gratia vobis benefaciendo in eadem auctoritate presencium et nostri generalis capituli confirmamus, approbamus et ratificamus necnon pro uberiori dono gratie de novo conferimus, concedimus et donamus ad annos decem incipiendos in festo nativitatis sancti Iohannis baptiste proxime venturo et extunc continue secuturos et completos retento nobis et specialiter reservato, prout per mortem preceptorum evenire contingerit, vacantibus vel vacaturis baiulia vel baiuliis in dicto prioratu possumus anno quolibet providere secundum continenciam et seriem statuti et eciam retento et reservato nobis ordinacionibus omnibus per bone memorie dominum fratrem Raymundum Berengarii dicte sacre domus magistrum factis in generali capitulo per eum celebrato apud Avinionem de mense Marcii anno sexagesimosexto[1] nichilominus nobis retento et eciam reservato, quod si, quod absit, in solucione per vos statuto termino facienda annuarum responsionum vestrarum camerarum et baiuliarum, quas ad manus vestras habetis in premisso prioratu, deficere vos contingat, quod nos dictus magister de consilio fratrum baiuliorum et procerum nobis assistencium possimus disponere et ordinare de premisso prioratu secundum continenciam statutorum editorum in generali capitulo prelibato. Dantes et concedentes vobis auctoritatem et potestatem plenariam regendi, gubernandi et administrandi prioratum prefatum tam in capite quam in menbris in spiritualibus et temporalibus et quecumque alia agendi, celebrandi et excercendi, que ad prioris spectant officium et que pro utili regimine prioratus ipsius necessaria fuerint et eciam oportuna, insuper dandi, conferendi et distribuendi cum consilio fratrum et procerum dicti prioratus baiulias, castellanias atque domos vacaturas in iamdicto prioratu vestre spectantes donacioni secundum statuta nostre dicte domus editum super istis fratribus ydoneis et benemeritis domus nostre prioratus prefati per dictum tempus X annorum, prout melius et utilius videbitur expedire, nostris tamen retencionibus in omnibus semper salvis. Committentes vobis fiducialiter circa curam, regimen et administracionem ac gubernacionem[b] etcetera. Quocirca etcetera vobisque suum prebeant auxilium, consilium et favorem in omnibus, que ad curam, regimen et administracionem ac gubernacionem utilem prescripti prioratus pertinere noscuntur, quociens opus fuerit et eos duxeritis requirendos. Inhibentes vobis etcetera. In cuius rei testimonium etcetera. Datum Neap. durante nostro predicto capitulo generali die tercia mensis Aprilis anno incarnacionis Domini millesimo trecentesimo octuagesimo quarto.

In capitulo generali confirmatio prioratus Boemie *marg.* *a)* ut *praem. ante corr.* *b)* gubernaconem *MS*

*1) 1367 March 5: Delaville (1913), 161–2.*

## 130

*Decisions concerning the two Priories of* Alamania *and Bohemia taken in the chapter general of the Master Fr. Riccardo Caracciolo. (1) Presentation of the summons by Fr. Giovanni Vicheria that had been sent to* Alamania *by the two cardinals of Corfu and of S. Ciriaco. Appointment of [Fr. Duke Ziemovit of Teschen], Prior of Bohemia and Poland[!], to be lieutenant of the Master and the Treasurer in* Alamania, *Saxony, Brabant, in the County of Aynaldus, in Flanders and in the Dioceses of Liège and Cambrai. (2) Presentation of the credentials of the prior of Bohemia which are accepted. (3) Commission to Fr. Giovanni Vicheria to travel to the three Priories of Bohemia and Poland[!],* Alamania *and England. For his expenses he is entitled to 40 florins from the Priory of Bohemia and to 60 florins each from the Priories of* Alamania *and England.*

*Naples, 1384 March 28*

*AOM 281 fol. 1r-9r.*

(1) *Fol. 2r:* Item dicta die frater Iohannes de Viqueria presentavit suas litteras citatorias destinatas ad partes Alamanie per reverendissimos patres et cardinales Corfiensis et Ciriaci.[1)] <. . .> Item deliberatum fuit et obtentum per predictos magistrum et fratres capitulariter congregatos, quod prior Boemie et Polonie sit locumtenens magistri et thesaurarius in prioratibus Alamannie et Saxonie et Brabanzie necnon in comitatu Aynaldi et in Flandria et in tota diocesi Leodiensi et Cameracensi.[2)]

(2) *Fol. 2v:* Item dicta die producta fuerunt instrumenta procurationis per procuratores prioris Boemie et fratrum et fuerunt acceptata.

(3) *Fol. 7v:* Item deliberatum fuit, quod frater Iohannes de Viqueria[3)] vadat in serviciis religionis ad prioratum Boemie et Polonie, Almannie et Anglie. In prioratu Boemie habeat pro expensis florenos XL, in Almania LX et in Anglia LX.

## 131

*The Master Fr. R[iccardo Caracciolo] retains Fr. Giovanni Vicheria and orders payments to him as commissioner for* Alamania, *Bohemia and England.*

*Naples, [1384 April 12]*

*AOM 281 fol. 40r.*

1) *Two cardinals created by Urban VI in 1378, Nicolaus Misquinus seu Caracciolus (vulg. s. Cyriaci) and Johannes de Amelia, Archbishop of Corfu: Eubel 1 (1898), 23 nos. 27.8 and 27.10.*

2) *Bailiwick of Avalterre, Chantraine and Flanders: Legras (1987), 148–50.*

3) *Cf. Delaville (1913), 255 note 2. Fr. Giovanni de Vicheria was Preceptor of San Leonardo and receiver in the Priory of Venice: AOM 281, fol. 1r, 3r.*

Frater R. etcetera religioso in Christo nobis carissimo fratri Iohanni de Viqueria domus eiusdem etcetera salutem etcetera. Dum laudabilia etcetera igitur tuam volentes honorare personam, ut proinde tue fidei et devocionis zelus ad laudabiliora ferventius inantea animetur, te cum omnibus tuis rebus et graciis auctoritate presencium ad manus nostras de speciali gratia retinemus etcetera. Mandantes harum serie omnibus fratribus preceptoribus et prioribus ac aliis fratribus et confratribus domus nostre sub[a] virtute sancte obediencie, ne contra presentem nostre retencionis gratiam aliquatenus etcetera. Ac eciam mandamus omnibus ut supra, ut eundem fratrem Iohannem nostrum commissarium ad partes Almannie, Boemie et Anglie benigne recipiatis et tractetis eidem providendo in eundo, stando et redeundo in expensis necessariis ad victum. In cuius etcetera bulla nostra etcetera. Datum Neap. die quo supra proximo precedente[b].

In capitulo generali reservatio fratris Io. de Viqueria *marg.* *a)* ne contra *praem. ante corr.* *b)* presente *praem. ante corr.*

## 132

*The Master [Fr. Juan Fernández de Heredia] quits the honourable Konrad Stobeker from Freiburg for 300 florins of Germany. Konrad has paid this sum on behalf of Fr. Hesso Schlegelholz, Preceptor of Rottweil, who owed this to the Master for the Master's chamber he holds in the Priory of* Alamania.

*[Avignon, 1384] September 20*

*AOM 322 fol. 324r (313r$^{bis}$), under* assignaciones pecuniarum.

Die vicesima mensis Septembris dictus magister confessus fuit se recepisse in peccunia numerata florenos Alamanie trecentos ab honorabili viro Conrado Stobeker de Friburgo nomine fratris Hessonis Slegelholcz preceptoris de Rotuuil racione et ex causa camere ipsius,[1] quam habet in prioratu Alamanie. De quibus florenis CCC ipsum fratrem Hessonem et Conradum quitavit.

## 133

*The Master Fr. Riccardo [Caracciolo] appoints the priest Fr. Johann Sternberg to be his chaplain and household familiar.*

*Lucera, 1384 October 25*

*AOM 281 fol. 56r.*

*1) Buchsee: Helvetia Sacra (2006), 399.*

Frater Riccardus etcetera religioso in Christo nobis carissimo fratri Iohanni Sternebergh[a)] presbitero domus eiusdem salutem et sinceram in Domino caritatem. Vite et morum honestas aliaque laudabilia probitatis et virtutum merita, quibus personam tuam experimento nobis cognito iuvari percepimus, nos inducunt et non immerito promerentur, ut te, quem premissa exibent gratum atque dignum, nostris favoribus et honoribus attollamus. Ut igitur benevolentiam nostram, qua personam tuam ob premissorum intuitum prosequimur, per effectum operis sentias et cognoscas, te exnunc in cappellanum nostrum commensalem recipimus et aliorum cappellanorum nostrorum commensalium tenore presentium aggregamus volentes, ut de cetero ubique locorum et terrarum gratiis, emolumentis, libertatibus et privilegiis, quibus ceteri cappellani nostri commensales gaudent et utuntur, tu gaudeas et fruaris et in tuis agendis et promovendis negotiis secure habeas ad nos recursum cum fiducia speciali. In cuius rei testimonium bulla nostra plumbea presentibus est appensa. Data apud Luceriam Cristianorum die XXV mensis Octobris anno incarnacionis Domini M° CCC LXXXIIII°.

Littera cappellanie *marg.* *a)* Sterlinebergh *ante corr.*

## 134

*The Master Fr. Riccardo [Caracciolo] permits his chaplain Fr. Johann Sternberg to study canon law for five years. For his maintenance the Priors of Bohemia and* Dacia *are to contribute. He may also accept ecclesiastical benefices, including one with pastoral care.*

*Lucera, [13]84 October 25*

*AOM 281 fol. 56r-v; cf. Hatt Olsen (1962), 102 no. 7.*

Frater Riccardus etcetera religioso in Christo nobis carissimo fratri Iohanni Sternebergh presbitero domus eiusdem, cappellano nostro commensali salutem etcetera. Extimamus digne agere et rationabiliter operari, si quos ad abitum nostri ordinis evocavit, eos ad gratiam et prerogativam honoris attollamus. Attendentes itaque tuos laudabiles mores et animum, scientiam et virtutes adipiscendum nos inducunt, ut tibi iusta petita reddamur ad gratiam liberales. Igitur tuis supplicationibus inclinati tenore presencium tibi damus et concedimus licentiam et facultatem eundi ad studium privilegiatum ibidemque standi et in iure canonico per quinquennium studendi, quo termino finito ad obedientiam prioris Datie volumus te reverti rogantes et ortantes per presentes priores prioratuum nostrorum Boemie et Datie, ut in subsidium tui studii iuxta eorum bonas et pias voluntates et facultates tibi in tantum ministrent, ut huiusmodi studium eorum mediantibus auxiliis valeas cum effectu adimplere. Insuper tibi concedimus et donamus licentiam et auctoritatem recipiendi, acceptandi et retinendi quecumque benefitia ecclesiastica, etiam si curatum existat, tibi a quocumque rite et canonice collata absque alia nostra speciali licentia et mandato. Mandantes in virtute sancte obedientie firmiter et districte, qua nobis et nostre domui sunt astricti[a)], universis et singulis fratribus domus nostre quacumque auctoritate, dignitate vel offitio fulgentibus, presentibus et futuris, ne contra hanc nostram licentiam et gratiam aliquatenus venire presumant, quinimmo eam studeant iuxta eius mentem et seriem inviolabiliter observare. In cuius rei testimonium etcetera. Datum apud Luceriam christianorum die XXV mensis Octobris anno LXXXIIII°.

Concessio fratri Iohanni Sternebergh eundi ad studium *marg.* *a)* abstricti *MS*

## 135

*[The Master Fr. Juan Fernández de Heredia] informs the Priors of* Alamania *and Bohemia that, after consultation with six named and other brethren, he convokes an assembly at Valence on 6 April 1385 to discuss the reform of the Order. They are to participate, each of them with two preceptors in decent company of familiars and horses but without unseemly expenditures. They are to take with them sufficient letters of authorisation, all dues and arrears of dues to be paid. They are to inform the Master about the date when they receive the present letter. Furthermore, they are to take with them a detailed list of the chambers, offices and preceptories and the names of all brethren and donats. Finally, they are to send to Rhodes three preceptors who can be used on galleys or embassies or other missions, and three brethren fit for armed service; the date and place for the* passagium *of these brethren will be notified to the priors in due course of time.*

*Avignon, 1385 January 2*

*AOM 322 fol. 209r (199r), under* prioratus Alamanie et Boemie.

Sub eisdem tenore, anno, mense, die et data expressis supra folio XI°[!] quilibet scriptum fuit et mandatum priori Alamanie et Boemie pro assembleia ordinata tenere.

*AOM 322 fol. 18v-19r (9v-10r [IX-X!]) under* castellania Enposte, *Master Fr. Juan to the Castellan of Amposta Fr. Martin de Lihori:*

Frater Iohannes etcetera religioso in Christo nobis carissimo fratri Martino de Lyerhorl castellano Emposte domus eiusdem salutem et sinceram in Domino caritatem. Ad vestram harum serie noticiam adducimus, quoniam nostra ac dicte domus fratrum Petri Bussoni prioris nostri Rodi conventus eiusdem procuratoris, Roberti de Castronouo Aluernie, Girardi de Vienna Francie, Iohannis Garnerii Campanie prioratuum priorum, Petri de Prouinis thesaurarii, Iohannis Siffe Pisarum prioris et aliorum preceptorum et procerum zelatorum nostre religionis aliorumque preceptorum et procerum consulta deliberatio censuit et decrevit nos eosque fratres priores et proceres eiusdem domus pro expedienti et utili nostre religionis reformatione necnon conservatione ipsius in unum convenire, tenere et facere in Christi nomine assembleiam in Valencia supra Rodanum die decima sexta mensis Aprilis instantis. In qua assembleia nos cum ipsorum et vestro consilio disponamus disponenda expediencia queque utilia dicto domui auxiliante Domino et taliter, quod ob excequtionis ordinandorum accionem ipsa religio in augmento Christiane fidei, Christicolarum protectione favores salubres pociorum senciat nosque fratres ipsi et vos ab altissimo et prelatis ecclesiasticis necnon regibus, principibus, ceteris dominis temporalibus et tocius orbis Christi fidelibus de regiminis cura salutifera possimus et valeant merito comendari. Quapropter fraternitatem vestram, quam pro directione et expeditione agendorum expedientem existere agnoscimus, in Domino exortamur ac vobis et per vos depputandis et vestrum cuilibet districte precipiendo mandamus in virtute sancte obedientie districtius iniungentes, quatenus apud locum predictum die supra assignata, ubi tunc adesse disponimus Domino favente, cum duobus fratribus preceptoribus dicte castellanie proceritate et industria comprobatis, quos eligendos duxeritis, cum familiaribus[a] et equitaturis decentibus iuxta statutum pro sumptibus evitandis veniatis plena potestate vos et ipsi suffulti nomine acque vice fratrum aliorum preceptorum omnium et singulorum castellanie eiusdem necnon cum responsionibus[b], arreragiis, subsidiis, tailliis et aliis bonis, rebus, deneriis pertinentibus nobis et ipsius conventus thesauro communiter seu divisim intersitis presencialiter attencius precaventes, ne in premissis adimplendum committatis negligenciam, sed tanquam veri obediencie filii ex prompta et reverenti excequtione premissorum valeatis premiari a Domino. Aliter contra illos, que premissa recusaverint adimplere, nos, prout nostre religionis regula et statuta exhigunt, procedamus. Nichilominus nobis per vestras litteras rescribatis diem receptionis presencium, nam aliter relationi portitorum earum super ipsarum presentatione vobis facta nobis refferenda dabimus plenam fidem. Ceterum volumus et vobis harum serie precipiendo mandamus, quatenus particulariter et distincte die prescripta ad locum prefixum apportetis statum camerarum baiuliarum et domorum, nomina singulorum fratrum et donatorum dicte castellanie et veniatis instructi et informati de omnibus negociis castellanie eiusdem, ut suffragante Domino vestro et aliorum fratrum baillivorum procuratorum, priorum et procerum dicte domus in ipsa assemblaya presencium consilio [19r] et auxilio super hiis providere salubriter valeamus. Sane iuxta exhigenciam prefati nostri Rodi conventus et ordinata in nostro capitulo generali dudum Valencie supra Rodanum celebrato vobis tenore presencium precipimus sub virtute sancte obediencie, ut fratres dictarum domus et castellanie preceptorum tres, qui possint, sciant et valeant galleas ducere, ambaxiatas et alia excercenda incumbencia[c] supportare onera, ac fratres conventuales tres habiles ad armorum excercitia eligatis et ordinetis cum equis et armis sufficientibus, ut moris est et eorum decet statui, dispositos et paratos Rodi transfectare in brevi tempore, de quo et loco fiendi passagii eorum et aliorum vos et eos efficiemus et reddemus certo competenti et debito tempore cerciores.

In cuius etcetera. Data Avinione die secunda mensis Ianuarii anno incarnationis Domini M° CCC° LXXX IIII°.

*a)* famullo *praem. ante corr.* *b)* respontoribus *MS* *c)* incumbecia *MS*

## 136

*The Master Fr. Juan Fernández [de Heredia] orders all subjects of the Priory of* Alamania *to obey the lieutenants constituted by the Prior Fr. Konrad von Braunsberg because of his age and sickness.*

*Avignon, 1385 February 22*

*AOM 323 fol. 157v (149v), under* prioratus Alamanie et Boemie.

Frater Iohannes Ferdinandi etcetera religiosis etcetera fratribus ·· preceptoribus fratribusque aliis, sororibus, donatis, hominibus subditis et vassallis universis et singulis prioratus nostri Alamanie domus eiusdem etcetera. Cum dicte domus frater Cunradus de Brunsberg, dicti prioratus prior, qui virtuose et laudabiliter cum famose laudis preconio prioratus eiusdem presedit regimini, ea excercuit eciam agere nititur, que ad prioris spectant officium prepeditus et gravatus senili debilitate et gravi infirmitate intuens, ut opus foret et exhigit tempus vigentis conditio se non posse presentialiter vacare, adesse et intendere in salubri advectione et expeditione utili agendorum prioratus predicti suo more solito loco et tempore opportuno preservare cupiens prioratum ipsum inde religere a dispendiis, que ipse prioratus religio eius corporali absenciam possent incurere, horum consideratione domus nostre et prioratus predictorum fratrem seu fratres in prioratu eodem ipsius fratris Cunradi prioris vicesgerentes et locatenentes nostra impetita sibi licencia[a)] ordinaverit et quociens sibi placuerit ad dicti prioratus regimen deputare, ordinare et disponere intendat sufficienti et utili regimine comprobatis. Intencioni et proposito comendabilibus eiusdem prioris favorabiliter annuentes, ducti confidencia, quod solerti diligentia huiusmodi fratrum seu fratris vicesgerentium ab eodem priore deputatorum et ordinandorum prioratus idem dirigetur utiliter, vobis et cuilibet vestrum sub virtute sancte obedientie ac sacramento fidelitatis et homagii, quo nobis et nostre domui estis astricti, precipimus et mandamus districte iniungentes, quatenus domus eiusdem et prioratus predicti fratrem et fratres, quem et quos dictus prior frater Cunradus in dicto prioratu ordinavit seu deputandum ducxerit ipsius vicesgerentes seu locatenentes, suscipiatis iuxta locumtenencie tenorem et seriem ac ipsi vel ipsis fratri et fratribus locatenentibus obediatis et pareatis tamquam superiori et maiori et, prout a dicto priore fratre Cunrado habueritis in mandatum, quodque in omnibus concernentibus utilitatem dicti prioratus prebeatis opem et favorem, quociens fueritis requisiti, sic vos habentes in prompta et reverenti executione presencium, ut de vobis fiduciam gerimus, ne inhobediencie et rebellionis macula vos inculpet et puniendum propterea exponat per iusticiam domus nostre. In cuius etcetera. Data Avinione die XX[a]II[a] mensis Februarii anno LXXX quinto.

*a)* licentiam *MS*

*See no. 162.*

## 137

*Assignation [from the Master Fr. Juan Fernández de Heredia] of maintenance to Fr. Johann von Lech in the Preceptory of Mainz for his lifetime.*

*[Avignon, 1385] May 7*

*AOM 323 fol. 156v (148v), under* prioratus Alamanie et Boemie.

Anno quo supra et die septima mensis predicti fratri Iohanni de Lech fuit assignata stagia ad vitam in baiulia Maguncie.

*Fr. Johann von Lich was co-Preceptor of Mainz on 16 September 1391: Karlsruhe, Generallandesarchiv, Abt. 20 Joh.Orden Generalia Conv. 21. A citizen of Mainz named Konrad von Lyche appeared as witness on 4 and 10 June 1396: Dertsch 3 (1965), nos. 2554, 2564.*

## 138

*Assignation [from the Master Fr. Juan Fernández de Heredia] of maintenance to Fr. Konrad von Ehenheim in the Preceptory of Schlettstadt for his lifetime.*

*[Avignon, 1385] May 7*

*AOM 323 fol. 156v (148v), under* prioratus Alamanie et Boemie.

Anno quo supra et die septima dicti mensis fuit assignata stagia fratri Cůnrado de Ehenhem in baiulia de Schletstat ad ipsius vitam.

## 139

*Licence for Fr. Rudolf von Rüdigheim to leave the Convent to rule his Preceptory of Meisenheim.*

*[Avignon, 1385 May] 7*

*AOM 323 fol. 157r (149r), under* prioratus Alamanie et Boemie.

Die septima dicti mensis fratri Rodulfo de Rudekyn preceptori de Meysekeyn data fuit licentia recedendi de conventu et eundi ad prioratum Alamanie ad regendam[a)] dictam baiuliam.

*a)* rengedam *MS*

## 140

*The Master Fr. Juan Fernández [de Heredia] grants for ten years to Fr. Stephan Kluber the Preceptory of Laa (Priory of* Alamania *[recte Bohemia]), which is vacant following the death of Fr. Johann Rinderschink.*

*Avignon, 1385 May 12*

*AOM 323 fol. 153v-4r (145v-6r), under* prioratus Alamanie et Boemie.

Frater Iohannes Ferdinandi etcetera religioso in Christo nobis carissimo fratri Stephano Klůber domus eiusdem salutem et sinceram in Domino caritatem. Ad illos libenter gratiosum nostrum favorem extendimus, quos benemeritis reputamus, ut reffecti ex gratia et hexilarati ex honore suscepto ad promovendum religionis nostre commoda libencius invigilent et ad virtutum studia ferventius animentur. Grata igitur fidedigna relatione percepto[a], quod gratiarum largitor Dominus vos morum compositione vite mundiciam et naturali discretiam virtute dotavit, sperantes in commissa vobis regimine favente Domino fructus uberes allaturum preceptoriam seu baiuliam de Loch prioratus nostri Alamanie per obitum fratris Iohannis Rindersching vacantem et ad nostram dispositionem propterea devolutam cum omnibus et singulis suis membris, iuribus et pertinentiis universis ad eam spectantibus et pertinentibus ac spectare et pertinere debentibus, quoquomodo et cum quibus illam tenuit, habuit et possedit dictus condam frater Iohannes, habendam, tenendam, regendam, gubernandam, augmentandam et meliorandam in spiritualibus et temporalibus tam in capite quam in membris sub annua responsione et aliis oneribus impositis et imponendis rationabiliter secundum communem cursum aliarum baiuliarum prioratus predicti in capitulo provinciali prioratus ipsius per vos annis singulis infallibiliter exsolvendis – alias secundum continenciam et seriem statuti super deficientibus in responsionum solutione suarum editi in generali capitulo apud Avinionem mense Martii anno sexagesimo sexto celebrato[1] de premissa baiulia per religiosos in Christo nobis carissimos fratres ·· domus eiusdem quovis titulo regimini prioratus ipsius nunc et imposterum presidentem et receptores responsionum prioratus ipsius cum consilio quatuor fratrum preceptorum prioratus iamdicti suarum baiuliarum responsiones bene solvencium fratri alicui nostre dicte domus prioratus predicti puta sufficienti, utili et ydoneo ad regimen baiulie antedicte et qui illius respontiones et alia onera bene solvat et supportet expresse precipimus provideri gracia huiusmodi de dicta baiulia vobis facta in aliquo non obstante – ad requisitionem dicte domus fratrum ·· locumnostrumtenentis in ultramarinis, baillivorum et procerum nostri Rodi conventus de nostra certa scientia et speciali gratia, voluntate, consilio et assensu eiusdem domus fratrum ·· procuratorum ipsius conventus, preceptorum et procerum nobis assistentium vobis auctoritate

1) *1367 March 5: Delaville (1913), 161–2.*

presentium hinc ad annos decem continuos et completos conferimus et donamus benefaciendo in eadem vosque preceptorem et comendatorem in dicta constituimus baiulia hac serie et eciam ordinamus. Comittentes vobis fiducialiter circa curam, regimen et administrationem accomodam dicte baiulie ac bonorum et iurium [154r] eius deffensionem et recuperationem tam in agendo quam deffendendo hac serie vices nostras. Quocirca universis et singulis fratribus, sororibus et donatis sub virtute sancte obediencie ac hominibus et vassallis et quibusvis aliis vobis subditis in dicta baiulia constitutis, presentibus et futuris sub sacramento fidelitatis et homagii, quo nobis et nostre domui sunt astricti, precipimus et mandamus, ut vobis tanquam eorum superiori, preceptori et maiori reverenter pareant, obediant et intendant vobisque suum prebeant auxilium, consilium et favorem in omnibus concernentibus utilitatem dicte baiulie, quociens opus fuerit et eos ducxeritis requirendos, necnon universis et singulis fratribus domus nostre quacumque auctoritate, dignitate vel officio fungentibus, presentibus et futuris, ne contra presentem nostram donationem et gratiam aliquatenus venire presumant, quinymo eam studeant iuxta eius mentem et seriem inviolabiliter observare, ac priori seu presidenti prefato, ut vos vel procuratorem vestrum in corporalem possessionem pacificam et quietam dicte baiulie inducat et conservet inductum omni contradictione remota amoto abinde quolibet detentore, si quis sit, quem nos amovemus per presentes et decernimus firmiter amovendum. Inhibentes vobis districtius sub virtute sancte obediencie supradicta, ne pretextu donationis et gratie nostre huiusmodi aliqua de bonis, rebus aut iuribus memorate baiulie vendatis, detis, obligetis, impignoretis, alienetis, distrahatis, permutetis seu in emphiteosim[b)] perpetuam concedatis vel quocumque alio colore quesito extra nostram religionem transferatis sine nostra speciali licencia et mandato. Et si, quod absit, contra inhibitionem nostram huiusmodi aliquid vel aliqua operari vel facere vos contingat, illud et illa exnunc prout extunc et extunc prout exnunc cassamus, anullamus ac decernimus irritum et inane nulliusque existere penitus efficacie vel valoris. In cuius etcetera. Data Avinione die duodecima Maii anno incarnationis etcetera M° CCC° LXXX V$^{to}$.

*a) ante corr.* preceptore, *recte* precepta. *b)* emphiteosum *MS*

## 141

*The Master Fr. Juan Fernández de Heredia, with consent of the procurators of the Convent and other brethren, grants for ten years to Fr. Ulrich von Weitersdorf the Preceptory of Bubikon (Priory of* Alamania*), which is vacant following the death of Fr. Werner Schürer.*

*Avignon, 1385 May 12*

*AOM 323 fol. 153r (145r), under* prioratus Alamanie et Boemie.

Frater Iohannes Ferdinandi de Redia etcetera religioso in Christo nobis carissimo fratri V̊lrico de Witerstorf[1] domus eiusdem salutem et sinceram in Domino caritatem. Dum professoribus religionis nostre benemeritis dexteram dapsillem aperimus, eorum serviciis et meritis premiis respondendo eosve dignis honoribus et condignis gratiis attollendo et ipsos ad virtutum excercitia annuamus et alios exemplariter ad consimilia invitamus. Hinc est, quoniam grata et accepta vestra obsequia Deo et nostre religioni diucius per vos prestita laudabiliter gratitudine placida prosequentes preceptoriam seu baiuliam de Bůbenkem prioratus nostri Alamanie per obitum fratris Wernheri Schinner[2] vacantem presencialiter et ad nostram dispositionem propterea devolutam cum omnibus et singulis suis membris, iuribus et pertinentiis universis ad eam spectantibus et pertinentibus ac spectare et pertinere debentibus, quoquomodo et cum quibus illam tenuit, habuit et possedit dictus condam frater Wernheri[!], habendam, tenendam, regendam, gubernandam, augmentandam et meliorandam in spiritualibus etenim in temporalibus tam in capite quam in membris sub annua respontione et aliis oneribus imposituris et imponendis rationabiliter secundum communem cursum aliarum baiuliarum prioratus predicti in capitulo provinciali prioratus ipsius per vos annis singulis infallibiliter exolvendis – alias secundum continenciam et seriem statuti super defficientibus in responsionum solutione suarum editi in generali capitulo apud Avinionem mense Martii anno sexagesimo sexto celebrato[3] de premissa baiulia per religiosos in Christo nobis carissimos fratres ·· domus eiusdem quovis titulo regimini prioratus ipsius nunc et imposterum presidentem et receptores responsionum prioratus ipsius cum consilio quatuor fratrum preceptorum prioratus iamdicti suarum baiuliarum respontiones bene solventium fratri alicui nostre dicte domus prioratus predicti puta sufficienti, utili et ydoneo ad regimen baiulie antedicte et qui illius respontiones et alia onera bene solvat et supportet expresse precipimus provideri gratia huiusmodi de dicta baiulia vobis facta in aliquo non obstante – de nostra certa scientia et speciali gratia, voluntate, consilio et assenssu eiusdem domus fratrum ·· procuratorum ipsius conventus, preceptorum et procerum nobis assistentium vobis auctoritate presencium hinc ad annos decem continuos et completos conferimus et donamus benefaciendo in eadem vosque etcetera. Comittentes etcetera. Quocirca etcetera necnon etcetera ac priori etcetera. Inhibentes etcetera. Dat. Avinione die duodecima mensis Maii anno incarnacionis Domini M° CCC° LXXX quinto.

1) *Fr. Ulrich von Weitersdorf, Preceptor of Münster, Altmühlmünster, 1377 March 16: Munich, Bayerisches Hauptstaatsarchiv, Ritterorden Urkunden 403.*

2) *Fr. Werner Schürer: Helvetia Sacra (2006), 153.*

3) *1367 March 5: Delaville (1913), 161–2.*

## 142

*The Master Fr. Juan Fernández [de Heredia], acting at the request of the Lieutenant Master and Convent on Rhodes, grants for ten years to Fr. Peter Kuttner the Preceptory of Fürstenfeld (Priory of Bohemia), which is vacant following the death of Fr. Johann Rinderschink.*

*Avignon, 1385 May 12*

*AOM 323 fol. 156r-v (148r-v), under* prioratus Alamanie et Boemie.

Frater Iohannes Ferdinandi etcetera religioso in Christo nobis carissimo fratri Petro Cutner domus eiusdem salutem et sinceram in Domino caritatem. Religionis decor, morum honestas et alia virtutum dona, quibus vos carismatis gratia insignivit, ad imparciendum vobis nostri favoris gratiam rationabiliter nos moventes, sperantes, quod in commisso vobis regimine effectus administrationis utilis favente Domino vos comendetis[a], preceptoriam Furstenvelt prioratus nostri Bohemie per obitum fratris Iohannis Rindersinch vacantem et ad nostram dispositionem propterea devolutam cum omnibus et singulis suis membris, iuribus et pertinentiis universis ad eam spectantibus et pertinentibus ac spectare et pertinere debentibus, quoquomodo et cum quibus illam tenuit, habuit et possedit dictus quondam frater Iohannes, habendam, tenendam, regendam, gubernandam, augmentandam et meliorandam in spiritualibus et in temporalibus tam in capite quam in membris sub annua respontione et aliis [156v] oneribus impositis et imponendis rationabiliter secundum communem cursum aliarum baiuliarum prioratus predicti in capitulo provinciali prioratus ipsius per vos annis singulis infallibiliter exsolvendis – alias secundum continenciam et seriem statuti super deficientibus in respontionum solutione suarum editi in generali capitulo apud Avinionem mense Martii anno sexagesimo sexto celebrato[1] de premissa baiulia per religiosos in Christo nobis carissimos fratres ·· domus eiusdem quovis titulo regimini prioratus ipsius nunc et imposterum presidentem et receptores respontionum prioratus ipsius cum consilio quatuor fratrum preceptorum prioratus iamdicti suarum baiuliarum respontiones bene solvencium[b] fratri alicui nostre dicte domus prioratus predicti puta sufficienti, utili et ydoneo ad regimen baiulie antedicte et[c] qui illius respontiones et alia onera bene solvat et supportet expresse precipimus provideri gratia huiusmodi de dicta baiulia vobis facta in aliquo non obstante – ad requisitionem dicte domus fratrum ·· locumnostrumtenentis in ultramarinis, baillivorum et procerum nostri Rodi conventus de nostra certa scientia et speciali gratia, voluntate, consilio et assensu eiusdem domus fratrum ·· procuratorum ipsius conventus, preceptorum et procerum nobis assistencium vobis auctoritate presencium hinc ad annos decem continuos et completos conferimus et donamus

1) *1367 March 5: Delaville (1913), 161–2.*

benefaciendo in eadem vosque etcetera. Comittentes etcetera. Quocirca etcetera necnon etcetera ac priori etcetera. Inhibentes etcetera. Et si, quod etcetera ut supra in foliis CXLV, CXLVI huius robure. In cuius etcetera. Dat. Avinione die XII[a] mensis Maii anno incarnationis Domini M° CCC° LXXXV[to].

Collatio commende Furstenuelt *marg. (saec. XVI). a)* comendet *MS b)* solvecium *MS c)* et *dupl.*

## 143

*The Master Fr. Juan Fernández [de Heredia], at the request of Fr. Heinrich von Wolfach, Preceptor of Grünenwörth, and with the consent of the procurators of the Convent and other brethren, confirms the incorporation of the Preceptory of Rheinau and other purchased possessions into the Preceptory of Grünenwörth. This incorporation was made by Fr. Konrad von Braunsberg, Prior of* Alamania, *and the Master was informed of it by Fr. Hesso Schlegelholz.*

*Avignon, 1385 May 12*

*AOM 323 fol. 154r-5v (146r-7v), under* prioratus Alamanie et Boemie.

Frater Iohannes[a)] Ferdinandi etcetera religioso in Christo nobis carissimo fratri Heinrico de Wolfach, baiulie de Grůnenwerd preceptori domus eiusdem salutem et sinceram in Domino caritatem. Instanter petencium desideriis libenter annuimus eaque favore prosequimur opportuno. Sane peticio pro parte vestra nobis exhibita continebat, quod dicte domus frater Cunradus de Brunsberg prior prioratus nostri Alamanie consulta [154v] deliberatione prehabita cum domus et prioratus predictorum fratribus, preceptoribus proceribusque agnoscens fructus, redditus, proventus et emolimenta dicte baiulie non posse ad status preceptoris ipsius decenciam et incumbencia supportanda onera sufficere, plena ad hec predecessoris nostri fratris Raymundi Berengarii et fratrum ·· procuratorum nostri[b)] Rodi conventus, baillivorum conventus eiusdem, priorum, preceptorum et procerum in hiis partibus in eorum capitulo generali apud Avinionem celebrato existencium potestate suffultus,[1)] dicte baiulie de Grůnenwerd univit, adiuncxit et submisit domum de Rynow ac bona quedam per ipsum priorem empta et acquisita cum suis pertinentiis ut membra perpetuis temporibus habenda, tenenda et possidenda per dicte baiulie preceptores domus nostre fratres cum debita respontione et supportacione onerum, quem

1) *March 1367: Delaville (1913), 162. – Fr. Heinrich von Wolfach was Preceptor of Grünenwörth in 1374: Krieger 2 (1905), col. 1497; his tombstone in Freiburg:* Anno domini 1404 in die Ambrosii *[April 4]* obiit Henricus Mesenus de Wolfach, commendator in Argentina*: Ruppert (1889), 295.*

domum et bona membra baiulie eiusdem tenetis et possidetis, subiungens ipsa petitio, ut pro habundanciori firmitate domus et bonorum huiusmodi unioni nostrum impartiri assensum et vobis nichilominus dictam baiuliam cum dicto domo et bonis membris unitis et aliis confirmare dignaremur[c]. Porro quia de prescripto potestate et unione nobis constitit assertione fidedigna eiusdem domus fratris Hessonis Slegelholcz, castellani Rodi, procuratoris dicti conventus et preceptoris de Rotwil, cui plenam fidem adhibemus, volentes que provida et laudabili dicte domus fratrum ordinatione sunt facta observari irrefragabiliter unionem, adiuccionem et submissionem huiusmodi ratas, gratas et firmas habentes valituras perpetuo baiuliam supradictam de Grůnenwerd cum domo de Rynow bonisque emptis et acquisitis eidem baiulie, ut prefertur, membris unitis, ipsorum iuribus, pertinentiis et aliis omnibus et singulis ad eam spectantibus et pertinentibus ac spectare et pertinere debentibus, quoquomodo et cum quibus illam tenetis, habetis et possidetis, habendam, tenendam, regendam, gubernandam, augmentandam et meliorandam in spiritualibus et temporalibus tam in capite quam in membris sub annua respontione et aliis oneribus impositis et imponendis rationabiliter secundum communem cursum aliarum baiuliarum prioratus predicti in capitulo provinciali prioratus ipsius annis singulis infallibiliter exolvendis – alias secundum continenciam [155r] et seriem statuti super defficientibus in respontionum solutione suarum editi in generali capitulo apud Avinionem de mense Martii anno sexagesimo sexto celebrato[1] de premissa baiulia per religiosos in Christo nobis carissimos fratres ·· domus eiusdem quovis titulo dicti prioratus regimini nunc vel imposterum presidentem et receptores respontionum prioratus ipsius cum consilio quatuor fratrum preceptorum prioratus iamdicti suarum baiuliarum respontiones bene solventium[d] fratri alicui nostre dicte domus prioratus predicti puta sufficienti, utili et ydoneo ad regimen baiulie antedicte et qui illius responsiones et alia onera bene solvat et supportet expresse precipimus provideri confirmatione et nova donatione huiusmodi de dicta baiulia vobis facta in aliquo non obstante – de voluntate, consilio et assensu dicte domus fratrum ·· procuratorum dicti[e] conventus, priorum, preceptorum et procerum nobis assistentium de nostra certa scientia vobis ad dictam et eidem baiulie de Grůnenwerd domum de Rynow et bona huiusmodi membra unita per imperpetuum auctoritate presentis assembleie confirmamus et ad maiorem cautelam concedimus et unimus vosque preceptorem et comendatorem in dicta constituimus baiulia hac serie et eciam ordinamus. Comittentes vobis fiducialiter circa curam, regimen et administrationem accomodam dicte baiulie ac dictorum membrorum bonorum et iurium eius deffentionem et recuperationem tam in agendo quam deffendendo hac serie vices nostras. Quocirca universis et singulis fratribus, sororibus et donatis sub virtute sancte obediencie ac hominibus et vassallis et quibusvis aliis vobis subditis in baiulia, membris et bonis predictis constitutis, presentibus et futuris sub sacramento fidelitatis et homagii, quo nobis et nostre domui sunt astricti, precipimus et mandamus, ut vobis tamquam eorum superiori, preceptori et maiori reverenter pareant, obediant et intendant vobisque suum prebeant auxilium, consilium et favorem in omnibus concernentibus utilitatem dictorum baiulie et membrorum, quociens opus fuerit et eos ducxeritis requirendos, necnon universis et singulis fratribus domus nostre quacumque auctoritate, dignitate vel officio fungentibus, presentibus et futuris, [155v] ne contra presentes nostras confirmationem, donationem, unionem, adiunctionem et submissionem seu coadunationem aliquatenus venire presumant, quinymo eas studeant iuxta earum mentem et seriem inviolabiliter observare. Inhibentes vobis districtius sub virtute sancte obedientie supradicta, ne pretextu confirmationis[f)], donationis et unionis nostre huiusmodi aliqua de bonis, rebus aut iuribus memorate baiulie vendatis, detis, obligetis, impignoretis, alienetis, distrahatis, permutetis seu in emphiteosim perpetuam concedatis vel quocumque alio colore quesito extra nostram religionem transferatis sine nostra speciali licentia et mandato. Et si, quod absit, contra inhibitionem nostram huiusmodi aliquid vel aliqua operari vel facere vos contingat, illud et illa exnunc prout extunc et extunc prout exnunc cassamus, anullamus ac decernimus irritum et inane nulliusque existere penitus efficacie vel valoris. In cuius etcetera. Data Avinione die duodecima Maii anno incarnacionis Domini M° CCC° LXXX quinto.

*a)* etcetera *del.* *b)* enim *del.* *c)* dugnaremur *MS* *d)* solventum *MS* *e)* dicti *dupl.* *f)* confirmatonis *MS*

## 144

*The Master Fr. Juan Fernández [de Heredia], with the consent of the procurators of the Convent and other brethren, grants for ten years to Fr. Bertrand Tobel the Preceptory of Tobel (Priory of* Alamania), *which is vacant following the death of an unnamed person.*

*Avignon, 1385 May 12*

*AOM 323 fol. 155v-6r (147v-8r), under* prioratus Alamanie et Boemie.

Frater Iohannes Ferdinandi etcetera religioso in Christo nobis carissimo fratri Berhtrando Duetil domus eiusdem salutem et sinceram in Domino caritatem. Vestrorum comendabilium gratia meritorum ac sperantes, quod in commisso vobis regimine effectus administrationis utilis dante Domino vos comendetis[a)], vobis ad gratiam redditi liberales, ut propterea de bono in melius vestre sinceritatis affectus fervencius animetur, preceptoriam seu baiuliam de Tueli prioratus nostri Alamanie per obitum fratris ·· ultimi preceptoris seu quovis alio modo vacantem et ad nostram dispositionem propterea devolutam cum omnibus et singulis suis membris, iuribus et pertinentiis universis ad eam spectantibus et pertinentibus ac spectare et pertinere debentibus, quoquomodo[b)] et cum quibus illam tenuit, habuit et possedit dictus quondam frater ··, habendam, tenendam, regendam, gubernandam, augmentandam et meliorandam in spiritualibus et in temporalibus tam in capite quam in membris sub annua respontione et aliis oneribus impositis et imponendis rationabiliter secundum communem cursum aliarum baiuliarum prioratus [156r] predicti in capitulo provinciali prioratus ipsius per vos annis singulis infallibiliter exsolvendis – alias secundum continenciam et seriem statuti super defficientibus in respontionum solutione suarum editi in generali capitulo apud Avinionem mense Martii anno sexagesimo sexto celebrato[1] de premissa baiulia per religiosos in Christo nobis carissimos fratres ·· domus eiusdem quovis titulo regimini prioratus ipsius nunc et imposterum presidentem et receptores respontionum prioratus ipsius cum consilio quatuor fratrum preceptorum prioratus iamdicti suarum baiuliarum respontiones bene solvencium fratri alicui nostre dicte domus prioratus predicti puta sufficienti, utili et ydoneo ad regimen baiulie antedicte et qui illius responsiones et alia onera bene solvat et supportet expresse precipimus provideri gratia huiusmodi de dicta baiulia vobis facta in aliquo non obstante – de nostra certa scientia et speciali gratia, voluntate, consilio et assensu eiusdem domus fratrum ·· procuratorum nostri Rodi conventus, preceptorum et procerum nobis assistencium vobis auctoritate presencium hinc ad annos decem continuos et completos conferimus et donamus benefaciendo in eadem vosque etcetera. Comittentes etcetera. Quocirca etcetera necnon etcetera ac priori etcetera. Inhibentes etcetera. Et si, quod etcetera ut supra in foliis CXLV, CXLVI huius robure. In cuius etcetera. Data Avinione die XII[a] Maii anno incarnationis Domini M° CCC° LXXXV[to].

*a)* comendet *MS* *b)* quoquio *ante corr.*

## 145

*The Master Fr. Riccardo [Caracciolo], after consultation with an assembly of brethren, attaches the preceptories in the March of Brandenburg and in Saxony to the Priory of Bohemia, Poland and Austria[!]. The reason is that some Hospitallers in Brandenburg and Saxony refuse to be obedient to the Prior of* Alamania, *who is unable to enforce obedience. What is worse, these Hospitallers have started to sell houses and castles of the Hospital to laymen. Now the Prior of Bohemia, Poland and Austria is to rule them.*

*Cicciano, 1385 May 16*

*AOM 281 fol. 68r-v.*

Frater Ricardus etcetera unacum fratribus etcetera[1] venerabili religioso in Christo nobis carissimo fratri Symovito duci Thasinensi priori prioratus nostri

1) *March 1367: Delaville (1913), 162. – Probably the Preceptory of Tobel, although Fr. Ulrich von Tettingen was its preceptor from 1378 to 1405: Helvetia Sacra (2006), 495.*

1) *The phrase* unacum fratribus etcetera *refers to a chapter general in nos. 129 and 153. But nos. 145, 146, 149 and 150 were not dated* durante nostro capitulo generali. *Cf. Delaville (1913), 255 with note 1. So the meeting here was probably more than just a consultation with counsellors and less than a chapter general.*

Boemie, Polonie et Austrie salutem etcetera. Cum nos ex declaracione fidedigna evidenter, quod singuli preceptores, commendatores, rectores, gubernatores et fratres domorum nostrarum in partibus marchionatus Brandeburgensis et Saxonie consistentes priori prioratus nostri Almanie, sub cuius prioratus regimine ab olim fuerunt constituti, aliquatenus[a)] obedire non curant nec intendant et quia dictus prior eos non potest ad sui obedienciam reducere nec eos propter eorum excessus condigne punire presumentes, quod deterius est, domos et castra in illis partibus nostre religioni subiectas et subiecta vendere secularibus et a nostra religione minus iuste alienare et auferre, unde nostra religio gravia et illicita patitur detrimenta et quibus non succurratur tempestive de die in diem pacietur graviora, ut manifestis indiciis experimur et sentimus. Nos vero intendentes, ut de remedio oportuno salubriter providere et ut dictorum fratrum compescatur temeritas, ne amplius similia attemptare[b)] presumant, ut et nostra religio in illis partibus non permittatur diminui, set pocius realiter augmentari, habito[c)] super predictis consilio et deliberatione matura cum fratribus nobis assistentibus domus eiusdem in ecclesia castri nostri Cizani ad sonum campane capitulariter congregatis, ut moris est, in unum convenientibus omnes et singulas preceptorias, domorum nostrarum villas, loca et castra in partibus marchionatus Brandeburgensis et Saxonie predictis consistentes et nostre domui subiectas exnunc prioratui nostro Boemie et Polonie predicto unimus[d)], anectimus et incorporamus ita et taliter, ut singuli fratres dictarum preceptoriarum exnunc[e)] et imperpetuum sub vera obedientia prioratus predicti existant et sub eius regimine, ut[f)] secundum aliarum preceptoriarum consuetudinem dicti prioratus debeant gubernari necnon preceptores et fratres domorum nostrarum predictarum elevantes a gubernacione priori prioratus nostri Almanie predicti et eius successorum eosdem ab eisdem realiter exemptos decernimus et declaramus. Vos autem priorem Boemie, Polonie et Austrie predictum propter vestra virtutum merita et circumspeccionis industriam et vestros legitimos successores in marchionatu Brandeburgensi et Saxonia tamquam eidem nostro prioratui predicto canonice annexis priorem[g)] predictarum parcium de nostra certa scientia et speciali gratia auctoritate presencium constituimus gratiose et ordinamus benefaciendo in eisdem. Committentes tibi fiducialiter circa curam, regimen et administracionem accomodam predictarum parcium defensionem et recuperacionem tam in agendo quam defendendo hac serie vices nostras. Quocirca universis et singulis fratribus etcetera in partibus marchionatus Brandeburgensis et Saxonie predictis constitutis, presentibus et futuris, ut vobis tamquam eorum superiori et maiori reverenter pareant, obediant et intendant vobisque suum prebeant consilium, auxilium et favorem in omnibus concernentibus utilitatem tocius prioratus predicti, quociens opus fuerit et eos duxeritis requirendos. Mandantes insuper omnibus et singulis preceptoribus et fratribus in dictis partibus marchionatus et Saxonie constitutis, presentibus et futuris sub virtute sancte obediencie predicta, ut prioratui nostro Boemie predicto eorum responsiones et alia debita singulis annis infallibiliter solvere procurent, prout prioratui nostro Almanie solvere tenebantur. Necnon universis etcetera, ne contra hanc unionem, incorporacionem, constitucionem et ordinacionem aliquatenus venire presumant etcetera ac religiosis in Christo nobis carissimis fratribus domus eiusdem Iohanni preceptori Vratislaviensi et Iohanni de Viqueria preceptori Sucioli,[2] ut vos vel procuratorem vestrum in possessionem publicam dictarum parcium marchionatus et Saxonie exnunc et inantea sub regimine dicti prioratus nostri Boemie pertinencium, ut decrevimus, inducant et conservent[h] inductum. Inhibentes vobis districtius etcetera. Datum in castro nostro Cizani[3] [i]Nolane diocesis[i] die XVI Maii anno incarnacionis Domini M° CCC^mo^ LXXXV.

Unio marchionatus Brandeburgensis prioratui Boemie *marg.* *a)* alioratinus *MS* *b)* pre *praem. ante corr.* *c)* habitio s *praem. ante corr.* *d)* anneximus *del. in lin.*, unimus *add. marg.* *e)* exnuc *MS* *f)* ut *supra lin.* *g)* priores *ante corr.* *h)* conservet *MS* *i-i) supra lin.*

## 146

*The Master Fr. Riccardo [Caracciolo], after consultation with an assembly of brethren, confirms Fr. Hugo von Wechingen for his lifetime in the Preceptory of Mailberg (Priory of Bohemia).*

*Cicciano, [13]85 May 16*

*AOM 281 fol. 68v-9r.*

Frater Ricardus etcetera unacum etcetera religioso in Christo nobis carissimo fratri Hugoni de Wechingen domus eiusdem preceptori domus nostre Maurpurg prioratus nostri Boemie districtus Austrie salutem etcetera. Extimamus digne agere etcetera. Attendentes itaque, quod in administracione dicte baiulie etcetera. Igitur preceptoriam predictam, quam hactenus digne tenuisti et tenes, cum omnibus et singulis suis menbris etcetera invicem deliberato consilio de nostra certa scientia et speciali gratia ad vitam tuam, quamdiu omnipotens tibi dederit in humanis, tibi tamquam digne et benemerite auctoritate presencium confirmamus et de uberiori dono gratie de novo conferimus, concedimus et gratiose donamus benefaciendo in eadem te quiete sine executore. In cuius etcetera. Datum in castro nostro Cizani Nolane diocesis die XVI mensis Maii anno LXXXV.

Confirmatio in prioratu Boemie fratris Hugonis *marg.*

*Dauber (1998), 583, mentions Fr. Haug von Wehing as Preceptor of Mailberg in 1387.*

2) *To the Preceptors of Breslau Fr. Johann and of Sacile (near Udine in the Priory of Venice) Fr. Giovanni Vicheria; cf. A. Strnad, s. v. Riccardo Caracciolo, DBI 19 (1976), 443–6.*

3) *Cicciano, 35 km north-east of Naples.*

## 147

*The Master Fr. Juan Fernández [de Heredia] assigns maintenance to Heimerin von Maastricht for his lifetime as a donat in Heitersheim, a member of the Preceptory of Freiburg.*

*Avignon, 1385 May 17*

*AOM 323 fol. 157r (149r), under* prioratus Alamanie et Boemie. *Cf. van Winter (1998), 32 no. 6.*

Frater Iohannes Ferdinandi etcetera dilecto nobis in Christo Heimerino de Mastricht salutem in Domino. Quia ex premio fides crescit et remunerata servitia ad obsequendum fervencius solicitant servitores, non indigne fidelia et accepta tua servicia nostre prestita religioni et que te prestiturum inantea speramus remuneratione prosequimur gratie specialis. Quamobrem victum[a)] et vestitum dari et assignari consuetum uni donato dicte domus et ab eodem percipi et haberi de nostra certa sciencia et speciali gratia, de voluntate et assensu domus eiusdem fratrum ·· nobis assistentium tibi, quamdiu vitam ducxeritis in humanis, in domo nostra de Heutershein membro baiulie de Friburgo tenore presencium assignamus, concedimus et donamus bene et fideliter serviendo in domo predicta. Quocirca religioso in Christo nobis carissimo fratri ·· baiulie et membri predictorum nunc et imposterum regimini presidenti quovis titulo sub virtute sancte obediencie precipimus districte iniungentes, quatenus tibi in tuis necessariis consuetis dari et assignari uni donato domus eiusdem provideat et administret secundum usus et consuetudines domus nostre. Mandantes sub dicta virtute sancte obediencie omnibus et singulis domus eiusdem fratribus presentibus et futuris quacumque dignitate vel officio fungentibus, ne contra assignationem, donacionem et gratiam nostram huiusmodi aliquatenus venire presumant, quinymo illam studeant inviolabiliter observare. In cuius etcetera. Dat. Avinione die XVII[a] Maii anno incarnationis Domini M° CCC° LXXXV[to].

*a)* vitum *MS*

## 148

*Licence [from the Master Fr. Juan Fernández de Heredia] for the Castellan of Rhodes and Preceptor of Rottweil Fr. Hesso Schlegelholz to receive two nobles as knight brethren into the Order, who are to travel to Rhodes.*

*[Avignon, 1385] May 17*

*AOM 323 fol. 157r (149r), under* prioratus Alamanie et Boemie.

Die XVII mensis Maii anno quo supra fratri Hessoni Slegelehoz, castellano Rodi et preceptori de Rotwil, data fuit licentia recipiendi viros duos in fratres religiosos, dum nobiles sint utroque parente[a)] thoro procreatos legitimo et habeant membrorum integritatem ipsos prius decoratos milicia, quibus receptis datur licentia eundi ad conventum cum equis et armis, ut moris est, requisita ab ipsorum superiore licentia.

*a)* parante *MS*

## 149

*The Master Fr. Riccardo [Caracciolo], after consultation with an assembly of brethren, confirms a donation made by Fr. Duke Ziemovit von Teschen, Prior of Bohemia and Poland, the Mark of Brandenburg and Saxony. For 2,000 marks of groats of Prague Polish style, Fr. Ziemovit has bought estates inherited from his father and ancestors. These estates, four villages which pay 123 marks and nine homesteads, he has incorporated into the Preceptory of Oels. So far there lived 13 persons at Oels with its church of St. Mary, one priest, the others knights and sergeants. From now on there are to be one preceptor, eight priests, four lay sergeants-at-office and six secular clerics for celebrating every day the canonical hours and three masses. The prior of the house at Oels is to receive 50 marks each year. From these revenues the prior is to pay 2 marks to each priest, one mark to each sergeant-at-office, and to each secular cleric 60 groats and one tunic, and 20 marks he has to distribute as a common* pitancia *among all these persons on 1 November.*

*Cicciano, 1385 May 20*

*AOM 281 fol. 67r-8r.*

Frater Riccardus etcetera venerabili religioso in Christo nobis carissimo fratri Symouito duci Thasinensi priori prioratus nostri Boemie, Polonie, Austrie, marchionatus Brandeburgensis et Saxonie salutem etcetera. Cum fidedignorum testimonio relatibus animo evidenti percepimus, quod vos ecclesiam domus nostre in Olsna Wratislaviensis diocesis prioratus nostri predicti, in qua ab olim tredecim persone, quorum erat frater presbiter et alii fratres milites et servientes, ad gubernandam dictam ecclesiam in honore beate Marie virginis fundatam et dedicatam esse consueverunt, considerantes de eius sufficienti et laudabili regimine parati detrimentum intendentes dictam domum nostram secundum bonos usus et laudabiles mores nostre religionis salubriter augmentare constituistis et ordinastis ab anno et citra, quod in eadem domo nostra sunt et debent esse omnibus[a)] temporibus tredecim fratres domus nostre, videlicet unus preceptor, octo sacerdotes et quatuor laici officiales et sex clerici seculares, qui dicte ecclesie domus nostre in Olsna die noctuque secundum laudabiles mores nostre religionis deserviunt et horas canonicas, primam missam beate Marie virginis in aurora, secundam vero missam pro fidelibus defunctis et terciam missam diei horis debitis et competentibus singulis diebus inibi celebrant per notas decantando et vos decernentes, quod redditus, fructus et facultas predicte domus nostre aliquibus annis propter hospitalitatem advenientem ibidem servatam minime sufficiebant, emistis et comparastis pro pecuniis duorum milium marcharum grossorum Pragensium mensure Polonicalium ad vos, ut asseritur, iure hereditario et paterna successione devolutis redditus et proventus perpetuos centum et viginti trium marcharum monete predicte in villis Mergenaw, Hermansdorf, Brositz et Czanctentzitz districtus Strolmensis Wratislaviensis diocesis,[1] que ad dominum ducem terre Strolmensi iure ducali antiquitus pertinebant, ac eciam allodium novem mansorum Swegoni nuncupatum,[2] que quidem redditus et proventus dicte domui nostre Olsne de novo incorporastis per eosdem preceptorem, fratres, clericos percipiendos, possidendos sub tali distributione, videlicet, quod prior dicte ecclesie domus nostre in Olsna primo et pre omnibus percipiat et recipiat singulis annis de eisdem redditibus quinquaginta marcas, de quibus quinquaginta marcis cuilibet sacerdoti due marce, cuilibet fratri laico servienti unam marcam pro usu et comparacione necessariorum suorum, sex vero clericis secularibus ibidem, ut predicitur, serviencibus cuilibet eorum una sexagena grossorum et una tunica[b] et pro communi pietantia fratrum et clericorum predictorum viginti marce singulis annis perpetuis temporibus absque contradicione in festo sancti Martini exsolvantur et quod residuum predictorum[c] reddituum et fructuum ac obvenciones et utilitates de predictis bonis provenientes, quocumque nomine, causa vel racione censeantur, ad manus predicti preceptoris perveniant pro utilitate domus predicte et necessariis fratribus benigne administrandis. Nos igitur super premissis ordinacione, constitucione et incorporacione habito consilio unacum fratribus nobis assistentibus domus eiusdem considerantes nostram religionem exinde laudabiliter augmentare de nostra certa scientia et speciali gratia auctoritate presencium predictam constitucionem, ordinacionem et incorporacionem confirmamus, ratificamus et approbamus decernentes eam perpetuo valituram. Mandantes universis et singulis fratribus domus nostre etcetera, ne contra hanc nostram confirmacionem, ratificacionem et approbacionem dictarum constitucionis, ordinacionis et incorporacionis aliquatenus venire presumant. In cuius etcetera. Datum in castro nostro Cizani die XX mensis Maii anno incarnacionis Domini millesimo trecentesimo octuagesimo quinto.

Confirmatio cuiusdam constitutionis facte per priorem Boemie *marg.* *a)* omnes *MS* *b) del.* *c)* per *praem. ante corr.*

## 150

*The Master Fr. Riccardo [Caracciolo], after consultation with an assembly of brethren, orders Fr. Konrad von Braunsberg, Prior of* Alamania, *to respond within one month of the presentation of the present letter to charges that he does not support Pope Urban VI.*

1) *Strehlen in the diocese of Breslau with the villages of Marienau, Hermsdorf, Brosewitz, and Tschammendorf in the district of Strehlen.*

2) *Not identified.*

*Three times Fr. Giovanni de Vicheria, who is constituted to reform the Order, has been sent with letters to procure Fr. Konrad's obedience. For the first time he presented letters of Urban VI and Cardinal Tommaso, protector of the Order, in July 1381 at Straßburg. But the brethren there continued to adhere to Robert [of Geneva, Clement VII], as did the pretended Master Fr. Juan Fernández de Heredia and many brethren in the Convent. Then Cardinal Tommaso died and Fr. Giovanni de Vicheria was reappointed by Cardinal [Nicola] of S. Ciriaco, protector of the Order. Again he presented his letters in September 1383 in Lower Alamania. And for the third time he presented letters of the Master Fr. Riccardo in July 1384 at Cologne. Now Fr. Konrad is peremptorily ordered to return to obedience within one month of the presentation of the present letter and to pay all responsions, arrears of responsions,* spolia, *pension payments for the Master's chamber and other dues.*

*Cicciano, [13]85 May 20*

*AOM 281 fol. 70v-71r.*

Frater Ricardus etcetera unacum fratribus etcetera venerabili religioso in Christo nobis carissimo fratri Conrado de Brunsberg domus eiusdem priori prioratus nostri Almanie salutem etcetera. Intenti magisterii incumbit officio subiectos sibi redditos vigili cura preservare a noxiis[a] et illa, si quando ingruerint, salubris remediis adhibicione amovere. Nuper siquidem non sine mentis perturbacione ad nostrum pervenit auditum[b], quod, cum frater Iohannes de Viqueria domus eiusdem veniens ad partes Almanie, scilicet anno LXXXI[mo] de mense Iulii litteras sanctissimi in Christo patris et domini nostri domini Urbani divina providentia pape VI[ti] necnon litteras reverendissimi patris et domini condam fratris Thome episcopi Tuscolani olim sacrosancte Romane ecclesie cardinalis protectoris, correctoris et reformatoris nostre religionis[1] a dicto domino nostro domino Urbano tunc specialiter deputati tamquam commissarius vobis in civitate Argentina personaliter presentavit inter cetera continentes, quod omnes et singuli priores, commendatores et fratres domus nostre in quibuscumque partibus consistentes Iohanni Ferdinandi de Heredia se pro magistro hospitalis tunc gerenti in reprobum sensum dato ac immitatori dampnati scismatis, qui dampnato Roberto antipape ausu temerario adherere et in omnibus quibus potuit favere presumpsit et presumit ac eciam fratribus conventus Rodi in aliquo non deberent obedire nec eisdem consilium, auxilium vel favorem aliquatenus exhibere, postea vero, sicud Deo placuit, demum reverendissimus pater frater Thomas diem suum clausit extremum,

1) *Tommaso da Fregnano, a Franciscan from Modena, on 18 September 1378 created by Urban VI cardinal priest of SS. Nereo e Achilleo, also called of Tusculum, died at Rome on 19 November 1381: Eubel 1 (1898), 23 no. 27/1.*

loco cuius reverendissimus pater et dominus dominus cardinalis sancti Ciriaci[2] a dicto domino nostro in protectorem nostre religionis ut supra specialiter fuit deputatus, cuius reverendissimi patris litteras tenore mandati ac inhibicionis ut supra dictus frater Iohannes de Viqueria tamquam commissarius iterato ad partes Almanie et Boemie veniens anno LXXXIII° de mense Septembris vobis in quadam terra ab inferioribus partibus Almanie iterum personaliter presentavit, quiquidem frater Iohannes vos in presentia fratrum domus nostre ex parte dicti nostri pape et cardinalis tamquam commissarius iuratus in quolibet predictarum presentacione videlicet anno LXXXI et LXXXIII in virtute sancte obedientie et sub pena privacionis dignitatis, ut moris est, requisivit, quod vos mandatis dicti domini nostri pape et cardinalis deberetis fideliter obedire, eorum litteras iuxta earum seriem et tenorem inviolabiliter observare, nichilominus nos, postquam per dictum dominum nostrum papam in magistrum hospitalis sancti Iohannis Ierosolimitani predicti fuimus creati legitime et assumpti, nostras litteras similiter vobis per dictum fratrem Iohannem personaliter duximus destinandas, quas vobis in civitate Coloniensi de mense Iulii anno LXXXIIII[to] iterum personaliter presentavit, vos autem indurato corde mandatis domini nostri pape, predicti cardinalis ac nostri numquam curastis obedire, ymo verius per omnem modum, quo potuistis, predictis tribus mandatis successive vobis presentatis ut prefertur requisicione semper mediante ausu temerario studuistis contraire ac eciam nobis de vestris responsionibus, arreragiis et aliis quibuscumque nobis et hospitali nostro debitis numquam curastis respondere in vestre anime preiudicium non modicum et gravamen. Quapropter non modicum cogimur ammirari, quoniam ad vestri officii dignitatem rationabiliter spectat nostram religionem augmentare, quod obscura temeritati suadente perpendere non valetis. Nos igitur volentes, ut similia presumentibus in exemplum precludatur vos ad nostram presenciam repellimus necnon tenore presencium vobis in virtute sancte obedientie pro primo, secundo, tercio, peremptorio termino districte precipiendo mandamus, quatenus infra unius mensis spacium a die presentacionis presencium vobis seu locumtenentibus aut procuratoribus vestris in cameris vestris constitutis presentandum computandum iter vestrum arripiatis ad veram obedientiam domini nostri predicti et nostri personaliter transiturus de predictis omnibus et singulis vos realiter excusantes nobisque de omnibus vestris responsionibus, arreragiis, spoliis et pecuniis camere nostre ac de aliis quibuscumque nobis et hospitali nostro debitis integre satisfacientes, que, si facere non curaveritis, contra vos ad graviora procedemus tamquam contra domino nostro predicto et nobis inobedientem, prout ordo iuris secundum nostre religionis statuta

2) *Nicola Moschino, a Dominican from Naples, through his mother perhaps related with the Caracciolo, on 18 September 1378 created by Urban VI cardinal priest of S. Ciriaco alle Terme, died on 29 July 1389: Eubel 1 (1898), 23 no. 27/7; G. Barone, s. v. Nicola Moschino Caracciolo, DBI 19 (1976), 435–7.*

postulat et requirit. In cuius etcetera bulla etcetera. Datum in castro nostro Cizani Nolane diocesis die XX mensis Maii anno etcetera LXXXV[to].

Bulla prioris Almanie *marg.* *a)* a nostis *praem. ante corr.* *b)* ad praem. *ante corr.*

## 151

*A note that Sulz is the Master's chamber in* Alamania *and is held by Fr. Reinhard Söler [from the registers of Fr. Riccardo Caracciolo].*

*[1385]*

*AOM 281 fol. 75r.*

Camera magistri in prioratu Alamanie vocatur Sultz et eam tenet frater Reynhardus Solre.

## 152

*The Preceptor of Mailberg Fr. Hugo von Wechingen is retained by the Master [Fr. Riccardo Caracciolo].*

*Genoa, [1386] January 11*

*AOM 281 fol. 80v.*

Item fuit facta littera retencionis pro fratre Hugone Wechingen preceptori Maurperg prioratus Boemie sub bulla data Ianue die undecima mensis Ianuarii ut supra.

## 153

*The Master Fr. Riccardo [Caracciolo] summons, at papal command, the Priors of Bohemia and* Alamania, *Fr. Duke Ziemovit von Teschen and Fr. Konrad von Braunsberg, with four preceptors each, to a chapter general at Genoa or elsewhere on 1 November 1386. They are to take with them the responsions, arrears of responsions*, spolia *and other dues to the Treasury plus full information about the state of their priories. If it is not safe for them to come, they may send a procurator.*

*Genoa, [13]86 April 10*

*AOM 281 fol. 85v-6r.*

Frater Riccardus etcetera venerabilibus et religiosis in Christo nobis carissimis fratribus domus eiusdem Symouito duci Tassinensi et Conrado de Brunsbergh, prioratuum nostrorum Boemie et Almanie prioribus, necnon universis et singulis prioribus, preceptoribus et fratribus domus eiusdem, ad quos presentes pervenerint seu certa noticia eorundem, salutem et sinceram in Domino caritatem. Cum sanctissimus in Christo pater et dominus noster dominus Urbanus divina providencia papa sextus ac reverendissimus pater et dominus dominus Nycolaus miseracione divina tituli sancti Ciriaci sacrosancte Romane ecclesie presbiter cardinalis[1] nostre religionis protector, corrector et reformator ab eodem domino nostro papa specialiter deputatus nobis vive vocis oraculo mandaverit et iunxerit, ut capitulum generale unacum singulis prioribus, preceptoribus et fratribus domus nostre dicto domino nostro et nobis subiectis, quibus interest seu interesse poterit quoquomodo, propter nonnulla nostra et nostre religionis negocia in Christo capitulo divina favente clemencia pro bono statu ipsius nostre religionis, ad quam prefatus sanctissimus dominus noster speciali devocione afficitur, salubriter ordinanda et necessaria reformanda celebrare curaremus, nos igitur volentes procedere ut tenemur premissa executioni debite, quantum ex alto nobis permittitur, demandando vos fratres Symouitum et Conradum priores predictos ac omnes et singulos priores dicte domus nostre ubilibet constitutis auctoritate presencium requirimus, monemus et hortamur attentius vobisque nichilominus et vestrum cuilibet in virtute sancte obediencie et sub pena suspensionis a vestris administracionibus districte, precise et peremptorie precipiendo mandamus, quatenus singuli vestrum cum quatuor saltem vestrorum prioratuum subiectis preceptoribus per vos eligendis, qui de statu ipsorum prioratuum plenarie sint informati, ac eadem auctoritate requirendis, monendis ad infrascripta et hortandis, quos vos eciam exnunc sub pena et virtute predictis requirimus, monemus et hortamur, Ianue vel alibi, ubi tunc dominum nostrum papam cum sua curia residere contingerit, in festo Omnium Sanctorum de mense Novembris proxime venturi personaliter legitimo impedimento cessante, alias per procuratores legitimos fratres domus nostre ydoneos cum pleno mandato specialiter ad supra- et infrascripta studeatis remoto cuilibet difficultatis obstaculo convenire. Responsiones quoque singulas, arreragia, spolia et alia quecumque nobis et thesauro nostro debitas et debita ac plenam informacionem de statu [a]et circumstanciis[a] ipsorum prioratuum ad ipsum capitulum vobiscum, si tute fieri poterit, apportetis seu per fidelem[b] procuratorem et nuncium destinare curetis ipsum generale capitulum legitime celebraturi, dispondituri et ordinaturi aliaque facturi ad reformacionem nostre religionis, prout in quibusdam litteris citatoriis super huiusmodi generalis capituli celebracione per dictum dominum cardinalem emanatis plenius et seriosius enarrantur. Alioquin contra vos et vestrum quemlibet inobedientem[c] seu rebellem ac premissa iuxta dicti domini cardinalis et nostri huiusmodi mandata adimplere non curantes ad graviora procedemus, prout secundum nostre religionis statuta dictaverit ordo racionis. In cuius rei etcetera. Datum Ianue die decima mensis Aprilis anno LXXX sexto.

*a-a) marg.* *b)* fidum *ante corr.* *c)* inobediencie *MS*

*1) No. 150 note 2.*

## 154

*The Master Fr. Riccardo [Caracciolo] orders the Priors of Bohemia, Fr. Duke Ziemovit von Teschen, and of* Alamania, *Fr. Konrad von Braunsberg, to pay 20 florins each to the Master's notary and familiar, master Gerard Enschede, for the delivery of his summons to the next chapter general.*

*Genoa, 1[3]86 April 11*

*AOM 281 fol. 85r.*

Frater Riccardus etcetera venerabilibus religiosis in Christo nobis carissimis fratribus domus eiusdem Symovito duci Tassinensi et Conrado de Brunsbergh, prioratuum nostrorum Boemie et Almanie prioribus, et eorum cuilibet insolidum salutem et sinceram in Domino caritatem. Cum discretum virum magistrum Gerardum Enschede, nostrum notarium et familiarem predilectum, nuncium iuratum a reverendissimo patre et domino domino Nycolao miseracione divina tituli sancti Ciriaci sacrosancte Romane ecclesie presbitero cardinali nostre religionis protectore[1)] ad infrascripta specialiter deputatum ad Boemie, Almanie et nonnullas alias partes pro nostris et nostre religionis negociis ac generali capitulo Ianue vel alibi, ubi tunc dominum nostrum papam cum sua curia residere contingerit, in festo Omnium Sanctorum de mense Novembris proxime venturi de mandato ipsius domini nostri pape celebrando fideliter exequendis, prout in litteris citatoriis per dictum dominum cardinalem ac nostris mandatis super hoc emanatis plenius continetur, duxerimus presencialiter destinandum, vos et vestrum quemlibet seriose rogamus, requirimus, monemus et hortamur attencius vobisque nichilominus tenore presencium et vestrum cuilibet in virtute sancte obediencie districte precipiendo mandamus, quatenus eundem Gerardum suscipientes propensius commendatum quilibet vestrum de suo prioratu eidem pro suo labore, sallario et expensis florenos viginti auri secundum bonos usus domus nostre ministretis, tradatis, solvatis realiter et assignetis dilectione qualibet penitus pretermissa, ut huiusmodi nostre religionis negocia per prefatum Gerardum ut premittitur exequenda debitum sortiantur effectum et occasione prorogationis vel dilacionis huiusmodi viginti florenorum per vos et vestrum quemlibet ad cuiuslibet tamen preceptoris sive commendatoris prioratuum predictorum debitam proporcionem sibi solvendorum impediri non valeant quomodolibet vel differri ipsumque Gerardum in eundo, stando et redeundo habeatis graciosius recommissum taliter facientes in premissis, quod de vestra vera et solita obediencia merito possitis in Domino commendari quodque deinde suo tempore vobis gratiam teneamur salubrius impartiri. In cuius rei testimonium bulla nostra plumbea presentibus est appensa. Data Ianue die undecima mensis Aprilis anno incarnacionis Domini millesimo LXXX sexto.

1) *No. 150 note 2. The following entry is the same order to the lieutenant of the Prior of England (fol. 85v).*

## 155

*The Master Fr. Riccardo [Caracciolo] issues a letter of safe-conduct to his notary and familiar, Gerard Enschede, who is being sent to Italy,* Alamania, *Bohemia and England.*
*Genoa, [1386] April 17*

*AOM 281 fol. 88v.*

Frater Riccardus etcetera universis et singulis magnatibus, dominis, prelatis, ducibus, comitibus, baronibus, militibus, nobilibus ac nobis sincere carissimis comitatibus, potestatibus, prioribus, rectoribus, capitaneis, vigeriis, bailivis, baiulis, castellanis, pedagiatoribus, lendariis, gabellatoribus et receptoribus rene seu redibencie ceterisque iusticiariis portuumque et passuum quorumcumque[a)] custodibus et aliis, ad quos presentes nostre littere pervenerint, salutem et sinceram in Domino caritatem. Cum dilectus notarius et familiaris noster Gerardus Enschede, presencium exhibitor, ad Ytalie, Almanie, Boemie et Anglie partes pro quibusdam nostris et[b)] nostre religionis peragendis negociis accedat, vos et vestrum quemlibet ac universitatem vestram attente rogamus, quatenus eundem Gerardum, familiarem nostrum, cum arnesiis, raubis et rebus suis quibuscumque ac[c)] personis in sua comitiva existentibus per loca, passus, portus, terras et districtus vestros quoscumque, in quibus ipsum Gerardum familiarem nostrum proficisci contingerit, absque solucione pedagii vel gabelle transitum facientem eundo et redeundo absque aliquo impedimento nostri contemplacione et amore transire libere permittatis sibique de salvo et securo conductu, si indiguerit, nichilominus graciose providentes taliter, ut idem Gerardus nobis, dum redierit Deo duce, de vestra benivolencia super premissis per vos signanter acceptis gratanter et admissis relacionem valeat benigniter exhibere, quodque vobis exinde reddere teneamur actiones condignas gratiarum. In cuius rei testimonium bulla nostra plumbea presentibus est appensa. Datum Ianue die XVII mensis Aprilis.

*a)* quorucumque *MS* *b)* p *praem.* *c) supra lin.*

## 156

*Accounts have been heard as presented by Fr. Hesso Schlegelholz, Preceptor of Kos and Rottweil. He has paid as the responsions of the Priory of* Alamania *1,000 florins each year for 1383 and 1384. Of this sum Hesso has paid 1,000 florins to Fr. Domenico d'Alamania for the Treasury and 526 florins he has kept for his own expenses on behalf of the Order. So Hesso still owes to the Treasury 474 florins for the two years of responsions from* Alamania.
*1386 August 3*

*AOM 323 fol. 236v (226v), under* assignaciones peccuniarum.

Mense et die predictis audito computo fratri[s] Hessonis Sleghoclg preceptoris Langonis [et] Ro[t]wiil de responsionibus prioratus Alamanie de duobus annus predictis octuagesimo tercio et quarto habitis per ipsum fratrem Hessonem pro anno quolibet florenos mille, de quibus ipse frater Hesso solvit fratri Dominico Dalamahna nomine thesauri florenos mille[a] et exposuit pro suis expensis in negotiis religionis florenos quingentos XXVI. Dominus magister relatione thesaurarii fratris Petri de Provinis hiis informatus de premissis florenis mille traditis dicto fratri Dominico et aliis quingentis XXVI expositis, ut prefertur, dictum fratrem Hessonem quitavit. Et ex hoc restat dictus frater Hesso teneri comuni thesauro de responsionibus dictorum duorum annorum, que ascendunt duo milia, in florenis trescentis[1] septuaginta quatuor.

*a)* florenos mille *supra lin.*

## 157

*The Master Fr. Riccardo [Caracciolo] grants for ten years to Fr. Count Hartmann von Werdenberg, Preceptor of Wädenswil, the Preceptory of Bubikon (Priory of* Alamania), *which is vacant following the death of Fr. Werner Schürer, and names as executors the Preceptor of Küsnacht and Fr. Rudolf Mülner.*

*Genoa, [13]86 September 22*

*AOM 281 fol. 94v.*

Frater Riccardus etcetera religioso in Christo nobis carissimo fratri Hartmanno domus eiusdem comiti de Werdenberg preceptori domus nostre sancti Iohannis in Wędiswil prioratus nostri Almanie salutem etcetera. Laudabilia probitatis et virtutum merita[a], quibus Altissimus personam tuam munivit, necnon considerantes tua servicia nostre domui impensa et laudabiles tuos mores nos inducunt etcetera. Eapropter baiuliam seu preceptoriam domus nostre in Bubicon prioratus nostri predicti vacantem ad presens per obitum quondam fratris Wernheri Schurer domus eiusdem ultimi dicte domus nostre preceptoris seu aliquovis modo vacet et propterea ad nostram disposicionem legitime devolutam etcetera invicem ad X annos tantummodo incipiendos in festo nativitatis sancti Iohannis baptiste proxime futuri etcetera ac religioso in Christo nobis carissimo preceptori domus nostre in Kussnach[1] prioratus nostri predicti et fratri Rudolfo Muller seu eorum alteri domus eiusdem, ut te vel procuratorem tuum in possessionem etcetera. Datum Ianue die XXII mensis Septembris anno LXXXVI.

*a) supra lin.*

*1) 400 would be correct.*

*1) Fr. Burkhard Bilgeri from 1383 to 1392, from a family of citizens in Zürich: Helvetia Sacra (2006), 287.*

## 158

*[The Master Fr. Juan Fernández de Heredia] orders Fr. Hesso Schlegelholz, Preceptor of Kos and Rottweil, to receive into the Order, at the request of Aubert Conffens, Dean of Angoulême and papal acolyte, as a knight brother Nikolaus Zenich, who is to travel to Rhodes with the next* passagium *in the following March or April; meanwhile, he is to be assigned his maintenance in a preceptory of the Priory of* Alamania.

*1386 October 26*

*AOM 323 fol. 158r (150r), under* prioratus Alamanie et Boemie.

Die XX[a]VI mensis Ottobris anno LXXX sexto commissum fuit et mandatum fratri Hessoni Slegelholtz preceptori Langonis et Rotwil ad instantiam domini Auberti Conffens decani Engolismensis, domini nostri pape acoliti, ut Nicolaum Zenich, dum tamen nobilis sit, ex utroque parente matrimonio legitimo[a)] natus, sanus et integer membris suis, ipso insignito prius milicia recipiat in fratrem religiosum servata forma servari consueta. Et ipsi Nicolao recepto data fuit licentia eundi ad conventum cum equis et armis et preceptum, ut vadat in primo passagio fiendo de mense Martii seu Aprilis, quo pendente tempore provideatur in suis neccessariis in altera baiuliarum prioratus Alamanie.

*a)* legitio *MS*

## 159

*The Master Fr. Juan Fernández [de Heredia] assigns maintenance for Fr. Johann von Lyech for his lifetime in the Preceptory of Cologne (Priory of* Alamania), *which is to be provided by the Preceptor Fr. Karl von Monreal and his successors.*

*Avignon, 1390 February 5*

*AOM 324 fol. 109r-v (100r-v), under* prioratus Alamanie, Boemie et Vngarie.

Frater Iohannes Ferdinandi etcetera religioso etcetera fratri Iohanni de Lyech domus eiusdem etcetera. Odor religiose vestre vite et fame cum aliorum suffrangancia laudabilium meritorum usque ad nos fidedignorum relatione perductus nobis nos liberales ad gratiam indigens vobis in preceptoria Coloniensi prioratus nostri Alamanie ad vitam vestram auctoritate presencium de nostra certa scientia et speciali gratia stagiam assignamus. Mandantes sub virtute sancte obediencie firmiter et districte religioso etcetera fratri Karolo de Munreal domus eiusdem, dicte preceptorie preceptori, et suis successoribus aut quovis alio titulo premisse preceptorie regimini presidenti nunc vel in futurum, ut vos ad dictam preceptoriam venientem moraturum pro stagia seu in ea residentem ad stagiam ipsam benigne admittat et[a)] [109v] caritative pertractet vobisque[b)], quamdiu vixeritis, in preceptoria ipsa in vestris neccessariis provideat secundum bonos usus et laudabiles consuetudines domus nostre. Quocirca universis et singulis fratribus domus nostre presentibus et futuris, cuiuscumque status, gradus vel conditionis existant, sub virtute sancte obedientie districte mandantes precipimus, quatenus contra predictam nostram assignationem stagie nullatenus venire presumant, quinymo efficaciter illam servent. In cuius rei etcetera. Data Avinione die quinta mensis Februarii anno incarnacionis Domini M° CCC° LXXX$^{mo}$ nono.

*a)* et *dupl.* *b)* -que *supra lin.*

## 160

*The Master Fr. Juan Fernández [de Heredia], with consent of brethren, confirms Fr. Karl von Monreal in the Preceptory of Cologne (Priory of* Alamania), *which has been granted him for his lifetime by Fr. Konrad von Braunsberg, Prior of* Alamania.

*Avignon, 1390 February 11*

*AOM 324 fol. 109r (100r), under* prioratus Alamanie, Boemie et Vngarie.

Frater Iohannes Ferdinandi etcetera religioso etcetera fratri Karolo de Munreal preceptori baiulie Coloniensis domus eiusdem salutem etcetera. Ob preclara vestre proceritatis merita et diuturna laboriosa obsequia per vos nostre prestita religioni et que solicitis studiis impendere non sinitis ac administrationem accomodam per vos habitam in vobis commissis regiminibus in nostro ordine, sicut fidedigno testimonio accepimus, illa vobis prompto affectu concedimus, que conservationem prosperi et transquilli status vestri concernere dignoscuntur. Hinc est, quod donationem et gratiam de dicta baiulia Coloniensi prioratus nostri Alamanie per domus eiusdem fratrem Cunradum de Brunsperg priorem dicti prioratus nuper vobis factas sub eisdem tenore, modo et forma expressis et contentis in litteris donationis et gratie huiusmodi proinde confectis dictorum prioris et prioratus sigilli impressione roboratis ratas, gratas et placidas de nostra certa scientia habentes, quarum litterarum tenorem hiis presentibus nostris volumus pro expressis haberi, supradictam baiuliam Coloniensem dicti prioratus cum omnibus et singulis suis membris, pertinenciis et iuribus ad eam spectantibus et pertinentibus ac spectare et pertinere debentibus, quoquomodo et cum quibus illam habetis et presentialiter possidetis, habendam, tenendam etcetera – alias etcetera – de voluntate, consilio et assensu dicte domus fratrum ·· preceptorum et procerum nobis assistencium de nostra certa scientia et speciali gratia vobis auctoritate presencium ad vitam vestram confirmamus et ad uberiorem vestram cautelam de novo conferimus et donamus benefaciendo in eadem ·· vosque etcetera. Comittentes etcetera. Quocirca etcetera necnon etcetera. Inhibentes etcetera. In cuius etcetera. Data Avinione die undecima mensis Febroarii anno incarnacionis Domini M° CCC$^{mo}$ LXXX$^{mo}$ nono.

## 161

*The Master Fr. Juan Fernández [de Heredia], with consent of brethren, confirms to Fr. Johann von Lyech alias von Mainz the incomes from the Preceptory of Worms, guaranteed to him for his lifetime in recognition of his services, by Fr. Konrad von Braunsberg, Prior of* Alamania.

*Avignon, 1390 February 11*

*AOM 324 fol. 109v (100v), under* prioratus Alamanie, Boemie et Vngarie.

Frater Iohannes Ferdinandi etcetera religioso etcetera fratri Iohanni de Lyech alias de Maguncia domus eiusdem etcetera. Ex vestre sufficiencie meritis et acceptis serviciis fidelibus per vos dicte domui eiusque fratri Cunrado de Brunsperg priori Alamanie impensis, et que vos inantea prestiturum speramus, susceptum testimonium comendabile nos inducit, ut vos favore specialis gratie prosequamur, presertim ubi circa iam vobis concessa aliquid exhigitis, per quod ea pleniori robore fulciantur. Quamobrem donationes et gratias simul et successive nuper per dictum priorem fratrem Cunradum de certis redditibus, peccuniis et bonis, in quibuscumque rebus consistant, per vos percipiendis et habendis, quamdiu vicxeritis, super baiulia Wormaciensi vobis factas sub quovis verborum tenore ac modo et forma expressis in certis proinde confectis litteris impressione sigilli dictorum prioris et prioratus roboratis, quas hiis nostris presentibus pro expressis volumus haberi, de voluntate, consilio et assensu dicte domus fratrum ·· preceptorum et procerum nobis assistencium auctoritate presencium de nostra certa scientia et speciali gratia confirmamus. Mandantes eiusdem domus fratri ··, dicte baiulie Wormaciensis preceptori, eiusque successoribus seu quovis alio titulo premisse preceptorie regimini nunc vel in futurum presidenti sub virtute sancte obedientie necnon universis et singulis dicte domus fratribus ·· presentibus et futuris quacumque dignitate vel officio fungentibus, ne contra nostram presentem confirmationem aliquatenus venire presumant, quinymo illam inviolabiliter habeant observare. In cuius etcetera. Data Avinione die undecima mensis Febroarii anno incarnacionis Domini M° CCC° LXXX$^{mo}$ nono.

## 162

*The Master Fr. Juan Fernández [de Heredia] permits Fr. Konrad von Braunsberg, Prior of* Alamania, *to appoint lieutenants because Konrad is now old and sick.*

*Avignon, [1390] February 11*

*AOM 324 fol. 110r (101r), under* prioratus Alamanie, Boemie et Vngarie.

Frater Iohannes Ferdinandi etcetera religioso etcetera fratri Cunrado de Brunsperg priori Alamanie domus eiusdem etcetera. Antique proceritatis vestre et aliorum vestrorum exhigencia meritorum, quibus persona vestra dignoscitur insignita, promeretur, ut petitiones vestras, illas presertim, que vestre quietis comoda, conscientie pacem et anime salutem prospiciunt, quantum possumus comode admictamus. Cum itaque, sicut accepimus ex vestrarum serie litterarum et plurimorum fidedignorum assertiva relatione, circa administrationem accomodam dicti prioratus per vosmet ob vestri corporis debilitatem, que ex senio et infirmitate gravi procedit, prepeditus vacare, intendere et ipsius regimini prioratus preesse, prout expediret, nullatenus potestis absque conscientie scrupulo et anime vestre periculo, pro qua re a nobis pro vestri parte supplicatum extitit, ut opportuno super hec vobis remedio providere dignaremur, nos itaque vestris supplicationibus inclinati, quod unum vel plures dicte domus fratres prioratus eiusdem ad hec sufficientes locumvestrumtenentes in ipso prioratu, tociens vobis placuerit, ad regimen dicti prioratus vestro nomine cum potestate, que ad prioris spectat officium seu cum qua vobis videbitur, constituere possitis, vobis de nostra certa scientia auctoritate presencium facultatem et licenciam concedimus, quem et quos dum constituendos et ordinandos ducxeritis, ut prefertur, sufficientes eo casu vos deffectu negligencie dumtaxat harum serie ab onere regiminis ipsius prioratus in foro conscientie relevamus, supportamus et vestram conscientiam exoneramus conscientias fratris seu fratrum huiusmodi sic constitutorum nomine vestro ad dicti prioratus regimen penitus onerantes, usquequo in premissis aliud ducxerimus ordinandum. Data Avinione die XI[a] mensis Febroarii anno quo supra.

*See no. 136.*

## 163

*[The Master Fr. Juan Fernández de Heredia] orders the Preceptors of Frankfurt Fr. Helfrich von Rüdigheim and of Erdlingen Fr. [Konrad von] Wolfsdorf to receive into the Order as knight brother a noble man nominated by Fr. Johann Merklin, Preceptor of Würzburg. He assigns him his maintenance in Würzburg and licenses him to travel to Rhodes.*

*[Avignon,] 1390 February 12*

*AOM 324 fol. 109v (100v), under* prioratus Alamanie, Boemie et Vngarie.

Die duodecima mensis Febroarii anno incarnacionis Domini M° CCC[mo] LXXX[mo] nono commissum fuit et mandatum fratribus Helfrico de Rudeleyn[!] in Frankenfordia et Wolfersdorffer in Erningen baiuliis preceptoribus et eorum cuilibet, ut ad requisitionem fratris Iohannis Merklin[a)] preceptoris baiulie Herbipolensis virum unum nobilem ex utroque parente matrimonio procreatus[!] legitimo, aptum, sanum et integrum suis membris, quem nominandum ducxit, ipso prius decorato militia recipiant in fratrem religiosum prioratus Alamanie, ipsique recepto assignent stagium in dicta baiulia dicti fratris Iohannis Merklin, in qua sibi provideatur in suis neccessariis, ut moris est. Ac eidem recepto in fratrem data fuit licentia eundi ad conventum, quando voluerit, cum equis et armis sufficientibus a suo superiore licentia requisita.

*a)* i *praem. ante corr.*

## 164

*Licence for Fr. Johann Merklin, Preceptor of Würzburg, to receive one sergeant into the Order who is to be maintained in Würzburg.*

*[Avignon, 1390 February 12]*

*AOM 324 fol. 110r (101r), under* prioratus Alamanie, Boemie et Vngarie.

Anno, mense et die predictis data fuit licentia fratri Iohanni Merklin preceptori baiulie Herbipolensis recipiendi fratrem unum servientem nostre religionis, quo asserit pro regimine baiulie sue [indigere]. Et assignet sibi stagiam in dicta baiulia, in qua sibi provideat in suis neccessariis, ut moris est.

## 165

*Licence for Fr. Johann Merklin, Preceptor of Würzburg, to travel to Rhodes and to the Holy Sepulchre and to return to Würzburg.*

*[Avignon, 1390] February 12*

*AOM 324 fol. 110r (101r), under* prioratus Alamanie, Boemie et Vngarie.

Die XII$^{ma}$ mensis Febroarii anno quo supra data fuit licentia fratri Iohanni Merklin preceptori Herbipolensi eundi ad conventum Rodi et deinde ad sanctum sepulcrum, quando sibi placuerit, et inde redeundi ad dictam baiuliam.

## 166

*The Master Fr. Juan Fernández [de Heredia], after consultation with brethren and in view of the difficult times, constitutes Fr. Guillaume de Munte, Preceptor of Flanders and lieutenant of the Prior of* Francia, *and Fr. Pierre de Provins, Treasurer and Receiver General, as visitors with full powers in the Priory of* Alamania. *They are to act as lieutenants of the Master who cannot be present himself in all parts of the world. They are to visit, correct and reform the Priory of* Alamania *with its brethren, sisters, donats, leaseholders and lieutenants, with its chambers, offices, houses, its castles, villages and subjects. He may accept from Fr. Konrad von Braunsberg, Prior of* Alamania, *his preceptors, chambers, preceptories and houses their responsions, arrears of responsions,* mortuaria *and other dues to the Master and Convent. The visitors are to audit accounts and issue receipts. They are to dispense justice. They can convoke assemblies. With the counsel of the prior and the senior brethren of the priory they are to rule the priory, to redeem alienated goods, to act inside and outside law courts and to accept oaths as if the Master himself were present. The Hospital's brethren and subjects are ordered to be obedient to them. Without the Master's special licence the visitors may not alienate goods of the Hospital nor admit brethren or donats into the Order.*

*Avignon, 1390 February 15*

*AOM 324 fol. 110r-11v (101r-2v), under* prioratus Alamanie, Boemie et Vngarie.

Noverint universi et singuli presentem constitutionem et ordinationem locuntenentium, visitatorum et reformatorum visuri et audituri, quoniam considerantes attento, quod, dum nos frater Iohannes Ferdinandi etcetera erga salubrem directionem agendorum nostre religionis, conservationem status illius prosperum administrationemve in ea iusticie et sublevationem professorum eius a perplexis laboribus et gravibus sumptuosis expensis nostre solicitudinis studia adhibemus, euisdem nostre religionis regiminis exequimur impositum nobis onus. Attendentes itaque, quod per universas mundi partes adesse personaliter non valemus et quod, si fratres ipsius nostre domus prioratus nostri Alamanie presertim attenta inordinata dispositione temporis et alii nobis et ipsi domui subditi prioratus prefati pro petenda et obtinenda iusticia et aliis querendis remediis [110v] super questionibus et controversiis et aliis casibus, que et qui possent accidere inter eos, ad nostram oporteret venire presenciam, sumptuosum et laboriosum admodum eis esset et propterea expediens et neccessarium existeret, ut loco nostri fratres aliquos dicte domus exemplaris vite, mature providencie proceritatisque famose in partem nostre solicitudinis nostre potestatis auctoritate sufultos deputemus in prioratu Alamanie prelibato, quorum discretiva virtute fratribus et subdittis prelibatis, cum ad eos[a] pro predictis et aliis ipsos continget recurrere, iustitia et congrua remedia, prout casus exigerint, ministrentur et rursum consolidentur confracta, corrigenda corrigantur et refformanda faciente Domino in melius reformentur, que consolidatione, correctione et reformatione indigere in eodem prioratu noscentur. Quamobrem de religiosorum in Christo nobis carissimorum dicte domus fratrum Guillelmi de Munto preceptoris Flandrie et prioris Francie locu[m]tenentis[1] et Petri de Provinis thesaurarii et receptoris generalis circumspectione, industria[b], fide et probitate legali plenam in Domino fiduciam obtinentes nos prefatus magister consulta deliberatione prehabita cum domus eiusdem fratribus ·· baillivis, prioribus, preceptoribus et proceribus aliis nobis assistentibus eosdem fratres Guillelmum et Petrum et eorum quemlibet insolidum absentes tanquam presentes de nostra certa scientia nostro et dicte domus nomine acque vice tenore presencium locuntenentes, visitatores, correctores et reformatores in dicto prioratu Alamanie facimus, creamus, constitutimus et solemniter ordinamus. Dantes et concedentes harum serie predictis et eorum cuilibet nostro et dicte domus locuntenentibus, visitatoribus, correctoribus et reformatoribus licenciam, potestatem et auctoritatem plenariam prioratum prefatum eiusque omnes et singulos fratres ··, sorores, donatos, firmarios, rendarios et eorum locatenentes ac ipsorum et cuiuslibet cameras, baiulias, domos, administrationes et regimina ac loca, castra, villas, homines et vassallos visitandi, reformandi, corrigendi et meliorandi in spiritualibus et temporalibus tam in capitibus[!] quam in

1) *On him, Legras (1987), 437–8.*

membris necnon petendi, recipiendi et habendi a dicte domus fratre Cunrado de Brunsperg priore dicti prioratus et fratribus ·· preceptoribus ceterisque prioratus ipsius camerarum, preceptoriarum et domorum suarum responsiones, arreragia responsionum, mortuaria, peccunias, res, bona et alia omnia et singula quovis titulo, ratione sive causa per eos et quemlibet ipsorum debita et debenda nobis et conventui nostro Rodi communiter vel divisim et ad nos, conventum eundem Rodi communiter vel divisim spectancia[c] et debencia pervenire et huiusmodi fratres ·· priorem, preceptores, firmarios, rendarios ad ea[d] solvenda compellendi et ab eisdem et quolibet eorum computa et rationes audiendi et de computis redditis necnon habitis et receptis ab ipsis fratribus ·· priore, preceptoribus et aliis prioratus ipsius eos et quemlibet ipsorum quictandi et litteras quictationis valituras perpetuo faciendi, inter fratres, sorores, donatos, homines et vassallos nostros et domus nostre dicti prioratus, quociens oporteat, iusticiam ministrandi et faciendi, plantam et plantas fratrum esgardia petendi et tenendi et mandari, teneri faciendi, capitulum et capitula et assembleyas et congregationes fratrum in dicto prioratu mandandi et tenendi, quociens dictis locumtenentibus, visitatoribus et reformatoribus et eorum cuilibet super quibuscumque [111r] domus nostre dicti prioratus negociis emergentibus visum fuerit expedire, et in illis disponendi et ordinandi cum consilio fratrum ·· prioris iamdicti et procerum dicti prioratus ibidem tunc astancium omnia et singula concernencia utilitatem et honorem domus et prioratus predittorum, castra, loca, bona, iura et res quasvis alias eorundem domus et prioratus alienata et alienatas et per personas ecclesiasticas vel seculares occupatas et occupata, detenta et detentas petendi, recuperandi et ad ius et proprietatem nostre dicte domus revocandi et reducendi, pro nobis et dicta nostra domo quibuscumque[e] dominis et personis ecclesiasticis vel mundanis supplicandi et ab eis et eorum quolibet litteras gratie et simplicis iusticie ac indulgencias et privilegia quecumque impetrandi ac impetratis et impetrandis contra nos et dictam nostram domum et personas illius et loca obiciendi et contradicendi, homagia et fidelitatis sacramenta petendi et recipiendi, si expediat, a[f] nostris et domus nostre hominibus et vassallis ac omnia et singula insuper dependencia et emergencia ex eis et eorum quolibet ac ipsis et eorum alteri quoquomodo connexa, ut dictis locumtenentibus, visitatoribus et reformatoribus et eorum cuilibet pro utiliori visum fuerit, excercendi, exequendi, faciendi, disponendi et ordinandi cum consilio fratrum ·· prioris predicti et procerum dicti prioratus, que nos ipsi visitare, reformare, facere et exercere possemus, si in dicto prioratu personaliter adessemus. Mandantes insuper prefatis fratribus ·· priori et preceptoribus ceterisque domus nostre prioratus Alamanie predicti presentibus et futuris, cuiuscumque status, gradus vel conditionis existant, sub virtute sancte obediencie firmiter et districte, ac hominibus et vassallis nobis et dicte domui subdictis, in dicto prioratu constitutis sub sacramento fidelitatis et homagii, quo nobis et eidem domui sunt astricti, precipimus, ut in premissis et quolibet premissorum prenominatis nostris visitatoribus[g], locumtenentibus et reformatoribus et ipsorum cuilibet reverenter pareant, obediant et intendant tanquam nobis imparciendo eisdem et eorum cuilibet consilium et favorem veritati testimonium perhibendo in omnibus, super quibus eos aut eorum alterum ducxerint requirendos, non obstante, si aliqui ex dictis fratribus ad manus nostras sint retenti aliasve exempti, quibus in hiis casibus retentionem aut exemptionem aliquam nolumus de certa scientia sufragare, necnon ut ad dictorum locumnostrumtenentium, visitatorum et reformatorum et cuiuslibet eorum vocationem et mandatum ad locum et loca, ad quem et que ipsos vel aliquem aut aliquos ex eis semel et pluries evocaverint seu evocaverit, veniant contradictione et[h] excusatione remotis. Super quibus omnibus et singulis predictis nostris locumnostrumtenentibus et visiatoribus et cuilibet eorum committimus plenarie vices nostras inhibentes dictis nostris[i] locumnostrumtenentibus, visitatoribus et cuilibet eorum sub virtute sancte obediencie firmiter et districte, ne pretextu locumtenentie et visitationis predictarum nec alias aliqua de bonis, rebus et iuribus dicte nostre domus donent, vendant, alienent, permutent[j], impignorent, distrahant seu in emphiteosum perpetuam concedant aut quocumque alio colore quesito extra nostram religionem transferant nec fratres nec donatos faciant seu faciat nec aliis faciendi licenciam tribuant sine nostra speciali licencia et mandato. Et si, quod absit, contra inhibitionem nostram huiusmodi aliquid vel aliqua eos vel eorum alterum facere vel operari contingerit, illud et illa exnunc prout extunc et extunc prout [111v] exnunc cassamus, anullamus ac decernimus irritum et inane nulliusque existere penitus efficacie vel valoris. In cuius etcetera. Data Avinione die XV mensis Febroarii anno incarnationis Domini M° CCC° LXXX$^{mo}$ nono.

*a)* eum *ante corr.* *b)* industia *MS* *c)* spectantiam *MS* *d)* a *praem. ante corr.* *e)* et *praem. ante corr.* *f)* n *add. ante corr.* *g)* visitatorebus *MS* *h)* et *supra lin.* *i)* de *praem. ante corr.* *j)* permittent *MS*

## 167

*The Master Fr. Riccardo Caracciolo issues, through a notarial act, a decision concerning the resignation of the Preceptory of Bubikon (Priory of* Alamania*) and its member of Küsnacht by Fr. Hermann von Werdenberg, Preceptor of Wädenswil and Feldkirch, granting it to Fr. Hugo von Bregenz in whose favour Fr. Hermann von Werdenberg had resigned it.*

*Rome, [1391] May 14*

*AOM 281 fol. 96v.*

Die XIIII mensis Maii XIIII indictione[1] Rome in palacio apostolico in aula videlicet reverendissimi patris et domini domini R. Carazoli magistri hospitalis sancti Iohannis Ierosolimitani constitutus coram me, notario publico, et testibus infrascriptis venerabilis vir magister Iohannes Greci canonicus ecclesie

1) *The 14th indiction is 1391. On 1 December 1393 the Master Fr. Riccardo Caracciolo granted to Fr. Hugo von Bregenz the Preceptories of Bubikon and Küsnacht: Helvetia Sacra (2006), 154 with note 4 according to the original, Zürich, Staatsarchiv, C II 4 Urkunden Klosteramt Küsnacht no. 49.*

sancti Martini Columbar. Bas(iliensis) diocesis,[2] procurator religiosi viri fratris Hartmani Werdenberg preceptoris domorum Wediswilr Veltkilch et in Bubicon prioratus Almanie ordinis sancti Iohannis Ierosolimitani, de cuius procuratione plene michi, notario infrascripto, constat, renuntiavit nomine et pro parte dicti fratris Hartmanni domui seu preceptorie in Bubicokon cum membro eius dicto Kussnach cum universis iuribus et pertinentiis suis in manibus dicti domini magistri iurans, quod nec dolo nec fraude huiusmodi renunciacionem faceret quodque frater Ingo[!] de Bregencz. ordinis eiusdem, pro quo eciam tunc supplicavit, quod dictus dominus magister sibi de domo sive preceptoria ut premittitur renunciata provideret, esset bonus catholicus et obediens frater. Super quibus omnibus et singulis idem reverendissimus pater et dominus ·· magister de Rodis sibi petiit per me Angelillum notarium publicum fieri publicum instrumentum ad dictamen cuiuslibet sapientis corrigendum substantia facti non mutata. Presentibus venerabilibus et religiosis viris fratribus Iacobo de Olecis[!] de Lucca ac Leonardo de Bonafede de Florencia eiusdem ordinis mecum magistro Iohanne Bocholt testibus[3] ad premissa vocatis specialiter et rogatis.

Renunciatio domus in Bubichon prioratus Almanie *marg.*

## 168

*The Master Fr. Juan Fernández [de Heredia] orders his procurator Dragonetto Clavelli, citizen of Rhodes, to pay on behalf of Fr. Hesso Schlegelholz, Preceptor of Kos, 20 florins annually, which so far had been paid to the late Fr. Bertrand von Tobel, from now on to Fr. Gaspal de Curuet until Gaspal secures a preceptory.*

*Avignon, 1391 August 29*

*AOM 325 fol. 169v (175v), under* prioratus Alamanie et Boemie.

Frater Iohannes etcetera venerabili et provido viro Dragoneto Clavelli, civi et procuratori nostro Rodi, salutem in Domino et presentibus dare fidem. Ecce vestre noticie deducimus harum serie, quod nos contemplatione dicte domus fratris Hessonis Slegelholtz preceptoris Langonis concessimus, eciam damus per presentes domus eiusdem fratri Gaspal de Curuet lingue Alamanie loco quondam fratris Bertrandi de Totil florenos viginti anno quolibet per vos sibi exolvendos, usquequo eidem fuerit de aliqua baiulia provisum. Quapropter

2) *Johannes Greci, canon of St. Martin in Colmar, in the Diocese of Basel.*

3) *Fr. Jacopo degli Obizzi from Lucca, Fr. Leonardo di Buonafede from Florence, both Hospitallers; magister Johann Bocholt, papal familiar and abbreviator: Rep. Germ. 2 (1933), col. 269, 570–1, 952. On Lionardo Bonafedi cf. De Palma (2010).*

vobis tenore presentium committimus et mandamus, quatenus dicto fratri Gaspal quolibet anno et termino consueto de bonis[a)] et peccuniis nostris per vos receptis et habendis florenos viginti detis et solvatis, quibus florenis viginti sic, ut prescribitur, solutis eos reputamus pro habitis et nobis solutis et in vestris computationibus et rationibus volumus apponi. In cuius etcetera. Data Avinione die XXIX[a] mensis Augusti anno quo supra nonagesimo primo.

*a)* p *praem. ante corr.*

## 169

*The Master Fr. Juan Fernández [de Heredia] orders Dragonetto Clavelli to pay on behalf of Fr. Hesso Schlegelholz, Preceptor of Kos, 20 florins annually, which so far has been paid to the late Fr. Erwin, from now on to Fr. Hermann von Ow.*

*Avignon, 1391 August 29*

*AOM 325 fol. 169v (175v), under* prioratus Alamanie et Boemie.

Frater Iohannes etcetera venerabili et provido viro Dragoneto Clavelli etcetera salutem etcetera. Ecce vestre noticie deducimus harum serie, quod nos contemplatione dicte domus fratris Hessonis Slegelholcz preceptoris Langonis concessimus, eciam damus per presentes domus eiusdem fratri Alamano de Owe lingue Alamanie loco quondam fratris Eruyn florenos viginti etcetera ut in precedenti.

*This was Fr. Hermann von Ow the Younger. An elder Hospitaller of the same name was Preceptor of Hemmendorf and Rohrdorf, who died on 1 November 1390: Rupert (1889), 295.*

## 170

*The Master Fr. Juan Fernández [de Heredia], with consent of brethren, confirms Fr. Hesso Schlegelholz, Preceptor of Rottweil, an old and high-ranking Hospitaller, for his lifetime in the Preceptory (here* baiulia*) of Kos with the islands of Kalymnos and Leros. Fr. Hesso is to pay a responsion of 100 florins a year on 24 June. He is to provide the churches on these islands with divine services and lights. He is to maintain at his own expense 25 brethren, that is 15 knights, two chaplains, six sergeants-at-arms and two sergeants-at-office with their servants. He is to transport these brethren, their servants, horses and armour from Rhodes to Kos and back at his own expense. He is to maintain at his own expense 10 free-born men-at-arms from the East with their armour and animals and more than 100 turcopoles or sergeants with their usual salary and expense. He is to provide donats with the usual clothing and other necessities, and the ten men-at-arms are not among these donats. He may permit donats sent from Rhodes to return, but while such donats serve him Fr. Hesso is to provide them with clothing* *and other necessities. He is to maintain a physician and a pharmacist on Kos. Each year in April he is to open a sluice gate and to let in fresh sea water into the lagoon. He may not sell grain, horses or other animals outside of Rhodes, except with special licence from the Master or the Master's lieutenant. For their own use, however, the brethren may buy light horses and other pack animals from* francomati. *Fr. Hesso is to uphold the liberties of the islands' peasants and to practice justice for them. In order to protect the islands, he is to maintain a ship with 20 benches of oarsmen, as may be necessary. He is to keep in their present state or to improve all castles and lodgings* (hospitia) *on the islands. He is to observe all truces accepted by the Master. The grant is made with the consent of Fr. Domenico d'Alamania, Preceptor of Naples and of Santo Stefano di Monopoli, and of other brethren. Fr. Hesso is granted full powers to administer the islands and to rule his subjects. The Hospital's brethren and subjects are ordered to obey him. He may not alienate properties without the Master's special licence; in case of default such action will be null and void.*

*Avignon, 1391 August 29*

*AOM 325 fol. 180r-81r (186r-7r)*, under libertates marinarum et receptiones officii et terrarum.

Frater Iohannes etcetera fratri Hessoni Slegelholtz preceptori Langoni domus eiusdem etcetera. Morem laudabilem nostre religionis sequentes, secundum quem, nedum ipsa religio antiquos et proceres fratres promovere, verum eos in suis conservare statibus consuevit, sperantes, quod in premisse vestre baiulie comisso vobis regimine eritis faciente Domino comendabiliter fructuosus et tanquam oliva fructifera vos in eadem fructus uberes allaturus, baiuliam ipsam Langoni una cum insulis de Calamo et de Lerro et omnibus et singulis earum et cuiuslibet ipsarum membris, pertinenciis et iuribus ad eas et ipsarum quamlibet spectantibus et pertinentibus ac spectare et pertinere debentibus quoquo modo, et cum quibus illas tenetis, habetis et possidetis, habendam, tenendam, regendam, gubernandam, augmentandam et meliorandam in spiritualibus et temporalibus tam in capitis quam in membis ad vitam vestram sub pactis et condicionibus subsequentibus – primo videlicet, quod anno quolibet solvere teneamini dicte domus conventus Rodi thesauro comuni in festi nativitatis beati Iohannis babtiste pro ispius responsione florenos centum. Item quod teneamini deserviri et illuminari facere capellas insularum predictarum, sicut convenit, bene et decenter et ad divinum servicium exercendum in ipsis capellanos necessarios tenere. Item quod teneamini tenere ad omnes vestras expensas in preceptoria predicta fratres domus nostre viginti quinque, scilicet fratres milites quindecim, fratres capellanos duos, fratres servientes armorum sex et fratres servientes officii duos, cum ipsorum familiis ita, quod tam pro predictis fratribus quam pro eorum familiis dictus thesaurus nichil dare vobis neque ipsis teneatur. Item quod dicti fratres cum ipsorum familiis, equis et armis eundo ad Langonem et redeundo de Langone ad Rodum eant et veniant ad expensas vestras. Item quod teneamini tenere ad omnes expensas vestras in preceptoria predicta continuo homines armorum decem francos in partibus cismarinis natos bene armatos et bene montatos et ultra homines centum inter tricoplos et sergentes ad stipendia solita et ad expensas alias omnes vestras per vos eis solvenda[s] et faciendas. Item quod recepti in donatos domus nostre in Langone ibidem teneantur et debeant remanere et vos ipsis teneamini providere de vestiario solito et aliis expensis neccessariis iuxta domus nostre bonos usus, et dicti donati in numero dictorum decem hominum armatorum nullatenus computantur. Item quod donatis missis de Rodo ad Langonem possitis conferre licenciam redeundi ad Rodum. Verunptamen quod ispis teneamini eorum vestiaria solvere et in aliis neccessariis iuxta domus nostre bonos usus providere, quamdiu residebunt in Langone. Item quod teneamini tenere in Langone vestris expensis pro fratribus et donatis medicum et apothecarium et apothecam neccessariis munitam. Item quod teneamini anno quolibet in mense Aprilis ad vestras expensas facere aperiri bucam latus sic, quod mare [180v] ingredi et egredi inde possit. Item quod non debatis neque possitis mittere ad vendendum alibi quam in Rodum blada aliqua nec bestias cavalinas nec quodcunque bestiare aliud sine licencia nostri prelibati magistri seu nostrorum locumtenentis nobis absentibus. Item quod fratres ad usum ipsorum possint emere ab hominibus francomatis roncinos turcamanos et animalia alia saumagii. Item quod teneamini incolis et habitatoribus insularum predictarum eorum libertates servare et iusticiam ministrare. Item quod teneamini tenere unum lignum bancorum viginti fornitum neccessariis ad tuicionem insularum predictarum, cum fuerit oportunum. Item quod teneamini tenere et manutenere dictarum preceptorie et insularum castra et hospicia reparata et illa relinquere in eo statu, in quo nunc sunt vel in meliori. Item quod teneamini servare sacramentale cum omnibus, cum quibus treugas facere et inhire nos contingat – de voluntate, consilio et assensu dicte domus fratris Dominici de Alamania preceptoris Neapolis et sancti Stephani de Monopolo et aliorum fratrum nobis assistencium vobis tenore presencium de nostra certa scientia et speciali gratia insimul cum baiulia de Rotwil confirmamus et ad uberiorem cauthelam vestram[a)] de novo ad vitam vestram concedimus et donamus benefaciendo in eisdem. Dantes et concedentes vobis auctoritate presencium licenciam, potestatem et auctoritatem regendi, gubernandi et administrandi preceptoriam prefatam una cum insulis de Calamo et de Lerro prefatis in spiritualibus et temporalibus tam in capite quam in membris ac inter fratres et donatos et homines et vassallos et stipendiarios insularum premissarum super quibuscunque casibus iusticiam ministrandi et facere ministrari, fratrum esgardia tenendi et mandare teneri, plantam et plantas faciendi, quociens oporteat, et rebelles et inhobedientes seu alias delinquentes secundum statuta nostre domus ducendi per iusticiam domus nostre iuxta statuta et consuetudines prefate domus nostre. Quocirca universis et singulis fratribus domus nostre presentibus et futuris, cuiuscunque status, gradus vel condicionis existant, et donatis sub virtute sancte obediencie ac hominibus et vassallis et stipendiariis aliis in dictis insulis residentibus, presentibus et futuris sub sacramento fidelitatis et homagii, quo nobis et nostre dicte religioni tenentur, districte precipiendo mandamus, ut vobis tanquam eorum preceptori, superiori et maiori, quamdiu vicxeritis, tanquam nobis reverenter pareant, obediant et intendant in[b)] omnibus[c)] et singulis utilitatem et bonum regimen concernentibus insularum predictarum, super eis vobis prebeant consilium, auxilium et favorem tociens, quociens eos vel eorum alterum ducxeritis requirendos. Inhibentes vobis districtius sub virtute sancte obediencie firmiter et districte, ne aliqua de bonis, rebus et iuribus memorate baiulie pretextu donationis et gratie nostre huiusmodi vendatis, detis, obligetis, impignoretis, distrahatis, alienetis, permutetis [181r] seu in emphiteosim perpetuam concedatis vel quocunque alio colore quesito extra nostram religionem transferatis sine nostra speciali licencia et mandato. Et si, quod absit, contra inhibicionem nostram huiusmodi aliquid vel aliqua operari vel facere vos contingat, illud et illa exnunc prout extunc et extunc prout exnunc cassamus, annullamus ac decernimus irritum et inane nulliusque existere efficacie vel valoris. In cuius etcetera. Data Avinione die XXIX[a] mensis Augusti anno incarnationis Domini M[o] CCC[mo] nonagesimo primo.

Ista littera deberet registrari in partibus ultramarinis *marg.* *a)* concedimus et donamus *add. ante corr.* *b)* in *praem. ante corr.* *c)* reverenter in *add. ante corr.*

## 171

*Licence for Fr. Hesso Schlegelholz, Preceptor of Kos, to travel to the Priory of* Alamania *and to return to Kos or to the Master.*

*1392 January 16*

*AOM 325 fol. 134v (140v), under* prioratus Alamanie et Boemie.

Die XVI mensis Ianuarii anno incarnacionis Domini M[mo] CCC[mo] nonagesimo primo data fuit licentia fratri Hessoni Sleglholtz preceptori Langonis recedendi de dicta baiulia et eundi ad prioratum Alamanie ex certis causis et de dicto prioratu redeundi[a)] ad dictam baiuliam seu ad dominum magistrum, quando sibi placuerit.

*a)* rev *praem. ante corr.*

## 172

*The Master Fr. Juan Fernández [de Heredia], with consent of the procurator of the Convent, four named and other brethren, constitutes Fr. Friedrich von Zollern until further notice as his lieutenant in the Priory of* Alamania*, which is vacant following the death of Fr. Konrad von Braunsberg. Fr. Friedrich is to rule the priory, to convoke assemblies and chapters, to appoint officers to vacant offices, to dispense justice and to punish brethren* *in the same way as if the Master himself were present. The brethren in the priory have to obey him as the Master's lieutenant. But Fr. Friedrich may not alienate goods of the Hospital without the Master's special licence.*

*Avignon, 1392 January 23*

*AOM 325 fol. 134r-v (140r-v), under* prioratus Alamanie et Boemie. *Cf. van Winter (1998), 32 no. 7, with the year 1390 in the text and 1391 as the date.*

Frater Iohannes Ferdinandi etcetera religioso in Christo nobis carissimo fratri Friderico de Zolra preceptori ·· domus eiusdem salutem et sinceram in Domino caritatem. Illos, inquam, deliberato proposito ad regimina administrationum notabilium domus nostre libenter assumimus, quos proceritatis decorat titulus et sollicite gubernationis accommode effectus approbat fructuosus. Sane fidedignorum fratrum procerum domus nostre relatibus intellecto, quod vobis digna laude merita suffragantur et experiencia vos exibuit et exibet industrem et utilem in regiminibus nostre commissis sollercie in eadem nostra domo, quia prioratus noster Alamanie per obitum fratris Cunradi de Brunsperg prioris ultimi priore et superiore est noviter destitutus, ne destitutione huiusmodi superioris carencia prioratus ipse exponi, quod absit, valeat noxiis detrimentis, confidencia ducti, quod nostra solerti diligencia prioratus idem sub nostra administratione provida dirigetur utiliter et administrabitur fructuose, idcirco in prioratu supradicto de voluntate, consilio et assensu dicte domus fratrum Palamides Iohannis admirati nostri Rodi conventus ipsiusque procuratoris, Hugonis Giraudi magni comendatoris, Petri Brios Montis Pesullani, Guillelmi de Vierges sancti Petri de Calanda, Iohannis Sancti Averini baiuliarum preceptorum[1] et aliorum nobis assistencium vos locu[m]tenentem nostrum usque ad beneplacitum nostrum auctoritate presencium de nostra certa scientia creamus, facimus ac eciam ordinamus. Dantes vobis et concedentes hac serie potestatem, auctoritatem et licenciam regendi, gubernandi et administrandi prioratum prefatum in spiritualibus et temporalibus tam in capite quam in membris ut locumnostrumtenens necnon in illo celebrandi et tenendi assembleyas et capitula vel fratrum congregationes alias, quociens vobis pro prioratu predicto videbitur opportunum, et in illis et sine illis disponendi et ordinandi cum consilio fratrum et procerum domus nostre prioratus ipsius, que ad ipsius prioratus redundent comodum et honorem, ac eciam baiulias in iamdicto prioratu vacantes et vacaturas recomendandi usque ad nostrum beneplacitum fratribus memorati prioratus ydoneis et regiminis fructuosi, inter fratres, sorores et donatos ac homines et vassallos nostros ac dicte nostre domus iamdicti prioratus, quociens oporteat, iusticiam ministrandi et ducendi culpabiles, si expediat, per

1) *The Admiral and procurator of the Convent Fr. Palamedo di Giovanni, the Grand Commander Fr. Hugues Giraud, and the Preceptors Fr. Pierre Brès of Montpellier, Fr. Guillem de Verges of Samper de Calanda and Fr. Jean of* Sanctus Averinus, *perhaps Saint-Aubin or Saverin.*

iusticiam nostre dicte domus secundum statuta et consuetudines ipsius domus, fratrum esgardia tenendi et mandare teneri, inobedientes quoque et rebelles ad nostram citra mare presenciam repellandi et generaliter et specialiter omnia et singula alia faciendi et excercendi et operandi in ipso prioratu, que nos in eo, si personaliter adessemus, facere et excercere possemus. Super quibus omnibus et singulis [134v] ac dependentibus et emergentibus ex eis et eorum quolibet vobis tenore presencium committimus vices nostras. Mandantes universis et singulis fratribus preceptoribus et baillivis et aliis fratribus, confratribus, sororibus et donatis sub virtute sancte obediencie ac hominibus et vassallis et quibusvis aliis vobis subditis in prioratu prefato existentibus sub sacramento fidelitatis et homagii, quo nobis et eidem domui sunt astricti, precipimus et mandamus harum serie districtius, ut vobis tanquam locu[m]tenenti nostro eorumque superiori et maiori reverenter pareant, obediant et intendant vobisque suum prebeant consilium, auxilium et favorem in omnibus, que ad curam, regimen et administrationem et gubernationem utilem prefati prioratus pertinere noscentur, quociens opus fuerit et eos duxeritis requirendos. Inhibentes vobis sub dicta virtute sancte obedientie, ne pretextu locumtenencie nostre huiusmodi aliqua de bonis, rebus aut iuribus dicti prioratus vendatis, alienetis, obligetis, detis seu extra nostram religionem transferatis sine nostra speciali licentia et mandato. Et si, quod absit, contra inhibitionem nostram huiusmodi aliquid operari vel facere vos contingat, illud et illa exnunc prout extunc et extunc prout exnunc cassamus, anullamus nulliusque volumus existere penitus efficacie vel valoris. In cuius rei etcetera. Data Avinione die XXIII$^{ma}$ mensis Ianuarii anno incarnacionis Domini M$^{o}$ CCC$^{mo}$ nonagesimo [primo].[2)]

## 173

*The Master Fr. Juan Fernández [de Heredia] confirms Fr. Wilhelm Velga in the Preceptory of Freiburg im Üchtland (Priory of* Alamania), *which is vacant following the death of Fr. Wilhelm Huser. The Preceptory has been given to Wilhelm by Fr. Pierre de Culant, Marshal and Lieutenant Master in the East, and the Convent at Rhodes for ten years, in a document corroborated with the seal of the Marshal's office.*

*Avignon, 1392 March 8*

*AOM 325 fol. 134v-5r (140v-41r), under* prioratus Alamanie et Boemie.

Frater Iohannes Ferdinandi etcetera religioso in Christo etcetera fratri Guillelmo Velguen preceptori de Friburgo Hottellandie[1)] domus eiusdem salutem

2) *Judging by other documents in AOM 325,* primo *was omitted erroneously.*

1) *Wilhelm Velga and his late predecessor Wilhelm Huser came from families of citizens in Freiburg: Zeininger (1946), 286–7.*

etcetera. Dum famose antique proceritatis vestre notam consideranter attendimus et diuturna laboriosa obsequia per vos nostre prestita religioni et que vos prestiturum inantea speramus quidquid alia virtuosa vestra merita, quibus, prout fidedignorum relatione nobis innotuit, largitor gratiarum Dominus vos insignivit, non indigne vota nostra prosequentes favorabiliter vos benemeritis gratiis amplectimur eaque vobis concedimus, per que vester status transquille pacis munimine fulciatur. Hinc est, quod donationem et gratiam de dicta baiulia de Friburgo prioratus nostri Alamanie tunc vacante per [135r] obitum fratris Guillelmi Huser per dicte domus fratres Petrum de Culento, marescallum et nostrum locumtenentem in ultramarinis, ac conventum nostrum Rodi ad annos decem vobis factas, sicut continetur latius in litteris donationis et gratie huiusmodi proinde confectis nobis exhibitis impressione sigilli officii marescallie appositis in appenso roboratis, quarum tenorem hiis presentibus volumus pro expresso haberi, ratas, gratas et placidas de nostra certa scientia habentes supradictam baiuliam de Friburgo dicti prioratus cum omnibus et singulis suis membris, pertinenciis et iuribus ad eam spectantibus et pertinentibus ac spectare et pertinere debentibus, quoquomodo et cum quibus illam dictus quondam frater Guillelmus Huser tenuit, habuit et possedit, habendam, tenendam etcetera – alias etcetera – de voluntate, consilio et assensu dicte domus fratrum nobis assistencium vobis ad dictum tempus annorum decem auctoritate presencium de nostra certa scientia et speciali gratia confirmamus et ad uberiorem vestram cauthelam de novo confermius et donamus benefaciendo in eadem vosque etcetera. Comittentes vobis etcetera. Quocirca etcetera necnon etcetera ac priori etcetera. Inhibentes vobis etcetera. In cuius etcetera. Data Avinione die octava mensis Marcii anno incarnacionis Domini M^mo^ CCC^mo^ nonagesmio primo.

## 174

*Licence for Fr. Wilhelm Velga, Preceptor of Freiburg, to receive two men who can become priests into the Order and to maintain them in Freiburg.*

*[Avignon], 1392 December 26*

*AOM 326 fol. 114r (106r), under* prioratus Alamanie, Boemie et Vngarie.

Die XXVI^ta^ mensis Decembris anno incarnacionis Domini M° CCC^mo^ nonagesimo secundo data fuit licencia fratri Wilhelmo Velgen preceptori de Friburgo recipiendi viros duos aptos, sufficientes et ydoneos in sacerdotali ordine constitutos, [a]quibus pro divino officio asserit se indigere[a], in fratres religionis ipsisque receptis assignandi stagias in dicta baiulia, in qua sibi provideatur in eorum neccessariis secundum usus et consuetudines dicte domus.

*a-a)* quibus – indigere *add. et corr. in fine.*

## 175

*Licence for Fr. Thomas von Buchheim to travel to the Convent on Rhodes.*

*[Avignon], 1393 July 9*

*AOM 327 fol. 103r (92r), under* prioratus Alamanie et Boemie.

Die nona mensis Iulii anno incarnacionis Domini M$^{mo}$ CCC$^{mo}$ nonagesimo tercio data fuit licencia fratri Thome de Bůchkemheim eundi ad conventum Rodi, quando sibi placuerit, a suo superiore licencia requisita.

## 176

*Licence for Fr. Peter Rod to travel to the Convent on Rhodes.*

*[Avignon, 1393 July 9]*

*AOM 327 fol. 103r (92r), under* prioratus Alamanie et Boemie.

Anno, mense et die quibus supra fuit data licentia fratri Petro Rodi eundi ad conventum Rodi, quando sibi placuerit, a suo superiore licentia requisita.

## 177

*The Master Fr. Juan [Fernández de Heredia], with consent of brethren, confirms Fr. Wilhelm Velga for his lifetime in the Preceptory of Freiburg im Üchtland (Priory of* Alamania).

*Avignon, [139]3 September 12*

*AOM 327 fol. 103r-v (92r-v), under* prioratus Alamanie et Boemie.

Frater Iohannes etcetera religioso in Christo nobis carissimo fratri Guillelmo Velguen preceptori de Friburgo Hoctellandie domus eiusdem salutem et sinceram in Domino caritatem. Propter probitatis vestre merita et administracionem accomodam, quam in commissis vobis regiminibus in nostro ordine, sicut fidedigno testimonio accepimus, habuistis, illa vobis libenter annuymus, que conservacionem vestri status concernere dignoscuntur. Hinc est, quod preceptoriam sive baiuliam de Friburgo prioratus nostri Alamannie supradictam cum omnibus et singulis suis membris, pertinenciis et iuribus ad eam spectantibus et pertinentibus ac spectare et pertinere debentibus, quoquomodo et cum quibus illam habetis et presencialiter possidetis, habendam, tenendam, regendam, gubernandam, augmentandam et meliorandam in spiritualibus et temporalibus tam in capite quam in membris sub annua responcione et aliis oneribus impositis et imponendis racionabiliter secundum comunem cursum aliarum baiuliarum prioratus predicti in capitulo provinciali prioratus ipsius annis singulis infallibiliter exolvendis – [103v] alias secundum continenciam et seriem statuti super defficientibus in responcionum solucione suarum editi in generali capitulo apud Avinionem de mense Marcii anno sexagesimo sexto celebrato[1] de premissa baiulia per religiosos in Christo nobis carissimos fratres ·· domus eiusdem quovis titulo dicti prioratus regimini nunc vel imposterum[a] presidentem et receptores responcionum prioratus ipsius cum consilio quatuor fratrum preceptorum prioratus iamdicti suarum baiuliarum bene solvencium fratri alicui nostre dicte domus prioratus predicti puta sufficienti, utili et ydoneo ad regimen baiulie antedicte et qui illius responciones et alia onera bene solvat et supportet expresse precipimus provideri confirmacione et nova donacione huiusmodi de dicta baiulia vobis facta in aliquo non obstante – de voluntate, consilio et assensu dicte domus fratrum ·· priorum, preceptorum et procerum nobis assistencium de nostra certa scientia et speciali gratia ad vitam vestram confirmamus et pro uberiori nostra cautela de novo concedimus et donamus benefaciendo in eadem ·· vosque preceptorem et comendatorem in dicta constituimus baiulia hac serie et eciam ordinamus. Comittentes vobis fiducialiter circa curam, regimen et administracionem accomodam dicte baiulie ac bonorum et iurium eius deffencionem ac recuperacionem tam in agendo quam deffendendo hac serie vices nostras. Quocirca universis et singulis fratribus, sororibus et donatis sub virtute sancte obediencie[b] ac hominibus et vassallis et quibusvis aliis nobis subdictis in dicta baiulia constitutis, presentibus et futuris sub sacramento fidelitatis et homagii, quo nobis et nostre domui sunt astricti, precipimus et mandamus, ut vobis tamquam eorum superiori, preceptori et maiori reverenter pareant, obediant et intendant vobisque suum prebeant auxilium, consilium et favorem in omnibus concernentibus utilitatem dicte baiulie, quociens opus fuerit et eos duxeritis requirendos, necnon universis et singulis fratribus domus nostre quacumque auctoritate, dignitate vel officio fungentibus, presentibus et futuris, ne contra presentem nostram donacionem et gratiam aliquatenus venire presumant, quinymmo eam studeant iuxta eius mentem et seriem inviollabiliter observare. Inhibentes vobis districtius sub virtute sancte obediencie supradicta, ne pretextu confirmationis, donationis et gratie nostre huiusmodi aliqua de bonis, rebus aut iuribus memorate baiulie vendatis, detis, obligetis, impignoretis, alienetis, distrahatis seu in emphiteosim perpetuam concedatis vel quocumque alio colore quesito extra nostram religionem transferatis sine nostra speciali licencia et mandato. Et si, quod absit, contra inhibitionem nostram huiusmodi aliquid vel aliqua operari vel facere vos contingat, illud et illa exnunc prout extunc et extunc prout exnunc cassamus, anullamus ac decernimus[c] irritum et inane nulliusque existere penitus efficacie vel valoris. In cuius etcetera. Data Avinione die duodecima mensis Septembris anno tercio.

*a)* imposterim *MS* *b)* obodiencie *MS* *c)* decernibus *praem. ante corr.*

1) *1367 March 5: Delaville (1913), 161–2.*

## 178

*Licence for Fr. Wilhelm Velga, Preceptor of Freiburg im Üchtland, to receive two men as chaplains into the Order.*

*[Avignon, 1393 September 12]*

*AOM 327 fol. 104r (93r), under* prioratus Alamanie et Boemie.

Anno, mense et die quibus supra data fuit licentia fratri Guillelmo Velguen preceptori de Friburgo Hoctellandie faciendi duos fratres capellanos.

## 179

*Mandate for Fr. Hesso [Schlegelholz], Preceptor of Kos, to receive Matthäus Stoweil as knight brother into the Priory of* Alamania, *provided that he be knighted, apt, sound, of legitimate birth. After his reception into the Order, Matthäus is to come to the Convent on Rhodes with his horses and armour.*

*[Avignon,] 1394 July 4*

*AOM 328 fol. 132r (130r), under* prioratus Vngarie, Alamanie et Boemie.

Die IIII mensis Iullii anno presenti nonagesimo quarto comissa fuit fratri Hessoni preceptori Langoni, ut Macheum de Scouiulo recipiat in fratrem religionis prioratus Alamanie, ipso prius insingito milicia, dum tamen nobilis sit ex utroque parente matrimonio natus legitimo, sanus et integer suis membris, et cum equis et armis vadat ad conventum Rodi, ad quem conventum, dum receptus fuerit, eidem Macheo data licencia.

Scouiulo *may by* Stouuilo, *meaning Stoweil. A document dated Avignon, 1394 June 16, mentioned Fr.* Anthonio Stobail *[Stoweil?] as a chaplain in the Conventual church of St. John in Rhodes: AOM 328 fol. 162r (160r), under* partes cismarine.

## 180

*The Master Fr. Juan Fernández de Heredia retains Fr. Kaspar Ederli for his lifetime with all his possessions, including the two churches in Gündlingen and St. Peter in Alt-Kenzingen and the two villages in Gündlingen and Bremgarten, which Kaspar has bought for the Order. Kaspar is to hold these churches for his lifetime. After his death they are to pass to the Preceptory (here* baiulia*) of Freiburg. No person in charge of the Priory of* Alamania *may violate this decision of the Master.*

*Avignon, 1394 August 8*

*AOM 328 fol. 132r (130r), under* prioratus Vngarie, Alamanie et Boemie.

Frater Iohannes etcetera religioso in Christo nobis carissimo fratri Caspar Ederli domus eiusdem salutem et sinceram in Domino caritatem. Dum[a)] laudabilia antique proceritatis vestre merita in consideracionis nostre aciem recensemus, digne agimus, cum vos inter alios domus nostre fratres proceres attolimus et prosequimur prerogativaspecialis gratie et honoris, illa presertim, per quem possitis malignis conatibus obviare. Huiusmodi consideracione ducti vestram volentes honorare personam, ut proinde vestre devocionis et fidei zelus ad laudabiliora inantea ferventibus animetur, vos et ecclesias in Gundlingen et sancti Petri in Aldenkenneziegenn vobis, ut asseritis, ad vitam et post vestrum decessum nostro ordini ac villas in Gundlingen et in Bremgarten prioratus nostri Almanie a baiulia de Friburg dependentes cum suis pertinenciis per vos emptis et bona alia vestra quecunque ad manus nostras retinemus tenore presencium de speciali gratia et sub protectione nostra quamdieu[!] vicxeritis suscepimus[b)] necnon a dicte domus fratris nostrum locumtenentis in dicto prioratu et quocunque al[i]orum fratrum domus eiusdem quovis titulo prioratus Alamanie regimini nunc vel imposterum presidentis potestate, iurisdictione, domin[i]o, punicione, correctione et visitacione omnimodis totaliter ex nostra certa scientia et de gratia speciali eximimus[c)] et etiam liberamus. Quocirca universis et singulis domus eiusdem fratribus quascunque[!][d)] dignitate vel officio fungentibus, presentibus et futuris sub virtute sancte obediencie districte mandamus, ne contra nostras huiusmodi retencionem, susceptionem, exemptionem et liberacionem aliquid attemptare seu facere presumant, quynimo efficaciter illas servent[e)]. Quod, si secus eum vel eos in contrarium opperiri vel facere contingat, illud et ea exnunc pro[ut] extunc cassamus, revocamus et nullius existere volumus efficacie vel valoris. In cuius rei testimonium bulla nostra plumbea presentibus est appensa. Dat. Avinione die octava mensis Augusti anno incarnacionis Domini millesimo CCC° nonagesimo quarto.

*a)* i *add. MS* *b)* succe *praem. ante corr.* *c)* exininus *MS* *d)* quacun *praem. ante corr.* *e)* serrient *MS*

## 181

*The Master Fr. Juan Fernández de Heredia absolves Fr. Kaspar Ederli from a contract forced upon him by the pretended Prior of* Alamania *Fr. Friedrich von Zollern and orders the restoration of the parish churches and villages of Gündlingen, Alt-Kenzingen and Bremgarten. This contract has been confirmed by an oath and guaranteed by bailsmen, but Kaspar now refused to leave the obedience of Pope Clement VII.*

*[Avignon, 1394 August 8]*

*AOM 328 fol. 132v-3r (130v-31r), under* prioratus Vngarie, Alamanie et Boemie.

Frater Iohannes Ferdinandi de Redia Dei gratia sacre domus hospitalis etcetera religioso in Christo nobis carissimo fratri Caspari Ederli domus eiusdem salutem et sinceram in Domino caritatem. Quia oppressis in iusticia dedecet provisionis debite remedium denegari denotato siquidem nobis per vos, quod dudum dicte domus frater Fredericus de Zolre[a] prior pretensus prioratus Alamanie vos absque iusta et racionabili causa voluntarie et de facto cepit captum, carceribus mancipavit, detinuit aquibus, vos liberare recusavit, nisi prius per vos violenter et de facto eidem fratri Frederico de ecclesiis in Grundlingen et sancti Petri in Aldenkentzingen et in Bremgarten[1] prioratus predicti, quas iusto titulo possedistis et habuistis[b], facta resignacione iuramento et fideiussoribus super hec per vos prestitis huiusmodi ecclesias et villas non receptere illa dumtaxat occasione pretensa, quod in obedientia beatissimi domini nostri pape Clementis septimi ac fidelitate et devocione sancte Romane ecclesie et nostri dicti magistri iugiter permansistis, eciam de presenti permanetis quodque subiuncto suppliciter humilitate[c] devota, ut ecclesias et villas predictas vobis reddere, restituere vosque in eorum possessionem inducere ac eas confirmare cum ipsarum iuribus et pertinenciis dignaremur. Nosque premissorum consideracione necnon propter susceptum de famosa et antiqua proceritate vestra ac fructuoso vestro regimine testimonium laudabile vota vestra exaudientes benigne ac volentes ea, que indebite gesta sunt, ad statum reduci debitum, si denotacio supradicta veritatem contineat, vobis ab dicto iuramento, ut asseritis, absoluto ecclesias parrochiales et villas supradictas cum earum et cuiuslibet iuribus, menbris et pertinenciis ad eas et quamlibet ipsarum spectantibus et pertinentibus et debentibus pertinere et cum quibus illas tenuistis et possedistis, tenebatis, possidebatis tempore dicte resignacionis habendas, tenendas[d] et gubernandas cum oneribus annexis et supportari consuetis, quamdiu vicxeritis, tenore presencium de nostra certa scientia reddimus, restituimus vosque in ipsarum possessionem per tradicionem litterarum presencium inducimus et pro habundanciori[e] cautela [133r] huiusmodi ecclesias et villas prenominatas vobis ad vitam vestram harum serie de speciali gratia confirmamus. Quocirca universis et singulis fratribus, sororibus et donatis sub virtute sancte obedientie ac hominibus et vassallis et quibusvis aliis nobis subdictis in dictis ecclesiis et villis constitutis, presentibus et futuris sub sacramento fidelitatis et homagii, quo nobis et dicte domui sunt astricti, precipimus et mandamus, ut vobis tamquam eorum superiori et maiori reverenter pareant, obediant et intendant vobisque suum prebeant auxilium, consilium et favorem in omnibus concernentibus utilitatem dictarum ecclesiarum et villarum, quociens opus fuerit et eos ducxeritis requirendos, necnon universis et singulis fratribus domus nostre quacumque auctoritate, dignitate vel officio fungentibus, presentibus et futuris, ne contra presentes venire presumant, quinymo efficaciter illas servent.

*a)* deso *praem. ante corr.* *b)* habuisti *MS* *c)* dev *praem. ante corr.* *d)* tenendas *praem.* *e)* habundancioni *MS*

*1) No. 180.*

## 182

*The Master Fr. Juan [Fernández de Heredia] orders the restoration to Fr. Dietrich von Keppenbach of the Preceptory (here* baiulia) *of Neuenburg with the parish churches in Schlatt and Schliengen unlawfully detained by the pretended Prior of* Alamania *Fr. Friedrich von Zollern.*

*Avignon, 1394 August 8*

*AOM 328 fol. 133r-v (131r-v), under* prioratus Vngarie, Alamanie et Boemie.

Frater Iohannes etcetera religioso in Christo nobis carissimo fratri Dyetrico de Keppenbach preceptori baiulie Novicastri domus eiusdem salutem et sinceram in Domino caritatem. Quia oppressis in iusticia non[a] decet provisionis debite remedium denegari exposito nobis siquidem pro parte vestra, quod dudum dicte domus frater Fredericus de Zolre[b] pretensus prior prioratus nostri Alamanie absque iusta et rationabili causa voluntarie et de facto vos suppliavit[c] et abiexit de baiulia predicta Novicastri, quam in dicto prioratu iusto et legitimo titulo obtinebatis, illa dumtaxat occasione pretensa, quod in obediencia beatissimi domini nostri pape Clementis septimi ac fidelitate et devocione sancte Romane ecclesie et nostri dicti magistri iugiter[d] permansistis, eciam de presenti permanetis quodque subiuncto suppliciter humilitate devota, ut dictam baiuliam vobis reddere, restituere vosque in eius possessiones inducere et ipsam baiuliam unacum preceptoriis sive ecclesiis parrochialibus de Slat et in Singen[1] cum ipsarum et cuiuslibet iuribus et pertinenciis vobis ad vitam de novo concedere dignaremur. Nosque premissorum consideracione necnon propter susceptum[e] de famosa et antiqua proceritate vestra ac utili vestro regimine testimonium laudabile vota vestra exaudientes benigne [133v] ac volentes ea, que indebite gesta sunt, ad statum redduci debitum, si exposicio supradicta veritatem contineat, baiuliam Novicastri supradictam[f] cum suis menbris, iuribus et pertinentiis ad eam spectantibus et pertinentibus et debentibus pertinere, quoquomodo et cum quibus illam tenuistis et possedistis, tenebatis et possidebatis tempore huiusmodi supplicacionis habendam, tenendam et gubernandam, quamdiu vicxeritis, sub annua responcione et aliis oneribus exolvendis anno quolibet loco et termino consuetis tenore presencium de nostra certa sciencia reddimus, restituimus vosque in ipsius possessionem per tradicionem litterarum presencium inducimus et pro habundanciori cautela vestra huiusmodi baiuliam Novicastri unacum dictis preceptoriis seu ecclesiis parrochialibus de Slat et in

1) *In Schlatt Fr. Dietrich von Keppenbach, Preceptor of Freiburg, bought in 1362 from the Lazarites their preceptory and in 1371 the village from the Landgraf im Breisgau Count Egeno von Freiburg: Krieger 2 (1905), col. 847–9. In Schliengen the Prior Fr. Helwich von Randersacker bought in 1300 the parish church from the patrician family in Freiburg called Schnewli: ibid. 856.*

Singen vobis ad vitam de speciali gratia harum serie contulimus et donamus. Quocirca universis et singulis fratribus, sororibus et donatis sub virtute sancte obediencie ac hominibus et vassallis et quibusvis aliis nobis subdictis in dictis baiulia et ecclesiis constitutis, presentibus et futuris sub sacramento fidelitatis et homagii, quo nobis et nostre domui sunt astricti, precipimus et mandamus, ut tamquam eorum superiori, preceptori et maiori reverenter pareant, obediant et intendant vobisque suum prebeant auxilium, consilium et favorem in omnibus concernentibus[g] utilitatem dictarum baiulie et ecclesiarum[h], quociens opus fuerit et eos duxeritis requirendos, necnon universis et singulis fratribus domus nostre quacumque auctoritate, dignitate vel officio fungentibus, presentibus et futuris, ne contra presentes venire presumant, quinymo efficaciter illas servent. In cuius rei testimonium bulla nostra plumbea presentibus est appensa. Datum Avinione die octava mensis Augusti anno incarnacionis Domini millesimo CCC° nonagesimo quarto.

*a)* non *repetit.* *b)* Solre *praem. ante corr.* *c)* spoliavit *forsan.* *d)* ius *praem. ante corr.* *e)* suspectum *MS* *f)* suprad *praem. ante corr.* *g)* concertibus *MS* *h)* ecclesiarum *praem. ante corr.*

## 183

*The Master Fr. Juan [Fernández de Heredia] retains Fr. Dietrich von Keppenbach, Preceptor of Neuenburg, together with his preceptory (here* baiulia*) and the parish churches of Schlatt and Schliengen.*

*Avignon, 1394 August 8*

*AOM 328 fol. 133v-4r (131v-2r), under* prioratus Vngarie, Alamanie et Boemie.

Frater Iohannes etcetera religioso in Christo nobis carissimo fratri Dyetrico de Keppenbach preceptori baiulie Novicastri[a] domus eiusdem salutem et sinceram in Domino caritatem. Dum laudabilia antique proceritatis vestre merita in consideracionis [134r] nostre aciem recensemus, digne agimus, cum vos inter alios domus nostre fratres proceres atollimus[b] et prosequamur prerogativa specialis gracie et honoris illa presertim, per quam possitis malignis conatibus obviare. Huiusmodi consideracione ducti, vestram volentes honorare personam et proinde vestre devocionis et fidei zelus ad laudabiliora inantea fervencius animetur vos et ecclesias parrochiales seu preceptorias de Slat et in Singen[1] prioratus Alamanie[c] et bona alia vestra quecumque solutis termino consueto integre per vos animus earundem in domorum et ecclesiarum responcionibus et oneribus quibuslibet impositis et imponendis supportatis ad manus nostras retinemus tenore presencium de speciali gracia sub protectione nostra, quamdiu

*1) No. 182.*

vicxeritis, suscepimus necnon a dicte domus fratris nostrumlocumtenentis in dicto prioratu et quorumlibet aliorum fratrum domus eiusdem quovis titulo dicti prioratus Alamanie regimini nunc vel imposterum presidentium potestate, iurisdictione, dominio, punitione, correctione et visitacione omnimodis totaliter ex nostra certa scientia et de gratia speciali eximimus et eciam liberamus. Quocirca universis et singulis domus eiusdem fratribus quacumque dignitate vel officio fungentibus, presentibus et futuris sub virtute sancte obedientie districte[d)] mandamus, ne contra nostras huiusmodi retencionem, susceptionem, exempcionem et liberacionem aliquid atemptare seu facere presumant, quinymmo efficaciter illas servent. Quod, si secus eum vel eos in contrarium opperari vel facere contingat, illud et ea exnunc prout extunc cassamus, revocamus et nullius existere volumus efficacie vel valoris. In cuius rei testimonium bulla nostra plumbea presentibus est appenssa. Datum Avinione die octava mensis Augusti anno incarnacionis Domini millesimo CCC° nonagesimo quarto.

*a)* Nouist *praem. ante corr.* *b)* et a *praem. ante corr.* *c)* Alamania *MS* *d)* discripte *MS*

## 181

*The Master Fr. Juan [Fernández de Heredia] orders his lieutenant in the Priory of* Alamania *Fr. Friedrich von Zollern to restore to Fr. Kaspar Ederli the churches in Gündlingen and St. Peter in Alt-Kenzingen and the villages of Gündlingen and Bremgarten. Fr. Kaspar has served for a long time in the Order.*

*Avignon, 1394 August 8*

*AOM 328 fol. 134r-v (132r-v), under* prioratus Vngarie, Alamanie et Boemie.

Frater Iohannes etcetera religioso in Christo nobis carissimo fratri Frederico de Zolre, in prioratu Alamanie nostrumlocumtenenti domus eiusdem, salutem et sinceram in Domino caritatem. Vos scire supponimus, quod religio nostra regitur regula, statutis et usibus approbatis, secundum que ipsa religio eius professores, fratres benemeritos ad honores promovere et promotos in eorum statibus conservare consuevit, nisi racionabilis causa subsit, ob quam abinde debeant removeri. Cum itaque, sicut accepimus, [134v] vos fratrem Caspar Ederli, qui in nostro ordine per longa[a)] tempora vitam ducxit laudabilem, ecclesiis in Gundlingen et sancti Petri in Aldenkenczingen et villis in Gundlingen et in Bremgarten[1)] prioratus predicti, quas iusto possedit titulo, spoliastis et deiecistis[b)] violenter et de facto nulla subeunte causa et absque fratrum esgardis tamquam immemor regule statutorum et usuum religionis in dedecus vestrum et non modicum dispendium[c)]

*1) Krieger 1 (1904), col. 283–4, 790, 1147.*

dicti fratris Caspari suplicantis a nobis super hiis debito iusticie remedio provideri[d]. Et quia nos debitores iusticie cunctas exposcentes existere agnoscimus, dicta supplicacione admissa vobis tenore presentium sub virtute sancte obediencie precipimus et mandamus, quatenus dictum fratrem Caspar ad dictas ecclesias et villas per nos restitutum, prout in litteris inde confectis bullatis bulla nostra plumbea continetur, et in earum possessionem inductum habeatis, ad eas gratanter admittere permicttatis et faciatis ipsum gaudere ecclesiis et villis huiusmodi earumque iuribus et emolumentis eatenus retrolapsis temporibus ante spoliacionem et deiectionem earundem facere consuevit, ut vos in prompta et reverenti executione dictarum litterarum et presencium huiusmodi, ne inobediencie macula vos vituperet et propterea vos tanquam inobedientem et rebellem exponat puniendum per iusticiam domus nostre. Datum Avinione die octava mensis Augusti anno incarnacionis Domini millesimo CCC° nonagesimo quarto.

*a)* longua *MS* *b)* devecistis *MS* *c)* dispenduum *MS* *d)* Et quia nos debitores iusticie remedio provideri *dupl. (homoiotel.)*

## 185

*Licence for Fr. Dietrich von Keppenbach, Preceptor of Neuenburg, and for Fr. Kaspar Ederli to travel to the Convent on Rhodes.*

*[Avignon, 13]94 August 29*

*AOM 328 fol. 134v (132v), under* prioratus Vngarie, Alamanie et Boemie.

Anno quo supra nonagesimo quarto et die vicesimo nona mensis Augusti fratribus Diectrico de Keppenbach preceptori Novicastri et Caspar Ederli fuit data licentia in statu sibi decenti eundi ad conventum Rodi.

## 186

*Licence for Fr. Hermann Ow, Preceptor of Villingen, to leave the Convent on Rhodes for the Priory of* Alamania *and to return whenever he wishes.*

*[Rhodes, 1400] February 21*

*AOM 330 fol. 81r (82r), under* prioratus Alamanie, Boemie et Vngarie.

Anno quo supra et die vicesima prima mensis Februarii[a] data fuit licensia fratri Hermando[b] Oub preceptori baiullie Fillingen prioratus Almanie recedendi de conventu Rodi et eundi ad dictum prioratum et pariter redeundi ad dictum conventum, quando voluerit.

*a)* Frebruarii *MS* *b)* Armando *praem. ante corr.*

## 187

*The Master Fr. Philibert de Naillac and the Convent grant for ten years to Fr. Ulrich Tripscher the Preceptory of Überlingen (Priory of* Alamania), *which is vacant following the death of Fr. Johann von Hegi.*

*Rhodes, 1400 July 6*

*AOM 330 fol. 81r (82r), under* prioratus Alamanie, Boemie et Vngarie.

Frater Philibertus de Nailhaco etcetera et nos conventus etcetera religioso in Christo nobis carissimo fratri Uolrich Tripschr dicte domus salutem etcetera. Dum ad ydoneitatis et sufficiencie vestre notam et alia virtuosa vestra merita obsequiave per vos prestita Deo et nostre religioni zelo fidei, contra cuius emulos sepius velud intrepidus Christi milles exponendo personam[a)] consideracionem reflectimus, racione duce credimus operari, cum vos dono prosequimur gratie specialis. Hinc est, quod baiuliam de Uberlingen prioratus nostri Alamanie vacantem per mortem fratris Iohannis de Hegi et ad nostram disposicionem propterea devolutam cum omnibus et singulis suis membris, pertinenciis et iuribus ad eam spectantibus et pertinentibus ac spectare et pertinere debentibus, quoquomodo et cum quibus illam condam dictus frater Iohannes tenuit, habuit et possedit, habendam etcetera invice[b)] deliberato consilio de nostra certa sciencia et speciali gratia hinc ad annos decem continuos et completos salvo iure communis thesauri pro una annata ratione vacantie vobis auctoritate presencium conferimus et donamus benefaciendo in eadem vosque preceptorem etcetera. Comittentes etcetera. Quocirca etcetera necnon etcetera ac priori seu presidenti etcetera. Inhibentes etcetera. Et si, quod absit, etcetera. In cuius rey testimonium bulla nostra communis plumbea presentibus est apensa. Datum Rodi die sexta mensis Iulii anno incarnacionis Domini M° quatercentesimo.

*a)* personem *MS* *b)* invicem *forsan.*

## 188

*The Master Fr. Philibert [de Naillac] and the Convent grant to Fr. Hesso Schlegelholz, Prior of* Alamania *and Preceptor of Kos, as his fifth preceptory the houses of Frankfurt and Mosbach (Priory of* Alamania), *which are vacant following the death of Fr. Helfrich von Rüdigheim, called Rückingen. This grant is made according to a decision of the Tongue reported by the Pilier Fr. Ulrich Tripscher.*

*Rhodes, 1400 July 6*

*AOM 330 fol. 81r-v (82r-v), under* prioratus Alamanie, Boemie et Vngarie. *Partial ed. van Winter (1998), 32–3 no. 8.*

Frater Philibertus etcetera et nos conventus etcetera religioso in Christo nobis carissimo fratri Hessoni Slegelholtz priori Alamanie et preceptori Lengonis dicte domus salutem etcetera. Sequentes, ut tenemur, nostre religionis statuta, secundum que dicte domus fratres priores et castellani omnes et singuli in ipsorum prioratibus et castellaniis pro statu et oneribus suis supportandis quatuor baiulias pro suis cameris ipsorum iure ordinario et quintam baiuliam eorum tamen collacioni pertinentem debent habere in recompensationem certorum iurium, que ipsi solebant percipere et habere de bonis fratrum preceptorum prioratuum et castellaniarum suarum decedencium, quodque quintam baiuliam, ut prefertur, vobis debitam in dicto prioratu nondum[a)] fueritis assecutus et ad [81v] presens in eodem prioratu domus de Frankenfort et de Moesbach[b)] per obitum dicte domus fratris Halfridi de Ruckingen nostre pertinentes collacioni fratribus conventus dicti prioratus per nos conferendi vacare noscantur, huiusmodi domos de Frankenfort et de Moesbach, ut predicitur, vacantes et ad nostram collationem devolutam dicti prioratus lingue Allamanie fratribus consentientibus[c)], prout dicte lingue pilerius frater V̊lricus Trischer nobis retulit, cum omnibus et singulis eorum membris, iuribus et pertinentiis ad eas et earum quemlibet spetantibus et pertinentibus ac spectare debentibus, quoquomodo et cum quibus dictus condam frater Helfridus illas habuit, tenuit et possedit, habendam etcetera invicem deliberato consilio de nostra certa scientia et speciali gratia vobis concedimus et donamus auctoritate presencium benefaciendo in eisdem vosque preceptorem etcetera. Committentes etcetera. Quocirca etcetera. Inhibentes etcetera. Et si, quod absit, etcetera. In cuius rey testimonium bulla nostra communis plumbea presentibus est appensa. Datum Rodi die sexta mensis Iullii anno incarnacionis Domini M° quatercentesimo.

*a)* nundum *MS* *b)* Most *praem. ante corr.* *c)* consensientibus *MS*

## 189

*Licence for Fr. Stephan Kluber to leave the Convent for the Priory of* Alamania *and to return.*

*[Rhodes, 1400] August 28*

*AOM 330 fol. 81v (82v), under* prioratus Alamanie, Boemie et Vngarie.

Anno quo supra et die XXVIII[a] mensis Augusti fratri Stephano Klober fuit data licencia recedendi de conventu Rodi et eundi ad prioratum et partes Alamanie et inde redeundi ad conventum, quando voluerit, a superiore suo requisita licentia.

## 190

*The Master Fr. Philibert de Naillac and the Convent at Rhodes confirm Fr. Stephen Kluber for ten years in the Preceptory of Laa (Priory of Bohemia), which was granted to him by the former Master Fr. Juan Fernández de Heredia (no. 140).*

*Rhodes, 1400 October 26*

*AOM 330 fol. 81v (82v), under* prioratus Alamanie, Boemie et Vngarie.

Frater Philibertus de Nailhaco etcetera et nos conventus Rodi domus eiusdem religioso in Christo nobis carissimo fratri Stephano Kluber preceptori baiulie de Lo̊ch dicte domus salutem etcetera. Propter susceptum de vobis testimonium comendabile ac sperantes, quod in commisso vobis regimine effectus administracionis utilis faciente divina gratia vos comendet, donacionem et collationem de dicta baiulia de Loach prioratus Boemie per inmediatum predecessorem nostrum fratrem Iohannem Ferdinandi de Redia vobis factam gratam, placidam habentes et acceptam preceptoriam sive baiuliam predictam de Loach cum omnibus et singulis suis membris, pertinentiis et iuribus ad eam spectantibus et pertinentibus ac spectare et pertinere debentibus, quoquomodo habendam etcetera invicem deliberato consilio de nostra certa scientia et speciali gratia hinc ad annos decem continuos et completos vobis auctoritate presencium confirmamus et ad uberiorem vestram cautelam de novo conferimus et donamus benefaciendo in eadem vosque etcetera. Comittentes etcetera. Quocirca etcetera necnon etcetera ac priori etcetera. Inhibentes etcetera. Et si, quod etcetera. In cuius etcetera. Datum Rodi die vicesima sexta mensis Octobris anno incarnacionis Domini millesimo quatercentesimo.

## 191

*The Master Fr. Philibert de Naillac and the Convent grant for ten years to Fr. Henman von Küssaberg the Preceptory of Hohenrain (Priory of* Alamania), *which is vacant following the death of Fr. Johann Züricher.*

*Rhodes, 1402 January 3*

*AOM 331 fol. 120r (120r), under* prioratus Alamanie et Boemie.

Frater Philibertus de Nailhaco etcetera et nos conventus Rodi etcetera religioso in Christo nobis carissimo fratri Hermanys de Kuissaberg dicte domus salutem et sinceram in Domino caritatem. Ad illos libenter[a] gratiosum nostrum favorem extendimus, quos benemeritos reputamus, ut reffecti ex gratia et exhilarati ex honore suscepto ad promovenda religionis nostre commoda libencius invigilent et ad virtutum studia fervencius animentur. Grata igitur fidedigna relatione percepto, quod gratiarum largitor Dominus vos morum composicione, vite mundicia et naturali discretiva virtute dotavit, sperantes in commisso vobis regimine favente Domino vos fructus uberes allaturus preceptoriam seu baiuliam Hŏnrain prioratus nostri Alamanie vacantem per obitum dicte domus fratris Iohannis Zůrycher vakat et ad nostram collationem propterea devolutam cum omnibus et singulis suis membris, pertinenciis et iuribus ad eam spectantibus et pertinentibus ac spectare et pertinere debentibus, quoquomodo et cum quibus illam dictus quondam frater Iohannes tenuit, habuit et possedit, habendam etcetera invicem deliberato consilio de nostra certa scientia et speciali gratia ad annos decem continuos et completos salvo iure communis thesauri ratione vacationis pro una annata vobis auctoritate presencium conferimus, concedimus et donamus benefaciendo in eadem vosque etcetera. Comittentes etcetera. Quocirca etcetera necnon etcetera ac priori etcetera. Inhibentes etcetera. Et si, quod etcetera. In cuius etcetera. Data Rodi die tercia mensis Ianuarii anno incarnacionis Domini millesimo quatercentesimo primo.

*a)* li *supra lin.*

## 192

*Fr. Ulrich Tripscher, Pilier of the Tongue of* Alamania *and Preceptor of [Villingen], is appointed lieutenant of Fr. Hesso Schlegelholz, Preceptor of Kos, until further notice. When Fr. Iñigo d'Alfaro arrives, Fr. Ulrich has to give up this lieutenancy.*

*[Rhodes, 1402] January 3*

*AOM 331 fol. 120r (120r), under* prioratus Alamanie et Boemie.

Anno quo supra et die tercia mensis Ianuarii frater Ulricus Trypscher, pilerius lingue Almanie et preceptor ··, fuit per magistrum cum consilio fratrum ·· baillivorum, preceptorum et procerum conventus deputatus[a)] locumtenens in baiulia Langoni usque ad magistri beneplacitum et alias fuerit super hoc ordinatum per preceptorem Langoni fratrem Hessonem priorem[b)] Alamanie. Itaque in accessu fratris Eugenio Dalfara[1)] purgatur officio locumtenentis.

*a)* fuit *praem. ante corr.* *b)* priore *MS*

## 193

*The Master Fr. Philibert de Naillac and the Convent quit Fr. Domenico d'Alamania, Preceptor of Naples, Santo Stefano di Monopoli and Avignon, for 1,700 florins of Rhodes. They order Fr. Hesso Schlegelholz, Prior of* Alamania *and Preceptor of Kos, to pay this sum to Fr. Domenico in satisfaction of a debt of 1,800 florins of Germany.*

*Rhodes, 1402 January 3*

*1) Fr. Iñigo d'Alfaro.*

*AOM 331 fol. 173v (174v), under* assignaciones peccuniarum.

Frater Philibertus de Nailhaco etcetera et nos conventus Rodi domus eiusdem ·· universis et singulis dicte domus fratribus ·· et quibusvis aliis inspecturis et audituris presentes nostras litteras notum facimus, recognoscimus et in verbo veritatis testamur, quoniam religiosus in Christo nobis carissimus frater Dominicus de Alamania preceptor Neapolis, sancti Stephani Monopolitani et Avinionensis baiuliarum nobis pro nostris supportandis neccessitatibus tradidit, consignavit mille septingentos florenos Rodi currentes seu ipsorum valorem, quos sibi per presentes assignamus per eum vel eius procuratorem recipiendos et habendos de et super mille octingentis florenis Alamanie de peccuniis nostris receptis et habitis per dicte domus fratrem Hessonem Slegelholtz priorem Alamanie et preceptorem baiulie Langonis, prout dictus prior et preceptor nobis scripsit. Quapropter [a)]cupientes eidem fratri Dominico de dicta quantitate mille septingentorum florenorum Rodi currentium satisfieri[a)] prefato fratri Hessoni priori et preceptori ipsiusque locumtenentibus et procuratoribus [b)]et eorum cuilibet insolidum[b)] ubilibet constitutis sub virtute sancte obedientie tenore presencium precipimus et mandamus, ut dicto fratri Dominico seu eius procuratori et ab eo mandatum sufficiens habenti dictos mille septingentos florenos Rodi currentes vel eorum valorem presentibus receptis dent, solvant, tradant et assignent in deducione dicte quantitatis mille octingentorum florenorum Alamanie. Quibus mille septingentis florenis Rodi currentibus vel ipsorum valore solutis et traditis, ut prefertur, illos pro receptis et habitis reputamus et [b)]inde contenti tenore presencium[b)] eosdem[c)] priorem et [d)]preceptorem eiusque locatenentes et procuratores[e)] et[d)] quos tangat absolvimus et quictamus. In cuius rei testimonium bulla nostra communis plumbea presentibus est appensa. Data Rodi die tercia mensis Ianuarii anno incarnacionis Domini millesimo quatercentesimo primo.

*a-a) marg.* *b-b) marg.* *c)* dictum *praem. ante corr.* *d-d) supra lin.* *e)* procuratoribus *MS*

*See no. 195.*

## 194

*Licence for Fr. Henman von Küssaberg, Preceptor of Hohenrain, to leave the Convent on Rhodes for his preceptory and to return.*

*[Rhodes, 1402] January 8*

*AOM 331 fol. 120r (120r), under* prioratus Alamanie et Boemie.

Anno quo supra et die VIII[a] mensis Ianuarii data fuit licentia fratri Henmanys de Kuissaberg preceptori baiulie de Hůnrain recedendi de nostro conventu Rodi et eundi ad regendum dictam baiuliam et de dictis prioratu Alamanie et baiulia[a)] reddeundi ad ipsum conventum, quando voluerit, a superiore suo requisita licentia.

*a)* baiulie *MS*

## 195

*The Master Fr. Philibert de Naillac and the Convent order [Fr. Hesso Schlegelholz], Prior of* Alamania *and Preceptor of Kos, and his lieutenant to deduct from 1,800 florins of Germany they owe to Fr. Domenico d'Alamania 820 florins of Rhodes for Nicholaus Belloch, citizen and inhabitant of Rhodes. This leaves a debt of 1,700 florins of Rhodes they owe to Fr. Domenico.*

*Rhodes, 1402 January 10*

*AOM 331 fol. 174r (175r), under* assignaciones peccuniarum.

Frater Philibertus de Nailhaco etcetera et nos conventus Rodi domus eiusdem universis et singulis dicte domus fratribus ·· priori Alamanie, preceptori Langonis eiusque locatenentibus et procuratoribus ubilibet constitutis notum facimus, testamur et in verbo veritatis publice tenore presencium recognoscimus nos teneri et ex vera causa dare debere discreto viro Nicolao Beluche, civi et habitatori nostro Rodi, mille florenos Rodi currentes, de quibus eidem Nicolao satisfieri volentes, ut tenemur, sibi in deducione et defalcacione dicte quantitatis mille florenorum assignamus florenos octingentos viginti Rodi currentes per dictorum prioratus Alamanie et baiulie Langoni dicte domus fratrem ·· priorem et preceptorem de summa et quantitate mille octingentorum florenorum Alamanie per ipsum priorem et preceptorem habitorum de peccuniis nostris nobis debitos et restantes ad solvendum computata assignacione per nos facta super hec dicte domus fratri Dominico de Alamania de florenis Rodi currentibus mille et septingentis. Quapropter vobis dicte domus fratribus ·· priori et preceptori necnon locatenentibus et procuratoribus vestris et eorum cuilibet insolidum tenore presencium precipimus et mandamus sub virtute sancte obedientie, ut dicto Nicolao Beluche seu eius procuratori dictos octingentos et viginti florenos Rodi currentibus infra mensem a presentacione presencium vobis facta computandum tradatis et solvatis, quibus octingentis viginti florenis Rodi currentibus solutis, ut prefertur, illos pro habitis et receptis reputamus et nos inde contenti vos priorem et preceptorem et quos tangit tenore presencium absolvimus et quictamus. In cuius rei testimonium bulla nostra communis plumbea presentibus est appensa. Data Rodi die decima mensis Ianuarii anno incarnacionis Domini millesimo quatercentesimo primo.

*See no. 193. On Belloch, Countryside (2019), 37, 59, 128 with note, 206–7, 279.*

## 196

*The Master Fr. Philibert de Naillac and the Convent quit Fr. Iñigo d'Alfaro as lieutenant of Fr. Hesso Schlegelholz, Prior of* Alamania *and Preceptor of Kos, for 1,800 florins as the responsions of the priory.*

*Rhodes, 1402 February 17*

*AOM 331 fol. 175r (176r), under* assignaciones peccuniarum.

Noverint universi et singuli presentes recognicionis[a] et quictacionis litteras visuri et audituri, quod nos frater Philibertus de Nailhaco etcetera et nos conventus Rodi etcetera tenore presencium fatemur et in verbo veritatis recognoscimus nos habuisse et recepisse per manus dicte domus fratris Oneygo Dalfara[1] vice et nomine religiosi in Christo nobis carissimi fratris Hessonis Slegelholtz prioris Alamanie et preceptoris baiulie Langonis mille et octingentos florenos Alamanie pro responsione dicti prioratus, de quibus mille et octingentis florenis Alamanie nobis solutis et traditis, ut prefertur, contenti dictum priorem et quos tangit tenore presencium invicem deliberato consilio de nostra certa scientia quictamus. In cuius rei testimonium bulla nostra communis plumbea presentibus est appensa. Data Rodi die decima septima mensis Februarii anno incarnacionis Domini millesimo quatercentesimo primo.

*a)* regnicionis *MS*

## 197

*Assignation to pay to Fr. Ulrich [Tripscher], Pilier [of the Tongue of* Alamania*], 166 florins of Germany from the Priory of* Alamania.

*[Rhodes, 1402] February 20*

*AOM 331 fol. 174r (175r), under* assignaciones peccuniarum.

Anno quo supra et die XX mensis Februarii fuit facta assignacio fratri Ulrico pilerio lingue Alamanie super ipso prioratu de centum LX sex florenis Alamanie.

## 198

*The Master Fr. Philibert de Naillac and the Convent order Fr. Hesso Schlegelholz, Prior of* Alamania *and Preceptor of Kos, to deduct from the responsions which Fr. Ulrich Tripscher owes for his preceptory 166 florins which Fr. Ulrich is to receive from the Treasury.*

*Rhodes, 1402 February 20*

*1) No. 193.*

*AOM 331 fol. 173v (174v), under* assignaciones peccuniarum.

Frater Philibertus de Nailhaco etcetera et nos conventus Rodi etcetera religioso in Christo nobis carissimo fratri Hessoni Slegelholcz priori Alamanie et preceptori Langonis dicte domus salutem etcetera. Ecce vobis tenore presencium notum facimus, quoniam dicte domus frater Ulricus Trippscher pilerius lingue Alamanie debet recipere et habere a communi thesauro nostre religionis centum sexaginta sex florenos Alamanie, de quibus sibi satisfieri volentes vobis tenore presencium comittimus et mandamus, quatenus de et super responsione baiulie dicti fratris Ulrici dictam quantitatem florenorum deducatis eidem seu alias contentetis eundem de responsionibus prioratus predicti. In cuius rei testimonium bulla nostra communis plumbea presentibus est appensa. Data Rodi die vicesima mensis Februarii anno incarnacionis Domini millesimo quatercentesimo primo.

## 199

*The Master Fr. Philibert [de Naillac] and the Convent grant for a further ten years to Fr. Ulrich Tripscher, Preceptor of Überlingen, the Preceptory of Sulz (Priory of* Alamania), *which is vacant following the death of Fr. Johann Ulrich [von Masmünster].*

*Rhodes, 1403 May 17*

*AOM 332 fol. 120r (120r), under* prioratus Alamanie et Boemie.

Frater Philibertus etcetera et nos conventus Rodi domus eiusdem religioso in Christo nobis carissimo fratri Ulrico Tripscher preceptori de Uberlinghen dicte domus salutem [et] sinceram in Domino caritatem. Duce ratione dirigi credimus, [si] quos laudande prospicuitatis illustrant merita et experta utilia regimina nostre domui exhibent fructuosos, talium vota liberali favore prosequimur gratiose, ut, dum votivis gratiis se reffectos prospexerint, merita meritis et virtutes virtutibus studeant cumulare et ad eiusdem nostre domus compendia eorum studia iugiter fervenciora convertant. Meritorum igitur comendabilium consideratione vestrorum et obsequiorum notabilium in promotione catholice fidei adversus eius emulos per vos prestitorum respectu, et quia in eadem nostra domo venustate morum, religiosa vita et conversacione placida continua claruistis, non indigne, prout meruistis, merito in graciarum largicionibus erga vos reddimur liberales, itaque non obstante, quod dictam baiuliam de Uberlinghen obtinere noscamini, preceptoriam seu baiuliam de Sulcz[a)] prioratus nostri Alamanie per obitum dicte domus fratris Iohannis Vͤlin vacantem presentialiter et ad nostram collationem propterea devolutam cum omnibus et singulis suis membris, pertinenciis[b)] et iuribus ad eam spectantibus et pertinentibus ac spectare et pertinere debentibus, quoquomodo et cum quibus illam dictus frater Iohannes tenuit, habuit et possedit, habendam etcetera invicem deliberato consilio de nostra certa scientia et speciali gratia ad annos decem continuos et completos insimul cum predicta baiulia de Uberlinghen vobis auctoritate presencium conferimus, concedimus et donamus benefaciendo in eadem vosque etcetera. Committentes etcetera. Quocirca etcetera necnon etcetera ac priori etcetera. Inhibentes etcetera. In cuius etcetera. Data Rodi die decima septima mensis Madii anno incarnacionis Domini millesimo quatercentesimo tercio.

*a)* Sulem *praem. ante corr.* *b)* pro *praem. ante corr.*

*See the grant to Fr. Dietrich von Keppenbach on 18 November 1403, no. 201.*

## 200

*Licence for Fr. Friedrich Huber to travel to Fr. Hesso [Schlegelholz], Prior of* Alamania, *and to return to Rhodes whenever he wishes.*

*[Rhodes, 1403] June 15*

*AOM 332 fol. 120r (120r), under* prioratus Alamanie et Boemie.

Anno quo supra et die XV mensis Iunii data fuit licencia fratri Frederico Hůbert eundi ad priorem Alamanie fratrem Hessonem et redire ad conventum, quando voluerit.

## 201

*The Master Fr. Philibert de Naillac and the Convent grant for ten years to Fr. Dietrich von Keppenbach the Preceptory of Sulz (Priory of* Alamania), *which is vacant following the death of Fr. Johann Ulrich von Masmünster.*

*Rhodes, 1403 November 18*

*AOM 332 fol. 120v (120v), under* prioratus Alamanie et Boemie.

Frater Philibertus de Nailhaco etcetera et nos conventus Rodi domus eiusdem religioso in Christo nobis carissimo fratri Theoderico de Keppenbach dicte domus salutem etcetera. Ad illos libenter gratiosum nostrum favorem extendimus, quos benemeritos reputamus, ut reffecti ex gratia et exhilarati ex honore suscepto ad promovenda religionis nostre commoda libencius invigilent et ad virtutum studia fervencius animentur. Grata igitur fidedigna relatione percepto, quod gratiarum largitor Dominus vos morum composicione, vite mundicia et naturali discretiva virtute dotavit, sperantes in commisso vobis regimine favente Domino vos fructus uberes allaturos, preceptoriam seu baiuliam nostram de Sulcz prioratus nostri Alamanie per obitum dicte domus fratris Iohannis Vͤlin de Masemunster vacantem presencialiter, seu quovis alio modo vacet, et ad nostram collationem propterea devolutam cum omnibus et singulis suis membris, pertinenciis et iuribus ad eam spectantibus et pertinentibus ac spectare et pertinere debentibus, quoquomodo et cum quibus illam dictus quondam frater Iohannes habuit, tenuit et possedit, habendam etcetera invicem deliberato consilio de nostra certa scientia et speciali gratia ad annos decem continuos et completos vobis auctoritate presencium conferimus, concedimus et donamus benefaciendo in eadem vosque etcetera. Comittentes etcetera. Quocirca etcetera necnon etcetera ac priori etcetera. Inhibentes etcetera. Et si, quod etcetera. In cuius etcetera. Data Rodi die decima octava mensis Novembris anno incarnacionis Domini millesimo quatercentesimo tercio.

*See the grant to Fr. Ulrich Tripscher on 17 May 1403, no. 199.*

## 202

*Licence for Fr. Dietrich von Keppenbach, Preceptor of Sulz, to travel to his preceptory and to return to Rhodes, with his superior's licence.*

*[Rhodes, 1404] April 5*

*AOM 333 fol. 80r (80r), under* prioratus Alamanie et Boemie.

Die quinta mensis Aprilis[a] anno suprascripto data fuit licencia[b] fratri Theodorico de Keppenbach preceptori baiulie de Sulcz[c] eundi ad regendum dictam baiuliam et redeundi ad Rodi conventum, quando voluerit, requisita a[d] suo superiori licentia.

*a)* apris *praem. ante corr.* *b)* licentiam *MS* *c)* Sulcz *praem. ante corr.* *d)* a *om.*

## 203

*The Master Fr. Philibert de Naillac and the Convent grant for ten years to Fr. Johann von Ow the Preceptory of Hemmendorf and its members (Priory of* Alamania), *which are vacant following the death of Fr. Heinrich Burler von Tettingen.*

*Rhodes, 1404 April 12*

*AOM 333 fol. 80r-v (80r-v), under* prioratus Alamanie et Boemie.

Frater Philibertus etcetera et nos conventus Rodi domus eiusdem religioso in Christo nobis[a] carissimo fratri Iohanni de Ouw dicte domus salutem et sinceram in Domino caritatem. Meritorum commendabilium vestrorum vos specialis favoris gratia prosequentes ·· preceptoriam seu domum Hemmendorf prioratus nostri Alamanie vacantem per mortem fratris Henrici Burler dicti de Tettingen et ad nostram collacionem propterea devolutam cum omnibus et singulis suis menbris, pertinentiis et iuribus ad eam spectantibus et pertinentibus ac spectare et pertinere debentibus habendam etcetera non obstante invicem deliberato consilio de nostra certa scientia et speciali gratia ad annos decem continuos et completos vobis auctoritate presencium conferimus, concedimus et donamus benefaciendo in eadem vosque preceptorem et comendatorem in dicta baiulia constituimus hac serie et eciam ordinamus vobis fiducialiter circa curam, regimen et administracionem accomodam dicte baiulie ac bonorum et iurium eius deffensionem et recuperacionem tam in agendo quam deffendendo hac serie vices nostras. Quocirca universis et singulis fratribus, sororibus et donatis sub virtute sancte obediencie ac hominibus et vassallis et quibusvis aliis nobis subditis in dicta baiulia constitutis, presentibus et futuris sub sacramento fidelitatis et homagii, quo nobis et nostre domui sunt astricti, precipimus et mandamus, ut vobis tanquam eorum superiori, preceptori et maiori reverenter pareant, obediant et intendant vobisque suum prebeant auxilium, consilium et favorem in omnibus concernentibus utilitatem dicte baiulie, quociens opus fuerit et eos duceritis requirendos, necnon universis et singulis fratribus domus nostre quacumque auctoritate, dignitate vel officio fungentibus, presentibus et futuris, ne contra presentem nostram donacionem et gratiam aliquatenus venire presumant, quinymo eam studeant iuxta eius mentem et seriem[b)] inviolabiliter observare, ac priori seu presidenti [80v] prefato, ut vos vel procuratorem vestrum in corporalem possessionem pacificam et quietam dicte baiulie inducat et conservet inductum omni contradicione remota amoto abinde quolibet detentore, si quis sit, quem amovemus per presentes et decernimus firmiter amovendum. Ceterum vos ampliori gratia prosequentes volumus et vobis de gratia concedimus speciali, quod omnes et singule grangie et domus aut quevis alie possessiones et bona, que[c)] ab olim seu antiquitus menbra fuerint[d)] preceptorie prefate, nunc illas et illa tenentibus illis cedentibus aut decedentibus reducantur et revertantur[e)] ad preceptoriam prefatam tanquam ad caput eorundem omni contradictione remota, in quem casum eas et ea nos ad illam extunc prout exnunc et exnunc prout extunc reducimus et reductas esse decernimus per presentes. Inhibentes etcetera. In cuius rei etcetera. Data Rodi die duodecima mensis Aprilis anno incarnationis Domini millesimo quatercentesimo quarto.

*a)* nobis *supra lin.* *b)* serie *MS* *c)* et *praem. ante corr.* *d)* fuerit *MS* *e)* ne *praem. ante corr.*

*Heinrich von Tettingen was on 16 November 1382 together with Hermann von Ow the Elder (died 1390) preceptor in Hemmendorf: Wunder (1972), 377. Fr. Johann von Ow is not mentioned by Stälin (1883), 109.*

## 204

*Licence for Fr. Johann von Ow to leave the Convent on Rhodes and return, with his superior's licence.*

*[Rhodes, 1404] July 20*

*AOM 333 fol. 80v (80v), under* prioratus Alamanie et Boemie.

Vicesima die mensis Iulii anno predicto data fuit licentia dicto fratri Iohanni de Ouw recedendi de conventu et redeundi, quando voluerit, requisita licentia a[a)] suo superiore.

*a)* a *supra lin.*

*Fr. Johann von Ow the Elder died in Freiburg on 2 April 1408: Ruppert (1889), 296; from 1393 to his death he had been Preceptor of Freiburg: Krieger 1 (1904), col. 641–2. See also no. 211.*

## 205

*Fr. Ulrich Tripscher, Preceptor of Überlingen, is retained.*

*[Rhodes, 1405] February 1*

*AOM 333 fol. 80v (80v), under* prioratus Alamanie et Boemie.

Die prima mensis Februarii anno predicto retentus fuit ad manus magistri frater V̊lricus Tribscher preceptor baiulie de Verberlingen.

*Ulrich Tripscher was Preceptor of Überlingen in 1408: Krieger 2 (1905), col. 1220.*

## 206

*Assignation of maintenance to Fr. Ulrich Weibler from Überlingen for his lifetime in the Preceptory of Überlingen at the request of its Preceptor, Fr. Ulrich Tripscher.*

*[Rhodes, 1405] February 1*

*AOM 333 fol. 80v (80v), under* prioratus Alamanie et Boemie.

Anno et die predictis data fuit stagia fratri V̊lrico Baibler[a)] de Verberlingen in[b)] preceptoria seu baiulia de Verberlingen prioratus nostri Alamanie ad requisitionem dicte domus fratris V̊lrici Tribscher, dicte preceptoris.

*a)* ad vitam suam *ante corr.* *b)* in *dupl.*

## 207

*Licence for Fr. Ulrich Tripscher, Preceptor of Überlingen, to leave the Convent on Rhodes and return, with his superior's licence.*

*[Rhodes, 1405 February 1]*

*AOM 333 fol. 80v (80v), under* prioratus Alamanie et Boemie.

Anno et die predictis data fuit licentia fratri V̊lrico Tribscher preceptori de Verberlingen recedendi de conventu et redeundi, quando voluerit, a superiore requisita[a)] licentia.

*a)* v *praem. ante corr.*

## 208

*Licence for Fr. Johann von Masmünster to travel whenever he wishes with horses and armour to the Convent on Rhodes.*

*1405 November 10*

*AOM 333 fol. 81r (81r), under* prioratus Alamanie et Boemie.

Die X[ma] Novembris anno incarnationis Domini M[o] CCCC[mo] quinto data fuit licentia fratri Iohanni de Masmustre veniendi ad conventum cum equis et armis sufficientibus, quando voluerit, a suo superiore requisita licentia.

## 209

*Licence for Fr. Henry, Duke of Silesia, from the* curia *or grange of Oels to travel to the Convent on Rhodes with two brethren.*

*1407 May 29*

*AOM 334 fol. 113r (112r), under* prioratus Alamanie et Boemie.

Die XXIX[a] Maii anno incarnacionis Domini M[o] CCCC[o] septimo data fuit licencia fratri Henrico duci Slezie curie Olsne dicte domus veniendi ad conventum cum equis et armis sufficientibus secundum statuta etcetera et quod duo fratres[a)] ad conventum venire optantes, quos eligere voluerit, ad ipsum conventum in sua commitiva veniant cum equis et armis, prout decet, a suo tamen superiore requisita licentia eis licencia tributa.

*a)* quos eligere voluerit *dupl. ante corr. (homoiotel.).*

*Probably Duke Henry IX (d. 1419/20) whose infant son Duke Rupert was attested as Preceptor of Oels from 1402 onwards and later became Prior of Bohemia. Contrary to the text Duke Henry was not a Hospitaller. Cf. Europäische Stammtafeln 3/1 (1984), no. 10.*

## 210

*Licence for Fr. Dietrich von Keppenbach, Preceptor of Sulz, to travel to his preceptory and to return to the Convent, with his superior's licence.*

*[Rhodes, 1407] August 25*

*AOM 334 fol. 113r (112r), under* prioratus Alamanie et Boemie.

Die XXV[a] Augusti anno predicto data fuit licentia fratri Dietrich de Kapenbach preceptori de Sulcz[a)] recedendi de conventu et eundi ad regendum dictam baiuliam et redeundi ad ipsum conventum, quando voluerit, a suo superiore requisita licentia.

*a)* Sulchz *praem. ante corr.*

## 211

*The Master Fr. Philibert [de Naillac] and the Convent grant for ten years to Fr. Johann von Ow the Preceptory of Rottweil (Priory of* Alamania*), which is vacant following the death of Fr. Johann von Ow.*

*Rhodes, 1408 November 5*

*AOM 334 fol. 113r (112r), under* prioratus Alamanie et Boemie.

Frater Philibertus etcetera et nos conventus Rodi religioso etcetera fratri Iohanni de Ow dicte domus salutem etcetera. Ad illos libenter nostrum gratiosum favorem extendimus, quos benemeritos reputamus, ut reffecti ex gratia et exhilerati ex honore suscepto ad promovenda nostre religionis commoda libencius invigilent et ad virtutum studia fervencius animentur. Grata igitur fidedigna relatione percepto[a)], quod gratiarum largitor Dominus vos morum composicione, vite mundicia et discretiva naturali virtute dotavit, sperantes in comisso vobis regimine fructus uberes allaturos preceptoriam seu baiuliam de Rotwyl prioratus nostri Alamanie per obitum dicte domus fratris Iohannis de Ow vacantem presencialiter et ad nostram dispositionem etcetera cum omnibus et singulis [suis] membris, pertinentiis etcetera et cum quibus illam dictus quondam frater habuit etcetera habendam etcetera invicem deliberato consilio de nostra certa sciencia et speciali gratia ad annos decem continuos etcetera salvo iure communis thesauri ratione vacancie pro una annata vobis auctoritate presencium conferimus, concedimus et donamus benefaciendo in eadem vosque etcetera. Committentes etcetera. Quocirca etcetera necnon etcetera ac priori etcetera. Inhibentes etcetera. Data Rodi die[b)] quinta mensis Novembris[c)] anno incarnacionis Domini millesimo CCCC° octavo.

*a)* proce *praem. ante corr.* *b)* de *praem. ante corr.* *c)* nob *praem. ante corr.*

*This was Fr. Johann von Ow the Younger. See nos. 203–4.*

## 212

*The Master Fr. Philibert [de Naillac] and the Convent grant for ten years to Fr. Henman zu Rhein the Priory of* Alamania*, including the prioral chambers of Klingnau,*

*Rheinfelden, Utrecht and Cologne, which is vacant following its resignation by Fr. Hesso Schlegelholz, Preceptor of Kos.*

*Rhodes, 1408 November 5*

*AOM 334 fol. 113v (112v), under* prioratus Alamanie et Boemie. *Partial ed. van Winter (1998), 33–4 no. 9.*

Frater Philibertus etcetera et nos conventus Rodi domus eiusdem religioso etcetera fratri Hanmanno ze Ryn dicte domus salutem etcetera. Preeminenciorum meritorum prerogativa pollentes domus[a] nostre fratres non indigne ad multiplicia domus eiusdem notabilia regimina evocamus, ut retribuciones respondeant meritis et virtuosorum[b] remunerate virtutes incrementis proficiant et ad promovenda dicte domus accomoda eorum perpense solicitudinis continua studia attentiora convertant. Sane fidedignorum relatione percepto, quod gratiarum infasor Dominus vos morum composicione, discretiva naturali virtute ac[c] solicita gubernacione dotavit, merito, prout meruistis, in gratiarum largicionibus erga vos reddimur liberales. Igitur prioratum nostrum Alamanie per resignacionem per dicte domus fratrem Hessonem Schlegeholtz preceptorem Langonis et dicti prioratus priorem ultimum de eo sua spontanea voluntate in manibus nostris factam et per nos acceptam vacantem presencialiter et ad nostram disposicionem racionabiliter propterea devolutum cum omnibus et singulis suis membris, pertinentiis et iuribus ad prioratum ipsum spectantibus et pertinentibus ac spectare et pertinere debentibus quoquomodo cum omni onere, emolumentis et honore et cum preceptoriis de Clingenow[d], Riuelden, Traiectensis[e] et Coloniensis cameris suis, et quas vobis pro cameris assignamus cum omnibus et singulis earum et cuiuslibet earum membris, pertinentiis et iuribus universis, habendum, tenendum, regendum, gubernandum, augmentandum et meliorandum in spiritualibus et temporalibus tam in capite quam in membris vobis tanquam digno et benemerito invicem deliberato consilio auctoritate presencium sub responsione annua ·· florenorum auri[f] de Florencia et boni ponderis per vos, prout pro cameris vestris vos continget, et per preceptores preceptoriarum dicti prioratus, prout pro preceptoriis suis pro rata eis pertinebit, receptoribus deputatis vel deputandis per nos ad recipiendum responsiones in prioratu prefato aut alii vel aliis, quibus et ubi ordinaverimus[g] et mandaverimus, in festo nativitatis sancti Iohannis baptiste annis singulis ex pacto expresso infallibiliter exsolvenda[h] et quibuscunque aliis oneribus dicto prioratui qualitercunque et quomodocunque incumbentibus et incumbendis[i], impositis et imponendis per vos et dictos preceptores[j], ut predicitur, ex pacto eciam ultra responsionem predictam supportandis de nostra certa scientia et speciali gratia benefaciendo in eadem conferimus, concedimus et donamus ad annos decem continuos et completos salvo iure communis thesauri ratione vacantie pro una annata retento nobis et specialiter reservato etcetera ac eciam etcetera nichilominus etcetera rursum etcetera. Dantes etcetera. Insuper etcetera. Comittentes etcetera. Quocirca etcetera. Inhibentes etcetera. Data Rodi die quinta mensis Novembris anno incarnacionis Domini millesimo CCCC° octavo[k].

*a) dupl. b)* virt *praem. ante corr. c)* et *praem. ante corr. d)* Clingn *praem. ante corr. e)* Trec *praem. ante corr. f)* auri *supra lin. g)* mandaverimus *praem. ante corr. h)* exsoluen. *praem. ante corr. i)* incumbendus *MS j)* pre *praem. ante corr. k)* ut *praem. ante corr.*

## 213

*The Master Fr. Philibert [de Naillac] and the Convent grant for ten years to Fr. Peter Mersner the Preceptory of Rothenburg (Priory of* Alamania), *which is vacant following its resignation by Fr. Johann Crudrat.*

*Rhodes, 1408 November 5*

*AOM 334 fol. 114r (113r), under* prioratus Alamanie et Boemie.

Frater Philibertus etcetera et nos conventus Rodi etcetera religioso etcetera fratri Petro Merschner dicte domus salutem etcetera. Vestre prospicuitatis meritis comendabilis titulus atributus nos inducit, ut vos dono specialis gratie prosequamur. Hinc est, quod preceptoriam seu baiuliam de Rottembourg prioratus nostri Alamanie per resignacionem spontaneam per dicte domus fratrem Iohannem Crudrat[a] de ea factam et per nos acceptam vacantem presencialiter et ad nostram dispositionem etcetera cum omnibus et singulis suis membris, pertinentiis et iuribus ad eam spectantibus etcetera et cum quibus illam dictus frater Iohannes habuit etcetera habendam etcetera invicem deliberato consilio de nostra certa scientia et speciali gratia ad annos decem continuos et completos salvo iure communis thesauri ratione vacantie pro[b] annata vobis auctoritate presencium conferimus, concedimus ac donamus benefaciendo in eadem vosque etcetera. Comittentes etcetera. Quocirca etcetera necnon etcetera ac priori etcetera. Inhibentes etcetera. Data Rodi die quinta mensis Novembris anno incarnacionis Domini M° CCCC° octavo.

*a)* co *praem. ante corr. b)* u *praem. ante corr.*

*Borchardt 1 (1988), 532–3 nos. 121, 124.*

## 214

*Licence for Fr. Johann von Monreal, Preceptor of Cologne and Adenau, to travel with one brother to the Convent on Rhodes, with horses and armour and with his superior's licence.*

*[Rhodes, 1408] November 10*

*AOM 334 fol. 114r (113r), under* prioratus Alamanie et Boemie.

Die decima Novembris anno predicto data fuit licentia fratri Iohanni de Montreal preceptori domorum Colonie et in Adenowe veniendi ad conventum et in sua commitiva ducendi fratrem unum cum equis et armis sufficientibus secundum statuta etcetera, quando voluerit, a suo superiore requisita licentia.

## 215

*The Master Fr. Philibert [de Naillac] orders Fr. Henman zu Rhein, Prior of* Alamania, *to decide the lawsuit brought by Fr. Hermann von Ow, Preceptor of Villingen, against Fr. Hugo von Montfort, Preceptor of Bubikon, concerning undischarged guarantees to laymen from Freiburg.*

*Rhodes, [1408] November 13*

*AOM 334 fol. 114r (113r), under* prioratus Alamanie et Boemie.

Frater Philibertus etcetera[a)] religioso etcetera fratri Hanmanno ze Ryn priori prioratus nostri Alamanie dicte domus salutem etcetera. Religiosus in Christo nobis carissimus frater Hermannus de Ow preceptor baiulie de Villingen nobis exposuit, quod, cum diu baiulia de Buobikon prioratus predicti ex certis causis anno quolibet teneatur obligata quibusdam personis secularibus de Fribourc in certa pecunie quantitate, pro qua pecunie quantitate anno quolibet exsolvenda pro tunc dicta baiulia de Villingen tanquam fideiussor ad reddendum et solvendum dictam pecunie quantitatem dictis secularibus personis anno quolibet obligata extiterit, ita tamen, quod preceptor dicte baiulie de Buobikon, qui tunc erat et qui pro tempore foret, teneretur dictam baiuliam de Villingen et ipsius preceptores servare indempnes, ob cuius obligacionis causam dictus frater Hermannus et eius baiulia compulsi fuerunt dictam pecunie quantitatem reddere et solvere dictis secularibus personis a certo tempore citra loco et tempore declarando, quod fecerunt. Et hoc dicte domus fratri Hugoni de Montfort preceptori dicte baiulie de Buobikon pluries ex parte dicti fratris Hermanni fuit notificatum ipsum requirendo, ut dictum fratrem Hermannum et eius baiuliam de predicta quantitate pecunie, ut tenebatur, indampnes servaret, quod facere recusavit in dictorum fratris Hermani et eius baiulie dampnum non modicum et gravamen. Unde nobis humiliter suplicavit, ut sibi super hec providere dignaremur de remedio opportuno. Hinc est, quod vobis tenore presencium committimus et mandamus, quatenus, si res ita se habet, partibus seu eorum procuratoribus hinc inde auditis causam huiusmodi fine debito terminetis. Data Rodi die XIII[a] mensis Novembris anno predicto.

*a)* et nos conventus Rodi *add. ante corr.*

## 216

*The Master Fr. Philibert [de Naillac] licenses Fr. Johann [Söler von] Richtenberg, Preceptor of Mainz, to receive three brethren and to maintain them in Mainz.*

*Rhodes, 1408 November 13*

*AOM 334 fol. 114v (113v), under* prioratus Alamanie et Boemie.

Frater Philibertus etcetera religioso etcetera fratri Iohanni Rihtemberg[a)] preceptori Magoncie dicte domus [b)]salutem etcetera[b)]. Peticioni vestra[c)] parte nobis exhibite continenti, quod, cum fratribus ad directionem administracionis[d)] utiliorem dicte baiulie indigeatis, recipiendi viros ·· tres in domus nostre[e)] fratres vobis licenciam impertiri dignaremur, in hac[f)] parte deflexi vestra proceritate interveniente[g)], quod viros ·· tres, qui apti sint sanique et integri suis membris existant, secundum statutorum domus nostre mentem et seriem in domus nostre fratres recipere possitis eisque in dicta vestra baiulia stagias assignandi, in qua ipsis provideri in eorum neccessariis ffaciatis secundum bonos usus et laudabiles consuetudines domus nostre, vobis tenore presencium licentiam impertimur. Data Rodi die XIII[a] mensis Novembris anno incarnacionis Domini M° CCCC° octavo.

*a)* Rihten *praem. ante corr.* *b-b) repetit.* *c)* vestri *MS* *d)* v *praem. ante corr.* *e)* nr *praem. ante corr.* *f)* hec *MS* *g)* interute *MS*

*Fr. Johann Söler von Richtenberg is not mentioned by Hartmann (1981), 106–7.*

## 217

*Licence for Fr. Markward Stahler, Preceptor of [Schwäbisch] Hall, to receive one noble man as a knight brother of the Priory of* Alamania *into the Order who is to travel to the Convent on Rhodes.*

*[Rhodes, 1408 November 13]*

*AOM 334 fol. 114v (113v), under* prioratus Alamanie et Boemie.

Anno et die predictis data fuit licencia fratri Marquardo[a)] Stalher preceptori de Hall recipiendi virum ·· unum in domus nostre fratrem prioratus Alamanie secundum mentem et seriem statutorum domus nostre, dum nobilis sit etcetera legitimo matrimonio etcetera sanusque etcetera ipso prius per vos vel alios etcetera milicie cingulo insignito, ita tamen et non aliter, quod ad nostrum Rodi conventum veniat cum equis et armis sufficientibus etcetera.

*a)* s *praem. ante corr.*

*According to Stälin, Komthure 108 mentioned from 1405 to 1408.*

## 218

*At the request of Fr. Hermann von Ow, Preceptor of Villingen and Pilier of the Tongue of* Alamania, *the two Preceptors of Mainz Fr. Johann [Söler] von Richtenberg and of Rottweil Fr. Johann von Ow are ordered each to receive one brother from Hermann's kin on Hermann's nomination, one into the Preceptoy of Mainz, the other into the Preceptory of Rottweil; the two new brethren are to travel to the Convent on Rhodes.*

*[Rhodes, 1408 November 13]*

*AOM 334 fol. 114v (113v), under* prioratus Alamanie et Boemie.

Die et anno predictis ad suplicacionem fratris Hermanni de Ow preceptoris de Villingen, pillerii lingue Alamanie commissum fuit fratribus Iohanni de Rihtemberg de Mencz et Iohanni de Ow de Rotwyl preceptoribus, ut recipient in domus nostre[a)] fratrem militem unum virum de genere dicti fratris Hermanni, quem idem frater Hermannus[b)] duxerit nominandum, dum nobilis sit etcetera matrimonio[c)] legitimo etcetera sanusque etcetera ipso prius per eos vel alium milicie cingulo insignito, ita tamen et non aliter, quod ad nostrum Rodi conventum veniat cum equis et armis sufficientibus.

*a)* fratre *praem. ante corr.* *b)* Hermannus *praem. ante corr.* *c)* s *praem. ante corr.*

## 219

*Licence for the Preceptors of Rottweil Fr. Johann von Ow and of Rothenburg Fr. Peter Mersner to travel to their preceptories and to return to the Convent on Rhodes.*

*[Rhodes, 1408 November 13]*

*AOM 334 fol. 114v (113v), under* prioratus Alamanie et Boemie.

Die et anno predictis data fuit licencia fratribus Iohanni de Ow de Rotwyl et Petro Merschener de Rottinbourc preceptoribus recedendi de conventu et eundi ad regendum baiulias suas et de ipsis redeundi ad conventum ipsum, quando voluerint, a suo[a)] superiore requisita licentia.

*a) supra lin.;* vestro *in lin. ante corr.*

## 220

*The Master Fr. Philibert [de Naillac] and the Convent order Fr. Henman zu Rhein, Prior of* Alamania, *to pay 60 florins of Germany to Fr. Peter Mersner, Preceptor of Rothenburg.*

*Rhodes, 1408 November 14*

*AOM 334 fol. 174v (172v), under* assignationes peccuniarum.

Frater Philibertus etcetera et nos conventus Rodi etcetera[a)] religioso etcetera fratri Hanmanno[b)] ze Ryn priori Alamanie dicte domus salutem etcetera. Ecce[c)] sinceritati vestre adducimus per presentes, quando facto finali computo cum dicte domus fratre Petro Merschner preceptore de Rottembourg noster communis thesaurus tenetur eidem fratri Petro dare et solvere florenos auri Alamanie sexaginta, quas eidem[d)] fratri Petro promisimus per vos dari et consignari. Eapropter vobis tenore presencium committimus et mandamus, ut eidem fratri seu eius procuratori legitimo aut ab eo causam habenti predictos sexaginta florenos Alamanie ad ipsius requisitionem de pecuniis nostris per vos receptis et recipiendis[e)] detis, solvatis et consignetis, quibus solutis recipiatis recognicionem, que nobis et vobis sufficiat ad cautelam. In cuius rei etcetera. Data Rodi die XIIII mensis Novembris anno incarnacionis Domini M° CCCC° ottavo.

*a)* etcetera *supra lin.* *b)* Hamanno *praem. ante corr.* *c)* Eccce *MS* *d)* sibi *praem. ante corr.* *e)* rec *praem. ante corr.*

## 221

*The Master Fr. Philibert [de Naillac] orders, after consultation with brethren of the Convent, Fr. Henman zu Rhein, Prior of* Alamania, *to send five* fratres conventuales *to the Convent on Rhodes.*

*Rhodes, 1408 November 17*

*AOM 334 fol. 115r (114r), under* prioratus Alamanie et Boemie.

Frater Philibertus etcetera religioso etcetera fratri Hanmanno ze Ryn priori Alamanie dicte domus salutem etcetera. Quia ad promocionem fidei catholice, ad quam nostra professio specialiter nos deducit, disponit et nostre religionis agenda salubriter dirigenda in hiis cismarinis partibus domus nostre fratribus opus presencialiter habemus, igitur vestre sinceritati tenore presencium de consilio fratrum ·· bailhivorum, priorum et procerum nostri Rodi conventus comittimus et mandamus, quatenus, cicius fieri poterit, quinque fratres[a)] conventuales prioratus vestri sufficientes et ydoneos ad Dei et nostre[b)] religionis servicia cum equis et armis sufficientibus et non alias ad nostrum Rodi conventum iuxta statuta domus nostre venire faciatis eisdem et eorum cuilibet firmiter et districte iniungendo, ut ad dictum conventum veniant omni dilacione postposita vobis in hac parte[c)] vices nostrum committendo quibus fratribus et eorum cuilibet veniendi ad dictum conventum, ut prefertur, harum serie licentia tributa. Data Rodi die XVII[a] Novembris anno incarnationis Domini M° CCCC° octavo.

*a)* prior *add. ante corr.* *b) add. ante corr.* *c)* partes *ante corr.*

## 222

*Licence for Fr. Ulrich Tripscher, Preceptor of Überlingen, to travel to the Priory of* Alamania *and to return to the Convent on Rhodes, with his superior's licence.*

*[Rhodes, 1408 November 17]*

*AOM 334 fol. 115r (114r), under* prioratus Alamanie et Boemie.

Anno et die predictis data fuit licencia fratri Ulrico Tripcher preceptori baiulie in Uberlingen[a] ex certis causis nobis et domui nostre utilibus recedendi de conventu et eundi[b] ad partes prioratus Alamanie et de ipsis partibus redeundi ad dictum conventum, quando voluerit, a suo superiore requisita licentia.

*a)* Uber *et* Ubb *praem. ante corr.* *b) add. ante corr.*

## 223

*The Master Fr. Philibert [de Naillac] and the Convent confirm to the brethren of the Tongue of* Alamania *living in the Convent an annual pension payment or rent of 30 florins for their* pitancia; *the money is due from the Preceptory of Rottweil through its Preceptor Fr. Johann von Ow.*

*Rhodes, 1408 November 17*

*AOM 334 fol. 115r-v (114r-v), under* prioratus Alamanie et Boemie.

Frater Philibertus etcetera et nos conventus Rodi universis et singulis domus nostre fratribus ·· lingue Alamanie in dicto conventu ad Dei servicia residentibus salutem etcetera. Suplicatoria peticioni vestre continenti, quod, cum diu super preceptoria seu baiulia de Rotwil prioratus nostri Alamanie pro pictanciis vestris singulis annis[a] haberetis et perciperetis florenos Alamanie auri boni et legalis ponderis triginta, quos preceptor dicte baiulie, qui pro tunc erat et pro tempore foret, annuatim vobis seu procuratoribus vestris reddere et solvere tenebatur, prout in litteris a predecessore nostri, dicti magistri, et a nobis, conventu predicto, ut asseritis, vobis concessis liquidius dicitur contineri, quas pro nunc reperire non valetis, et quod a pluribus annis[b] citra de dictis florenis auri triginta vobis minime extitit satisfactum, ut pensionem annuam dictorum florenorum auri triginta pro pictanciis vestris super dicta baiulia anno quolibet assignare dignaremur benigne annuentes, igitur invicem deliberato consilio [115v] de nostra certa scientia et speciali gratia predictam pensionem annuam dictorum triginta florenorum Alamanie auri boni et legalis ponderis super dicta baiulia de Rotwil fratre Iohanne de Ow, dicte baiulie preceptore, presente premissa confitente et in ipsis et infrascriptis consentiente nostri dicti magistri auctoritate interveniente pro pictanciis vestris anno quolibet in capitulo promissis prioratus predicti reddendam et solvendam procuratoribus[c] vestris seu a vobis[d] deputatis et deputandis perpetuo assignamus solutis prius per vos dictum preceptorem et successores annuis dicte baiulie responsionibus et aliis supportacionum[e] oneribus mandantes et tenore presencium precipientes dicto preceptori et eius successoribus dicte baiulie preceptoribus sub virtute sancte obediencie, ut dictam pensionem pro dictis pictanciis vestris super dicta baiulia, ut prefertur, assignatis anno quolibet ad dictum capitulum dictis procuratoribus vestris seu a vobis deputatis et deputandis omni contradicione remota realiter et cum effectu dent, liberent, redderent et solvant necnon universis et singulis fratribus domus nostre quacumque auctoritate, dignitate vel officio fungentibus, presentibus et futuris, ne contra presentem nostram assignacionem[f] et gratiam aliquathenus facere vel venire presumant, quinymo eam studeant iuxta eius mentem et seriem inviolabiliter observare. In cuius rei testimonium etcetera. Data Rodi die XVII^a^ mensis Novembris anno incarnacionis Domini M° CCCC° ottavo.

*a)* perciperetis et *add. ante corr.* *b)* anis *MS* *c)* procuribus *MS* *d)* a vobis *supra lin.* *e)* supportacium *MS* *f)* ab *add. ante corr.*

## 224

*Commission to Domenico Contarini, citizen of Venice, to receive responsions and other payments from the Priory of* Alamania *through Fr. Ulrich Tripscher and to transmit them to Fr. Domenico d'Alamania in Rhodes.*

*[Rhodes, 1408] November 22*

*AOM 334 fol. 115v (114v), under* prioratus Alamanie et Boemie.

Die XXII[a] Novembris anno predicto ordinatus fuit ad recipiendum responsiones et sibi[a] rogatum per quandam epistolam clausam nobilis vir Dominicus Contarin, Veneciarum civis, quas responsiones et alias pecunias dominis magistro et conventui debitas frater W̊lricus Tripcher, lator dictarum litterarum, seu alius[b] fratri Dominico de prioratu Alamanie asportabunt, et litteras quictatorias de receptis dandum et recepta huc Rodum fideliter transmictendum.

*a)* et alias delata *praem. supra lin. ante corr.* *b)* ad *add. MS*

## 225

*The Master Fr. Philibert [de Naillac] receives Fr. Heinrich Rugeman as a familiar into his household. In future, Fr. Heinrich is to enjoy the prerogatives of the Master's familiars, wherever he lives.*

*Pisa, 1409 July 9*

*AOM 335 fol. 117r (118r), under* prioratus Alamanie et Boemie.

Frater Philibertus etcetera religioso etcetera fratri Henrico Rugeman dicte domus salutem. Probitatis merita, morum decor et religionis honestas, [a]quibus persona vestra laudabiliter decoratur[a], sicut testimonio accepimus fidedigno, nos merito induxerunt, ut vos, quem dignum honore dignoscimus, favore specialis benivolentie prosequamur. Ut igitur affectum nostrum evidencius agnoscatis et nostram vobis sentiatis benivolentiam fructuosam, vos exnunc in familiarem nostrum domesticum comensalem recepimus et familiarium nostrorum consorcio liberaliter agregamus volentes [b)]et vobis plenarie presencium tenore concedentes, ut decetero omnibus et singulis privilegiis, libertatibus, immunitatibus, exempcionibus, prerogativis et graciis ubique locorum uti et gaudere valeatis sicut ceteri familiares nostri domestici comensales et continui uti et gaudere possint, ut[b)], ubicumque fueritis, deinceps tanquam nostrum et inter nostros familiares ascriptum vos nostre protectionis et tuicionis presidio confoveri ac ad nostram presenciam, ubicumque fuerimus, pro vestris agendis, cum expedierit, cum fiducia accessum libere vos habere. Data Pisis die IX[a] mensis Iulii anno incarnacionis Domini M° CCCC° [c)] IX°.

*a-a) dupl. b-b) infra textum. c)* CCC *praem. ante corr.*

## 226

*The Master Fr. Philibert de Naillac allows Fr. Heinrich Rugeman for his lifetime to stay outside his* baiulia *or office.*

*Pisa, 1409 August 20*

*AOM 335 fol. 117r (118r), under* prioratus Alamanie et Boemie.

Frater Philibertus de Nailhaco Dei gratia sacre domus hospitalis sancti Iohannis Iherosolimitani magister humilis et pauperum Christi custos religioso in Christo nobis karissimo fratri Henrico Rugeman dicte domus salutem et sinceram in Domino caritatem. Religionis decor, morum honestas et alia virtutum dona, quibus, prout fidedigno accepimus testimonio, vos carismatis gratia insignivit, non inmerito nos inducunt, ut personam vestram congruis, quibus possumus, benivolenciis et graciis prosequamur[a)]. Ideo, ut affectum nostrum vobis senciatis existire fructuosum, in bailliva vestra vel extra ipsam, quamdiu vitam duxeritis in humanis, ubi vobis melius et congruencius in Dei laudem, anime vestre salutem et religionis nostre honestatem placuerit et videretur expedire, libere et licite commorandi, perseverandi, standi, eundi, redeundi et pro vestris eciam licitis peragendis negociis, quociens opus fuerit, vobis tenore presencium de nostra certa scientia et speciali gratia licenciam concedimus et donamus, cuiuscumque super hoc licencia minime requisita. Datum Pisis die XX[a] mensis Augusti anno nativitatis Domini nostri Ihesu Christi millesimo CCCC[mo] nono indiccione secunda.

*a)* prosequantur *MS*

## 227

*The Master Fr. Philibert [de Naillac], who had been guardian of the papal conclave, summons, on orders of the new pope Alexander V, Fr. Heinrich von Neuhaus, Prior of Bohemia, with three or four preceptors to the next chapter general at Nicei near Savona on 1 April 1410. The new pope has united the Hospital under the Master Fr. Philibert and wants to defend it. The chapter general is to discuss the reform of the Order and to restore fraternal love.*

*Pisa, 1409 August 22*

*AOM 335 fol. 117v-8v (118v-9v), under* prioratus Alamanie et Boemie.

Frater Philibertus etcetera religioso etcetera Henrico de Novadomo priori Boemie dictique prioratus preceptoribus salutem etcetera. Iam pervenit ad mundi terminos, quo labore diu vexata nostre fuerit religionis milicia, que pro fide sancta et Christi nomine se periculis opposuit et opponit incessanter, contra quam clipeum paravit effrenata pharaonis malicia, scilicet Turchorum nephanda protervia[a] causantibusque scismate pestifero, guerris, mortalitatibus hominumque maliciis – proch dolor! – et peccatis tot et tantum in suis tribulationibus, oppressionibus, neccessitatibus ac paupertate depressa est et inenarrabilibus affliccionibus perturbata, quod velut sine remige navis in medio procellarum derelicta quasi nauffragium passa est. Scitis equidem, quod inimico hominis inter filios pacis zizaniam seminante hiis, qui pie volunt vivere, parantur insidie, angustie imminent, proximus obiurgat[b], odio lacerat, invidia contabescit, fraude decipit, violenciis invalescit, murmuracionibus stridet, detractacionibus mordet, accusacionibus stimulat ac pre depressionibus acquiescit. Hac autem peccatis hominum exigentibus Deus de summis afflictiones dimictit[c] quid plura fulgure fulminat, tonitruo percutit, grandine vastat, confundit guerra, tremore concutit, morte dispendit et pestilencia comminatur, lapides frangunt, devorant voragines, erugo devastat, denigrat rubigo predanturque vispiliones. Nolunt siquidem homines Deo decimas solvere nec cesari censum reddere, scilicet responsiones annuas conventui debitas. Modo autem totum tollitur, hoc tollit fiscus, quod non accipit Christus, que omnia peccante populo frequencius eveniunt et in predicacionem universos hominum labores deducunt. Et quoniam tucius est ante discrimina resilire quam se discriminibus inexplicabilibus implicare cauciusque videtur morborum principia previdenti remedio prevenire quam post invalescenciam egritudinum infructuosa medicamina manducare, attendentes, quod circumspecti pastoris prudencia gregis sui periculis libenter occurrit ipsumque decet vigilare, ut grex, quem habet, regimine suo permaneat semper in vigore pacique subiaceat inconcusse ac considerantes, quod ex preteritorum memoria, que racionem probabiliter solet inducere, de futuris quam prudentis annuis tribus temporibus dispensatur, ordinat namque presencia, futuris previdet ac preterita recordatur, quantum nobis ab alto conceditur circa futura nostre religionis accomoda sedule cogitantes ad ipsius regimen salutiferum, ut felici amodo ducta regimine preservetur a noxiis et optatis semper proficiat incrementis, dominum nostrum papam Alexandrum quintum divina providencia vepribus scismatum deiectis ab ambobus collegiis in unum prius unitis et congregatis auctoritate concilii generalis Pisis congregati unanimiter et concorditer electum, in cuius electione conclavis custos, licet immeriti, fuimus, indilate post ipsius electionem et coronacionem adivimus eidem humilius supplicando, quatenus amore Dei, fidei favore et nostre religionis contemplacione circa dicte nostre religionis propter scisma et alias multipharie et cum importabili iactura lacerate vesperacionem de remedio providere[d] dignaretur opportuno. Qui sua viscerali misericordia more pii patris eidem compaciens fideique catholice ecclesie sancte Dei ac ipsi religioni et nobis omnibus, quantum cum Deo posset, subvenire desiderans ipsam religionem sic, ut est dictum, propter scisma divisam et laceratam auctoritate apostolica reunivit, reintegravit et reincorporavit nosque per conventum alias iuxta et secundum statuta et stabilimenta religionis [118r] concorditer in magistrum hospitalis electum, nominatum et creatum in magistrum tocius hospitalis confirmavit mandans et in virtute sancte obedientie precipiens omnibus et singulis prioribus etcetera, quatenus nobis magistro generali hospitalis omnes reverenter pareant, obediant et intendant cum effectu, prioratus, castellanias, preceptorias et alia religionis beneficia decetero a nobis tanquam a magistro et a conventui iuxta stabilimenta, ut est dictum, recipiant, responsiones integre et alia iura conventui solvant[e] et ad conventum secundum stabilimentorum[f] predictorum ordinacionem Deo et religioni servituri veniant et nichilominus, ut melius et cicius religio tam in capite quam in membris refformetur, prescindenda prescindantur, restauranda restaurentur et corrigenda corrigantur et inantea omnes nos non in invio, set in via salutis ambulemus, mandavit nostre religionis capitulum generale celebrari eadem auctoritate apostolica in civitate Niciensi prope Saonam[1] im prima die mensis Aprilis proximo futuri anni a nativitate Domini millesimi quadringentesimi decimi,[2] que civitas utique est omnibus prioribus etcetera nostre religionis quarumcumque nacionum quasi communis. In quo mandat eadem auctoritate omnes priores et[g] castellanos singulorumque prioratuum et castellaniarum unacum tribus vel quatuor fratribus preceptoribus notabilibus de quolibet prioratu et castellania comparere personaliter vel per locumtenentem in casu legitime excusacionis et cum procuratore sufficienti pro attentendo, approbando, auctorisando et complendo realiter et

1) *Nice according to Delaville (1913), 308–9. Nice is 150 km south-west of Savona. There is, however, a place called Nicei, 1 km near Magliolo, 30 km south-west of Savona. Magliolo belonged to the Del Carretto family, margraves of Savona at Finale and prominent Hospitallers.*

2) *Convocation for 1 April 1410, announced by Alexander V on 20 August 1409: Delaville (1913), 309 note 1, from the Libri Bullarum. In fact, the chapter general met at Aix on 19 April 1410, ibid. 311.*

cum effectu omnia et singula, que pro utilitate et conservacione religionis ad Dei honorem, fidei Christiane deffensionem et ipsius religionis et nostrum animum conservacionem ibidem ordinabuntur, statuentur, refformabuntur seu diffinientur. Et nos cupientes, quantum nobis permissum fuerit ab alto iuxta preceptum et ordinacionem domini nostri pape circa premissa realiter et cum effectu Deo semper propicio vacare diligenter, vos omnes et singulos etcetera hortamur in Domino nichilominus in virtute sancte obedientie districtius iniungentes, quatenus iuxta disposicionem et ordinacionem domini nostri pape ad dictos locum et diem nobiscum ad capitulum generale ibidem celebrandum et ea, que Deo sunt, placita et nostre religioni conservativa promovenda, tractanda et concludenda personaliter vel in casu legitime excusacionis per vestrum locumtenentem unacum tribus vel quatuor preceptoribus prudentibus, probis et antiquis viris in religione et cum procuratoribus, ut est dictum, legitime compareatis realiter et sufficienter de omnibus et singulis reparacione seu refformacione indigentibus in nostro prioratu predicto tam in capite quam in membris, tam circa spiritualia quam temporalia etcetera instructi et muniti, ut sic nos et religionem nostram tam in capite quam in membris, tam circa spiritualia quam temporalia, circa mores et conversacionem religiosam et alia omnia et singula refformacione indigentia refformare et tandem sic disponere de directore[h)] valeamus, quod nos omnes unanimos et hiis, qui nos et religionem nostram diligunt, et hiis, qui forsan nos diligere non videntur, caritatis affectum exhibeamus et sicut per hoc in nobis est et esse debet una fides, unus habitus unaque religionis professio, [118v] ita sit unus spiritus, una bene agendi voluntas, una caritas, una animorum coherencia, morum concordia, cultus virtutum, conformitas mencium et pietas actionum et sic inantea animetur[i)] nostri amator innocencie, pacis amicus, cultor fraternitatis pacientibus compaciens ut sic duce Deo glorie servicionis eterne metham nostrum quilibet cursu contingat feliciter consummato. Data Pisis sub sigillo nostro in absencia bulle nostre[j)] plumbee die XXII[a] mensis Augusti anno incarnacionis Domini millesimo quadringentesimo nono.

*a)* pertervia *MS* *b)* obirigat *praem. ante corr.* *c)* dinictit *MS* *d)* dignaretur *praem. ante corr.* *e)* debita *praem. ante corr.* *f)* stabilimetorum *MS* *g)* et *supra lin.* *h)* directore *marg.*, semper *ante corr.* *i)* animus *MS* *j)* nostre *supra lin.*

## 228

*Idem to Fr. Henman zu Rhein, Prior of* Alamania.

*[Pisa, 1409 August 22]*

*AOM 335 fol. 118v (119v), under* prioratus Alamanie et Boemie.

Sub eidem tenore et data mandatum fuit fratribus Hermanno ze Rin priori Alamanie et preceptoribus ipsius prioratus.

## 229

*The Master Fr. Philibert [de Naillac], with consent of three procurators of the Convent, constitutes Fr. Leonardo de Buonafede from Florence, Preceptor of Albarese, as visitor in the Priories of* Alamania, *Bohemia, Hungary, Venice and Pisa. As the Master's lieutenant he is to visit, correct, restore and reform the Hospital in these priories. He may constitute one or more Hospitaller brethren as his substitutes. The priors, vicepriors, preceptors, vicepreceptors, leaseholders and lieutenants, the priories, preceptories, houses and offices, the castles, villages and subjects of the Order are to be visited, reformed, corrected and meliorated both in spiritual and temporal affairs. Fr. Leonardo may accept one office in each priory for himself as the Master's chamber and rule it. He may accept from the priors, vicepriors, preceptors, vicepreceptors, leaseholders and lieutenants their responsions, arrears of responsions, pension payments of the Master's chambers*, procrassia, mortuaria *and other dues to the Treasury. In case of default he may summon them to the next chapter general in order to face trial. He may dispense justice, audit accounts, issue receipts, convoke assemblies and constitute one or more brethren as his substitutes. With the counsel of senior brethren he may redeem alienated goods and act inside and outside law courts as if the Master himself were present. The Hospital's brethren and subjects are ordered to be obedient to him, even if they had been retained by the Master. Without the Master's special licence he may not pawn or alienate goods nor admit brethren or donats into the Order.*

*Pisa, 1409 September 5*

*AOM 335 fol. 137r-8r (138r-9r), under* prioratus Veneciarum, Lombarde, Vngarie, Vrbis et Pisarum.

Noverint universi et singuli presentes litteras visuri et audituri, quod nos frater Philibertus de Nailhaco[a] etcetera, cum a multis iam retrolapsis temporibus causantibus scismate pestifero, quod diu in ecclesia sancta Dei viguit, guerris, mortalitatibus invalescenciaque potestatis inimicorum fidei catholice perfidorum in catholicos Domino permittente solus solito seviencium religio nostra in lapsum facultatum quamplurimum declinaverit et declinet, attendentes, quod magisterii sarcina servitutis nobis licet immeritis Domino disponente commissa nos ea reddit vigili exquisicione solicitos, ut circa direttivam conservacionem salubrem administracionem prioratuum et baiuliarum religionis nostre presertim prioratuum Alamanie, Boemie, Ungarie, Veneciarum et Pisarum et administracionem iusticie in illis nobis subditis efficacem operam impendamus, ut ea, que correctione, restauratione et reformacione indigent, in melius corrigantur, restaurentur et reformentur et propterea considerantes expediens et necessarium existere, ut loco nostri fratrem aliquem nostre dicte domus vite mature, providencie proceritatisque famose in partem nostre solicitudinis, nostre potestatis auctoritate suffultum deputemus in partibus memoratis. Quamobrem de religiosi in Christo nobis carissimi fratris Leonardi de Bonafedis de Florencia preceptoris Albarensis,[1]

1) *Albarese near Grosseto in Tuscany.*

fidelis consiliarii et socii nostri ac in dictis prioratibus Alamanie, Boemie, Ungarie, Veneciarum et Pisarum ambaxiatoris nostri circumspectione industri fideque et probitate legali plenam in Domino fiduciam obtinentes de voluntate, consilio et assensu religiosorum in Christo nobis carissimorum fratrum Galteri Crassi decretorum doctoris prioris[b)] ecclesie, Lucii de Vaillinis marescalli et Iohannis Grivelli preceptoris Chamborelli, procuratorum nostri Rodi conventus dicte domus,[2)] de nostra certa scientia eundum fratrem Leonardum auctoritate presencium facimus, creamus, constituimus et solemniter ordinamus nostrum ambaxiatorem et nuncium specialem, visitatorem, correctorem et refformatorem negociorumque gestorem generalem et specialem in partibus et prioratibus predictis. Dantes et concedentes harum serie dicto ambaxiatori nostro et nuncio licenciam, potestatem et auctoritatem plenariam per se vel alium seu alios domus nostre fratres ad talia sufficientes et ydoneos deputandi et deputatum seu deputatos per eum revocandi tociens, quociens sibi videbitur oportunum, omnes et singulos fratres domus nostre priores, vicepriores, preceptores, vicepreceptores, firmarios, rendarios et eorum locatenentes ac ipsorum et cuiusque ipsorum prioratus, preceptorias et domos, administraciones et regimina ac loca, castra, villas, homines et vassallos nostre dicte domus prioratuum et parcium predictarum visitandi, reformandi, corrigendi et meliorandi in spiritualibus et temporalibus tam in capite quam in membris tociens, quotiens opus fuerit et dicto nostro ambaxiatori videbitur expedire, necnon in quolibet dictorum prioratuum baiuliam unam pro camera nostra nomine nostro et pro nobis acceptandi ipiusque possessionem nomine quo supra intrandi, adipiscendi et assequendi ipsamque cameram nostram regendi, gubernandi et administrandi seu regi, gubernari et administrari faciendi nomine nostro et pro nobis tam in spiritualibus quam temporalibus et tam in capite quam in membris ac ipsam arrendandi [137v] et affictandi seu in arrendamentum et affictum tradendi, insuper predictos priores, vicepriores, preceptores, vicepreceptores, arrendarios, firmarios et eorum locatenentes et eorum quemlibet efficaciter compellendi per omnem cohercionis modum racionabilem et visum ad solvendum responsiones suas, arreragia[c)] responsionum, camerarum pensiones nostrarum procrassiave et mortuaria et quevis bona alia fratrum domus nostre deffunctorum et decedendorum inantea, quorum bona, res et iura in toto vel in parte ad nos et communem thesaurum domus nostre communiter vel divisim pertinencia ipsaque recipiendi, recuperandi, levandi et habendi nostro procuratorio nomine et dicti conventus atque vice, rebelles quoque et inobedientes et solvere per eos debita et debenda recusantes ad ipsius presenciam evocandi et eum et eos secundum statuta et consuetudines domus nostre, prout demeruerint, puniandi et ducendi per iusticiam nostre dicte domus seu eum et eos ad nostram in proximo generali

2) *Fr. Gautier le Gras, Prior of the Convent, Fr. Luce de Vallins, Marshal, and Fr. Jean Grivel, Preceptor of Chamberaud, as procurators of the Convent on Rhodes accompanying the Master in Europe.*

religionis capitulo[d)] presenciam repellandi et trasmictandi nostri fratres, sorores et donatos homines et vassallos nostros et dicte nostre domus parcium et prioratuum predictorum quotiens oporteat iusticiam ministrandi et faciendi super demeritis,[e)] causis, litibus et aliis casibus quibuscumque plantam et plantas faciendi fratrum esgardia petendi et tenendi et mandare teneri faciendi, raciones et computa audiendi et per alios audiri faciendi et que recipientur nobis et dicto nostro communi thesauro communiter vel divisim deberi recuperandi, levandi, habendi et recipiendi litterasque quictatorias et alias super premissis et infrascriptis ad faciendum et concedendum necessarias cum clausulis opportunis dandi et concedendi, assembleiam et assembleias et fratrum congregaciones in partibus et prioratibus predictis mandandi et tenendi, quociens dicto ambaxiatori et consiliario nostro super premissis et infrascriptis emergentibus visum fuerit expedire, et in illis et sine illis disponendi et ordinandi cum consilio fratrum et procerum domus nostre ibidem tunc astancium omnia et singula concernencia utilitatem dicte nostre domus, castra, loca, bona, domus, iura et res quasvis alias eiusdem nostre domus alienata[f)] et alienatas per personas ecclesiasticas vel seculares iniuste occupata vel occupatas, detenta et detentas petendi et recuperandi et ad ius et proprietatem nostre dicte domus revocandi et reducendi, pro nobis dictoque nostro conventu communiter vel divisim in dicta nostra domo quibuscumque dominis et personis ecclesiasticis vel mundanis supplicandi et ab eis et eorum quolibet litteras gracie et simplicis iusticie ac indulgencias et privilegia quecumque a quibuscumque dominis, regibus et principibus et aliis impetrandi et obtinendi et impetratis ac impetrandis contra nos et religionem nostram communiter vel divisim et personas illius et loca obiciendi et contradicendi ac omnia et singula insuper dependencia et emergencia ex eis et eorum quolibet ac ipsis et eorum alteri quomodolibet connexa, ut dicto nostro ambaxiatori, visitatori et reformatori pro utiliori visum fuerit, excercendi, exequendi, faciendi, disponendi cum consilio fratrum et procerum nostre domus in partibus et prioratibus memoratis, que nos ipsi visitare, refformare et excercere possemus, si in illis personaliter adessemus, insuper nostre religionis negocia ad utilitatem et honorem ipsius in quibuscumque curiis et coram dominis ecclesiasticis vel secularibus proponendi, promovendi et exequendi aut proponi, promoveri et exequi per alium seu alios faciendi, quociens fuerit oportunum. Mandantes insuper universis et singulis fratribus domus nostre presentibus et futuris, cuiuscumque status, gradus aut condicionis existant, sub virtute sancte obedientie firmiter et districte ac hominibus et vassallis [138r] nobis et nostre domui subditis in partibus memoratis sub sacramento fidelitatis et homagii, quo nobis et nostre dicte domui sunt astricti[g)], expresse precipimus[h)], ut in premissis et quolibet premissorum prenominato nostro ambaxiatori, visitatori et reffformatori et cui vel quibus fratri seu fratribus domus nostre pro premissis et eorum altero subrogato vel subrogatis aut mandato vel[i)] mandatis per eum loco ipsius reverenter pareant, obediant et intendant tamquam nobis imparciendo eisdem et eorum cuilibet consilium et favorem veritati se testimonium perhibendo in omnibus, super quibus eos aut eorum alterum duxerit requirendos, non obstante, si aliqui ex dictis fratribus ad manus dicti nostri magistri sint retenti aliasve[j] exempti, quibus in hiis casibus retencionem aut exempcionem aliquam nolumus de certa scientia in aliquo sufragare, necnon, ut ad dicti ambaxiatoris, visitatoris et refformatoris vocacionem[k] et mandatum ad locum et loca, ad quem et que ipsos vel aliquem aut aliquos ex eis semel et pluries evocaverit, veniant contradicione et excusacione remotis. Super quibus omnibus et singulis predicto ambaxiatori et visitatori committimus plenarie vices nostras inhibentes dicto ambaxiatori et visitatori nostro et subrogando vel subrogandis ab eo firmiter et districte sub virtute sancte obedientie, ne pretextu litterarum nostrarum nec alias aliqua de bonis, rebus et iuribus dicte nostre domus donent, vendant, alienent, permutent, impignorent, distrahant seu in amphiteosim perpetuam concedant aut quocumque alio colore quesito extra nostram religionem transferant nec fratres nec donatos faciant nec aliis licenciam faciendi tribuant, sed pocius prioribus et preceptoribus prioratuum et parcium predictarum ex parte nostra sub virtute sancte obedientie supradicta idem ambaxiator noster et deputati et deputandi ab eo inhibeant, ne ipsi priores ipsos preceptores fratres seu donatos faciant sine nostra speciali licencia et mandato. Et si, quod absit, contra inhibicionem nostram huiusmodi aliquid vel aliqua eos vel eorum alterum facere operari contingat, illud et illa exnunc prout extunc et extunc prout exnunc cassamus, anullamus ac decernimus irritum et inane nulliusque existere penitus efficacie vel valoris. In cuius rei testimonium bulla nostra plumbea presentibus est appensa. Data Pisis die quinta mensis Septembris anno incarnacionis Domini millesimo quatercentesimo nono.

*a)* Nailha *praem. ante corr.* *b)* priaris *MS* *c)* arregagia *ante corr.* *d)* consilio *praem. ante corr.* *e)* demendis *MS* *f)* aliena *praem. ante corr.* *g)* astricte *ante corr.* *h)* ex *praem. ante corr.* *i)* ve *MS* *j)* *add. corr.* *k)* visitacionem *praem. ante corr.*

## 230

*The Master Fr. Philibert de Naillac, with consent of three procurators of the Convent and of the Procurator General at the Roman curia, assigns to Fr. Leonardo de Buonafede, visitor in the Priories of* Alamania, *Bohemia, Hungary, Venice and Pisa, 2 ducats per day and commits to him the administration of the indulgence granted by Pope Alexander V.*

*Pisa, 1409 September 5*

*AOM 335 fol. 138v (139v), under* prioratus Veneciarum, Lombardie, Vngarie, Vrbis et Pisarum.

Noverint universi presentes litteras visuri et audituri, quod, cum nos frater Philibertus de Nailhaco Dei gratia sacre domus hospitalis sancti Iohannis Iherosolimitani magister humilis et pauperum Christi custos pro nonnullis arduis negociis promocionem fidei catholice, religionis nostre commodum et honorem et ipsius status conservacionem concernentibus ad partes Alamanie, Boemie, Ungarie, Veneciarum et Pisarum religiosum in Christo nobis carissimum fratrem Leonardum de Bonafedis de Florencia preceptorem Albarensem, fidelem ambaxiatorem, consiliarium et socium nostrum commensalem presencialiter destinamus et, quia nullus tenetur propriis stipendiis militare, nos de voluntate, consilio et assensu religiosorum in Christo nobis carissimorum fratrum Galteri Crassi prioris ecclesie, Lucii de Vailhins marescalli, Iohannis Grivelli preceptoris Chamberelli, procuratorum nostri Rodi conventus dicte domus, et Iohannis de Mayronis preceptoris Vazonicensis, procuratoris generalis religionis nostre in curia Romana,[1] tenore presencium de nostra certa scientia pro die qualibet, quamdiu idem ambaxiator in dicta ambaxiata vacaverit eundo, stando et redeundo a die, qua iter suum arripiet, pro suo viagio continuando et complendo computandi pro stipendiis et expensis suis ducatos auri duos eidem assignamus per ipsum ambaxiatorem nostrum habendos et percipiendos super peccuniis nostro communi thesauro partibus in illis debitis et debendis per ipsum ambaxiatorem nostrum recipiendis, quos duos ducatos auri eidem ambaxiatori, ut prefertur, assignatos de recipiendis racionibus et computis suis deduci ac ipsum ambaxiatorem eiusque bona et res de ipsis quictum et liberum ess volumus. Rursum cum sanctissimus dominus noster papa Alexander quintus plenissimam indulgenciam videlicet a pena et culpa omnibus vere penitentibus et confessis, qui secundum facultatem bonorum suorum a Deo sibi collatorum manus suas ad sustentacionem dicti conventus trans mare[a] et custodiam castri sancti Petri noviter in Turquia constructi[2] porrexerint adiutrices, dederit et concesserit, volumus et de voluntate et consilio quibus supra concedimus, quod idem frater Leonardus omnes et singulas expensas ac omnia et singula alia prosecutionem dicte indulgencie continencia, super quo suam oneramus conscienciam, de pecuniis occasione ipsius indulgencie recipiendis fieri et prosequi valeat. Data Pisis die quinta mensis Septembris anno incarnationis Domini millesimo quatercentesimo nono.

*a)* trans mare] I(e)hsu Marie *post corr.*

## 231

*The Master Fr. Philibert [de Naillac] authorises his counsellor,* socius *and familiar* commensalis *Fr. Leonardo de Buonafede, visitor in the Priories of* Alamania, *Bohemia, Hungary, Venice and Pisa, to receive knight brethren, sergeants and donats into the Order and to assign them their maintenance in the five priories*

*Pisa, 1409 September 5*

1) *Fr. Gautier le Gras, Prior of the Conventual churc on Rhodes, Fr. Luce de Vallins, Marshal, Fr. Jean Grivel, Preceptor of Chamberaud, Fr. Jean de Meyronés, Preceptor of Gap.*

2) *No. 261.*

*AOM 335 fol. 138v-9r (139v-40r), under* prioratus Veneciarum, Lombardie, Vngarie, Vrbis et Pisarum.

Frater Philibertus etcetera religioso etcetera fratri Leonardo de Bonafedis de Florencia preceptori etcetera consiliario et socio nostro commensali ac in prioratibus Alamanie, Boemie, Ungarie, Veneciarum et Pisarum ambaxiatori nostro et nuncio speciali, salutem etcetera. De vestris industri circumspectione, probitate et fidelitate plenam fiduciam in Domino obtinentes vos ambaxiatorem nostrum, visitatorem, refformatorem, negociorum gestorem et nuncium specialem et generalem in dictis prioratibus presentialiter destinamus, ut corrigenda corrigantur, restauranda[a)] restaurentur et refformanda in melius refformentur, prout in nostris inde confectis litteris plenius continetur, timentes, ne causantibus scismate pestifero, quod[b)] diu in ecclesia sancta Dei viguit, et divisione, qua nostra religio tamdiu fuit lacerata, temporumque et hominum maliciis preceptorie, baiulie sive domus fratrum religionis nostre [139r] carencia ab ecclesiasticis seu secularibus personis detineantur occupate, cupientes inde pravitati ipsarum celebri remedio providere volumus et vobis tenore presencium committimus et mandamus, quatenus viros sufficientes et ydoneos in fratres religionis nostre milites, servientes et donatos pro regimine baiuliarum, preceptoriarum et domorum prioratuum predictorum et camerarum, quas in ipsis obtinemus et nobis contingerit obtinere, videlicet milites, dum nobiles fuerint ex utroque parente legittimo matrimonio nati sanique et integri suis membris, necnon fratres servientes et donatos sufficientes et ydoneos, ut moris est, recipiatis, quociens vobis pro regimine predictarum baiuliarum, preceptoriarum et domorum ac eciam camerarum nostrarum videbitur expedire, eisque et eorum cuilibet in baiuliis dictorum prioratuum stagias assignatis[c)], in quibus sibi et eorum cuilibet in suis neccessariis provideri faciatis secundum bonos usus et laudabiles consuetudines domus nostre. Data Pisis die quinta mensis Septembris anno incarnacionis Domini millesimo quatercentesimo nono.

*a)* restaurenda *MS* *b)* quo *MS* *c)* assignantas *MS*

## 232

*The Lieutenant Master Fr. Domenico d'Alamania and the Convent on Rhodos order Fr. Henman zu Rhein, Prior of* Alamania, *to pay 100 florins as an annual pension payment to Fr. Hermann von Ow in compensation for Fr. Hermann's resignation of the priory, which has been made either by Fr. Hermann or by his procurator Fr. Heinrich Tripscher, Preceptor of Überlingen, or to compel him to come to Rhodes to face trial.*

*Rhodes, 1409 November 2*

*AOM 339 fol. 232v (198v), under* littere diversorum negotiorum.

[a]Venerabili religioso viro domino fratri Hamati Rin priori Alamanie in Christo nobis carissimo detur[a]. In Christo nobis carissime, salutem et sinceram in Domino caritatem. Notum vobis facimus, sicut frater Armandus de Ow comparuit in auditorio nostro et coram nobis et proceribus conventus nostri exposuit et significavit, quatenus frater Henricus Tripter preceptor Vberling existens in conventu Rodi ut procurator vester procuratorio nomine vestri[b] petens prioratum Alamanie vacantem a reverendissimo domino nostro magistro et conventu[c] vobis conferri et ipse frater Armandus similiter existebat ad colationem sibi fiendam dicti prioratus et, ne dictus frater Armandus impedimentum daret dicto fratri Henrico ad obtinendum dictum prioratum vestri nomine et aliis causis vobis utilibus, dictus frater Henricus ut procurator vester promisit procuratorio nomine eciam simplem se facturum et curaturum, quod vos dabitis omni anno et solvebitis eidem fratri Armando centum florenos auri in vita sua, de qua promisione constat quedam privata scriptura coram nobis exibita, ubi lacius ista continetur. Quem dictum prioratum cessante dicto fratre Armando ex dictis paxcionibus dictus frater Henricus dicto nomine obtinuit seu vobis conferri fecit duxitque. Et exposuit dictus frater Armandus vos nolle solvere dictos centum florenos eidem fratri Armando promissos per dictum fratrem Henricum dicto nomine dictis de causis vobis asserente dictum fratrem Henricum non esse procuratorem vestrum nec fuisse in predictis nec ratohabente per eum gesta petens a nobis iusticiam ministrandam in predictis a nobis requirendo, ut vos vel dictum fratrem Henricum iuris[d] remediis opportunis cogeremus ad solutionem fiendam dictorum centum florenorum secundum dicta pacta in dicto instrumento contenta. Quapropter, cum iuste petentibus tribuendus[e] sit assensus, vos in Christo rogamus et atencius ortamur, ut dicto fratri Armando solvatis seu solvere faciatis dictos centum florenos annuatim secundum pacta facta et inita per dictum fratrem Henricum vestro nomine, si procurator vester erat vel eciam si non erat, cum utiliter gesta vestri nomine debetis habere rata, quod debitum et honestum est vos habere rata. Si autem nolueritis solvere dictos centum florenos annuos ex eo, quod ille non erat procurator, ut dicitis, nec vult habere rata gesta per ipsum, tenore presencium vobis precipimus et mandamus in virtute sancte obedientie, quatenus dictum fratrem Henricum compellatis et cogatis ad realem solutionem dictorum centum florenorum fiendam dicto fratri Armando secundum dicta pacta vel, si resistat dicens se non teneri, eidem fratri Henrico expresse precipiatis in virtute sancte obedientie visis presentibus infra debitum tempus, quo possit, Rodum accedere coram nobis studeat comparere responsuro de iure dicto fratri Armando in predictis et iusticiam recepturo taliter vos habentes et ipse frater Henricus, ne inobedientie macula aspergamini, quod haberemus causam contra vos et eundem tamquam contra inobedientes procedere rigorose. Valete in Christo, qui est omnium vera salus. Data in prefato conventu Rodi die II[a] Novembris anno a nativitate Domini M° IIII$^{C}$ IX°. [f]Frater Dominicus de Alamania, locumtenens etcetera, ceterique baylivi, priores et proceres dicti conventus Rodi[f].

*a-a) supra lin.* *b)* det *praem. ante corr.* *c)* conventum *MS* *d)* iuniis *MS* *e)* tribuendum *ante corr.* *f-f) infrascript.*

## 233

*Fr. Domenico d'Alamania, Preceptor of Santo Stefano di Monopoli and Lieutenant of the Master Fr. Philibert de Naillac, and the Convent at Rhodos summon Fr. Heinrich Tripscher, Preceptor of Überlingen, because he had not paid 100 florins as an annual pension payment to Fr. Hermann von Ow.*

*Rhodes, 1409 November 2*

*AOM 339 fol. 233r (199r), under* littere diversorum negotiorum.

Frater Dominicus de Alamania sacre domus hospitalis sancti Iohannis Ierosolimitani preceptor sancti Stephani prope Monopolim, locumtenens reverendissimi in Christo patris domini et domini fratris Philiberti de Nalhaco eiusdem sacre domus dignissimi magistri et pauperum Christi custodis, et nos conventus Rodi religioso in Christo nobis carissimo fratri Henrico Tripter preceptori Vberling salutem et obedientiam presentibus adhibere. Cum frater Armandus de Ow coram nobis et consilio nostro[a] baylivorum et procerum nostri conventus conquestus sit dicens et significans, quatenus vos de anno elapso ut procurator religiosi in Christo nobis carissimi fratris Hamantis Rin nunc prioris Alamanie pro dicto prioratu obtinendo sine aliquorum impedimento et ex aliis causis dicto fratri Hamanti utilibus promisistis eidem fratri Armando vos facturum et curaturum, quatenus dictus frater Hamans dabit et solvet eidem fratri Armando annuatim florenos auri centum in vita ipsius fratris Armandi, ut patet quadam[b] privata scriptura per vos facta coram nobis exibita, dicensque eciam dictum[c] fratrem Hamantem, nunc priorem Alamanie[d], dictos centum florenos per vos promissos solvere nolle asserentem vos non fuisse procuratorem eius neque ratum[e] habuisse per vos gestum in hac parte, ex quibus requisivit nobis sibi iustitiam ministrari. Quapropter tenore presencium vobis in virtute sancte obedientie districte precipimus et mandamus, quatenus visis presentibus talia[f] faciatis, ut dictus frater Hamans solvat dictos centum florenos annuos per vos promissos iusta seriem vestre scripture vel vos solvatis eosdem, si dictus prior solvere noluerit seu non teneatur, eidem fratri Armando seu eius procuratori vel, si sencieritis vos ex predictis gravatum asserentem non teneri ad presentacionem dictarum litterarum, ipsis visis infra congruum tempus, quo Rodum posibile sit accedere, coram nobis infallibiliter studeamini comparere de iure responsurus in predictis dicto fratri Armando recepturus iusticie complementum taliter vos habendo, ut in predictis et circa predicta de inobedientia argui non possitis, ne habeamus causam contra vos ex aliqua inobedientia procedere rigorose, quod procederemus, si incideretis in eadem. In cuius rey testimonium bulla nostra cerea, qua utimur, presentibus est inpensa. Data in prefato conventu Rodi die II[a] Novembris anno a nativitate Domini M° IIII[C] IX°.

*a)* nostri *praem. ante corr.* *b)* quandam *MS* *c)* vestrum *praem. ante corr.* *d)* Alamanie *add. ante corr.* *e)* tali *MS* *f)* rationi *MS*

## 234

*The Priors Fr. Jacques Tivelli of Auvergne, Fr. Raymond de Lescure of Toulouse and Fr. Filippo de Langueglia of Lombardy as lieutenants of the Master Fr. Philibert de Naillac confirm to Fr. Johann von Monreal, Preceptor of Cologne and Adenau, the licence given by the same Master to travel with one brother to Rhodes, with licence of the Prior of* Alamania.

*Aix, 1410 May 2*

*AOM 336 fol. 142r (142r), under* prioratus Alamanie et Boemie.

Fratres Iacobus Tivelli Alvernie, Raymondus de Lescure Tholose et Phillipus de Languilhia Lombardie priores, reverendissimi in Christo patris ac domini fratris Philiberti de Nailliaco Dei gratia sacre domus hospitalis sancti Iohannis Iherosolemitani magistri dignissimi et pauperum Christi custodis locumtenentes, religioso in Christo nobis carissimo fratri Iohanni de Montreal[a] preceptori domorum Colonie et in Addenowe dicte domus salutem et sinceram in Domino caritatem. Cum nobis per litteras dicti reverendissimi domini nostri magistri sigillo suo in cera nigra sigillatas constiterit prefatum dominum nostrum magistrum vobis licentiam concessisse ad nostrum Rodi conventum eundi Deo et nostre religioni serviturum necnon in vestra commitiva unum fratrem prioratus nostri[b] Alamanie cum equis et armis sufficientibus secundum nostre religionis statuta ducendi a vestro superiore requisita licentia et pro priore Alamanie, superiore vestro, eundi et vobiscum unum fratrem ducendi ad dictum conventum cum equis et armis, ut prefertur, vobis tenore presencium licenciam impertitam declaramus. In cuius rei testimonium sigilla nostra litteris presentibus duximus apponenda. Data in capitulo generali in ecclesia nostra sancti Iohannis extra muros civitatis Aquensis celebrato die II[a] mensis Maii anno Domini millesimo quadringentesimo decymo.

*a)* d *praem. ante corr.* *b)* nostre *MS*

## 235

*The three lieutenants of the Master (as no. 234), three procurators of the Convent, 14 named and other brethren forming the chapter general permit Fr. Henman zu Rhein, Prior of* Alamania, *to choose another prioral chamber in lieu of the Preceptory of Rheinfelden, which has been destroyed by fire.*

*Aix, 1410 May 10*

*AOM 336 fol. 146v-7v (146v-7v), under* prioratus Alamanie et Boemie.

Fratres Iacobus Tivelli Alvernie, Raymundus de Lescure Tholose et Philippus de Languillia Lombardie priores, reverendissimi in Christo patris et domini domini Philiberti de Nailhaco Dei gracia sacre domus hospitalis sancti Iohannis Iherosolomitani[!] magistri dignissimi et pauperum Christi custodis locumtenentes generale capitulum celebrantes religioso in Christo nobis carissimo fratri Hammano ze Rin priori Ala[147r]manie dicte domus salutem et sinceram in Domino caritatem. Supplicatoriam peticionem vestram recepimus continentem, quod, cum preceptoria Ridedensi prioratus vestri predicti in collatione prioratus ipsius per dictum reverendissimum dominum nostrum magistrum et Rodi conventum vobis facta pro una quatuor vestrarum camerarum ordinariorum vobis assignata extiterit, verum quod a sex mensibus circa casu fortuito igne fuerit concremata taliter, quod domus preceptorie istius et omnia in ipsis existencia conversa fuerunt in cinerem et favillam et quod tam propter combustionem predictam quam propter guerras, mortalitates, que partibus in illius diucius viguerunt, redditus, proventus et exitus preceptorie prescripte taliter attenuati sunt, quod solutis responsionibus annuis et aliis oneribus supportatis redditus ipsi non suppetunt pro vices fratrum in ea degencium. Unde nobis supplicastis, quod attentis statum prioris Alamanie oneribusque per eum supportandis et aliis supradictis de gratia speciali vobis auctoritate presentis generalis capituli, quod aliam preceptoriam in dicto prioratu vestre spectantem donacioni, quam eligere malueritis, dum vacare contingerit, vobis retinendi et acceptandi pro una dictarum vestrarum IIII$^{or}$ camerarum loco preceptorie antedicte licentiam, facultatem et auctoritatem concedere dignaremur. Igitur propter vestrorum exigenciam meritorum illa libenter vobis annuimus, per que vobis possit comoditas pervenire, vestris supplicacionibus inclinati vobis retinendi et acceptandi preceptoriam unam cum suis membris, iuribus et pertinentiis pro una dictarum quatuor camerarum vestrarum ordinariarum loco dicte preceptorie Rinfeldens., quam exnunc prout extunc et extunc prout exnunc vacare decernimus et declaramus possessione pacifica dicte preceptorie, dum vacabit, unacum fructuum percepcione per vos prius assequta de voluntate [et] consilio religiosorum in Christo nobis carissimorum fratrum Galterii Crassi decretorum doctoris prioris ecclesie conventualis Rodi, Lucii de Vailhins marescalli, Iohannis Greuelli preceptoris Chambarelli, procuratorum nostrorum Rodi conventus, Iohannis Flote sancti Egidii, Aymonis de Monteauium Acquitanie et Priami de Gambacurtis Pizarum priorum, Petri de Tilio preceptoris de Gelesio locumtenentis magni preceptoris, Petri de Pruvinis thezaurarii et receptoris generalis, Tossani de Berneuille preceptoris de Boncort locumtenentis prioris Francie, Gallinni Petri de Petrusio preceptoris procuratoris prioratus sancti Egidii, Anthonii de Berneyo Forensis [147v] et Petri Carrel Caluie preceptorum procuratorum prioratus Alvernie, Iohannis Soubaudi prioris de Corbelio, Hugonis de Sartiis preceptoris de Oscomonte, procuratorum prioratus Francie, Helye Arnaudi Eodrie et Hemerici Danyet de Equitayo preceptorum, procuratorum prioratus Acquitanie, et aliorum fratrum in capitulo generali predicto astancium de nostra certa scientia et speciali gratia auctoritate presentis generalis capituli vobis licentiam, auctoritatem et facultatem concedimus et donamus. Mandantes et tenore presentium precipientes sub virtute sancte obedientie omnibus et singulis fratribus domus nostre quacunque dignitate, auctoritate vel officio fungentibus, presentibus et futuris, ne contra premissa vel premissorum aliqua facere vel venire presumant, quinymo illa[a)] studeant iuxta eorum mentem et seriem inviolabiliter observare. In cuius rei testimonium ad maiorem predictorum roboris firmitatem bulla dicti reverendissimi domini nostri magistri plumbea in absentia bulle communis plumbee presentibus est appensa. Data in dicto capitulo generali in ecclesia nostra sancti Iohannis extra muros civitatis Aquensis in Provincia celebrato die X$^{a}$ mensis Maii anno incarnacionis Domini millesimo CCCC$^{o}$ decimo.

*a)* ille *MS*

*The Priors Fr. Jean Flote of Saint-Gilles, Fr. Aymon de Oiselay of Aquitaine and Fr. Priamo Gambacorte of Pisa, the Treasurer and Receiver General Fr. Pierre de Provins, the lieutenant of the Grand Preceptor and Preceptor of Jallès Fr. Pierre de Theil, the lieutenant of the prior of* Francia *and Preceptor of Boncourt Fr. Tossanus de Berneville, the lieutenant of the Priory of Saint-Gilles and Preceptor Fr. Pierre de Petrusio, the lieutenant of the Priory of Venice and Preceptor of Bologna Fr. Pietro de Schapis, the procurators of the Priory of Auvergne and Preceptors of Forez Fr. Guy de Vernay and of Lachal* (Calvie) *Fr. Pierre Carrel, the procurators of the Priory of* Francia, *i.e. the Prior of Corbeil Fr. Jean Sobaudi and the Preceptor of Oisemont Fr. Hugues de Sarciis, the procurators of the Priory of Aquitaine and Preceptors of Vedrie Fr. Élie Arnaud and of Saint-Quitago Fr. Aimery Danyet.*

## 236

*The brethren forming the the chapter general (as no. 235) order the preceptors in the Priory of* Alamania *to pay to their Prior Fr. Henman zu Rhein a tax for his participation at the chapter general.*

*Aix, 1410 May 12*

*AOM 336 fol. 147v-8v (147v-8v), under* prioratus Alamanie et Boemie.

Fratres Iacobus Tivelli Alvernie, Raymundus de Lescure Tholose et Philippus de Languillia Lombardie priores[a)], reverendissimi in Christo patris et domini domini fratris Philiberti de Nailhaco Dei gratia sacre domus hospitalis sancti Iohannis Iherosolimitani magistri dignissimi et pauperum Christi custodis locumtenentes generale capitulum celebrantes universis et singulis fratribus bailivis et preceptoribus prioratus nostri Alamanie dicte domus salutem. Cum ex mandato speciali et expresso sanctissimi domini nostri Alexandri pape quinti generale capitulum religionis nostre in civitate Nicie prope Saonam celebrandum ordinatum extiterit, pro cuius celebracione dictus reverendus dominus noster magister inter alios domus nostre priores fratrem Hamanum ze Rin priorem prioratus nostri Alamanie unacum tribus vel IIII^or preceptoribus dicti prioratus per suas litteras sigillo suo sigillatas mandandum duxerit et postmodum certis de causis arduissimis vigentibus [148r] et neccessariis[b)] de dicta civitate Nicie ad civitatem Aquensem in Prouincia translatum extiterit, ad quod capitulum dictus prior cum preceptoribus antedictis honoriffice, sicut decuit, statui et ibi in dicto capitulo usque ad ipsius finem ipse et dicti preceptores indesinanter interfuerunt non sine magnis laboribus et expensis, hinc est, quod nos attendentes dictos priorem et preceptores ad huiusmodi capitulum pro utilitate, comodo, refformacione et directione prioratus ipsius personaliter accessisse et quod nemo propriis stipendiis tenetur militare, de voluntate, consilio et assensu religiosorum in Christo nobis carissimorum fratrum Galteri Crassi decretorum doctoris prioris ecclesie conventualis Rodi, Lucii de Vailhins marescalli Rodi, Iohannis Griuelli preceptoris Chambarelli, procuratorum Rodi conventus, Iohanis Flote sancti Egidii, Aymonis de Monteauium Acquitanie et Priami de Gambacurtis Pizarum priorum, Petri de Prouinis thezaurarii et receptoris generalis, Petri de Tilio preceptoris de Pelesio locumtenentis magni preceptoris, Tossani de Berneuille preceptoris de Boncourt locumtenentis prioris Francie, Galuini Petri de Petrusio preceptoris procuratoris prioratus sancti Egidii, Anthonii[c)] de Verneyo Forensis et Petri Carrelli Caluie preceptorum, procuratorum prioratus Alvernie, Iohannis Sobaudi prioris de Corbolio, Hugonis de Sarciis preceptoris de Ostromonte, procuratorum prioratus Francie, Helye Arnauldi Vodrie et Hemerici Danyet de Equitayo preceptorum, procuratorum Acquitanie et aliorum fratrum in dicto generali capitulo nobis astancium de nostra certa scientia, auctoritate presentis generalis capituli vobis tenore presencium sub virtute sancte obedientie precipimus et mandamus, quatenus vestram tailliam super ipso priore et vobismet ipsis imponatam usque ad summam florenorum auri partibus in illis currentium, prout aliis prioribus et prioratibus mandavimus, per ipsos priorem et preceptores expositam in eundo ad dictum capitulum, stando et redeundo assignetis, quam talliam per dictum priorem preceptoresque predictos et vos omnes et singulos prioratus ipsius, prout dictum priorem pro cameris suis, dictos preceptores et vos omnes et singulos prout[d)] vestrum quemlibet pro rata continget, eisdem priori et preceptoribus, prout ipsorum quemlibet tangit et tangere potest, reddi et solvi ac eisdem pro suis sumptibus et expensis satisfieri volumus, super qua tallie assignacione per vos super cameris dicti prioris baiuliarum et preceptoriarum dictorum preceptorum et vestrarum vestras oneramus consciencias. Quocirca priori prefato tenore presencium committimus et mandamus sub virtute sancte obedientie qua supra auctoritate presentis generalis capituli, quatenus vos preceptores prioratus[e)] [148v] iamdicti secundum ratam et porcionem dicte tallie impositam seu imponendam compellat per capcionem et vestrorum[f)] vendicionem et exibet racionem et alias omnem modum cohercionis racionabilem, prout sibi visum fuerit. In cuius rei testimonium ad maiorem omnium predictorum roboris firmitatem bulla dicti reverendissimi domini nostri magistri plumbea presentibus est appensa. Data in dicto generali capitulo in ecclesia nostra sancti Iohannis extra muros civitatis Aquensis in Prouincia celebrato die duodecima mensis Maii anno incarnacionis Domini millesimo quadringentesimo decimo.

*a)* prioris *MS* *b)* neccessius *MS* *c)* Anthonio *MS* *d) supra lin.* *e) dupl.* *f)* bonorum *MS*

## 237

*The brethren forming the chapter general (as no. 235) confirm to the preceptors in the Priory of* Alamania *the right to elect a prior, since there are too few brethren of their tongue in the Convent on Rhodes.*

*Aix, 1410 May 12*

*AOM 336 fol. 148v-9r (148v-9r), under* prioratus Alamanie et Boemie.

Fratres Iacobus Tivelli Alvernie, Raymundus de Lescure Tholose et Philippus de Languillia Lombardie priores, reverendissimi in Christo patris et domini domini fratris Philiberti de Nailhaco Dei gratia sacre domus hospitalis sancti Iohannis Iherosolimitani magistri dignissimi et pauperum Christi custodis locumtenentes generale capitulum celebrantes universis et singulis fratribus preceptoribus prioratus nostri Alamanie dicte domus presentibus et futuris salutem. Cum in cunctis religionis nostre prioratuum[a] regiminibus etatis maturitas morumque gravitas perstictetur et maxime, ubi inanis potest imminere periculum, ibi caucius est indagandum, et ideo in prioratus nostri predicti regimine[b] talis debet preponi prior, qui virtutum donis multipliciter prefulgeat et per eius solertiam idem prioratus in spiritualibus et temporalibus tam in capite quam in membris regatur utiliter et promovetur accomode. Sane cum pauci dicti prioratus fratres in nostro Roddi conventu resideant et in statutis domus nostre caveatur, quod, quando prioratus vel preceptorie ad dicti domini nostri magistri reverendissimi et Rodi conventus collacionem vaccant, si in lingua, in qua dictus prioratus vel [baiuli]a vacare noscitur, non sint fratres sufficientes ad regimen ipsorum prioratus et baiulie, tunc prior de baiuliis ex mandato dicti domini nostri magistri disponere debet et similiter de prioratu fratres preceptores prioratus prefati tenentur eligere unum fratrem ex ipsis utiliorem et sufficientiorem ad regendum prioratum prefatum, igitur premissis attentis et aliis attendendis pro utilitate et confirmacione prioratus ipsius eligendi vobis in priorem et pastorem unum fratrem de fratribus dicti prioratus in nostro Roddi conventu degentem, si ibi [149r] reperiatur sufficiens et ydoneus, aut alium in dicto prioratu residentem, prout pro utiliori regimine prioratus ipsius vobis videbitur expedire, de voluntate, consilio et assensu religiosorum in Christo nobis carissimorum fratrum Galteri Crassi decretorum doctoris prioris ecclesie conventualis Rodi, Lucii de Vailhins marescalli, Iohannis Griuelli preceptoris Chambarelli, procuratorum nostri Rodi conventus, Iohannis Flote sancti Egidii, Aymonis de

Monteauium Acquitanie, Hamanni ze Rin Alamanie et Priami de Gambacurtis Pizarum priorum, Petri de Pruuinis thesaurarii et receptoris generalis, Petri de Tilio preceptoris de Gelesio locumtenentis magni preceptoris, Tossani de Berneuille preceptoris de Boncort locumtenentis prioris Francie, Galuini Petri de Petrusio preceptoris procuratoris prioratus sancti Egidii, Anthomii[!] de Verneyo Forensis, Petri Carrelli Caluie preceptorum procuratorum prioratus [c)]Alvernie, Iohannis Sobaudi prioris de Corbolio, Hugonis de Serciis[d)] preceptoris procuratorum Francie, Helye Arnaudi Vodrie et Hemerici Danyet de Equitayo preceptorum procuratorum prioratus Acquitanie[c)] et aliorum fratrum in dicto generali capitulo nobis astancium de nostra certa scientia et speciali gratia auctoritate presentis generalis capituli auctoritatem, potestatem, facultatem et licentiam concedimus et donamus confirmacione tamen[e)] huiusmodi electionis dicto reverendissimo domino magistro nostro et[f)] suis successoribus semper reservata. Mandantes et tenore presencium precipientes sub virtute sancte obedientie universis et singulis fratribus domus nostre quacunque dignitate, auctoritate vel officio fungentibus, presentibus et futuris, ne contra presentem nostram confirmacionem aliquathenus facere vel venire presumant, quinymo illam servent. In cuius rei testimonium ad maiorem roboris firmitatem bulla dicti reverendissimi domini nostri magistri plumbea in absencia bulle communis plumbee presentibus est appensa. Data in generali predicto capitulo in ecclesia nostra sancti Iohannis extra muros civitatis Aquensis in Prouincia celebrato die duodecima mensis Maii anno incarnacionis Domini millesimo quadringentesimo decimo.

*a)* prioratum *corr.* *b)* regimen *corr.* *c-c) dupl. ante corr.* *d)* Sarciis *supra lin.* *e)* tn *supra lin.* *f)* et *supra lin.*

## 238

*The brethren forming the chapter general (as no. 235) confirm Fr. Johann Cruze for his lifetime in the Bailiwick of Westphalia, which he has been granted him by the former Prior of* Alamania *Fr. Hesso Schlegelholz.*

*Aix, 1410 May 12*

*AOM 336 fol. 142v (142v), under* prioratus Alamanie et Boemie. *Cf. van Winter (1998), 34 nr. 10.*

Fratres Iacobus Tivelli Alvernie, Raymundus de Lescure Tholose et Philippus de Longui Lombardie priores etcetera locumtenentes generale capitulum celebrantes religioso in Christo nobis carissimo fratri Iohanni Cruze baiulo seu preceptori baiulie seu preceptorie Westphale dicte domus salutem et sinceram in Domino caritatem. Vestrorum commendabilium gratia meritorum et ob administrationem accommodam per vos habitam in commisso vobis regimine in nostra religione illa vobis libenter annuimus, que conservacionem vestri status concernere dignoscuntur. Idcirco donationem et concessionem per dicte domus fratrem Hessonem Slegelholcz olim prioratus nostri Alamanie[a)] priorem de dicta baiulia vobis factas ratas, gratas et[b)] placidas habentes baiuliam ipsam cum omnibus et singulis suis menbris, pertinentiis et iuribus ad eam spectantibus et pertinentibus ac spectare et[c)] pertinere debentibus quoquomodo, prout ipsam tenetis presencialiter et habetis, habendam etcetera de voluntate etcetera ut in consimilibus[d)] litteris infra registratis et aliorum etcetera ad vitam etcetera vosque etcetera. Committentes etcetera. Quocirca etcetera necnon etcetera. Inhibentes etcetera. In cuius rei testimonium ad maiorem predictorum roboris firmitatem bulla dicti reverendissimi domini magistri plumbea in absencia bulle communis plumbee presentibus est appensa. Data in dicto generali capitulo in ecclesia nostra sancti Iohannis extra muros civitatis Aquensis in Provincia celebrato die duodecima mensis Maii anno incarnacionis[e)] Domini millesimo CCCC[mo] decimo.

*a)* Alvernie *MS* *b)* habentes *praem. ante corr.* *c)* de *praem. ante corr.* *d)* confratribus *praem. ante corr.* *e)* Domini millesimo CCCC° dec *praem. ante corr.*

## 239

*The brethren forming the chapter general (as no. 235) order, at the request of Fr. Henman zu Rhein, Prior of* Alamania, *that no brethren are to be received into the Order without the prior's knowledge. No brother is to be licensed to travel to the Convent on Rhodes without the prior's permission, unless he is retained. The prior and his chapter are entitled to increase or decrease the number of brethren and donats in the various preceptories according to their wealth. Laymen are not to be appointed procurators for disputes between brethren, contrary to what had occurred in the lawsuits between the Preceptors of Villingen Fr. Hermann von Ow and of Rottweil Fr. Johann von Ow.*

*Aix, 1410 May 12*

*AOM 336 fol. 142v-3r (142v-3r), under* prioratus Alamanie et Boemie. *Cf. Delaville (1913), 332 with note 3.*

Fratres Iacobus Tivelli Alvernie, Raymundus de Lescure Tholose et Philippus de Langui Lombardie priores etcetera locumtenentes generale capitulum celebrantes religioso in Christo nobis carissimo fratri Hamanno ze Rin priori prioratus nostri Alamanie dicte domus salutem. Supplicaciones vestras recepimus continentes, quod, cum dictus reverendissimus dominus noster magister de gratia speciali alicui fratri seu fratribus prioratus vestri predicti recipiendi viros aliquos in domus[a)] nostre fratres licenciam concesserit, ipsi fratres talem gratiam habentes sine aliqua reverencia vobis exhibenda[b)] et noticia aliqua recipiendorum viros nonnullos in domus nostre fratres recipiunt, quod facere non possunt nec debent per et secundum domus nostre statuta, in quibus cavetur, quod non obstante quibuscunque litteris per dictum dominum nostrum magistrum sub quocunque verborum tenore concessis frater, qui aliquem in domus nostre fratrem sine reverencia suo priori exhibenda nominisque desi[g]natione et persone noticia receperit propter personas inhabiles et minus ydoneas personas, que recepte fuerunt, debet amictere[c)] habitum et puniri[d)] pena in dictis statutis contenta auctoritate presentis generalis capituli de voluntate et consilio religiosorum in Christo nobis carissimorum fratrum Galteri Crassi etcetera ut in consimilibus litteris infra registratis et aliorum fratrum in dicto generali capitulo nobis astancium omnibus et singulis fratribus domus nostre prioratus predicti talem graciam habentibus et habituris sub virtute sancte obedientie et sub penis in dictis statutis contentis prohibemus, ne inantea fratres faciant seu recipiant sine[e)] vestra licencia et persone vel personarum noticia vobis facienda et casu, quo contra inhibicionem nostram huiusmodi attemptare presumpserint, per vos iuxta[f)] seriem [143r] dictorum statutorum predictorum auctoritate qua supra puniri precipimus et mandamus. Item, cum prefatus dominus noster magister alicui fratri vel fratribus licenciam veniendi ad conventum concedit propter hoc, quod idem dominus noster magister nullam habet noticiam personarum, semper cavetur in ipsis, quod veniant ad conventum a suo superiore requisita licencia et quod propter tales causas et fratrum inobedientias in dicto prioratu multa mala et scandala orta fuere, idem prioratus dispendia non modica sustinuit et sustinet, cupientes talibus obviare de voluntate, consilio et assensu ac auctoritate quibus supra statuimus, precipimus et ordinamus, ne decetero quicunque frater volens ad conventum transfretare quacunque licencia sibi concessa non obstante, nisi tales sint fratres, qui retenti sint ad manus dicti nostri magistri, de vestro prioratu sine licencia a vobis requisita sub penis privacionis baiulliarum et domorum, quas in vestro prioratu obtinent et inposterum obtinebunt, de dicto prioratu recedere non possint nec valeant, et quicunque contra fecerit, pena predicta puniatur. Item cum in pluribus baiuliis prioratus predicti sint ultra numerum statutum fratres et donati, propter quorum onus preceptores baiuliarum seu preceptoriarum ipsarum responsiones et alia sibi imposita onera exsolvere non possunt nec valent in preiudicium dicti Rodi conventus, et in aliis baiuliis seu preceptoriis dicti prioratus, quamvis redditibus habundent, nulli[g)] sint vel quasi, vobis de consilio et auctoritate predictis in baiuliis seu preceptoriis vestri prioratus de et cum consilio fratrum baillivorum[h)] et procerum prioratus[i)] ipsius numerum fratrum augendum et diminuendum, prout pro commodo et utilitate dictarum baiuliarum vobis videbitur expedire, auctoritatem, licenciam et facultatem harum serie impartimur. Item, cum per statuta dicte nostre domus prohibeatur, ne in controversiis[j)] de fratre contra fratrem motis et movendis frater constituere procuratores possit nec valeat nisi fratrem, et domus noster frater Hermannus de Ow preceptor de Vilingen et frater Iohannes de Ow preceptor de Raetvoila nonnullos procuratores seculares constituerint contra dictorum statutorum seriem, unde iurgia et controversie orte fuerunt in grave preiudicium dicti prioratus et perniciosum exemplum aliorum, de voluntate, consilio et assensu et auctoritate predictorum dictos procuratores seculares sic per dictos procuratores seculares constituant decernentes exnunc prout extunc et extunc prout exnunc irritum et inane omne et quicquid per dictos procuratores seculares dictum, actum, procuratum fuerit sive gestum. In cuius rei testimonium ad maiorem roboris firmitatem premissorum bulla dicti reverendissimi domini magistri plumbea in absencia bulle communis plumbee presentibus est appensa. Data in dicto capitulo generali in ecclesia nostra sancti Iohannis extra muros civitatis Aquensis celebrato die duodecima mensis Maii anno quo supra.

*a)* dominos *praem. ante corr.* *b)* hui *praem. ante corr.* *c)* admictere *MS* *d)* pium *MS* *e) dupl.* *f)* iust *praem. ante corr.* *g)* null *praem. ante corr.* *h)* baiul *praem. ante corr.* *i)* prioratus *add. ante corr.* *j)* dicte *add. ante corr.*

## 240

*The brethren forming the chapter general (as no. 235) constitute Fr. Henman zu Rhein, Prior of* Alamania, *as procurator of the Master and Convent and receiver in the Priory of* Alamania. *He is to collect the responsions and arrears of responsions from preceptories, offices and houses, the pension payments from the Master's chamber in this priory, the* procrassia, mortuaria, iocalia *and other dues from dead Hospitallers according to the 1367 statute, and all monies and other dues to the Master and Convent. He is to audit accounts of preceptors, vice-preceptors, leaseholders and lieutenants on their responsions, arrears of responsions, the pension payments of the Master's chamber, the* procrassia, mortuaria *and other dues to the Master and Convent. In case of default he may depose and reinstate or punish them according to the Hospital's statutes. He may audit accounts and issue receipts. If offices, preceptories, houses or members fell vacant in this way, he may grant them to new officers, with the counsel of the officers, preceptors and senior brethren. He may unite and separate preceptories and other offices to ensure the payment of responsions according to the statutes. He has full powers for all necessary legal acts, inside and outside law courts, as if the Master himself were present. He may constitute and destitute one or more Hospitaller brethren as his substitutes. What he does and they do is valid, and the Master will abide by it. The Hospital's brethren and subjects are ordered to be obedient to Fr. Henman zu Rhein and his substitutes.*

*Aix, [1410] May 12*

*AOM 336 fol. 143r-v (143r-4v), under* prioratus Alamanie et Boemie.

Noverint universi[a)] et singuli presens procuratorium visuri et audituri, [143v] quoniam nos fratres Iacobus Tivelli Alvernie, Raymondus de Lescure Tholose et Philippus de Langui Lombardie priores etcetera locumtenentes generale capitulum celebrantes confisi de fidei legalitate etcetera circuspectionis industria religiosi in Christo nobis carissimi fratris Hammani ze Rin prioris prioratus nostri Almanie domus eiusdem de voluntate, consilio et assensu religiosorum in Christo nobis carissimorum fratrum Galteri Crassi etcetera ut in litteris infra registratis et aliorum fratrum in dicto capitulo generali astancium eundem fratrem Hermannum ze Rin presentem et onus procurationis huiusmodi in se suscipientem de nostra certa scientia auctoritate presentis generalis capituli facimus, creamus, constituimus et sollempniter ordinamus dicti reverendissimi domini nostri magistri conventus nostri in nostre domus procuratorem, receptorem, sindicum, yconomum et nuncium specialem et generalem negociorumque gestorem ad petendum, recipiendum et recuperandum et habendum dictorum dominorum magistri et conventus nomine procuratorio atque vestro omnes et singulas responsiones et arreragia responsionum omnium et singularum preceptoriarum, baiuliarum et domorum prioratus nostri predicti pensionesque camere dicti nostri magistri, quam in dicto prioratu obtinet seu ipsum contingerit inposterum obtinere. Item ad petendum, recipiendum et habendum quibus supra nominibus tam tallias et alia onera inposita et imponenda tam de preterito tempore quam presenti et futuro procrassia, mortuaria, iocalia, res et bona alia, quecunque sint et quocunque alio nomine nuncupata et in quibuscunque consistant, omnium et singulorum fratrum domus nostre priorum seu[b)] preceptorum seu quorumvis aliorum mortuorum iam et inantea moriturorum in predicto prioratu ad dictos dominos magistrum et conventum pertinentes et debencia pervenire secundum statutum promulgatum et factum super istis in generali capitulo apud Avinionem de mense Marcii anno sexagesimo sexto[1)] celebrato seu quovis alio nomine. Item ad petendum et habendum quibus supra nominibus omnes et singulas pecunie summas ac bona, res et iura alia quecunque fuerint et quocunque nomine nuncupata dictis dominis magistro et conventui communiter vel divisim debitas vel debita, debendas vel debenda et sibi debencia racionabiliter pervenire quovis titulo, ratione sive causa tam per domus nostre fratres quam per personas alias quaslibet[c)] aliarum religionum religiosas seu ecclesiasticas et mundanas. Item ad petendum et audiendum quibus supra nominibus computa et raciones de predictis et altero eorundem ab omnibus et singulis, ad quos de premissis computa et raciones competabit et quomodolibet pertinebit et ad ponendum dicta computa et raciones eos et eorum quemlibet auctoritate presentis generalis capituli efficaciter compellendum, prout et quocunque dicto procuratori et responsionum receptori videbitur expedire, et que dictis domino magistro et conventui communiter vel divisim predicta computa deberi et pervenire debere, competere necnon preceptores[d)], vicepreceptores, firmarios, rendarios et eorum locatenentes ac eorum quemlibet in dicto prioratu efficaciter compellendum per omnem cohercionis modum racionabilem dicto procuratori[e)] et responsionum receptori visum fuerit[f)] expedire ad solvendum responsiones suas, arreragia responsionum, pensiones camere dicti domini magistri procrassiave, mortuaria et alia per eos quovis nomine dictis magistro et conventui communiter vel divisim [144r] debita et debenda. Eciam eos et eorum quemlibet tam pro deffectu solucionis responsionum suarum

*1) 1367 March 5: Delvaille (1913), 261–2.*

quam pro inutili regimine, bonorum alienacione, prodigalitate et dilapidacione baiuliarum, domorum et administrationum suarum et si eorum culpa et contumacia exegerint a suis administrationibus eciam si per dictos magistrum et conventum sibi collate et concesse fuerint, secundum religionis nostre statuta de et [cum] consilio fratrum baillivorum, preceptorum et procerum dicti prioratus destituendum et destitutos seu destituendos huiusmodi ad ipsorum restituendum regimina si earum satisfactio et eorum debita paratis meruerint. Rebelles quoque et inobedientes et per eos debita et debenda solvere recusantes[g)] ad ipsius presenciam evocandum et eum et eos secundum statuta et consuetudines domus nostre, prout demeruerunt, puniendum et ducendum per iustitiam dicte[h)] nostre domus seu eum et eos ad dicti magistri nostri presentiam reppellendum et transmictendum. Item ad faciendum quibus supra nominibus de receptis computis et racionibus auditis quittancias perpetuo valituras. Item baiullias, preceptorias sive domos ac membra vacantes vel vacancia in et cum aliis baiulliis prioratus predicti, si expediat, cum consilio et assensu baillivorum, preceptorum et procerum dicti prioratus annexandum, uniendum, incorporandum et inserendum[i)] et econtra dividendi et[j)] separandi ipsisque sic annexis, unitis, incorporatis et insertis fratri seu fratribus memorati prioratus sufficienti vel sufficientibus atque ydoneo vel ydoneis et regiminis fructuosis sub annuis responsionibus et aliis oneribus[k)] impositis et imponendis rationabiliter usque ad dicti domini nostri beneplacitum secundum statuta domus nostre religionis dandum. Dantes et concedentes predicto nostro procuratori et responsionum receptori licenciam, potestatem et auctoritatem cum plena, libera et generali[l)] administratione pro omnibus et singulis supra et infra scriptis ac dependentibus et emergentibus ex eisdem et altero eorundem aut ipsis et eorum cuilibet qualitercunque connexis coram quibuscunque iudicibus et curiis ecclesiasticis et mundanis semel et quociens oporteat et domino nostro procuratori et receptori responsionum videbitur expedire quibus supra nominibus occuparendi, proponendi, agendi et deffendendi, libellum seu libellos et quascunque summarias petitiones dandi et offerendi, litem seu lites contestandi, de calumpnia et de veritate dicendi, in animas dictorum magistri et conventus iurandi et subeundi cuiuslibet alterius communis licitum iuramentum ponendi, proponendi et articulandi, posicionibus et articulis[m)] alterius partis respondendi et datis per eum responderi, petendi[n)], excipiendi, excepciones dandi, replicandi, duplicandi, triplicandi, testes, instrumenta, litteras et quecunque alia probationum genera producendi et productis per partem adversam obiciendi, testes iurare videndi et in eos eorumque dicta dicendi, crimina et deffectus opponendi, beneficium absolutionis a quacunque sententia excommunicationis lata vel ferenda et restituciones in integrum semel et pluries, simpliciter et ad cautellam petendi et obtinendi, sententiam seu sententias tam interlocutorias quam diffinitivas ferri, petendi et audiendi et, si opus esset, eas variandi et ab ea vel eis et quocunque alio gravamine illato vel inferendo appellandi, apostolos et litteras dimissorias cum instantia semel [144v] et pluries petendi[o)] et appellacionum causas prosequendi, expensas et interesse petendi[p)], impetrandi quascunque litteras tam simplices quam loquendas gratiam seu iusticiam continentes et impetratis per partem adversam contradicendi, procuratores unum vel plures domus nostre fratres ad predicta et subscripta et eorum quodlibet loco sui semel vel pluries substituendi et eciam seculares personas ad lites et causas, tantummodo et eum seu eos revocandi et in se procurationis officium reassumendi et generaliter omnia alia et singula faciendi, dicendi, procurandi et exercendi, que in premissis et premissorum quolibet neccessaria fuerint seu eciam oportuna et que quilibet verus et legittimus procurator negociorum gestorum petitor et receptor facere potest et debet et que ipsi domini magister et conventus facere possent, si personaliter adessent, eciam si talia sint, in quibus[q)] requiratur mandatum speciale[r)]. Et relevantes dictum procuratorem et receptorem et substituendum et[s)] substituendos ab eo ab omni onere satisdandi, promittimus bona fide dictos dominos magistrum et conventum ratum, gratum et firmum habere perpetuo et tenere quicquid per dictum procuratorem et receptorem etcetera ac substitutum et substituendos ab eo actum, gestum, dictum, petitum, receptum et habitum, quictatum et prenotatum fuerit in premissis et quolibet premissorum ac iudicio sisti et iudicatum solvi cum omnibus et singulis suis clausulis opportunis sub ypotecha et obligatione omnium bonorum dicti prioratus nostri presencium pariter et futurorum. Mandantes per presens procuratorium sub virtute sancte obediencie firmiter[t)] et districte universis et singulis fratribus domus nostre prioratus predicti et preceptoriarum predictarum cuiuscunque gradus[u)] et condicionis existant et aliis quibuscunque, quibus predicta seu eo quodlibet pertinebunt et poterunt quomodolibet pertinere[v)], ut premisso nostro receptori et procuratori aut deputando vel deputandis ab[w)] eo super camerarum, domorum et baiulliarum responsiones et arreragia responsionum tam preteriti temporis quam presentis et futuri et omnia alia dictis magistro et conventui communiter vel divisim spectantes et debencia racionabiliter pervenire[x)] tradant et exhibent contradictione remota. In cuius rei testimonium ad maiorem predictorum roboris firmitatem bulla dicti reverendissimi magistri nostri plumbea in absentia bulle communis plumbee presentibus est appensa[y)]. Data in nostro generali capitulo in ecclesia nostra sancti Iohannis extra muros civitatis Aquensis[z)] in Provincia celebrato die duodecima[aa)] mensis Maii anno quo supra.

*a)* presentes *add. ante corr.* *b)* et *corr.* *c)* quelibet *praem. ante corr.* *d)* prec *praem. ante corr.* *e)* p *praem. ante corr.* *f)* ad *praem. ante corr.* *g)* recup *praem. ante corr.* *h)* de *add. ante corr.* *i)* inserun *praem. ante corr.* *j)* segregandi *praem. ante corr.* *k)* ho *praem. ante corr.* *l)* adm *add. ante corr.* *m)* art *praem. ante corr.* *n)* tenendi *praem. ante corr.* *o)* et audiendi *add. ante corr.* *p)* peten *praem. ante corr.* *q)* reperiatur man *add. ante corr.* *r)* spal *praem. ante corr.* *s)* se *praem. ante corr.* *t)* d *add. ante corr.* *u)* *dupl.* *v)* expedire *praem. ante corr.* *w)* su *praem. ante corr.* *x)* pertinere *praem. ante corr.* *y)* annexa. Data *praem. ante corr.* *z)* pro *praem. ante corr.* *aa)* de *praem. ante corr.*

## 241

*The brethren forming the chapter general (as no. 235) confirm Fr. Henman zu Rhein for his lifetime in the Priory of* Alamania. *He is to rule the priory, to pay the responsions of his prioral chambers and of the priory's preceptories on 24 June each year and all other dues to the receivers constituted by the Master and Convent or to others who are ordered to receive them. The Master and Convent reserve their right to grant one or more offices which are vacant following the death of the officer or preceptor according to the statute of 1367. In case that Fr. Henman zu Rhein fails to pay his dues on the date mentioned in the statute they reserve their right to depose him with the counsel of senior brethren according to the same statute. Following another statute of the 1367 chapter general certain death duties were transferred from the brethren in the priory to the Convent, and in recompensation the prior received the right to have one additional chamber in his priory. So Fr. Henman may choose one vacant office in the priory that he can grant to the next officer as his additional chamber. He may rule the priory but has to respect all rights of the Master and Convent. During ten years[!] and with the counsel of preceptors he may appoint suitable officers to vacant offices, castellanies and houses according to the Hospital's statutes. The Hospital's brethren,* confratres, *sisters and donats and subjects are to be obedient to him. Without the Master's special licence he may not pawn or alienate goods of the Order.*

*Aix, 1410 May 12*

*AOM 336 fol. 145r-6v (145r-6v), under* prioratus Alamanie et Boemie.

Fratres Iacobus Tivelli Alvernie, Raymundus de Lescure Tholose et Philippus de Languillia Lombardie priores, reverendissimi in Christo patris et domini domini fratris Philiberti de Nailhaco Dei gratia sacre domus hospitalis sancti Iohannis Iherosolimitani magistri dignissimi et pauperum Christi custodis locumtenentes generale capitulum celebrantes religioso in Christo nobis carissimo fratri Hammano ze Rin priori prioratus nostri Almanie dicte domus salutem et sinceram in Domino caritatem. Digne credimus agere et racionabiliter operari, si quos domus nostre fratres meritorum excellentia ad celsos gradus nostri ordinis evocavit, eos in suis, cum deposcunt, statibus conservamus, ut dum digne fructus dulcedine se reffectos conspiciunt et senciunt honoratos ad queque nostre religionis accomoda industrie eorum studia ingeri fervenciora comittant. Attendentes itaque, quod in administratione prioratus nostri Alamanie predicti estis fructuosus utiliter comprobatus, prioratum ipsum cum omnibus et singulis suis membris, iuribus et pertinenciis universis ad prioratum ipsum spectantibus et pertinentibus ac spectare et pertinere debentibus quoquomodo cum omni onere, emolumentis et honore et cum preceptoris cameris suis pro cameris assignatis cum omnibus et singulis earum et cuiuslibet earum membris, iuribus et pertinentiis universis habendum, [145v] tenendum, regendum, gubernandum, augmentandum et meliorandum in spiritualibus et temporalibus tam in capite quam in membris vobis tamquam digno et benemerito de consilio et assensu religiosorum in Christo nobis carissimorum fratrum Galteri Crassi decretorum doctoris prioris ecclesie conventualis Rodi, Lucii de Vailhins marescalli, Iohannis Griuelli preceptoris Chambacelli, procuratorum Rodi conventus, Iohannis Flote sancti Egidii, Aymonis de Monte Auium Acquitanie et Priami de Gambacurtis Pizarum priorum, Petri de Penninis thesaurarii et receptoris generalis, Petri de Thilio preceptoris de Gelesio locumtenentis magni[a)] preceptoris, Tossani de Berneuille preceptoris de Boncourt locumtenentis prioris Francie, Galuini Petri de Petrusio preceptoris procuratoris prioratus sancti Egidii, Petri de Stapis preceptoris Bononie locumtenentis prioris Veneciarum, Guionii de Verneyo Forensis et Petri Carrelli Caluie preceptorum, procuratorum prioratus Alvernie, Iohannis Sobaudi prioris de Corbolio, Hugonis de Sarciis preceptoris de Ostromonte procuratoris prioratus Francie, Helye Arnaudi Vodrie, Hemerici Danyet de Sancto Quitayo preceptorum procuratorum prioratus Acquitanie et aliorum fratrum in dicto generali capitulo astantium de nostra certa scientia et speciali gracia auctoritate presentis generalis capituli sub responsione annua [··] florenorum auri de Florencia et boni ponderis per vos, prout pro cameris vestris vos continget, et per preceptores preceptoriarum dicti prioratus, prout pro preceptoriis suis pro rata eis pertinebit, receptoribus deputatis vel deputandis per dictos dominos magistrum et conventum ad recipiendum responciones in prioratu prefato aut alii vel aliis, quibus et ubi prefati domini magister et conventus ordinaverint et mandaverint, in festo sancti Iohannis baptiste annis singulis ex pacto expresso infallibiliter exsolvenda et quibuscunque aliis oneribus dicto prioratui qualitercunque et quomodocunque incumbentiis, incumbendis, impositis et imponendis per vos et dictos preceptores, ut predicitur, ex pacto eciam veram responsionem predictam supportandum benefaciendo in eadem ad vitam vestram confirmamus retentis dictis dominis magistro et conventui et specialiter reservato, quod de una vel pluribus, prout per mortem preceptoris evenire contingerit, vacantis vel vacaturis baiulia vel baiuliis in dicto prioratu possint anno quolibet dicti domini magister et conventus providere secundum continenciam statuti, ac eciam retentis et reservatis dicto domino magistro ordinacionibus omnibus per bone memorie dominum fratrem Raymundum Berengarii dicte sacre domus magistrum predecessorem [146r] dicti domini nostri magistri factis[b)] et reservatis in generali capitulo per eum anno sexagesimo sexto[1)] in Avinione celebrato, nichilominus dicto domino magistro retento et eciam reservato, ut si, quod absit, in solucione per vos statuto termino facienda annuarum responsionum vestrarum camerarum et baiuliarum, quas ad manus vestras habetis vel habebitis in premisso prioratu, defficere vos contingat, quod dictus dominus magister cum consilio fratrum et procerum dicte domus possit disponere et ordinare de premisso prioratu secundum continenciam statuti edicti in prelibato capitulo

*1) 1367 March 5: Delaville (1913), 161–2.*

generali. Rursum cum ante celebracionem dicti capituli priores domus nostre supra bona et arnesia[c] preceptorum morientium haberent et reciperent certa iura et iura huiusmodi fuerint ex ordinacione et statuto in iamdicto capitulo promulgatis vigenti neccessitate applicata et reservata nostro communi thezauro nostre dicte domus et propterea ex dictis ordinacione et statuto fuerit concessum et provisum prioribus, ut in recompensacione iurium premissorum et eorum cuiuslibet ultra suas ordinarias cameras haberet et habere posset in suo prioratu unam aliam baiuliam despectantem et pertinentem videlicet sue donacioni, iuxta quas ordinacionem et statutum retinendum vobis in iurium recompensacionem premissorum ultra vestras ordinarias cameras unam aliam baiuliam, cum vacabit in vestro prioratu, vestre collacioni pertinentem potestatem et licentiam indulgemus. Dantes et concedentes vobis auctoritatem et potestatem plenariam regendi, gubernandi et administrandi prioratum prefatum tam in capite quam in membris, in spiritualibus et temporalibus et quecunque alia agendi, celebrandi et exercendi, que ad prioris spectant officium et que pro utili regimine prioratus ipsius neccessaria fuerint et eciam opportuna, insuper dandi et conferendi cum consilio fratrum et preceptorum dicti prioratus baiulias, castellanias atque domos vacaturas in iamdicto prioratu vestre spectantes donacioni secundum statutum nostre dicte domus edictum super istis fratribus ydoneis et benemeritis domus nostre prioratus prefati per dictum tempus decem annorum, prout melius et utilius vobis videbitur expedire, dicti tamen domini magister et conventus predictis retencionibus et omnibus semper salvis. Committentes vobis fiducialiter circa curam, regimen et administracionem ac gubernacionem accomodam dicti prioratus ac bonorum et iurium eiusdem deffensionem et recuperacionem tam in agendo quam defendendo hac serie vices nostras. Quocirca universis et singulis fratribus, preceptoribus et baiulis et aliis fratribus, confratribus, sororibus et donatis sub virtute [146v] sancte obedientie et [h]ominibus et vassallis et quibuscunque aliis nobis et nostre domui prefate subditis in dicto prioratu constitutis, presentibus et futuris sub sacramento fidelitatis et homagii, quo nobis et nostre domui sunt astricti, precipimus et mandamus harum serie districte, ut vobis tamquam eorum superiori, priori et maiori reverenter pareant, obediant et intendant vobisque suam prebeant auxilium, consilium et favorem in omnibus, que ad curam, regimen et administracionem ac gubernacionem utilem prescripti prioratus pertinere noscuntur, quociens opus fuerit et eos duxeritis requirendos. Inhibentes vobis districtius sub virtute sancte obedientie supradicta, ne pretextu confirmacionis et gracie nostre huiusmodi alique de bonis, rebus et iuribus prioratus predicti vendatis, detis, obligetis, impignoretis, permutetis, alienetis, distrahatis seu in emphiteosim perpetuam concedatis aut quocunque alio colore quesito extra nostram religionem transferatis sine nostra speciali licentia et mandato. Et si, quod absit, contra inhibicionem nostram huiusmodi aliquid vel aliqua operari vel facere vos contingat, illud et illa exnunc prout extunc et extunc prout exnunc cassamus, adnullamus ac decernimus irritum et inane nulliusque existere penitus efficacie vel valoris. In cuius rei testimonium ad maiorem predictorum roboris firmitatem bulla dicti reverendissimi domini nostri magistri plumbea in absentia bulle communis plumbee presentibus est appensa. Data in dicto generali capitulo in ecclesia nostra sancti Iohannis extra muros civitatis Aquensis in Provincia celebrato die duodecima mensis Maii anno incarnacionis Domini millesimo CCCC$^{mo}$ decimo.

*a)* generalis *praem. ante corr.* *b)* fratris *praem. ante corr.* *c)* anesia *praem. ante corr.*

## 242

*The brethren forming the chapter general (as no. 235) confirm to Fr. Wolf Schuck, Preceptor of Sulz, the licence granted him by the former Prior of* Alamania *Fr. Hesso Schlegelholz to receive eight chaplains and ten* scolares iuvenes *as pupils of the Order in his preceptory.*

*[Aix, 1410] May 15*

*AOM 336 fol. 144v-5r (144v-5r), under* prioratus Alamanie et Boemie.

Fratres Iacobus Tivelli etcetera religioso in Christo nobis carissimo fratri Wolf Schuck preceptori de Sulcz prioratus nostri Alamanie dicte domus salutem etcetera. Supplicatoriam peticionem nobis pro parte vestra exhibitam recepimus continentem, quod, cum per domus nostre fratrem Hessonem Slegelholcz[a)], olim priorem Almanie, per baiullos, preceptores et proceres dicti prioratus sibi tunc astantes ordinatum extiterit, quod in dicta baiullia de Sulcz, in qua ad Dei servicia degere debent prout degunt octo fratres cappellani et decem scolares iuvenes fratres semper foret studium sive scole ibidem perpetue tenentur, [145r] ut dicti fratres iuvenes litterarum scientiam addierent, bonos[b)] mores exterarem vitamque religiosam secundum domus nostre regulam, statuta et laudabiles consuetudines ducerent, unde nobis pro parte vestra extitit suplicatum, ut premissa auctoritate generalis capituli confirmare dignaremur. Hinc est, quod nos cupientes illa, que provida et laudabili deliberacione per domus nostre fratres ordinata, deliberata sunt et statuta, presertim ea, que divinum cultum et conservationem vestre religiose[c)] conversationis honeste concernere dignoscuntur, et servare ilesa[d)] premissa omnia et singula prout per dictos fratres Hessonem, olim priorem, ut prestitur, et baillivos et preceptores et proceres prioratus predicti facta sunt et inita, rata, grata et placida habentes baiuliam ipsam cum omnibus et singulis suis membris, pertinentiis et iuribus ad eam spectantibus et pertinentibus ac spectare et pertinere debentibus quoquomodo, prout ipsas habetis presencialiter et tenetis, habendam etcetera de voluntate etcetera et aliarum etcetera perpetuo confirmamus etcetera vosque etcetera. Committentes etcetera. Quocirca etcetera necnon etcetera. Inhibentes etcetera. In cuius etcetera bulla etcetera. Data etcetera die XV$^{a}$ mensis Maii anno quo supra.

*a)* Slegh *praem. ante corr.* *b)* bonum *corr.* *c) post corr.* *d)* ilasa *MS*

## 243

*The Lieutenant Master Fr. Domenico d'Alamania and the Convent write to Fr. Henman zu Rhein, Prior of* Alamania, *that they have opened his letter to the Master Fr. Philibert de Naillac. They ask Fr. Henman to treat with benivolence brothers doing penance, as decided in the chapter general currently held at Aix, and to pay 100 florins promised by Fr. Heinrich Tripscher, although he was not a procurator of Fr. Hermann von Ow, Preceptor of Villingen.*

*Rhodes, 1410 October 22*

*AOM 339 fol. 254r (220r), under* littere diversorum negotiorum.

[a)]Venerabili religioso in Christo nobis carissimo fratri Hermano[!] ze Ryn sacre domus hospitalis sancti Iohannis Iherosolemitani priori nostro in Alamania[a)]. Religiose in Christo nobis carissime, salutem et sinceram in Domino caritatem. Vestras recepimus litteras dirigentes verssus reverendissimum dominum dominum fratrem Philibertum de Nelihaco, magistrum dignissimum, superiorem nostrum, et in defectu ipsius versus nos locu[m]tenente, ut in dorso ipsorum lacius continetur, quorum tenorem diligenter inspeximus et vidimus ordinacionem et declaracionem inde securam in capitulo generali actualiter in Ax celebrato, quam declaracionem habemus nos eciam pro rata et firma, super facto illorum nostrorum fratrum vos estis superior ipsorum et pius pater, si penitenter veniunt[b)] procedi et sic vos rogamus ortantes in Domino[c)] facere sicut verus et verbus religiosus in omnibus peragendis nostre religionis sicut confidimus et speramus totiens quociens. Insuper requisitus pro parte fratris Armandis de Owe preceptoris in Vinlingen de C florenis premisis[d)] pro parte fratris Henrici Dupsich procuratorio nomine vestri, licet non fuerat vester procurator, velitis eidem cogi et compelli ad[e)] satisfaccionem et solucionem congruam ipsius vel certi nuncii nomine procuratoris. Alia non scribimus quam valete in eo, qui omnium est vera salus feliciter et longeve. Scripta Rodi die XXII Octobris M° IIII^c X. [f)]Frater Dominicus de Alamania locumtenens reverendissimi domini magistri ceterique bailivi, priores et procheres conventus Rodi[f)].

*a-a) suprascript.* *b)* venunt *MS* *c)* ortandes in Domini *MS* *d)* promises *corr.* *e)* ada *MS* *f-f) infrascript.*

## 244

*The Lieutenant Master Fr. Domenico d'Alamania and the Convent write to Fr. Count Hugo von Montfort, Preceptor of Bubikon and Tobel, that they have opened his letter to the Master Fr. Philibert de Naillac and have sent his proposals to the chapter general currently held at Aix.*

*Rhodes, 1410 October 22*

*AOM 339 fol. 254r (220r), under* littere diversorum negotiorum.

[a]Venerabili et religioso in Christo nobis carissimo fratri Hugoni de Mefort comitti preceptori baiuliarum[b] de Bubikon et Tobel in prioratu nostro Alamanie[a]. Religiose in Christo nobis carissime, salutem et sinceram in Domino caritatem. Vestras recepimus litteras dirigentes versus reverendissimum dominum dominum fratrem Philibertum de Nelihaco, magistrum dignissimum superiorem nostrum, et in defectu ipsius versus nos locu[m]tenente, ut in dorso ipsorum lacius continetur, quorum tenorem diligenter inspeximus et vidimus ordinacionem et declaracionem inde securam in capitulo generali actualiter in Ax celebrato, quam declaracionem habemus nos eciam pro rata et firma rogantes vos, ut facta nostre religionis sint vobis recomissa, prout confidimus. Alia non scribimus quam valete in eo, qui omnium est vera salus, feliciter et longeve. Scripta Rodi die XXII Octobris M IIII^C X. [c]Frater Dominicus de Alamania locumtenens reverendissimi domini magistri ceterique bailivi, priores et procheres conventus Rodi[c].

*a-a) suprascript.* *b)* bailivarum *MS* *c-c) infrascript.*

## 245

*The Lieutenant Master Fr. Domenico d'Alamania and the Convent complain to Fr. Henman zu Rhein, Prior of* Alamania, *that he has not paid his responsions as promised on his behalf by Fr. Heinrich Tripscher when Fr. Henman was appointed prior.*
*[Rhodes, 1410 without day]*

*AOM 339 fol. 236r (202r), under* littere diversorum negotiorum.

[a]Venerabili et religioso in Christo nobis carissimo fratri Hamanti Rin priori Alamanie detur[a]. In Christo nobis carissime, salutem et sinceram in Domino caritatem. Tenore presencium vobis intimamus, quod multa admiratione comovemur, quatenus responciones per vos debitas pro prioratu Alamanie nobis et thesauro nostro, ut promisit frater Henricus Tripter, qui hic pro vobis obtinuit dictum prioratum, nullatenus nobis transmisistis. Et cum subiacemus necessitatibus et nos opportet esse sollicitis in exaccionibus responcionum communi thesauro nostro debitarum pro subveniendis necessitatibus nostri conventus, ideo serie presencium vos ortamur in Christo et secundo vobis sub virtute sancte obedientie precipimus et districte mandamus, quatenus dictas responciones nobis et thesauro nostro hic in Rodo mittatis et nullathenus mitere tardetis, ne, si secus feceritis, quod absit, habeamus materiam contra vos procedere tamquam contra inobedientem. Speramus tamen vos taliter habere in predictis, quod nulla causa inobedientie vobis poterit ascribi, ex qua habeamus materiam contra vos procedere rigorose. Omnipotens Deus conservet vos. [b]Frater Dominicus de Alamania locumtenens etcetera et conventus Rodi[b].

*a-a) suprascript.* *b-b) infrascript.*

## 246

*The Lieutenant Master and Preceptor of Kos Fr. Hesso Schlegelholz and the Convent quit Dino di Giovanni,* burgensis *of Rhodes and scribe of the Treasury, for 669 ducats of Venice or 700 florins of Germany on behalf of Fr. Leonardo Buonafede, Preceptor of S. Giacomo in Florence and receiver in the Priory of Bohemia, for one year's responsions of that priory.*

*Rhodes, 1411 October 9*

*AOM 339 fol. 173r-v (148r-v), under* asegnationes pecuniarum.

Nos frater Hessonus Scleg. sacre domus hospitalis sancti Iohannis Iherosolimiani preceptor Langonis et reverendissimi in Christo patris et domini fratris Philiberti de Nailhaco Dei gratia eiusdem sacre domus magistri dignissimi et pauperum Christi custodis locumtenens et nos conventus Rodi domus prefate universis et singulis presentes recognitionis ac quitationis litteras visuris, lecturis et audituris per presentes fatemur et in verbo veritatis attestamur nos habuisse ac realiter atque de facto recepisse per manus discreti viri Dyni de Iohanne, burge[n]sis nostri[a] Rodi ac scribe nostri communis thesauri, ducatorum auri cugni Venetorum sexingentorum sexaginta novem equipollentium florenis septingentis de Alamania[b] ex parte religiosi[c] in Christo nobis carissimi fratris Leonardi de Bonafe eiusdem domus, preceptoris preceptorie sancti Iacobi de Florentia ac receptoris responsionum[d] prioratus nostri Boemie. Quamquidem summam dictus frater Leonardus recepit nomine nostri pro responsione dicti prioratus nostri Boemie anni finiti [173v] in festo resurrectionis Domini nostri Ihesu Christi proxime elapso de anno M° CCCC° undecimo,[1] de quibusquidem sexingentis sexaginta novem ducatis[e] auri cugni[f] Venetorum per nos, ut premittitur, habitis et realiter[g] ac manualiter receptis eosdem Dynum de Iohanne ac fratrem Leonardum, receptorem nostrum, de premissis et quemlibet ipsorum ac heredes et successores eorum et quelibet eorum bona mobilia et immobilia, presentia et futura de nostra certa scientia liberamus, absolvimus perpetue[h] et quitamus. In cuius rei testimonium et certitudinem pleniorem presentem recognicionem et quitanciam predictarum[i] inde fieri fecimus et appensione bulle nostre ceree, qua utimur ob defectum bulle plumbee nostri conventus, muniri. Dat. Rodi in prefato conventu die IX mensis Octobris anno a nativitate Domini M° CCCC° undecimo indictione quarta.

Duplicata *marg.* *a)* burgese nostro *corr.* *b)* equipollentium quos ad *add. ante corr.* *c)* religiosis *corr.* *d)* responsionum *supra lin.* *e)* duacatis *MS* *f)* de Venec. *praem. ante corr.* *g)* a *praem. ante corr.* *h)* perpetuo *MS* *i)* predictarum *supra lin.*

*1) 12 April 1411.*

## 247

*[The Lieutenant Master] Fr. Hesso Schlegelholz licenses, with the agreement of brethren of the Convent, Fr. Johann von Monreal, Preceptor of Cologne and Adenau, to leave the Convent and travel to the West.*

*Rhodes, 1411 October 9*

*AOM 339 fol. 203r-v (170r-v), under* littere licenciarum.

Frater Hessonus Scleghelholtz sacre domus etcetera religioso in Christo nobis carissimo fratri Iohanni de Mormeali preceptori preceptoriarum Colonie et Adenow prioratus nostri Alamanie[a)] salutem et sinceram in Domino caritatem. Sperantes per naturalem industriam a domino Deo vobis concessam, quod per vestram personalem presentiam prefatas preceptorias vestris meritis exigentibus vobis data[s] utilius in agendis [dirigi] et comodius gubernari, idcirco a conventu nostro Rodi [203v] [recedendi] et eundi ad predictum prioratum Alamanie ceterasque partes occidentales, ut eidem preceptorie utili gubernationi et regimini preesse valeatis et eidem modo debito intendere et vacare, et ad ipsum conventum redeundi, dum vestre placuerit voluntati, licentia tamen vestri superioris prius requisita, vobis tenore presentium de voluntate, consilio et assensu religiosorum in Christo nobis carissimorum fratrum dominorum baillivorum et procerum dicti conventus plenam licentiam concedimus pariter et donamus. Dat. in prefato conventu Rodi sub sigillo nostro, quo utimur, die nona mensis Octobris anno a nativitate Domini M° CCCC° undecimo.

Pro fratre Iohanne Monreal preceptori Colonie etcetera *marg.* *a)* Francie *praem. ante corr.*

## 248

*[The Lieutenant Master] Fr. Hesso Schlegelholz, with the agreement of brethren of the Convent, licenses Fr. Peter Mersner, Preceptor of Reichardsroth, to leave the Convent on Rhodes for his preceptory and return whenever he wishes, with his superior's licence.*

*Rhodes, 1411 October 16*

*AOM 339 fol. 204r (171r), under* littere licenciarum.

Frater Hesso Sleg. sacre domus etcetera religioso in Christo nobis carissimo fratri Petro Merscner preceptori de Rod prioratus nostri Alamanie salutem et sinceram caritatem in Domino. Sperantes per naturalem industriam a domino Deo vobis datam, quod per vestram personalem presenciam preceptoriam[a)] predictam per nos et conventum nostrum vestris meritis exigentibus nuper vobis datam utilius in agendis dirigi et comodius gubernari. Idcirco recedendi a conventu nostro Rodi et eundi ad predictum prioratum Alamanie et ad partes occidentales, ut eidem preceptorie utili gubernatione et regimine preesse valeatis et eidem modo debito intendere et vacare, et ad ipsum conventum redeundi, quando vestre placuerit voluntati, licentia tamen vestri superioris prius requisita vobis tenore presencium de voluntate, consilio et assensu religiosorum in Christo nobis carissimorum dominorum fratrum baillivorum et procerum nostri conventus plenam licentiam concedimus pariter et donamus. Dat. in prefato conventu die XVI mensis Octobris anno a nativitate Domini M° IIII[c] XI°.

Pro fratre Petro Merschner *marg.* *a)* presenciam *MS*

## 249

*The Lieutenant Master and Preceptor of Kos Fr. Hesso Schlegelholz and the Convent grant to Fr. Peter Mersner the Preceptory of Reichardsroth (Priory of* Alamania), *which is vacant following the death of Fr. Hermann Krantz.*

*Rhodes, 1411 October 22*

*AOM 339 fol. 155r (130r), under* prioratus Alamanie et Boemie.

Frater Hessonus Sclegelholtz sacre domus hospitalis sancti Iohannis Ierosolimitani preceptor Langonis et locumtenens reverendissimi in Christo patris et domini domini fratris Philiberti de Naylhaco Dei gratia eiusdem sacre domus magistri dignissimi et pauperum Christi custodis et nos conventus Rodi religioso in Christo nobis carissimo fratri Petro Merschner[1)] eiusdem domus salutem et sinceram in Domino caritatem. Dum ad ydoneitatem sufficiencie vestre et alia virtuosa vestra merita etcetera. Hinc est, quod preceptoriam de Rod prioratus nostri Alamanie vacantem per obitum condam fratris Hermanni Crance[2)] eiusdem domus presencialiter per eius mortem ad collationem et provisionem nostram devolutam cum omnibus et singulis suis membris, iuribus etcetera conferimus, concedimus et donamus etcetera. Comittentes vobis etcetera. Quocirca etcetera amoto abinde etcetera. Et si, quod absit, etcetera. In cuius rei testimonium etcetera. Dat. Rodi in prefato conventu die XXII[a] mensis Octobris anno a nativitate Domini M° CCCC° undecimo.

Pro fratre Petro Merschner *marg.*

## 250

*The Lieutenant Master Fr. Hesso Schlegelholz and the Convent answer a letter by Fr. Leonardo Buonafede, Preceptor of S. Giacomo in Florence and receiver of responsions*

*1) Borchardt 1 (1988), 533 no. 124.*
*2) Ibid. 532 no. 118.*

*in the Priory of Bohemia, which recently arrived with the Venetian galleys. They have received the Bohemian responsions from the scribe of the Treasury Dino Giovanni of Florence. About papal provisions of preceptories they will write to the Prior of Venice. They request Fr. Leonardo to help Fr. Pierre de Gaubert, Preceptor of Avignon, to secure possession of his preceptory.*

*Rhodes, [1]411 November 6*

*AOM 339 fol. 258r-v (224r-v), under* littere diversorum negotiorum.

Frater ac religiose nobis carissime. Pridie in adventu galearum Venetorum vestras litteras quamplura continentes alacri animo recepimus, quibus tale responsum prestare decrevimus reserientes vestre amicicie, quod responsiones prioratus Boemie integraliter recepimus a Dyno Iohannis de Florentia, scriba nostri communis thesauri, prout in quitancia ei facta liquide potest demonstrari, quas in futurum exigere et ad conventum nostrum destinare onus et laborem sumere non tedeat, quia omnes fratres hic residentes maximum consequenter gaudium et non solum in conventu commorantes, set eciam absentes comoda thesauri nostri bene pertractantes, qualis est vestra persona, non minus utilitates conferant, quam qui personaliter nostre religioni famulantur. De collacionibus autem [258v] preceptoriarum nostre religionis, que a domino nostro papa fiunt, sue sanctitati et dominis cardinalibus religionis nostre protectoribus circa talem materiam tangentibus plenarie scribimus ac priori Veneciarum, a quo poteritis plenarie informari. Alia non scribimus, nisi quod frater Petrus de Galbertis preceptor Avinionis sit vobis recomissus, cui prestare placeat auxilium, consilium et favorem, ut preceptorie sue possessionem possit pacificam obtinere, quod erit in maximum gaudium atque leticiam fratribus hic in conventu residentibus. Valete in Domino et sepius nos vestris litteris visitare[a)] de occurrentibus in partibus illis non tedeat. Rodi die VI[a] Novembris IIII[c] XI[o]. [b)]Venerabili et religioso viro fratri Leonardo de Bonafe preceptori sancti Iacobi de Florencia ac receptori responsionum prioratus nostri Boemie in Christo nobis carissimo[b)]. [b)]Frater Hesso Sleg. locumtenens domini nostri magistri ceterique fratres ballivi, priores et proceres conventus Rhodi[b)].

Fratri Leonardo preceptori sancti Iacobi de Florentia *marg.* *a)* visitando *praem. ante corr.* *b-b) infrascript.*

## 251

*The Lieutenant Master Fr. Hesso Schlegelholz and the Convent urge the Master Fr. Philibert de Naillac to return to Rhodes. With the Venetian galleys they have received letters from the Prior of Venice that the pope is destroying the Order by appointing preceptors, because the Master does not live in the Convent and has not visited the papal curia with presents, and that the Prior of Toulouse is neglecting the Order's affairs. The King of England and his Prior ordered the responsions to be sent only to Rhodes.*

*They received 5,876 ducats of Venice through the Alberti of Florence and for the responsions of Bohemia 669 ducats from Fr. Leonardo Buonafede, Preceptor of S. Giacomo in Florence, writing other priors to pay their dues.*

*Rhodes, [1]411 November 6*

*AOM 339 fol. 260r-v (226r-v), under* littere diversorum negotiorum. *Ed. Paoli (1737), 115.*

[a)]Reverendissimo in Christo patri et domino domino fratri Philiberto de Naylhaco Dei gratia sacre domus hospitalis sancti Iohannis Iherosolimitani magistro dignissimo et pauperum Christi custodi, patri et domino nostro metuendissimo[a)]. [a)]Vestre paternitatis frater Hesso Sleg., locumtenens, ceterique fratres baillivi, proceres et priores conventus vestri Rodi[a)]. Reverendissime pater ac domine metuendissime. Cum omni humilima recommendatione premissa. Cum absentia vestre magnifice dominationis conventum vestrum et quoslibet in eo commorantes[b)] orphanos quodammodo hactenus fecerit, et donec vestra metuendissima dominacio moram in aliis locis trahet, omnes vestri subditi cuiuslibet sexus alta voce clamant: "Sempiterne patre et domino nostro orbati erimus. O utinam pastor et dominus noster, sub cuius umbra regimur, eius accessus ad civitatem Rodi brevis esse dignoscatur, nam dominum nostrum et eius virtutes numquam cognovimus, cum ipsius presentiam cotidie corporaliter[c)] intuebamur[d)]. Nunc domini nostri distancia facit nos in anxietatibus[e)] et doloribus permanere." Istorum igitur, domine metuendissime, subditorum sermo communis talis existit, ut superius fuit prolatus. Placeat ergo versus civitatem vestram, ubi filii et vestri devotissimi servitores cum anxietate vos prestolantur, et quod affectant non mentaliter, set corporaliter valeant intueri, quod erit in maximum gaudium atque leticiam omnium in civitate Rhodi commorantium. Ceterum in adventu galearum Venetarum prior Veneciarum quasdam suas litteras destinavit, quarum tenore denotabat destructionem nostre religionis ex eo, quia dominus summus pontifex preceptorias conferebat, prout sue sanctitati placebat, et quod dominacio vestra non in conventu vestro[f)], set in partibus occidentalibus residebat, et quod summum pontificem et dominos cardinales vestra dominacio exeniis et muneribus hactenus non visitavit, cui domino nostro summo pontifici circa materiam seu illarum litterarum tenorum cum maxima humilitate aliquas litteras[g)] scribi fecimus vestram dominationem et nostram religionem sue sanctitati recommendandas. In prosecutione eciam illarum litterarum continebatur, qualiter dominus Tholosanus non vacabat [260v] circa facta sue religionis. Notificamus dominationi prelibate, qualiter rex Anglie et prior ac ceteri responsionum collectores ordinaverunt, quod prefate responsiones debent tantummodo ad conventum portari et non ad aliquem alium locum. Et per manus Albertoris[h)] de Florencia recepimus quantitatem ducatorum de Venec. quinque milium[i)] octingentorum septuaginta sex. Demum eciam per presentes notificamus, qualiter frater Leonardus de Bonafe preceptor sancti Iacobi de Florencia transmisit responsiones prioratus vestri Boemie ducatorum sexingentorum sexaginta novem. Ceteris vero prioribus generaliter scripsimus, quatenus sint in futurum soliciti[j] ad exigendum responsiones, taillas et mortuorum spolia et ad thesauro sollicitti esse debeant destinandum. Alia non scribimus nisi denuo obsecrando, ut vestros gressus desiderabiles[k] ad partes istas celeriter dirigere dignemini, quos hic prosperos perducat Altissimus feliciter et longeve conservet. Rodi in conventu vestro VI[a] die Novembris IIII[c] XI[o].

*a-a) suprascript.* *b)* comnorantes *MS* *c)* cop *praem. ante corr.* *d) dupl. ante corr.* *e)* anxietal *praem. ante corr.* *f)* Rodi *praem. ante corr.* *g)* et *praem. ante corr.* *h)* d *praem. ante corr.* *i)* V *praem. ante corr.* *j)* solu *praem. ante corr.* *k)* pros *praem. ante corr.*

## 252

*[The Lieutenant Master] Fr. Hesso Schlegelholz and the Convent on Rhodos grant for ten years to the chaplain Fr. Marcellus von Liechtenberg the Preceptory of Mülhausen (Priory of* Alamania), *which is vacant following the death of Fr. Kaspar Ederli.*

*Rhodes, 1412 April 18*

*AOM 339 fol. 155v-6r (130v-1r), under* prioratus Alamanie et Boemie.

Frater Hesso Sleg. sacre domus etcetera et nos conventus Rodi domus eiusdem religioso in Christo nobis carissimo fratri Marcello de Lichtenberg, capellano eiusdem domus prioratus nostri Alamanie, salutem et sinceram in Domino caritatem. Religionis decor, morum honestas, vite mundicia et alia virtutum[a] dona, quibus vos carismatis gratia insignivit, ad imparciendum vobis nostri favoris gratiam rationabiliter nos moventes, sperantes, quod vobis regimine effectus administrationis utilis favente Domino vos comendet. Hinc est, quod baiuliam seu preceptoriam de Merulnhusen dicti nostri prioratus Alamanie per obitum condam[b] fratris Caspar Ederly presencialiter vacantem et ad collationem et provisionem nostram propterea devolutam cum omnibus et singulis suis membris, iuribus et pertinentiis universis ad eam spectantibus et pertinentibus ac spectare et pertinere debentibus, quoquomodo et cum quibus illam habuit, tenuit et possedit dictus condam frater Caspar, habendam, tenendam, regendam etcetera invicem deliberato consilio de nostra certa scientia et speciali gratia ad annos decem incipiendos in festo nativitatis sancti Iohannis baptiste proximo et[c] extunc continue et integre secuturos vobis auctoritate presentium conferimus, concedimus et donamus benefaciendo in eadem[d] vosque preceptorem et comendatorem in dicta constituimus baiulia hac serie et eciam ordinamus. Comittentes vobis fiducialiter [156r] circa curam, regimen etcetera. Quocirca etcetera necnon universis et singulis etcetera ac priori seu presidenti prefato etcetera amoto abinde etcetera. Inhibentes vobis etcetera. Et si, quod absit, etcetera. In cuius rei testimonium bulla nostra cerea, qua utimur ob defectum bulle communis plumbee dicti nostri conventus, presentibus est appensa. Dat.

Rodi in prefato nostro[e)] conventu die decimaoctava mensis Aprilis anno a nativitate Domini M° IIII$^{C}$ duodecimo.

Pro fratre Marcello de Lietenberg *marg.* *a)* virtututum *MS* *b)* condam *dupl.* *c) dupl.* *d)* benefaciendo in eadem *supra lin.* *e)* nostre *MS*

*Ederli a family in Freiburg. Balthasar Ederli was mentioned in 1407: Krieger 1 (1904), col. 617. Kaspar is perhaps his brother, because it was a fashion of the time to name brothers after the Three Holy Kings Melchior, Kaspar and Balthasar.*

## 253

*[The Lieutenant Master] Fr. Hesso Schlegelholz and the Convent at Rhodes assign maintenance in the member of Heitersheim of the Preceptory of Freiburg im Breisgau to Michael de Polonia for his lifetime, because for more than 50 years Michael has been their domestic servant and familiar.*

*Rhodes, 1412 May 4*

*AOM 339 fol. 155r-v (130r-v), under* prioratus Alamanie et Boemie.

Frater Hesso Sclegelholtz sacre domus etcetera et nos conventus Rodi domus eiusdem in Christo nobis dilecto Michaeli de Polonia, servitori et familiari nostro domestico, salutem in Domino sempiternam. Grata tue familiaritatis et devotionis obsequia, que nobis hactenus et per spacium annorum quinquaginta et ultra ac nostre religioni[a)] fideliter impedisti et adhunc solicitis studiis impendere non desistis, nos inducunt, ut tibi tam gravitate annorum oppresso in et super membro de Heitersheim[b)] preceptorie de Friburgo[c)] prioratus nostri Alamanie tabullam ac mensam ad tuam vitam[d)] et omnia, quecumque pertinent unicuique donato nostre religionis[e)], non obstante, quod matrimonialiter sis copulatus, de nostra certa sciencia et speciali gratia invicem deliberato consilio in tuorum servitiorum retribucione damus, conferimus et assignamus. Quocirca universis et singulis fratribus domus nostre[f)] quacumque auctoritate[g)], [155v] dignitate vel officio fungentibus[h)], presentibus et futuris, ne contra presentem nostram donacionem ac gratiam sub virtute sancte obediencie aliquatenus venire presumant, quinymo eam iuxta mentem eius et seriem studeant inviolabiliter observare, ac priori seu presidenti dicti nostri prioratus ac preceptori dicte preceptorie, ut vobis tabullam antedictam[i)] et vitam et cetera necessaria modo predicto[j)] assignant et in possessionem corporalem eorundem inducant, precipimus et stricte mandamus. In cuius rey testimonium etcetera. Data Rodi die quarta mensis Maii anno a nativitate Domini M° IIII$^{C}$ duodecimo.

*a)* religionis *corr.* *b)* de Heitersheim *supra lin.* *c)* de Friburgo *supra lin.* *d)* sicuti viri fratri dicte preceptorie *add. ante corr.* *e)* et omnia – religionis *marg.* *f)* nostre *supra lin.* *g)* auctoritate *dupl. (nova pag.).* *h)* ne *add.* *i)* ante- *supra lin.* *j)* et vitam B predicto *supra lin.*

## 254

*[The Lieutenant Master] Fr. Luce de Vallins and the Convent order Fr. Hugo von Montfort, Prior of* Alamania, *to pay 100 florins of the Rhine to Fr. Dietrich von Keppenbach, to whom the Convent has promised this money.*

*[Rhodes, 1412/13]*

*AOM 339 fol. 181v (156v), under* littere assignationum seu cambiorum.

Frater Lucius de Valinis etcetera et nos[a] conventus Rodi domus eiusdem religiosis in Christo nobis carissimis fratri Hugoni de Monfordia prioratus nostri Alamanie seu cuicumque[b] receptori dicti nostri prioratus salutem[c] in Domino. Noveritis nostrum[d] communem thesaurum deberi religioso in Christo nobis carissimo fratri Theoderico de Keppenbach dicti prioratus in summa florenos de Reno centum, quos sibi per vos ibi solvi promisimus. Volentes igitur premissa complere, ut tenemur, mandamus[e], ut dicto fratri Theoderico dictos florenos de Reno centum integraliter solvatis atque detis etcetera. In cuius rei etcetera. Data in prefato nostro conventu etcetera.[1]

Pro fratre Theoderico de Keppenbach prioratus Alamanie *marg.* *a)* no *MS* *b)* cuicumcumque *MS* *c)* seualutem *corr.* *d)* nostri *corr.* *e)* vobis *praem. ante corr.*

## 255

*The Marshal Fr. Luce de Vallins as Lieutenant of the Master Fr. Philibert de Naillac and the Convent license their chaplain Fr. Marcellus von Liechtenberg, who has collected assets of the late Fr. Hesso Schlegelholz and of the late Fr. Henman zu Rhein for the Grand Preceptor Fr. Pierre du Theil and the vice-regent of the Treasury Fr. Jean de Patria, to travel to the Preceptory of Mülhausen (Priory of* Alamania), *which has been granted him by Fr. Hesso and the Convent.*

*Rhodes, 1412 June 1*

*AOM 339 fol. 207r-v (174r-v), under* littere licenciarum.

Frater Lucius de Valins sacre domus hospitalis sancti Iohannis Iherosolimitani humilis[a] marscalcus conventus Rodi domus eiusdem ac locumtenens reverendissimi in Christo patris et domini domini fratris Philiberti de Nailhaco Dei gratia eiusdem sacre domus magistri dignissimi et pauperum Christi custodis religioso in Christo nobis carissimo fratri Marcello dicto[a] de Lietenberg eiusdem domus cappellano, preceptori de Merulnhusen prioratus nostri Alamanie

1) *The date is probably 1412/13, not long after the death of Fr. Hesso Schlegelholz and the appointment of Fr. Luce de Vallins as Lieutenant Master.*

et procuratori nostro salutem in Domino. Sperantes, quod per naturalem industriam a domino Deo vobis collatam, quam circa exactionem et recuperacionem bonorum [207v] et iurium condam recolende memorie fratris Hessonis Sleg. continui predecessoris nostri ac eciam ipsius et[b)] condam fratris Hermanni Rin prioris dicti prioratus Alamanie per dilectos in[c)] Christo nobis carissimos fratres Petrum de Tillio, magnum preceptorem nostri[d)] conventus Rodi, et Iohannem de Patria, vicegerentem thesaurarii dicti nostri conventus, vobis comissas vigilabitis solicite ac prudenter vacabitis ac quod per[e)] vestram personalem presentiam preceptoriam predictam per condam bone memorie fratrem Hessonem Slegh. et conventum vobis nuper vestris meritis exigentibus datam utilius in agendis et comodius gubernari. Idcirco recedendi a conventu nostro Rodi etcetera ad ipsumque conventum redeundi et vobis licenciam etcetera. Dat. in prefato nostro conventu sub sigillo nostro, quo in talibus utimur, die I Iunii anno a nativitate Domini M° IIII$^{C}$ XII.

Pro fratre Marcello Lietenberg *marg.* (pro fratre *add. marg. ante corr.*) *a)* prehumilis *MS* *a)* dictum *MS* *b)* despo *praem. ante corr.* *c)* v *praem. ante corr.* *d)* dicti *praem. ante corr.* *e)* prefata preceptoria *praem. ante corr.*

## 256

*Licence for the chaplain Fr. Johann Frank (Priory of* Alamania) *to travel to the Convent.*

*[Rhodes, 1412 June 1]*

*AOM 339 fol. 207v (174v), under* littere licenciarum.

Item fuit data licentia [a)]eodem die[a)] fratri Iohanni Frank, capellano[b)] prioratus Alamanie, veniendi ad conventum, quando sibi placuerit[c)], reverentia tamen debita suo superiori exibita.

Pro fratre Iohanne Frank veniendi ad conventum prioratus Alamanie *marg.* *a-a) supra lin.* *b)* ven *in lin. ante corr.* *c)* vol *praem. ante corr.*

## 257

*The Marshal Fr. Luce de Vallins as Lieutenant of the Master Fr. Philibert de Naillac licenses, with the agreement brehtren of the Convent, Fr. Johann von Monreal, Preceptor of Adenau and Bailiff of Cologne, to receive four men as knight brethren into the Order and to assign them maintenance in his preceptories.*

*1412 June 1*

*AOM 339 fol. 207v-8r (174v-5r), under* littere licenciarum.

Frater Lucius de Valins sacre domus hospitalis sancti Iohannis Iher. humilis marscalcus conventus Rodi domus eiusdem ac locumtenens reverendissimi in Christo patris et domini domini fratris Philiberti de Naylhaco Dei gratia eiusdem sacre domus magistri dignissimi et pauperum Christi custodis religioso in Christo nobis carissimo fratri Iohanni de Montreali eiusdem domus preceptori de Adenay [a)]et baillivo Colonie salutem etcetera[a)]. Supplicatorie expositioni vestre exprimenti, quod, cum fratribus militibus[b)] ad presens indigeatis ad direccionem administrationis utilis vestrarum baiuliarum supradictarum, faciendi fratres [c)]milites nostre religionis[c)] vobis impertiri licentiam[d)] dignaremur, peticioni vestre in hac parte deflexImus vestra proceritate promerente, quod fratres IIII[or], si apti [c)]fuerint[c)], sani et integri suis membris, eis prius per vos vel alium cingulis[e)] milicie[f)] [208r] insignitis et decoratis, si eorum quilibet ex utroque parente nobilis fuerit de legittimo thoro natus, eisque stagiam assignandi in dictis preceptoriis vestris, in quibus eis provideri in eorum neccessariis secundum bonos usus et laudabiles consuetudines domus nostre faciatis, tenore presentium de voluntate, consilio et assensu religiosorum in Christo nobis carissimorum dominorum fratrum baillivorum, priorum et procerum dicti nostri conventus licentiam et plenam potestatem elargimur. Dat. sub sigillo nostro, quo in talibus utimur, die prima Iunii anno a nativitate Domini M° IIII[C] XII°.

Licentia fratris Iohannis de Montreal, ut possit accipere in religione quatuor milites *marg.* *a-a) marg.* *b)* quatuor *add. ante corr.* *c-c) supra lin.* *d)* d *praem. ante corr.* *e) cingulo corr.* *f)* miliciarum *corr.*

## 258

*[The Lieutenant Master] Fr. Luce de Vallins and the Convent on Rhodos notify to Fr. Hugo von Montfort, Prior of* Alamania, *the death of Fr. Hesso Schlegelholz on 20 May and send Fr. Marcellus von Liechtenberg, Preceptor of Mülhausen, to confiscate the debts and the assets of Fr. Hesso and of the also recently deceased Prior Fr. Henman zu Rhein. Moreover, Fr. Marcellus is to be inducted into possession of the Preceptory of Mülhausen granted him by Fr. Hesso. The prior is to support poor brethren of the Tongue of* Alamania *in the Convent and report dutifully on vacant preceptories.*

*Rhodes, 1412 June 1*

*AOM 339 fol. 276r (no old foliation), under* littere diversorum negotiorum. *Cf. Delaville (1913), 319, erroneously May 10; cf. Luttrell/Zachariadou (2008), note 353.*

Omne bonum pro salute, venerabilis frater. Tenor lacrimalis: Presenti themate vobis innotescat, qualiter die XX[a] Maii anni instantis venerandus et famosus religiosus dominus frater Hesso Sleg., olim reverendissimi domini nostri magistri locumtenens, diem suum[a)] clausit extremum. Ob cuius decessum ad partes illas religiosum in Christo nobis carissimum fratrem Marcellum dictum de Lietenberg preceptorem de Merulnhusen procuratorem nostrum nostrique communis thesauri et conventus ad recolligendum, recuperandum et obtinendum nomine nostro nostrique communis thesauri et conventus omnia et singula bona, iura, res et pecuniarum summas ad dictum condam fratrem Hessonem, similiter ad condam fratrem Hermannum Rin, continuum predecessorem vestrum, spectantes et pertinentes, que bona, res et pecuniarum summas ob eorum neceem ad nos nostrumque communem thesaurum et conventum sunt tam de iure quam de facto omnino devoluta eorumque despoillas, duximus presentialiter destinandum. Quapropter vestram in Domino ortamur fraternitatem, quatenus dicto fratri Marcello auxilium, consilium et favorem ad predicta nomine nostro nostrique communis thesauri et conventus prebere, quemadmodum teneri velitis recolligendum et recuperandum, ut noster communis thesaurus consequi valeat et possit, quod sui iuris dignoscitur esse, et maxime hodiernis temporibus, quo in summis inopiis et angustiis circumvenimur, necnon quatenus dictum fratrem Marcellum, quamquam bulla dicti condam reverendissimi domini locumtenentis et conventus in hac parte sufficiat, in dicte preceptorie de Merulnhusen corporalem[b)] possessionem pacificam et quietam inducatis et vestras manus semper in omnibus eidem incumbentibus porrigatis adiutrices. Ceterum, venerabilis frater, pauperculi fratres lingue Alamanie hic in conventu nostro degentes sunt vobis recommendati, ut habeant de pitantiis ibidem eis debitis in eorum refrigerium feliciter gaudere. Alio stilo presenti vobisve[c)] designamus nisi, quod preceptorias ibidem vacantes et vacaturas nobis notificare, quemadmodum teneri debeatis ceteraque nostre religionis negocia. Vestram Altissimus conservet fraternitatem fila. Rodi die I Iunii IIII$^{C}$ XII$^{o}$. [d)]Frater Lucius de Valinis, humilis marscallus conventus Rodi ac locumtenens reverendissimi domini magistri, ceterique baillivi, priores et proceres conventus Rodi venerabili religioso fratri Hugoni de Monfoert sacre domus etcetera priori prioratus Alamanie in Christo carissimo. Quasi similis tenor fuit scriptus preceptori Colonie etcetera[d)].[1)]

*a)* dies suos *corr.* *b)* in *praem. ante corr.* *c)* vobis de ve *corr.* *d-d) infrascript.*

## 259

*[The Lieutenant Master] Fr. Luce de Vallins and the Convent on Rhodes grant for ten years to Fr. Johann von Munzingen, Prior of Filerimos [on Rhodes], the Preceptory of Rheinfelden (Priory of* Alamania), *which is vacant following the death of the former Prior of* Alamania *Fr. Henman zu Rhein.*

*Rhodes, 1412 June 9*

*AOM 339 fol. 158r (133r), under* prioratus Alamanie et Boemie. *Ed. Countryside (2018), 267–8.*

1) *To the preceptor of Cologne.*

Frater Lucius de Vallinis etcetera et nos conventus Rodi domus eiusdem religioso in Christo nobis carissimo fratri Iohanni de Muntzingen cappellano, priori Philerme[2] eiusdem domus prioratus nostri Alamanie salutem et sinceram in Domino caritatem. Religionis decor, morum honestas et alia virtutum dona, quibus vos carismatis gratia insignivit, ad imparciendum vobis nostri favoris gratiam rationabiliter nos moventes, sperantes, quod in comisso vobis regimine effectus administrationis utilis favente Domino vos comendet. Hinc est, quod preceptoriam de Riuelden dicti prioratus presentialiter per obitum condam fratris Iohannis de Rin,[3] dudum dicti prioratus nostri Alamanie prioris, vacantem et ad nostram dispositionem et ordinationem ac collationem propterea rationabiliter devolutam cum omnibus et singulis membris, iuribus et pertinentiis ad eam spectantibus et pertinentibus ac spectare et pertinere debentibus, quoquomodo et cum quibus illam habuit, tenuit et possedit dictus condam frater Iohannes prior, habendam, tenendam, regendam, gubernandam, augmentandam et meliorandam[a] etiam invicem deliberato consilio de nostra certa scientia et speciali gratia ad annos decem incipiendos in festo nativitatis sancti Iohannis baptiste proximo et extunc continuo et integre secuturos vobis auctoritate presentium benefaciendo in eadem conferimus, concedimus et donamus vosque preceptorem et comendatorem in dicta constituimus baiulia hac serie et eciam ordinamus. Comittentes vobis fiducialiter circa curam etcetera. Quocirca universis et singulis fratribus domus[b] nostre quacumque etcetera necnon universis et singulis fratribus[c], sororibus et donatis ac priori seu presidenti prefato, ut vos vel procuratorem vestrum in etcetera amoto abinde quolibet alio detentore, si quis sit, quem nos etcetera. Inhibentes vobis districtius sub virtute sancte obedientie supradicte, ne etcetera. In cuius rei testimonium bulla nostra cerea, qua utimur ob defectum bulle communis plumbee dicti nostri conventus, presentibus est appensa. Dat. Rodi in prefato nostro conventu die nona mensis Iunii anno a nativitate Domini M° IIII$^{C}$ duodecimo.

Pro priori Philerime *marg.* *a)* melorandam *MS* *b)* do *praem. ante corr.* *c)* domus nostre *add. ante corr.*

## 260

*[The Lieutenant Master] Fr. Luce de Vallins and the Convent on Rhodes order Fr. Hugo von Montfort, Prior of* Alamania, *and the receiver in the Priory to pay 110 florins to Berthold Schlegelholz, nephew of the late Fr. Hesso Schlegelholz.*

*Rhodes, 1412 July 1*

*AOM 339 fol. 180r (155r), under* littere assignationum seu cambiorum.

2) *Filerimos on Rhodes was a* prioratus *or* capellania, *as in no. 275: Luttrell (2020), 120.*
3) *Henman zu Rhein.*

Frater Lucius de Valinis etcetera [a)]et nos conventus Rodi domus eiusdem[a)] religioso in Christo nobis carissimo fratri Hugoni de Mofort prioratus nostri Alamanie priori ac ·· receptori responsionum dicti prioratus salutem in Domino. Noveritis, quod noster communis thesaurus est[b)] obligatus in Christo nobis dilecto Bertoldo[c)] Slegelholtz, nepoti bone memorie reverendi in Christo patris et domini domini fratris Hessonis Sleg., immediati predecessoris nostri, de resta maioris summe florenorum de Alamania centum et decem, [c)]quos sibi ibidem per vos solvi promisimus[c)]. Quapropter vos in Domino hortamur precipiendo, quatenus dicto[d)] Bertrando immediate visis presentibus dictos C et X florenos de Almania integraliter solvatis et cum effectu consignetis. In cuius rei testimonium bulla nostra cerea, qua utimur loco bulle communis plumbee dicti nostri conventus, presentibus est appensa. Dat. Rodi in prefato conventu die prima mensis Iulii anno a nativitate Domini M° IIII$^{C}$ XII°.

Priori Alamanie *marg.* *a-a) supra lin.* *b)* ex *corr.* *c)* Bertrando *corr.* *c-c) add. in fine.* *d)* dicto *dupl.*

## 261

*The Marshal Fr. Luce de Vallins, Lieutenant of the Master Fr. Philibert de Naillac, and the Convent on Rhodes inform Fr. Heinrich von Neuhaus, Prior (here* prior generalis) *of Bohemia, that Fr. Johann Schweidler of Patzkorw, who has collected 1,090 florins for the Order by virtue of an indulgence accorded by Pope Alexander V, has been appointed chaplain of the Convent on Rhodes and visitor (here* visitator generalis) *in the Priories of Bohemia and Hungary. They quit Fr. Johann for the monies he has collected. Furthermore Fr. Johann is to be granted a preceptory (here* domus seu commenda) *in the Priory of Bohemia.*

*Rhodes, 1412 August 30*

*AOM 339 fol. 156r-v (131r-v), under* prioratus Alamanie et Boemie.

Frater Lucius de Valinis sacre domus hospitalis sancti Iohannis Iherosolimitani humilis marescallus et locumtenens reverendissimi in Christo patris et domini domini fratris Philiberti de Naylhaco Dei gratia eiusdem sacre domus magistri dignissimi et pauperum Christi custodis, et nos conventus Rodi domus eiusdem venerabili nobis in Christo dilecto Henrico de Novadomo priori generali regni Bohemie necnon omnibus preceptoribus et commendatoribus eiusdem prioratus salutem in Domino sempiternam. Cum in apice loci sancte religionis positi sumus et curam prefati reverendissimi domini nostri magistri ac domus et conventus Rodi facimus et indigne tenemus, ideo non immerito vigilare debemus, ut in quibus merita accrescunt, hos favor extollat et qui religioni fructum afferunt, illius suavitatis dulcedinem gustabunt. Set quem fidelitas et corporale servicium effectualiter et excellentius commendat tam in ordinis negociis et laboribus[a)] pro religione sancta fructificando exortacionibus et predicationibus per civitates et regna pertranseundo et benefaciendo recognoscimus fidelem collacionem factam, nos, qui sumus Rodi in sancta congregatione fratres et in castro sancti Petri,[1] hec nequaquam poterimus per oblivionem mentis supprimere et famam palliare et sic surdis auribus pertransire et, nisi merenti premium, fideli presidium, currenti bravium detur, argueremur, si non illi post laborem provideremus quietem. Devote vestre religiositati volumus per presentes insinuare, quod ad nostram accessit presentiam venerabilis nobis in Christo frater carissimus Iohannes Sweydeler de Paczkorw[b)], decretorum doctor, qui non modico solacio nos fecit iocundos, quod, quam pecuniam ex sua industria per gratiam indulgenciarum concessam ordini a sanctissimo patre domino Alexandro sacre memorie,[2] quam collegerat, coram nobis humiliter reposuit mille et nonaginta florenos. De hiis repositis eundem quitamus et absolvimus ab impeticione cuiuscumque hominis seu conditionis existit et amoris intuitu et fidelitatis. Nos[c)] eum cum deliberato et maturo consilio omnium bailivorum, priorum et procerum conventus Rodi ipsum fratrem Iohannem in specialem capellanum conventus nostri Rodi assumpsimus et visitatorem generalem prioratus Boehemie et Ungarie eum constituimus et omnem potestatem, que ad visitatorem pertineat nostri conventus Rodi, eidem concedimus et eodem titulo eum insigniri volumus. Eciam hoc latere vos nolumus, ut, sicut ad capitis reflexum videmus, quod ex naturali instinctu omnia membra comitantur, et nos omnes, qui in Christo unum corpus sumus et unius capitis membra, cuius imperio regulariter per obedientiam regimur, per eum proficimus et salvari credimus, ab illo erga discordari non [156v] patimur et non sit ergo baiulia, preceptoria seu commenda taliter per quemcumque priorem generalem solidata, que non possit dissolvi causa supervenienti, de nostra facultate omnique impedimento remoto et prefatum fratrem[d)] Iohannem nostrumque capellanum in illam vel in aliam domum seu commendam instituere poterimus auctoritate suffulta auctoritate prefati reverendissimi domini nostri magistri et balivorum et conventus Rodi, qua fungimur, vestre tamen in hoc venerabilitati sume honorem deferimus per presentes vestrisque convocatis balivis et congregatis predictum fratrem Iohannem conventus Rodi capellanum cordialiter inermi amore recommendamus submittentes eundem vestris providentiis in institutione et assignatione reali alicuius domus prioratus nostri Boehemie secundum statum et honoris sui et condigne dignitatis. In hoc scitote in eo, qui membrum est de capite, nos honorari et vos gratos recenseri et voluntati nobis conformes fieri per caritatem, que est in Christo Ihesu, sic indissolubili vinculo amoris vos pocius recognosci nobis esse coniunctos et de humilitate et obediencia debite subiectionis amplius[e)] valeamus vos virtuosius recomendari. Dat. Rodi in prefato nostro conventu sub sigillo nostro proprio, quo in talibus utimur, die penultima mensis Augusti[f)] anno a nativitate Domini M° IIII$^{C}$ duodecimo.

1) *Castle of St. Peter in Bodrum, Karia.*

2) *The indulgence was granted on 30 July 1409, and Alexander V died on 3 May 1410: Luttrell (1986), 146.*

Priori Boemie *marg.* *a)* i *praem. ante corr.* *b)* paser *praem. ante corr.* *c)* no *praem. ante corr.* *d)* pre *praem. ante corr.* *e)* ampleaius *praem. ante corr.* *f)* Augusti *dupl.*

## 262

*[The Lieutenant Master] Fr. Luce de Vallins and the Convent on Rhodes constitute Fr. Johann Schweidler of Patzkorw as domestic chaplain of the Convent on Rhodes and visitor and procurator of the Master and Convent in the Priories of Bohemia and Hungary with powers to receive five brethren into the Order and 50 persons of both sexes as* confratres *of the Order. Fr. Johann Schweidler has been commissioned to preach and announce the indulgences for St. Peter [in Bodrum] which the late Pope Alexander V has granted and which Pope John XXIII has confirmed. Through Fr. Johann the Convent has received large sums of monies. On behalf of the Master and Convent he may issue receipts. He may constitute one or more procurators. What he does and they do is to be valid as if the Master himself were present, even if it were momentuous enough to require the Master's special licence; the Master will abide by it.*

*Rhodes, 1412 August 30*

*AOM 339 fol. 156v-7r (131v-2r), under* prioratus Alamanie et Boemie.

Frater Lucius de Valinis etcetera et nos conventus Rodi domus eiusdem[a] universis et singulis presentibus inspecturis notum facimus, cum ad illorum subditorum premia et honores prelati et ceteri superiores instanter debeant vigilare, quorum virtutibus, sapientia et industria inter christicolarum genus fides catholica et eorum sancta religio premiis ac devocionibus augetur, datur ceteris subditis occasio, quos forsan inhercia non sinit labores tollerare, ut audaciores fiant omni ignavia expulsa premiorum atque honorum causa, ut que illorum devota religio exposcit, ferventiori animo seipsos prebeant tolleranda. Cum igitur venerabilis in Christo nobis carissimus frater Iohannes Sweydeler de Patzkorw, decretorum doctor, qui pro nostra sancta religione nequaquam formidavit diversas regionum partes personaliter peragrare indulgentias et remissiones peccatorum a summis Romane ecclesie pontificibus prefate nostre religioni concessas inter orthodoxe fidem cathalicos[!] suis predicationibus manifestare, ex quam causam ex ipsius fratris Iohannis predicationibus noster communis thesaurus conventus Rodi non modicas pecuniarum quantitates fuerit consecutus, ideoque, ut ardentiori animo inposterum seipsum prebeat labores pro augmentatione religionis substentare et ut verbum Dei et nostra privilegia specialiter noviter concessa ab Alexandro V. felicis recordationis, confirmata vero a summo pontifice Iohanne XXIII. in ecclesia Dei nostris temporibus presentibus militante pro augmentatione, reparatione et tuitione nostri castri sancti Petri, quod de novo per [157r] prefatum reverendissimum dominum nostrum magistrum et eius religionis milites manu forti cum non modica strage bonorum in visceribus Theucrorum noviter fuit fabricatum, inter Christianos quarumlibet nationum in Christo ardentium ardentius valeat predicare ad infrascriptas gratias de communi voluntate dominorum priorum, balivorum, procerum omniumque nostrorum fratrum in conventu degentium[b)] deliberato consilio prelibato fratri Iohanni faciendas unanimiter deliberavimus atque decernimus, videlicet ipsum fratrem Iohannem in specialem capellanum nostri conventus Rodi assumpsimus ipsumque visitatorem generalem prioratuum nostrorum Boemie et Ungarie constituimus et omnem potestatem, que ad visitorem pertineat nostri conventus Rodi, eidem concedimus per presentes et eodem titulo eum insigniri volumus ac eciam ad recipiendum in ordine nostro iuris ordine servato fratres quinque etiam[c)] ad recipiendum in confraternitatem ordinis nostri L personas honestas utriusque sexus necnon eundem fratrem Iohannem licet absentem tamquam presentem facimus, constituimus, creamus et solemniter ordinamus nostrum et dicte domus nostre in dictis prioratibus Boemie et Vngarie actorem, factorem, syndicum et yconomum et nuncium specialem et generalem in collectione facienda de gratia sancte memorie ab Alexandro papa quinto prefato castro nostro sancti Petri concessa ac eciam ad faciendum de receptis nomine nostre quitancias perpetuo valituras ac eciam procuratorem seu[d)] procuratores substituendi cum simili et plenaria potestate, dum et quando ei videbitur fore expediendum, et eum ac eos revocandi damus et concedimus per presentes dicto procuratori nostro licentiam, potestatem, auctoritatem plenariam cum plena, libera et generali administratione pro omnibus et singulis supradictis cum dependentibus, emergentibus et connexis ex eisdem seu altero eorundem coram quibuscumque[e)] iudicibus et curiis tam ecclesiasticis quam secularibus tociens, quociens opus fuerit, comparendum et ibidem agendum et defendendum et generaliter omnia alia singula faciendum, dicendum et exercendum, que[f)] nos ipse in illis facere, dicere et procurare possemus, si personaliter adessemus, eciamsi talia et tanta essent, que mandatum requirerent magis speciale. Promittimus bona fide habere ratum, gratum et firmum, quidquid in premissis per dictum procuratorem actum factumve fuerit sive quomodolibet procuratum etcetera. In cuius rei testimonium bulla nostra cerea, qua utimur ob defectum bulle communis plumbee dicti nostri conventus, presentibus est appensa. Dat. Rodi in prefato nostro conventu die penultima mensis Augusti anno a nativitate Domini M° IIII$^{C}$ duodecimo.

Pro fratre Iohanne Sweydeler *marg.* *a)* venerabili religioso in Christo nobis carissimo fratri Ioh. *del.* *b)* commune *praem. ante corr.* *c)* n *praem. ante corr.* *d)* procuratorem seu *supra lin.* *e)* quibuscunque *dupl.* *f)* in predictis et eorum quolibet *del.*

## 263

*Licence for Fr. Johann [Schweidler] to travel to the countries mentioned.*

*[Rhodes, 1412 August 30]*

*AOM 339 fol. 156r (132r), under* prioratus Alamanie et Boemie.

Item fuit eidem fratri Iohanni data licentia eundi ad dictas partes[a] et revertendi ad conventum, quando sue placuerit voluntati.

*a)* ad dictas partes *supra lin.*

## 264

*[The Lieutenant Master] Fr. Luce de Vallins and the Convent on Rhodes permit Fr. Johann zum Trübel to found at his own expenses a preceptory of the Prior of* Alamania. *The new preceptory has to maintain one knight, one chaplain and one or more sergeants, in case that there are enough revenues for them. These Hospitallers are to elect from themselves their first preceptor. The next preceptors can also be elected. But to save the rights of the Convent, it is stated that whenever the preceptory is granted to someone on Rhodes, this person has to be accepted as preceptor. For their buildings the Hospitallers may ask the faithful for alms (here* petitiones crucis). *As preceptories in* Alamania *pay only moderate responsions, the new preceptory is to pay only 3 florins of the Rhine each year. For taxes and* collecte *its contribution is also only 3 florins of the Rhine.*

*Rhodes, 1413 June 27*

*AOM 339 fol. 157v (132v), under* prioratus Alamanie et Boemie.

Frater Lucius de Vallinis etcetera et nos conventus Rodi domus eiusdem religioso in Christo nobis carissimo fratri Iohanni Zemtruuel eiusdem domus prioratus nostri Alamanie salutem in Domino. Merita vestre devotionis exposcunt, ut peticionibus vestris, quantum cum Deo possumus, favorabiliter annuamus. Exhibita nobis[a] siquidem pro parte vestra peticio continebat inter cetera capitula supplicatoria infrascripta, videlicet ut vobis concedere dignaremur, quod possitis Dei adiutorio vestrorumque parentum et amicorum de novo construere et edificare facere quandam preceptoriam cum suis membris pro religione nostra.[1] Item quod possitis recipere[b] in dicta preceptoria[c] fratres libenter ibidem degentes, militum unum, capellanum unum et fratrem servientem unum seu plures, si possint in eadem sustentari. Item et quod ipsi inter ipsos possint eligere unum fratrem religionis nostre non promotum ad aliquam preceptoriam in preceptorem et gubernatorem dicte preceptorie, qui libenter gubernationem ipsius acceptabit. Item et quod decedente dicto preceptore seu gubernatore ipsi fratres in eadem residentes valeant eligere unum ex eis vel[d] alium, qui eis utilis et magis proficuus videbitur, non tamen preiudicando fratribus conventualibus Rodi dicte prioratus, videlicet ut, si aliquis frater conventualis veniet cum bulla conventus nostri, quod eo tunc ille electus cederet alteri videlicet conventuali. Item et quod pro augmentanda

1) *Zum Trübel a family in Straßburg. Fr. Rembold zum Trübel, who died in 1439, was preceptor at Dorlisheim, Rottweil, and Hagenau. Probably Kenzingen, first mentioned in 1416 according to Krieger 1 (1904), col. 1148.*

devociones christifidelium edificando dictam preceptoriam possitis habere peticiones crucis. Item quia preceptorie Alamanie modicum solvunt nostro communi thesauro pro responsionibus, quod ipsa sit libera et franca de solvendo annuatim florenos de Reno tres. Item et quod pro taillis et collectis, dum necessitas urgeret seu casus eveniret, eciam solvent florenos de Reno tres. Nos igitur piis supplicationibus inclinati considerata magna affectione vestra, quam erga religionem nostram gessitis et geritis[e] de presenti et ut ferventi animo inposterum gerere valeatis, invicem deliberato consilio de nostra certa scientia et speciali gratia vobis, ut possitis exequi et facere ac complere omnia et singula in dictis capitulis supplicationis vestre contentis per vos supplicata, ut prescribitur, concedimus per presentes. Mandantes universis et singulis fratribus domus nostre quacunque auctoritate, dignitate vel officio fungentibus, ne contra presentem nostram concessionem et gratiam aliquatenus venire presumant, quinymo eam iuxta mentem eius et seriem studeant inviolabiliter observare sub virtute sancte obedientie vobisque suum prebeant auxilium, consilium et favorem in omnibus concernentibus utilitatem religionis nostre, quociens opus fuerit, et eos duxeritis requirendum. In cuius rei testimonium etcetera. Dat. Rodi in prefato nostro conventu die vigesimaseptima mensis Iunii anno a nativitate Domini M IIII$^{C}$ tredecimo.

Quadam littera pro fratre Iohanne Zemtruvel *marg.* *a)* nobis *supra lin.* *b)* recepere *MS* *c)* precepretoria *corr.* *d)* qui libenter *praem. ante corr.* *e)* gess *praem. ante corr.*

## 265

*[The Lieutenant Master] Fr. Luce de Vallins permits Fr. Johann zum Trübel (Priory of* Alamania) *to leave the Convent to live in the West and to return and to dispose of his possessions freely for the benefit of the Order.*

*Rhodes, 1413 June 27*

*AOM 339 fol. 215r (181r), under* littere licenciarum.

Frater Lucius de Vall. etcetera religioso in Christo nobis carissimo fratri Iohanni Zentruuel eiusdem domus prioratus nostri Alam. salutem in Domino. Vestre in hac parte supplicationi defleximus, ut ex causa per vos nobis exposita, quam ad recedendum de conventu nostro Rodi vobis expedientem agnovimus, ideo de dicto conventu nostro Rodi recedendi et eundi ad predictum prioratum Alamanie et ad ceteras partes occidentales et ibidem stagiam acceptandi et recipiendi sub preceptore aliquo domus nostre [a]dicti prioratus[a], ubi volueritis, qui libenter eos recipiat, si salubre intentum vestrum adimplere nequieritis, et deinde [b]de dicto prioratu ad nostrum conventum[b] Rodi redeundi, dum vestre placuerit voluntati, licentia tamen vestri superioris prius requisita vobis tenore presentium plenam licentiam concedimus pariter et donamus. Dat. Rodi sub sigillo nostro, quo in talibus utimur, in prefato nostro conventu die vigesima septima mensis Iunii anno a nativitate Domini M° IIII$^{C}$ tredecimo. Necnon quod possitis et valeatis uti bonis vestris propriis ad beneplacitum et voluntatem vestram in honore tamen et utilitate religionis nostre. Dat. ut supra.

*a-a) dupl.* *b-b)* ad dictum prioratus de nostro conventu *MS*

## 266

*[The Lieutenant Master] Fr. Luce de Vallins permits, with the agreement of Bailiffs of the Convent, Fr. Rembold zum Trübel (Priory of* Alamania) *to receive four men as knight brethren into the Order to serve and to be maintained in his preceptory. They follow a petition made on Rembold's behalf by Fr. Johann zum Trübel.*

*1413 June 27*

*AOM 339 fol. 215r (181r), under* littere licenciarum.

Frater Lucius etcetera religioso in Christo nobis carissimo fratri Reyboldo Zemtruuel dicte domus preceptori ·· [a] prioratus nostri Alamanie salutem in Domino. Pro parte vestra per religiosum in Christo nobis carissimum fratrem Iohannem Zentruůel extitit expositum ad presens pro directione administrationis dicte preceptorie[b] vestre fratribus militibus nostre religionis[c] indigetis ac eciam quod ibidem est defectus fratrum religionis nostre. Quapropter pro parte vestra extitit supplicatum, ut vobis[d] faciendi fratres milites nostri[e] ordinis concedere dignaremur licentiam. Peticioni vestre in hac parte deflexímus vestra probitate merente, ut quatuor fratres per prius tamen notificabitis religioso in Christo nobis carissimo fratri ·· priori prioratus nostri Alamanie, quos facere proponitis milites religionis nostre, si apti fuerint, sani et integri suis membris, eis prius per vos vel alium cingulis milicie insignitis et decoratis, si eorum quilibet ex utroque parente nobilis fuerit de legittimo thoro nati[f], eisque stagiam assignatis seu assignare faciatis in preceptoria vel alibi, ubi eis provideri faciatis, secundum bonos usus et laudabiles consuetudines domus nostre, vobis[g] tenore presentium de voluntate, consilio et assensu religiosorum in Christo nobis carissimorum dominorum fratrum balivorum etcetera. Dat. die XXVII mensis Iuni[i] anno a nativitate Domini M° [h] IIII$^{c}$ tredecimo.

*a) lac.* *b)* preceporie *MS* *c)* fr *praem. ante corr.* *d)* s *praem. ante corr.* *e)* nostre religionis *corr.* *f)* nati *corr.* *g) per praem. ante corr.* *h)* III$^{C}$ *praem. ante corr.*

## 267

*[The Lieutenant Master] Fr. Luce [de Vallins] licenses Fr. Johann von Munzingen, Preceptor of Rheinfelden (Priory of* Alamania) *and Prior of Filerimos, to travel to his preceptory and manage it and to return to the Convent in Rhodes whenever he pleases, but with permission of his superior.*

*Rhodes, 1413 October 15*

*AOM 339 fol. 216v (182v), under* littere licenciarum.

Frater Lucius etcetera religioso in Christo nobis carissimo fratri Iohanni de Muntzengen preceptori de Riuelden prioratus nostri Alamanie et priori Philerme salutem in Domino. Sperantes, quod naturalem industriam a domino Deo vobis collatam et quod per vestram personalem presentiam predictam preceptoriam[a)] nuper per nos et nostrum conventum vobis datam vestris meritis exigentibus utilius in agendis dirigi et comodius gubernari, idcirco recedendi a prefato nostro conventu et eundi ad predictum prioratum ceterasque partes occidentales et deinde de dicto prioratu et partibus ad nostram conventum Rodi redeundi, dum vobis placuerit, licentia tamen vestri superioris prius requisita de voluntate etcetera concedimus pariter et donamus. Dat. Rodi in prefato nostro conventu die XV mensis Octobris anno incarnationis Domini M° IIII^C XIII.

*a)* per nos *add. ante corr.*

## 268

*Order for Fr. Hugo von Montfort, Prior of* Alamania, *or any receiver of that priory to pay 28 florins of the Rhine, that is 41 florins of Rhodes, to Fr. Johann Munzingen, chaplain of that Priory, for his upkeep on Rhodes.*

*1413 October 27*

*AOM 339 fol. 185r (160r), under* littere assignationum seu cambiorum.

Die XXVII^a mensis Octobris fuerunt scripte littere assignatorie[b)] fratri Hugoni de Montfort priori Alamanie ac cuicunque receptori dicti prioratus, ut solverent fratri Iohanni Munzengen capellano[b)] prioratus Alamanie florenos de Reno viginti octo pro florenis currentibus Rodi XLI, quos recipere deberet hic in Rodo pro suo stipendio. Quibus solutis etcetera. M° IIII^C tredecimo die XXVII^a Octobris.

*a)* Septembris *corr.* *b) supra lin.*

## 269

*The Master Fr. Philibert de Naillac quits Fr. Count Hugo von Montfort, Prior of* Alamania, *for 500 francs of gold paid through the Conventual Prior on Rhodes Fr. Gautier le Gras and the curate of St-George in Lyons Fr. Jean Jossard.*

*Lyons, 1413 November 5*

*AOM 337 fol. 26r (77r), under* prioratus Alamanie et Boemie. *Cf. van Winter (1998), 35 n. 12.*

Noverint universi et singuli presentes recognicionis et quictationis litteras visuri et audituri, quod nos frater Philibertus de Nailliaco Dei gratia sacre domus hospitalis sancti Iohannis Iherosolemitani magister humilis et pauperum Christi custos fatemur, recognoscimus et in verbo veritatis testamur nos huc in civitate Lugduni habuisse et realiter recepisse per manus domus eiusdem fratris Iohannis Iossardi, curati sancti Georgii Lugd(unensis), a religioso in Christo nobis carissimo fratre Hugone comite de Montfort priore prioratus nostri Almanie quingentos francos auri seu ipsorum valorem, quos dictus prior nomine et pro communi thesauro domus nostre dederat et consignaverat domus eiusdem fratri Galtero Crassi decretorum doctori priori ecclesie conventualis Rodi, qui prior ecclesie de dicta summa litteras suas quictatorias predicto priori Almanie dedit et concessit et predictam summam dicto curato in custodia seu deposito tradidit et consignavit pro ipsis nobis dandis et consignandis in, de et super his, in quibus noster communis thesaurus nobis tenetur. De quibusquidem quingentis francis auri sic habitis et receptis contenti et bene pagati dictos priores ecclesie et Almanie et curatum eorumque[a)] bona et res et quos tangit et tangere potest et poterit in futurum quictamus, liberamus et absolvimus per presentes. Data Lugduni die quinta mensis Novembris anno incarnacionis Domini millesimo CCCC^mo^ decimo tercio.

*a)* eorumcunque *corr.*

## 270

*The Fr. Ailnardus de Doenen, Preceptor and Bailiff of Utrecht, is made chaplain and familiar of the Master.*

*Lyons, 1414 January 5*

*AOM 338 fol. 140r (140r), under* prioratus Alamanie et Boemie. *Ed. van Winter (1998), 35 no. 13, gives Arnold instead of Ailnardus.*

Die V^a^ Ianuarii anno incarnationis Domini M^o^ CCCC^o^ XIII^o^ Lugd(uni)[a)] admissus fuit in cappellanum et familiarem domini magistri frater Ailnardus de Doenen preceptor et bailhivus baiulie Traiectensis, cappellanus domus nostre[b)], ut in forma.

*a)* in *praem. ante corr.* *b)* et *praem. ante corr.*

## 271

*Licence for Fr. Lambert van Moerdijk, chaplain at St. Catherine in Utrecht, to travel from* Alamania *to the Convent on Rhodes.*

*[Lyons, 1414 January 5]*

*AOM 338 fol. 140r (140r), under* prioratus Alamanie et Boemie. *Ed. van Winter (1998), 35–6 no. 14.*

Anno, die et loco predictis data fuit licentia fratri Lamberto Wanmurdic[1] in sancta Katherina de Vtric commoranti cappellano domus eiusdem recedendi de prioratu nostro Alamania et eundi ad nostrum Rodi conventum, quando voluerit, Deo et nostre religioni serviturus a suo superiore requisita[a] licencia.

*a)* licen *praem. ante corr.*

## 272

*The Master Fr. Philibert [de Naillac] confirms the annulment of the illegal testament of the late Fr. Hesso Schlegelholz, Prior of* Alamania *and Preceptor of Kos, who had promised 2,300 florins of the Rhine to the Preceptory of Freiburg im Breisgau. The Convent had requested this through its procurator Fr. Marcellus von Liechtenberg. There have been discussions with Fr. Wilhelm von Landsberg, procurator of Fr. Marcellus, who came to the Master at Saint-Pourçain in the Diocese of Clermont, and with Fr. Hugo von Montfort, Prior of* Alamania, *who went to Lyon to see the Master, but the Master did not go to Lyon. Now Fr. Hugo has met the Master at Baden in the Diocese of Consatnce. The Master orders Fr. Erhard Thome, Preceptor of Straßburg, to pay 2,000 florins only to the Preceptory of Freiburg and to use the rest for expenses of Fr. Hugo and for the recovery of goods that had belonged to the late Fr. Hesso.*

*Baden, 1414 February 27*

*AOM 338 fol. 140r-41v (140r-41v), under* prioratus Alamanie et Boemie.

Noverint universi et singuli presentes litteras visuri et audituri, quod enim lis seu discordia coram nobis fratre Philiberto[a] etcetera oriri spereretur inter nostrum Rodi conventum ex una et priorem et prioratum nostrum Almanie ex altera parte in, de et super duobus millibus[b] trescentum florenis Renensibus[c] per deffunctum fratrem Hessonem Slegheholcz, quondam dicti prioratus priorem et preceptorem Langoni, tempore, quo vivebat, penes eiusdem domus fratrem Herodum Thome preceptorem Argentine depositis, quos unacum omnibus et singulis aliis bonis administracioni dicti deffuncti fratris Hessonis commissis dictus conventus ad nostrum communem thesaurum spectare et pertinere asserebat. Propter hoc idem[d] noster conventus ad has partes Theutonicas fratrem Marcellum Liehtemberg[e] unacum sufficienti procuratorio destinarunt, quod in presencia domus eiusdem fratris Hugonis comitis[f] de Montfort, dicti prioratus prioris, et nonnullorum ipsius prioratus preceptorum constituto et predictos duo mille

1) *Perhaps* wan Murdic.

trescentum florenos Renenses unacum aliis bonis dicti deffuncti fratris in partibus istis cum instantia nomine procuratorio dicti conventus atque vice petente dicti prior et preceptores obiciendo dixerunt dictos duo mille trescentum florenos unacum omnibus aliis bonis predictis vigore cuiusdam testamenti nuncupativi dicti deffuncti fratris Hessonis ad relevamen et restauracionem[g] baiulie Friburgi[h] in Brisgaudia, quam dictus[i] quondam frater Hessonus nomine et titutlo preceptoris per tempora longiora tenuerat et a debitis et erumpnis, quibus ipsa baiulia irretita[j] erat, ipsum indempnem servare promiserat, spectare et pertinere. Et propter hoc dicti prior et preceptores unanimi consensu, ut dicebant, procuratorem dicti conventus et fratrem Willemum de Lansperg[k], procuratorem suum, pro premissis decidendis[l] ad nostram presenciam ad villam sancti Porciani Claremontensis diocesis remiserunt. Qua causa per [140v] procuratorem dictorum prioris et preceptorum coram nobis ventilata et cartis, instrumentis et aliis probationum generibus ostensis et productis, quia ex tenore instrumentorum repperiebatur dictum deffunctum fratrem Hessonem more laicali verum condisse testamentum, quod facere non poterat, cum religiosus nichil possideat nec velle nec nolle habeat, dictum testamentum et quicquid in vim ipsius ex ob id dicti[m] prior et preceptores petebant, sicut debuimus, cassavimus, anullavimus et penitus irritavimus, ut lacius in litteris inde confectis, quas eisdem priori et preceptoribus misimus, continctur. Processu vero temporis dictus prior Almanie cum certis preceptoribus et quodam doctore sacri palatii auditore in civitate Lugd(unensi) ad certam diem per nos sibi assignatam comparuit, ad quam[n] nostris negociis prepediti[o] per dominios nostros de casa Francie comparere nequivimus et sic dicto priore de dicta civitate Lugd(unensi) recedente totum negocium remansit indiscussum. Nunc vero nobis per has partes transitum facientibus et ad nostrum Rodi conventum Deo semper directore proficiscentibus dictus prior cum suis certis preceptoribus pro premissis coram nobis in villa de Bada Constanciensis diocesis comparuit ibique parte sui et prioratus coram nobis[p] negocio ad longum[q] discusso ipsisque priore et preceptoribus dictum testamentum tanquam penitus invalidum reicientibus se gratiose nostri ordinacioni penitus submiserunt humiliter suplicantes, quatenus statum dicte domus Friburgensis desolate et ad nichilum reddacte intuitu pietatis compati dignaremur. Nos igitur eorum suplicationi tanquam iuste favorabiliter annuentes et[r], ut dicta baiulia preservetur a noxiis et servitiis floreat imposterum divinis, dictas anullacionem, irritacionem et anichilacionem ipsius testamenti et omnium[s], que ex ipso sequebantur et sequi sperabantur, sicut iustum fuit et est, apponentes ipsumque testamentum et omnium, que[t] ex ipso sequi sperabantur, iterato et de novo cassantes ipsis priori et prioratui Almanie gratiose ad usus dicte domus Friburgensis et eius membrorum, ut a ruynis relevctur et prosperis inantea proficiat incrementis, super dictis peccuniis in civitate Argentina depositis usque ad summam duorum milium florenorum ad usus dicte domus Friburgi et non alias nec aliter aplicandorum, residuum dictarum pecuniarum depositarum ibidem pro[u] sumptibus et[v] expensis ipsius prioris applicandum. Insuper omnia bona dicto fratri Hessoni in Almania debita ad usus predictos reparacionis dicte domus Friburgensis et non alios nec aliter ut supra applicanda ita [141r] tamen, quod ipsi teneantur recuperare suis sumptibus et expensis, si tamen poterunt recuperari quibus omnibus et singulis predictis ad usus predictos sint[w)] contenti nec quicquid de bonis dicti quondam fratris Hessonis reppetere seu exigere valeant, de voluntate, consilio et assensu religiosorum[x)] in Christo nobis carissimorum fratrum Galteri Crassi decretorum doctoris prioris ecclesie coventualis Rodi, Iohannis de Porta prioris Capue, Hugonis Darci de Cabilone, Natalis Lantequin[y)] de Villadei in Montana, Henrici de Bye hospitalis antiqui sancti Iohannis Parisiensis, Nicholai Weihyn Friburgi, Bertholdi de Altocastel in Columbaria et Henrici Cursor Welquerlt preceptorum et aliorum fratrum nobis assistencium de nostra certa sciencia et speciali gratia promisimus et duximus[z)] providendum. Mandantes et tenore presencium precipientes sub virtute sancte obediencie dicto preceptori Argentine et omnibus et singulis aliis subditis nostris, quos huiusmodi negocium tangit et tangere potest et poterit, quatenus predictos duo mille florenos et omnia alia bona dicti deffuncti fratris Hessonis pro ipsis ad dictos usus et non alios[aa)] aplicandos dent, tradent dicto priori et realiter et cum effectu consignent ac dicto preceptori Argentine, quatenus duos trescentum florenos preter[bb)] et ultra dictos duos mille florenos penes se, ut prefertur, depositos dicto priori aut eius certo mandato pro dictis[cc)] suis sumptibus et expensi[s] tradat et realiter consignet et quem fratrem Hugonem comitem de Montfort priorem dicti prioratus ad premissa omnia et singula recuperandum, levandum, habendum et recipiendum ad usus predictos[dd)] et non alios aplicandum et de receptis quittancias perpetuo valituras dandum et concedendum nostrum et domus nostre procuratorem, actorem, factorem negociorumque gestorem facimus, creamus, constituimus et solempniter ordinamus cum potestate unum vel plures procuratores loco sui ad premissa omnia et singula substituendum. Dantes et concedentes dicto[ee)] procuratori nostro et substituendo vel substituendis ab eo omnia et singula premissa et omnia alia faciendi, dicendi, gerendi[ff)], deffendendi et excercendi, que[gg)] in premissis et eorum quolibet necessaria[hh)] fuerint seu eciam opportuna et que nos ipsi faceremus et facere[ii)] possemus, si personaliter adessemus, ac ratum, gratum et firmum habere et perpetuo tenere omne et quicquid per dictum procuratorem nostrum et substituendum vel substituendos ab eo actum,[jj)] dictum, recuperatum, levatum, habitum, quittatum, receptum et procuratum fuerit sive gestum in premissis et quolibet premissorum ac iudicio sisti et iudicatum solvi cum omnibus et singulis suis[kk)] clausulis opportunis promittimus bona fide [141v] sub ypotheca et[ll)] obligacione omnium bonorum nostrorum et nostre dicte domus presentium pariter et futurorum. In cuius rei testimonium bulla nostra plumbea presentibus est appensa. Data in dicta villa de Bade die penultima mensis Februarii anno incarnacionis Domini M° CCCC° XIII°.

*a)* orta *add. ante corr.* *b)* militibus *corr.* *c)* Ren *praem. ante corr.* *d)* idem *supra lin.* *e)* temberg *supra lin.* *f)* remitis *corr.* *g)* restanciacionem *corr.* *h)* Friborge *corr.* *i)* dominus *in lin. ante corr.* *j)* soretita *in lin. ante corr.* *k)* Lansperg *in marg.* *l)* dicendis *in lin. ante corr.* *m)* dicte *corr.* *n)* iudiciis *add. ante corr.* *o)* pediti *in lin. ante corr.* *p)* ad longuum *add.*

*ante corr.* *q)* longuum *MS* *r)* et *supra lin.* *s)* dictum *corr.* *t)* que *supra lin.* *u)* qt *praem. ante corr.* *v) dupl. MS* *w)* sunt *corr.* *x)* reliquorum *in lin. ante corr.* *y)* Lantonin *corr.* *z)* duxis *add. ante corr.* *aa)* alios *supra lin.* *bb)* pt *in lin. ante corr.* *cc)* prodictis *corr.* *dd)* predictos *supra lin.* *ee)* dictos *corr.* *ff)* facere *praem. ante corr.* *gg)* que *supra lin.* *hh)* necc *praem. corr.* *ii)* faceremu *corr.* *jj)* actum *supra lin.* *kk)* suis *supra lin.* *ll) supra lin.*

*The Master was on his way from Bern to Meran. Baden is situated 20 km north-west of Zürich. Cf. Delaville (1913), 385.*

## 273

*The Master Fr. Philibert [de Naillac] permits Fr. Count Hugo von Montfort, Prior of* Alamania, *to donate 600 florins of the Rhine for religious purposes in churches or chapels of houses of the Order.*

*Meran, 1414 March 16*

*AOM 338 fol. 141v (141v), under* prioratus Alamanie et Boemie.

Frater Philibertus etcetera religioso in Christo nobis carissimo fratri Hugoni comiti de Montfort priori prioratus nostri Almanie domus eiusdem salutem et sinceram in Domino caritatem. Devocionis vestre sinceritas et alia preclara vestra merita, quibus fore dignoscimini insignitus, racionabiliter promerentur, ut peticionibus vestris in hiis presertim, que anime vestre salutem et divini cultus augmentum respiciunt, quantum cum Deo possumus, favorabiliter anuamus. Sane ex serie peticionis vestre percepimus[a], quod vos de salute propria cogitantes ac cupientes terrena pro celestibus et transitoria pro eternis felici commercio commutare de bonis administracioni vestre commissis usque ad summam sexcentum florenorum Renensum semel et dumtaxat in ecclesiis seu cappellis domus nostre ad cultus divini augmentum et alios pios usus convertere et de ipsis sexcentum florenis opitulante[b] Domino disponere intenditis suplicantes nostram super hoc impartiri licenciam. Hinc est, quod nos iustis petentium desideriis favorabiliter annuentes licentiam posterius postulatam de nostra certa scientia et speciali gratia vobis harum serie concedimus et donamus. Data in villa de Moranno die decimasexta mensis Marcii anno incarnacionis Domini M° CCCC° decimo tercio.

*a)* precepimus *MS* *b)* opitalante *MS*

## 274

*The Master Fr. Philibert [de Naillac] licenses Fr. Count Hugo von Montfort, Prior of* Alamania, *to receive two men as knight brethren into the Order until next June 24 and to send them to the Convent for four years.*

*Meran, 1414 March 16*

*AOM 338 fol. 141v-2r (141v-2r), under* prioratus Alamanie et Boemie.

Frater Philibertus etcetera religioso in Christo nobis carissimo fratri Hugoni comiti de Montfort priori prioratus nostri Almanie domus eiusdem salutem et sinceram in Domino caritatem. Vestrorum exigencia meritorum, quibus Altissimus vos insignivit, promeretur, ut peticiones vestras, illas presertim, per quas vos exhibere possitis aliis favorabilem et benignum, ad exaudicionis gratiam admittamus. Hinc est, quod nos vestris peticionibus inclinati licenciam recipiendi religionis nostre fratres prioratus predicti ipsis prius per vos vel alium seu alios militie cingulo insignitis, dum tamen et non aliter [142r] nobiles fuerint ex utroque parente matrimonio procreati legitimo, apti, sani et integri suis membris, a data presencium usque ad instans proximum festum nativitatis sancti Iohannis baptiste et exinde ad quatuor annos continuos et usus et laudabiles consuetudines domus[a] nostre aut quod nostrum conventum cum equis et armis sufficientibus secundum domus nostre statuta adeant, vobis damus. Data in villa de Maranno[b] die decimasexta mensis Marcii anno incarnationis Domini M° quadringentesimo decimo tercio.

*a)* domus *dupl.* *b)* Ro *praem. ante corr.*

## 275

*The Master Fr. Philibert [de Naillac] prolongs the licence granted by his Lieutenant, the Marshal Fr. Luce de Vallins, and the Convent to Fr. Johann von Muntzingen to travel to his Preceptory of Rheinfelden (Priory of* Alamania*) and to keep the chapel of Filerimos [on Rhodes], where he is prior, for another year until October 1415.*

*Trent, 1414 March 22*

*AOM 338 fol. 142r (142r), under* prioratus Alamanie et Boemie.

Frater Philibertus etcetera religioso etcetera fratri Iohanni de Mutzungen preceptori de Riuelden prioratus nostri Alamanie[a], priori[b] cappelle nostre de Filerme domus eiusdem salutem etcetera. Cum probitatis vestre merita et administracionem accomodam, quam in dicta cappella habuistis, sicut fidedigno[c] religiosi in Christo nobis carissimi fratres Lucius de Vailhinis, marescallius, nostrum locumtenens, et noster Rodi conventus domus eiusdem acceperunt testimonio et occulata fide prospexerunt, recedendi de dicto conventu et eundi ad dictum prioratum Alamanie ac gubernari faciendi dictam baiuliam de Riuelden et alias causas, quas vobis expedientes esse cognoverunt, licenciam benigne concessunt ita, quod per totum mensem Octobris proxime futurum inclusive ad dictum Conventum reverti deberetis dictam cappellam Filerme, cuius prior existis, vestri absencia non obstante vobis reservarunt et reservatam esse voluerunt, prout[d] per litteras dictorum nostrum locumtenentis et conventus sigillo ipsius locumtenentis sigillatas datas Rodi die secunda mensis Septembris anno a nativitate Domini M° CCCC° XIII° nobis liquidius apparuit. Et sicut nobis exposuistis propter locorum distanciam causantibus temporum infortuniis et quod tempore hyemale ad has partes de dicto conventu transfretastis tercia pars dicti anni est elapsa infra dictum mensem Octobris ad dictum conventum reverti cum adhuc[e)] possessionem dicte baiulie minime assequi et[f)] regimini ipsius baiulie providere commode non valetis, nobis humiliter suplicastis vobis per nos dictum terminum prorogari. Hinc est, quod vestris nos inducentibus meritis dictum terminum vobis prefixum a dicto proximo futuro mense Octobris inclusive usque per totum alium mensem Octobris, qui erit anno incarnationis Domini M° CCCC° XV° prorogamus et prorogatum esse volumus dictam cappellam seu prioratum Filerme usque ad dictum mensem Octobris anni millesimi CCCC[mi] XV vobis reservantes. Data Tridenti die XX[a] mensis Marcii anno incarnationis Domini millesimo CCCC° XIII°.

*a)* domus eiusdem salutem *add. ante corr.* *b)* prioratus *add. ante corr.* *c)* accepm *add. ante corr.* *d)* quod *praem. ante corr.* *e)* ad *praem. ante corr.* *f) dupl.*

## 276

*[The Lieutenant Master] Fr. Luce [de Vallins] and the Convent quit Fr. Hermann von Ow, Pilier of the Tongue of* Alamania, *for all payments due for his lieutenancy on Kos from 1 September 1411 to 31 August 1412.*

*Rhodes, 1414 April 2*

*AOM 339 fol. 186r-v (161r-v), under* littere assignationum et cambiorum.

Frater Lucius etcetera et nos conventus Rodi domus eiusdem universis et singulis presentes litteras inspecturis presentium tenore notum facimus et attestamur nos a religioso in Christo nobis carissimo fratre Hermanno de Ow, pillerio albergie lingue Alamanie ac locumtenente insule nostre Langoni, habuisse realiter atque de facto recepisse bonum ac legale computum, rationem et calculacionem et integram satisfactionem de omnibus rebus ac bonis ac granis et pecuniis, que ad eius manus ratione dignitatis locumtenentis de dicta insula de Langone et aliis locis sibi annexis videlicet a primo die mensis Septembris anni nativitatis Domini M IIII[c] undecimi usque per totum mensem Augusti inclusive anni nativitatis Domini M IIII[c] duodecimi. Et de quibus premissis omnibus et singulis fuimus et sumus contenti et integraliter satisfacti facientes sibi per presentes finem, quictacionem, remissionem et absolucionem perpetuam de premissis cum pacto perpetuo valituro de aliquod ulterius non petendo seu per aliquem peti[a)] faciendo. Mandantes universis et singulis dicte domus nostre fratribus [186v] presentibus et futuris, cuiuscunque status, gradus vel condicionis existant, sub virtute sancte obedientie, ne contra presentem nostram quitanciam, remissionem et absolucionem[b)] aliqualiter venire presumant, ymo pocius dictum fratrem Hermannum locumtenentem in predicta sua quitantia et absolucione indempnem firmiter et per imperpetuum conservare studeant.

In cuius rei etcetera. Data Rodi in prefato nostro conventu die secunda mensis Aprilis anno a nativitate Domini M° IIII$^{C}$ decimo quarto.

*a)* alium *praem. ante corr.* *b)* p *praem. ante corr.*, et absolutionem *dupl.*

## 277

*The Master Fr. Philibert [de Naillac], four named and other brethren confirm Fr. Heinrich Stehler for ten years in the Preceptory of Frankfurt (Priory of* Alamania).

*Bologna, 1414 May 12*

*AOM 338 fol. 142v (142v), under* prioratus Alamanie et Boemie.

Frater Philibertus etcetera religioso in Christo nobis carissimo fratri Henrico Streler preceptori domus seu baiulie in Francfordia prioratus nostri Alamanie salutem etcetera. Propter susceptum de vobis testimonium commendandum illa vobis libenter concedimus, que conservacionem vestri status concernere dignoscuntur. Igitur preceptoriam seu baiuliam in Francford. supradictam prioratus nostri Alamanie cum omnibus et singulis suis membris etcetera, prout illam iuste habetis presencialiter et tenetis habendam etcetera de voluntate[a], consilio et assensu religiosorum in Christo nobis carissimorum fratrum Galteri Crassi decretorum doctoris prioris ecclesie conventualis Rodi, Iohannis de Porta prioris Capue, Iohannis de Autuno Bellecombe, Natalis Lankequin de Villadei in Montana[1] et aliorum domus nostre fratrum nobis assistencium de nostra certa scientia et speciali gratia[b] ad annos decem continuos et completos[c] vobis auctoritate presencium confirmamus et ad uberiorem vestram cautelam de novo conferimus, concedimus et donamus benefaciendo in eadem vosque etcetera.[d] Comittentes etcetera necnon etcetera. Quocirca etcetera necnon. Inhibentes etcetera. In cuius rei testimonium bulla nostra in absencia bulle communis plumbee presentibus est appensa. Data Bononie die XII$^{a}$ mensis Maii anno incarnacionis Domini M° CCCC° XIIII°.

*a)* volunta *MS* *b)* vobis *add. ante corr.* *c)* complendos *MS* *d)* ordinantes etcetera *add. ante corr.*

## 278

*The Master Fr. Philibert [de Naillac] constitutes master Henricus Birnbaum (de Piro),* licenciatus in decretis *and Provost of St. Kunibert in Cologne, as the Order's procurator at the Roman curia. His salary of 25 florins of the papal chamber is due each year on 24 June.*

*Bologna, 1414 May 21*

1) *Fr. Gautier le Gras, Prior of the Conventual church, Fr. Jean de Porta, Prior of Capua, Fr. Jean d'Autun, Preceptor of Bellecombe, Fr. Natale Lantequin, Preceptor of Villedieu la Montagne.*

*AOM 337 fol. 35r (86r), under* prioratus Veneciarum, Lombardie, Vngarie, Vrbis et Pisarum.

Frater Philibertus etcetera venerabili et circumspecto viro magistro Henrico[a] de Piro licentciato in decretis, preposito ecclesie sancti Cuniberti Coloniensis,[1] in Romana curia procuratori salutem in Domino sempiternam. Attendentes sincere dilectionis affectum, quem ad nos et domum nostram fructuosi exhibitione operis experimur, vos habere et in futurm favento Domino hebebitis, tenemus et firma speramus fiducia nostra et religionis nostre peragenda negocia vestro provido mediante consilio directius et utilibus dirigi consiliis et a noxivis preservari. Harum consideratione ducti vos in procuratorem et consiliarium nostrum de nostra certa scientia, quantum nostre placuerit voluntati, retinemus et assumimus et cum stipendiis florenorum auri de camera viginti quinque, quos vobis annis singulis in festo nativitatis sancti Iohannis babtiste[b] reddere et solvere promittimus bona fide. In cuius rei testimonium bulla nostra plumbea presentibus est appensa. Data Bononie die vicesima prima mensis Maii anno incarnationis Domini millesimo quadringentesimo decimo quarto.

*a)* Hinrico *corr.* *b)* beate *praem. ante corr.*

## 279

*Licence for Fr. Gregor Brant (Priory of Bohemia) to leave the Convent.*
*[Rhodes, 1414] May 24*

*AOM 339 fol. 217r (183r), under* littere licenciarum.

Die XXIIII Madii dicti anni fuit data licentia fratri Gregorio Brant prioratus Bohemie ad recedendum de conventu Rodi pro suis negociis expediendis et revertendi, quando voluerit, etcetera.

## 280

*The Master Fr. Philibert [de Naillac] licenses the chaplain Fr. Trugillus Nicholai to leave the house of Andvorskov and live in another house of the Priory of* Alamania.
*Bologna, 1414 June 4*

*AOM 338 fol. 142v-3r (142v-3r), under* prioratus Alamanie et Boemie.

1) *Heinrich Birnbaum: Kürten (1985), 268, 270, 288. He was canon of St. Kunibert and* licentiatus in decretis *in 1389, when he registered as a student of the university of Cologne; he is known as Provost of St. Kunibert only from 1407 onwards: Repertorium Academicum Germanicum, http://d-nb.infoo/gnd/135661145*

Frater Philibertus etcetera religioso in Christo nobis carissimo Trugillo Nicholai cappellano domus eiusdem salutem et sinceram in Domino caritatem. Supplicatoriam petitionem nobis vestri parte exhibitam recepimus continentem, quod, cum[a] in domo nostra de Andworskow in domus nostre fratrem receptus fueritis et ibidem secundum domus[b] eiusdem statuta stagia vobis assignata extiterit [c]et extra domum predictam ad anime vestre salutem magis proficere valeretis[c], nobis humiliter extitit supplicatum, ut stagiam predictam[d] mutare dignaremur. Hinc est, quod nos [e]ex certis causis animum nostrum moventibus[e] vestris supplicationibus inclinati recedendi de dicta domo de Andworskow et eundi ad aliam baiuliam, preceptoriam sive domum prioratus Alamanie et ibidem moram trahendi, dummodo de preceptoris illius baiulie, preceptorie[f] sive domus processerit voluntate, vobis [143r] auctoritate presentium licenciam concedimus[g] et damus. Mandantes et tenore presentium precipientes preceptori baiulie, preceptorie sive domus, in qua[h] vos recipi contigerit, sub virtute sancte obedientie, quatenus vobis inibi recepto vos caritative pertractet [i]vobis necessaria ministrando seu ministrari faciendo[i] secundum bonos usus et laudabiles consuetudines domus nostre. Data Bononie die quarta mensis Iunii anno incarnationis Domini millesimo CCCC$^{mo}$ XIIII$^{to}$.

*a)* cum *supra lin.* *b)* statuta *praem. ante corr.* *c-c) marg.;* et ipse domus de Andworskow a partibus, quibus originem traxistis, non modicum sit remota, ex quo factum est, quod amicorum suffragiis estis penitus alienus *in lin. ante corr.* *d)* predictam *supra lin.* *e-e) marg.* *f)* preceptoris *MS* *g)* conces *praem. ante corr.* *h) quam corr.* *i-i) marg.;* vobisque in vestris necessariis provideat seu provideri faciat *in lin. ante corr.*

## 281

*The Master [Fr. Philibert de Naillac] orders Fr. Heinrich von Neuhaus, Prior of Bohemia, to send responsions and the incomes from the indulgences of Pope Alexander V to Antonio di Giovanni who lives in Prague. The monies are to be sent to Filippo dei Ricci, merchant at the papal curia, in order to repay a loan made by Francesco dei Ricci at Avignon.*

*Bologna, 1414 June 11*

*AOM 338 fol. 143r-v (143r-v), under* prioratus Alamanie et Boemie.

Carissime post salutem et animum ad grata paratum. Sicut vos credimus non ignorare, noster Rodi conventus a Turchis Christianorum inimicis hominibus in agro fidei catholice zizaniam seminare conantibus hiis – proch dolor! – diebus solito plus adeo deprimitur totque ac tantis laborum et expensarum concursibus enervatur tantasque ac tales expensas requirit omni die, que non possunt a paupere conventu sustineri nec poterunt ulterius ibidem vivere, nisi vestras et aliorum religionis ipsius priorum, preceptorum et bailhivorum manus viderint adiutrices. Hostes enim hii fidei regionem fidelium nuper ingressi assueta malicia Christianos trucidant, edes evacuant et thesauros Christianorum pauperizant. Et quia teste Seneca: "Consortium omnium rerum inter nos facit amicicia, nec secundum quidquam singulis est nec adversi, in commune enim vivitur amicicia, nec potest quisquam beate degere, qui se tantum intuetur, qui omnia ad utilitates suos vertit," et sequitur: "Alteri vivas oppertet, si vis tibi vivere,"[1] hec ille! Quas igitur vires habere poteritis nobiscum[a] ad ipsius fidei succursum conferatis, ut debachantibus in fidem catholicam Turchis occursuri triumphum letum [b]Dei auxilio[b] reportabimus. Iustis siquidem petitionibus gratum prebuisse favorem et meritorum stipendio alienas relevasse miserias a recte sapientibus virtuosum creditur. Scitis etenim, quod ipse noster Rodi conventus de prioratu vestro a longe retro temporibus de responsionibus annuis, mortuariis et vacantiis nichil vel modicum recepit in grave ipsius conventus[c] preiudicium et fidei catholice detrimentum. Hac autem de causa ad vos ipse conventus sperans a vobis et prioratu vestro predicta recuperare cum lacrimis clamat cum David: "Os petra mea et robur meum, salvator meus et fortis [143v] meus, scutum meum et cornu salutis mee, elevator[d] meus et refugium meum."[2] Igitur eidem conventui dicatis viceversa verbum eiusdem David: "Fratres mei vos, os meum et caro mea, vos omne, quod petieritis [b]a me[b] impetrabitis,"[3] ut scilicet responsiones annuas, mortuaria decedencium et vacancia preceptoriarum[e] unacum pecuniis indulgenciarum sancte memorie Alexandri pape quinti in prioratu vestro recollectas congregetis et recolligendas[f] colligatis omnes debitores per statuta religionis solvere compellendo omnesque predictas pecunias tam responsionum etcetera quam indulgenciarum congregatas indilate in manibus Antonii Iohannis in Pragensi civitate pro et nomine Philipi de Riciis mercatoris in curia Romana commorantis consignetis et de hiis, que eidem[g] Antonio nomine dicti Philipi pro nobis et nostro communi thesauro dederitis et consignaveritis recipiendo ab ipso Antonio litteras seu cedulam recognitionis et quittationis vos quittos et immunes esse volumus et iubemus per presentes. Sub spe etenim a vobis et vestro prioratu recuperandorum magnas pecunie summas a domino Francisco de Riciis Avinione commorante mutuo de presenti recipimus et ad conventum predictum mittimus, quas eidem domino Francisco de Riciis sub gravibus penis et infra tempus satis breve restituere tenemur. Unde in hiis nullathenus deficiatis, quantum Deo servire, religioni et conventui debitum facere et

1) *Seneca, Epistulae 48.2:* Consortium rerum omnium inter nos facit amicitia, nec secundi quicquam singulis est nec adversi, in commune vivitur, nec potest quisquam beate degere, qui se tantum intuetur, qui omnia ad utilitates suas convertit. Alteri vivas oportet, si vis tibi vivere.

2) *2. Reg. 19.12, 22.3.*

3) *Ps. 18.2, 2. Reg. 19.38.*

honorem vestrum servare cupitis et ad statim, ut est dictum. Et de hiis, que super hoc feceritis, nos indilate rescribatis, ut dictum mutuum attenuare valeamus. Et si que volueritis nos facturos, rescribatis confidenter, quia cordialiter adimplebimus. Et valete valenter in Christo feliciter semper. Scripta Bononie sub sigillo[h)] nostro et signo manuali domus eiusdem fratris Petri clerici, cancellarii nostri et domus nostre, in testimonium premissorum die XI[a] mensis Iunii anno incarnationis Domini M° CCCCXIIII[to]. – Religioso in Christo nobis carissimo fratri Henrico[i)] de Novadomo priori prioratus nostri Boemie magister hospitalis Iherusolimitani[j)].

*a)* nos *praem. ante corr.* *b-b) supra lin.* *c)* rel *praem. ante corr.* *d)* elel *praem. ante corr.* *e)* decedentium *praem. ante corr.* *f)* rel *praem. ante corr.* *g)* super *praem. ante corr.* *h)* stig *praem. ante corr.* *i) post corr.* *j) praem. corr.*

## 282

*The Master Fr. Philibert [de Naillac], six named and other brethren (as no. 277) constitute Anthonio di Ser Francesco of Florence, factor of Antonio di Giovanni di Ser Matheo in Prague, as procurator for the collection of revenues from Fr. Heinrich von Neuhaus and the Priory of Bohemia.*

*Venice, 1414 August 28*

*AOM 338 fol. 144r-v (143r-v), under* prioratus Alamanie et Boemie.

Noverint universi et singuli presens procuratorium visuri et audituri, quod nos frater Philibertus de Nailhaco Dei gratia sacre domus hospitalis sancti Iohannis Iherosolimitani magister et pauperum Christi custos, confisi de fidei legalitate et circumspectionis industria discreti viri Anthonii domini Francisci de Florencia factoris Anthonii de Iohanne de Ser Matheo in Praga commorantis, eundem Anthonium licet absentem tanquam presentem citra tamen revocationem aliorum procuratorium nostrorum ad quecunque nostra et domus nostre negocia ubicunque constitutorum de voluntate, consilio et assensu religiosorum in Christo nobis carissimorum fratrum Galteri Crassi decretorum doctoris prioris ecclesie conventualis Rodi, Iohannis de Porta prioris Capue, Iohannis de Autuno Bellecumbe, Iacobi de Alamania Neapolis, Henrici de Bye hospitalis sancti Iohannis Parisiensis, Natalis Lantequin de Villadei in Montana preceptorum[1)] et aliorum domus eiusdem fratrum nobis assistentium tenore presentium de nostra certa scientia facimus, creamus, constituimus et sollepniter ordinamus nostrum et dicte nostre[a)] domus procuratorem, actorem, sindicum, yconomum negociorumque gestorem ac

1) *For the revocation, see no. 286. As no. 277, plus Fr. Giacomo d'Alamania, Preceptor of Naples, and Fr. Henri de By, Preceptor of St-Jean in Paris.*

nuncium specialem et generalem ita tamen, quod specialitas generalitati non deroget nec econtra, ad petendum, recipiendum, recuperandum, levandum et habendum nostro et dicte domus nostre procuratorio nomine atque vice a religioso in Christo nobis carissimo fratre Henrico de Novadomo priore prioratus nostri Boemie et omnibus et singulis aliis, quorum interest seu interesse potest et poterit, omnes et singulas responsiones, arreragia[b)] responsionum omnium et singularum preceptoriarum, baiuliarum et domorum [c)]prioratus nostri predicti tam camerarum dicti prioris quam omnium et singularum baiuliarum et domorum[c)] aliarum quarumcunque prioratus eiusdem quamque pensiones camere nostre quam in dicto prioratu obtinemus, omnia p[r]ocrassiave et mortuaria ac iocalia, res et bona alia quecunque sint quocunque nomine nuncupata[d)] et in quibuscunque consistant omnium et singulorum fratrum domus nostre mortuorum seu deffunctorum in prioratu predicto ad nos et nostrum Rodi conventum seu communem thesaurum comuniter vel divisim pertinencia et debentia pervenire, item ad petendum, recipiendum, recuperandum, levandum et habendum nomine quo supra omnes et singulas pecuniarum summas ac bona, res et iura[e)] alia, quecunque fuerint et quovis nomine nuncupata, nobis et dicto conventui ac nostro comuni thesauro comuniter vel divisim debitas et debita et nobis dictisque[f)] conventui [144v] et[g)] comuni thesauro comuniter vel divisim pertinencia et debencia pervenire quovis titulo, ratione sive causa tam per domus nostre fratres quam per personas alias quaslibet aliarum religionum religiosas seu ecclesiasticas et mundanas, item ad faciendum quo supra nomine de receptis, recuperatis, levatis et habitis quictancias perpetuo valituras unacum pacto expresso de aliquid ulterius in futurum non petendo, et generaliter omnia alia et singula faciendum, dicendum, procurandum et exercendum, que in premissis et circa premissa necessaria fuerint seu etiam opportuna et que nos ipsi faceremus et facere possemus, si presentes personaliter adessemus, etiam si talia sint, in quibus requiratur mandatum maius et magis speciale. Et rellevantes dictum procuratorem nostrum[h)] ab omni onere satisdandi, promittimus bona fide ratum, gratum et firmum habere et perpetuo tenere omne et quicquid per dictum procuratorem nostrum actum, gestum, dictum, petitum, receptum, recuperatum, levatum, habitum, quittatum et procuratum fuerit in premissis et quolibet premissorum ac iudicio sisti et iudicatum solvi cum omnibus et singulis suis clausulis opportunis sub ypotheca et obligatione omnium bonorum nostrorum et nostre dicte domus presentium pariter et futurorum. In cuius rei testimonium bulla nostra plumbea in absentia bulle[i)] comunis plumbee presentibus est appensa. Data Veneciis die vicesima octava mensis Augusti anno incarnationis[j)] Domini millesimo quadringentesimo decimo quarto.

Revocata *marg.* *a)* do *praem. ante corr.* *b)* arregia *corr.* *c-c)* *marg.* *d)* no *praem. ante corr.* *e)* bona *in lin.* *f)* dis *praem. ante corr.* *g)* et *dupl. ante corr.* *h)* suum *praem. ante corr.* *i)* p *praem. ante corr.* *j)* Domini *praem. ante corr.*

## 283

*[The Lieutenant Master] Fr. Luce de Vallins and the Convent on Rhodes grant for ten years to Fr. Simon Berntvelde the Preceptory of Lage (Priory of* Alamania)*, which is vacant following the death of Fr. Hermann von Brandlecht.*

*Rhodes, 1414 October 18*

*AOM 339 fol. 158v (133v), under* prioratus Alamanie et Boemie. *Cf. van Winter (1998), 36 no. 15.*

Frater Lucius de Vallinis etcetera et nos conventus Rhodi domus eiusdem religioso in Christo nobis carissimo fratri Symoni Berntuelde eiusdem domus prioratus nostri Alamanie salutem[a)] et sinceram in Domino caritatis affectum. Dum ad ydoneitatis sufficientie vestre notam et alia virtuosa vestra merita obsequiave per vos Deo et religioni nostre prestita zelo fidei contra eius emulos sepius velut intrepidus Christi miles exponendo personam consideratione reflectimur et ratione duce credimus vos operari, cum vos dono speciali honoramus. Hinc est, quod preceptoriam seu baiuliam de Laghe dicti prioratus [b)]situatam in diocesi Osbrug.[b)1)] presentialiter et iamdiu per obitum condam fratris Hermanni de Brantlicht[2)] eiusdem domus vacantem et ad nostram dispositionem et ordinationem propterea rationabiliter devolutam cum omnibus et singulis suis membris, iuribus et pertinenciis ad eam spectantibus et pertinentibus ac spectare et pertinere debentibus, quoquomodo et cum quibus illam habuit, tenuit et possedit dictus condam frater Hermannus, habendam, tenendam, regendam, gubernandam etcetera invicem deliberato consilio de nostra certa scientia et speciali gratia ad annos decem incipiendos in festo nativitatis sancti Iohannis baptiste proximo et extunc continuo et integre secuturos vobis auctoritate presentium conferimus, concedimus et donamus benefaciendo[c)] in eadem vosque preceptorem et comendatorem in dicta constituimus baiulia hac serie et eciam ordinamus. Comittentes vobis fiducialiter circa curam, regimen et administrationem etcetera. Quocirca universis et singulis fratribus, sororibus et donatis etcetera necnon universis et singulis fratribus domus nostre quacumque auctoritate etcetera ac priori seu presidenti prefato, ut vos vel procuratorem vestrum etcetera amoto abinde quolibet alio detentore, si quis sit, quem nos amovemus etcetera. Inhibentes vobis districtius sub virtute sancte obedientie supradicta. Et si, quod absit, etcetera illud et illa exnunc prout extunc etcetera. In cuius rei

1) *Diocese of Osnabrück.*

2) *Apparently Fr. Simon did not get the preceptory, since Fr. Johann Cruze, Kruse, was Bailiff of Westphalia and Preceptor of Lage on 6 October 1412: Düsseldorf, Hauptstaatsarchiv, Wesel Johanniter Urkunden no. 244, and from 1413 to 1427: von Bruch (1982), 300. Fr. Simon Berntvelde was Preceptor of Münster in 1432/33: AOM 349 fol. 70v (note by van Winter).*

testimonium etcetera. Data Rodi in prefato nostro conventu die decimaoctava mensis Octobris anno a nativitate Domini M° IIII$^{C}$ decimo quarto.

Pro fratre Symone de Berntvelde *marg.* *a)* in *add. MS* *b-b) marg.* *c)* vos *praem. ante corr.*

## 284

*Licence for Fr. Simon Berntfelde, Preceptor of Lage (Priory of* Alamania), *to leave the Convent for his preceptory and return.*

*[Rhodes, 1414 October 18]*

*AOM 339 fol. 219r (185r), under* littere licenciarum.

Item dicto die fuit data licentia fratri Symoni Berntveld. preceptori de Laghe prioratus Alamanie eundi ad predictum prioratum ad regendum et gubernandum dictam preceptoriam etcetera et deinde revertendi etcetera.

## 285

*Licence for Fr. Johann Creps (Priory of* Alamania) *to leave the Convent and return.*

*[Rhodes, 1414 October 18]*

*AOM 339 fol. 219r (185r), under* littere licenciarum.

Item dicto die fuit data licentia fratri Iohanni Creps prioratus Almanie pro suis negociis expediendis et ad conventum redeundi etcetera.

## 286

*The Master Fr. Philibert [de Naillac and other brethren (as no. 282)] revoke the above letter for Antonio di Ser Francesco of Florence, factor of Antonio di Giovanni di ser Matheo in Prague (no. 282), since Fr. Heinrich von Neuhaus, Prior of Bohemia, wishes to come to Constance in person.*

*Constance, 1414 November 27*

*AOM 338 fol. 144ar (144r), under* prioratus Alamanie et Boemie.

Noverint universi et singuli presentes revocationis litteras visuri et audituri, quod nos frater Philibertus etcetera dudum a religioso in Christo nobis carissimo fratre Henrico de Novadomo priore prioratus nostri Boemie ceterisque domus nostre fratribus preceptoribus et aliis prioratus predicti, quorum interat, tam responsionum, arreragiorum ipsorum, mortuariorum[a)], vaccancium, indulgenciarum quam aliorum iurium nostro Rodi conventui ac comuni thesauro religionis debitorum et rationabiliter pervenire debentium pensionesque camere nostre peccunias recipere speraremus et propter hoc confisi de fidei legalitate et circumspectionis industria discreti viri Anthonii domini Francisci de Florencia factoris Anthonii de Johanne de Ser Matheo in Praga commorantis eundem Anthonium de consilio domus nostre fratrum tunc nobis assistencium nostrum et dicte domus nostre procuratorem, factorem, sindicum, yconomum et nuncium specialem et generalem cum clausulis opportunis ad premissa omnia et singula petendum, recuperandum, recipiendum, levandum ac de per eum receptis litteras quictatorias perpetuo valituras nostro et dicte domus nostre nomine[b)] procuratorio atque vice dandum, concedendum et passandum fecerimus, creaverimus, constituerimus et ordinaverimus, prout in litteris nostris procuratoriis bulla nostra plumbea bullatis datis Veneciis die vicesimaoctava mensis Augusti anno incarnacionis Domini millesimo CCCCXIIII° latius continetur.[1)] Et quia, sicut didiscimus, dictus[c)] prior et ceteri, quos huiusmodi negocium tangit, eidem Anthonio domini Francisci de Florencia, nostro procuratori predicto, de premissis nichil dederunt, tradiderunt seu consignaverunt seu tradi, dari aut consignari fecerunt, cum ipsi huc ad nos Constancie favente Domino sint accessuri, considerantes dictum procuratorium non suum sortitum fuisse effectum, ideo de voluntate, consilio et assensu religiosorum in Christo nobis carissimorum fratrum Galteri Crassi decretorum doctoris prioris ecclesie conventualis Rodi, Iohannis de Porta prioris Capue, Iohannis de Autuno preceptoris Bellecumbe et aliorum domus[d)] nostre fratrum nobis assistentium predictum Anthonium domini Francisci de Florencia procuratoriumque predictum sibi super hoc factum et concessum et omnia, que ex eo inantea sequi valerent, de nostra certa scientia tenore presentium melioribus modo et forma, quibus possumus et valemus, revocamus, cassamus, irritamus et penitus annullamus volentes et decernentes exnunc omnia et singula, que per sepedictum Anthonium in premissis vel eorum aliquo aut ex eis et eorum quolibet dependentibus, emergentibus et connexis fieri contigerit, esse nulla nulliusque valoris, efficacie vel momenti. In cuius rei testimonium bulla nostra plumbea in absencia bulle communis plumbee presentibus est appensa. Data Constancie die vicesimaseptima mensis Novembris anno incarnationis Domini M° CCCC XIIII°.

*a)* p *praem. ante corr.* *b)* fratrum tunc nobis *praem. ante corr.* *c)* litteris *praem. ante corr.* *d)* do *praem. ante corr.*

## 287

*The Master Fr. Philibert [de Naillac and other brethren (as no. 282)] quit Fr. Heinrich von Neuhaus, Prior of Bohemia, for 1,400 ducats he has paid to Fr. Gautier le Gras, Prior of the Conventual church on Rhodes, and Fr. Jean Meyronés, Preceptor of Gap,*

1) *No. 282.*

*for two years' responsions of his priory. This money was transferred from Constance by Giovanni dei Medici to Marco Morosini in Venice to repay a loan of 4,000 ducats contracted by the Order for its expenses in the papal curia.*

*Constance, 1414 December 6*

*AOM 338 fol. 144av-5r (144v-5r), under* prioratus Alamanie et Boemie.

Noverint universi et singuli presentes quictationis[a] litteras visuri et audituri, quod nos frater Philibertus etcetera fatemur, recognoscimus et in verbo veritatis testamur, quoniam religiosus in Christo nobis carissimus frater Henricus de Novadomo prior prioratus nostri Boemie huc in civitate Constancie in manibus religiosorum in Christo nobis carissimorum fratrum Galteri Crassi decretorum doctoris prioris ecclesie conventualis[b] Rodi et Iohannis de Maironis preceptoris Vapnicensis procuratorum nostri Rodi conventus solvit, tradidit et realiter consignavit in, de, pro et super responsionibus prioratus predicti duorum annorum finitorum in festo nativitatis sancti Iohannis baptiste proximo preterito[c] ducatos auri mille quatuorcentum, quos Iohanni de Medicis[1] mercatori et sociis in Constancia incontinentia dicti procuratoris nomine et pro communi thesauro ac[d] dicto conventu de et cum [145r] nostris auctoritate, voluntate et assensu in deduccionem et acquictacionem quatuor mille ducatorum auri a nobili viro domino Marcho Moresini Veneciis commorante pro negociis religionis nostre in curia Romana expediendis mutuo receptorum tradiderunt, solverunt et realiter consignaverunt, de quibus mille[e] quatuorcentum ducatis auri sic, ut prefertur, a dicto priore solutis et dicto mercatori[f] traditis dictum priorem eiusque bona et res et quos tangit et tangere potest et poterit in futurum quictamus, liberamus et absolvimus ac quictos, liberos et absolutos esse volumus et iubemus per presentes. In cuius rei testimonium bulla nostra plumbea[g] in absencia bulle communis plumbee presentibus[h] est appensa. Data Constancie die[i] sexta mensis Decembris anno incarnacionis Domini M° CCCC° XIIII°.

*a)* litteras recognicionis et *praem. ante corr.* *b)* nostre Rodi *praem. ante corr.* *c)* prot *praem. ante corr.* *d)* e *praem. corr.* *e)* mille *marg.* *f)* mar *praem. ante corr.* *g)* plubea *MS* *h)* presentes *MS* *i)* se *praem. ante corr.*

## 288

*The Master Fr. Philibert [de Naillac] quits Fr. Heinrich von Neuhaus, Prior of Bohemia, for 150 florins he has paid Fr. Henri de Bye, Preceptor of St-Jean at Paris, for the Master's chamber of Tinz, [as its annual pension payment] for three years.*

*Constance, 1414 December 6*

*1) Giovanni Averardi [detto di Bicci] dei Medici († 1429), father of Lorenzo († 1440) and Cosimo († 1464).*

*AOM 337 fol. 26r (77r), under* prioratus Alamanie et Boemie.

Noverint universi et singuli presentes recognicionis et quictacionis litteras visuri et audituri, quod nos frater Philibertus etcetera fatemur, recognoscimus et in verbo veritatis testamur nos[a] huc in civitate Constancie habuisse et realiter recepisse a religioso in Christo nobis carissimo fratre Henrico de Novadomo priore prioratus nostri Boemie per[b] manus domus eiusdem fratris Henrici de Bye preceptoris hospitalis[c] sancti Iohannis Parisensis in, de et super baiulia nostra de Tincia, quam in dicto prioratu Boemie pro camera obtinemus et pro tribus annis finitis in festo nativitatis sancti Iohannis baptiste proximo preterito summam centum quinquaginta florenorum auri, de quibus centum quinquaginta florenis auri sic habitis et receptis contenti et bene pagati dictos priorem et preceptorem [d]eorumque bona et res[d] et quos tangit et tangere potest et poterit in futurum quictamus, liberamus et absolvimus per presentes. In cuius rei testimonium bulla nostra plumbea presentibus est appensa. Data Constancie die sexta mensis Decembris anno incarnacionis Domini M° CCCC° XIIII°.

*a)* nos *dupl.* *b)* p *praem. ante corr.* *c) supra lin.* *d-d) supra lin.*

## 289

*The Master Fr. Philibert [de Naillac], with the consent of three named and other brethren, confirms Fr. Simon Berntfelde in the Preceptory of Lage (Priory of* Alamania)*, which has been granted him by the Lieutenant Master on Rhodes and the Convent (no. 283).*

*Constance, 1414 December 8*

*AOM 338 fol. 144av (144v), under* prioratus Alamanie et Boemie. *Cf. van Winter (1998), 36 no. 16.*

Frater Philibertus etcetera religioso in Christo nobis carissimo fratri Symoni Berntuelde preceptori baiulie[a] de Laghe domus eiusdem salutem etcetera. Exigunt vestra commendabilia merita et obsequia diuturna per vos Deo et nostre religioni in transmarinis partibus prestita, ut vos dono specialis gratie prosequamur in hiis presertim[b], que honorem vestrum et utilitatem ac vestri status augmentum concernere dignoscuntur. Igitur donacionem et concessionem de dicta baiulia de Laghe prioratus nostri Alamanie per religiosos in Christo nobis carissimos fratres Lucium de Vailhins humilem marescallum dicte domus, locumnostrumtenentem et nostrum Rodi conventum, prout[c] nobis per eorum litteras sigillo dicti marescalli[d] locumnostrumtenentis sigillatas datas Rodi in dicto conventu die[e] XIX[a] mensis Octobris[1)] anno a nativitate Domini

*1) Correct would be 18 October according to no. 283.*

M° CCCC° XIIII° latius apparuit, vobis factas ratas, gratas et placidas habentes predictam baiuliam de Laghe prioratus nostri predicti cum omnibus et singulis suis[f)] membris, pertinenciis et iuribus etcetera habendam etcetera sub annua responsione et aliis oneribus etcetera – alias etcetera – de voluntate, consilio et assensu religiosorum in Christo nobis carissimorum fratrum Galteri Crassi decretorum doctoris prioris ecclesie conventus Rodi, Iohannis de Porta prioris Capue, Henrici de Bye preceptoris sancti Iohannis Parisiensis[g) 2)] et aliorum domus nostre fratrum nobis assistentium de nostra certa scientia et speciali gratia ad annos decem continuos et completos[h)] salvo iure communis thesauri ratione vaccantie pro una annata vobis auctoritate presencium confirmamus et ad uberiorem[i)] vestram cautelam de novo conferimus, concedimus et donamus benefaciendo in eadem vosque etcetera. Committentes etcetera. Quocirca etcetera necnon etcetera[j)] ac priori etcetera. Inhibentes etcetera. In[k)] cuius [rei] testimonium bulla nostra plumbea presentibus est appensa. Data Constancie die octava mensis Decembris anno incarnationis Domini M° CCCC° XIIII°.

*a)* baulie *MS* *b)* presertim *supra lin.* *c)* per *corr.* *d)* hoc *add. ante corr.* *e)* die *dupl. ante corr.* *f)* suis *supra lin.* *g)* Pisien. *praem. ante corr.* *h)* complendos *MS* *i)* uberiorum *praem. ante corr.* *j)* etcetera *dupl.* *k)* d *praem. ante corr.*

## 290

*The Master Fr. Philibert [de Naillac] permits Fr. Heinrich von Neuhaus and the Priory of Bohemia to make payments to procurators of the Master, Convent or Treasury without the expenses of changing money in Prague or Nuremberg or other places within the priory.*

*Constance, [1414] December 21*

*AOM 338 fol. 145r (145r), under* prioratus Alamanie et Boemie.

Frater Philibertus etcetera religiosis in Christo nobis carissimis fratribus Henrico de Novadomo priori et preceptoribus prioratus nostri Boemie domus eiusdem salutem etcetera. Vestri parte nobis fuit expositum, quia ex eo, quod temporibus[a)] retroactis cui vel quibus, quo et ubi responsiones, mortuaria, vaccancia et alia iura in dicto prioratu nostro Rodi conventui pro deffensione fidei catholice, pauperum Christi alimentacione et eius conventus sustentacione pertinencia solvere ignorabatis, ipsa tradere et consignare distulistis subiungendo, quod dum ipsa nomine communis[b)] thesauri dare et consignare debebatis a vobis non modicam pro cambio peccunie quantitatem mercatores preter et ultra responsiones[c)]

2) *Fr. Gautier le Gras, Prior of the Conventual curch, Fr. Johannes de Porta, Prior of Capua, and Fr. Henri de Bye, Preceptor of St-Jean in Paris.*

et iura exigebant in vestri et dicti prioratus preiudicium non modicum et gravamen, unde nobis humiliter suplicastis super hoc per nos provideri remedio opportuno. Hinc est[d], quod nos indempnitatibus vestris et dicti prioratus pro viribus obviare cupientes volumus et vobis harum serie dicimus, quatenus predictas responsiones, arreragia ipsarum mortuariaque et vaccancia et alia iura ad dictum conventum spectancia et pertinencia et cetera, que eidem pertinere et competere poterunt, sine cambio vel alia exaccione a vobis solvenda procuratori vel procuratoribus nostris et dicti conventus ac communis thesauri premissa recipiendi potestatem habenti vel habentibus aut[e] ab[f] eis vel eorum altero substituto vel substitutis in Praga vel Noremberg aut alibi in dicto prioratu, ubi dictus [g]vel dicti[g] procurator vel procuratores aut substitutus vel substituti ab eis seu eorum altero vobis intimandum[h] duxerint, detis, solvatis et realiter consignetis, de quibus solutis, ut prefertur, recipiatis recognicionem, que nobis et vobis sufficiat ad cautelam. Data Constancie die XXI[a] mensis Decembris anno predicto.

*a)* tep *praem. ante corr.* *b)* conventus *praem. ante corr.* *c)* responsiones *dupl.;* dictas *praem. supra lin. ante corr.* *d)* q *praem. ante corr.* *e)* ab *praem.*, ab eo vel *add. ante corr.* *f)* ab *supra lin.* *g-g)* dictis *MS* *h)* inti *praem. ante corr.*

## 291

*The Master Fr. Philibert [de Naillac], six namend and other brethren (as no. 282) confirm Fr. Heinrich von Neuhaus for his lifetime in the Priory of Bohemia with its prioral chambers of Prague, Manětin, Ploskovice, Uhřiněves and Dub.*

*Constance, 1414 December 31*

*AOM 338 fol. 145v-6r (145v-6r), under* prioratus Alamanie et Boemie.

Frater Philibertus etcetera religioso in Christo nobis carissimo fratri Henrico de Novadomo priori prioratus nostri Boemie domus eiusdem salutem et sinceram in Domino caritatem. Morem laudabilem nostre religionis sequentes, secundum quem nedum ipsa religio antiquos promovere, verum eos in suis conservare statibus consuevit, sperantes, quod in premissi[a] nostri prioratus comisso vobis regimine eritis favento Domino commendabiliter fructuosus et tamquam oliva fructifera in eo vos fructus uberes allaturus prioratum ipsum Boemie, prout ipsum iuste habetis presencialiter et tenetis, cum omnibus et singulis suis membris, pertinenciis et iuribus universis ad prioratum ipsum spectantibus et pertinentibus ac spectare et pertinere debentibus quoquomodo cum omni onere, emolumentis et honore et cum preceptoriis seu baiuliis Pragensis, in Manetyn, in Ploskoloicz, in Vhizynaloess et Dub cameris[b] suis et quas vobis pro cameris assignamus cum omnibus et singulis earum et cuiusque earum membris, pertinenciis et iuribus universis habendum, tenendum, regendum, gubernandum, augmentandum et meliorandum in spiritualibus et temporalibus tam in capite quam in membris vobis tanquam digno et benemerito de voluntate, consilio et assensu religiosorum in Christo nobis carissimorum fratrum Galteri Crassi decretorum doctoris prioris ecclesie conventualis Rodi procuratoris nostri Rodi conventus, Iohannis de Porta prioris Capue, Iohannis de Autuno Bellecombe, Iohannis Clareti de Ternes, Emanionis de Montbrun de Caubin, Henrici de Bye hospitalis sancti Iohannis Parisiensis preceptorum[1] et aliorum domus nostre fratrum nobis assistencium auctoritate presentium sub[c] responsione annua florenorum ·· auri de Florentia et boni ponderis per vos, prout pro cameris vestris vos continget, et per preceptores preceptoriarum dicti prioratus, prout pro preceptoriis suis pro rata eis pertinebit, receptoribus deputatis vel deputandis per nos et dictum conventum ad recipiendum responsiones in prioratu prefato aut alii vel aliis, quibus et ubi ordinaverimus et mandaverimus in festo nativitatis sancti Iohannis baptiste annis singulis ex pacto expresso infallibiliter exsolvenda[d] et quibuscunque aliis oneribus dicto prioratui qualitercunque et quomodocunque incumbentibus et incumbendis, impositis et imponendis per vos et dictos preceptores, ut predicitur, ex pacto etiam ultra responsionem predictam supportandis de nostra certa scientia et speciali gratia benefaciendo in eadem ad vitam vestram confirmamus et ad uberiorem[e] vestram cautelam de novo conferimus, concedimus et donamus retento et specialiter reservato nobis et nostro dicto conventui, quod de una etcetera, ac[f] eciam retentis et reservatis nobis dicto magistro ordinationibus etcetera nichilominus etcetera. Dantes etcetera. Quocirca etcetera. Inhibentes etcetera. In cuius rei testimonium [146r] bulla nostra plumbea in[g] absencia bulle communis plumbee presentibus est appensa. Data Constancie die ultima mensis Decembris anno incarnacionis Domini millesimo CCCC XIIII[to].

*a)* premissis *corr.* *b)* cameris *dupl. ante corr.* *c)* de *praem. ante corr.* *d)* exsolvendis *praem. ante corr.* *e)* vobis *praem. ante corr.* *f)* nich *praem. ante corr.* *g)* pre *praem. ante corr.*

## 292

*The Master Fr. Philibert [de Naillac], six named and other brethren (as no. 291) constitute Giovanni Averardi dei Medici and Ilarione dei Bardi, merchants from Florence, as collectors of responsions in the Priories of Rome, Venice, Bohemia, Hungary and Pisa. Both merchants have exactly the same powers. What one of them begins can be continued and finished by the other. They are to collect the responsions and arrears of responsions of the preceptories and offices, the* procrassia, mortuaria *and other dues of deceased priors and preceptors due to the Master, Convent or Treasury and all other such dues. They may issue receipts. They may constitute and destitute one or more substitutes. They can do what the Master himself could do if he were present, and the Master will abide by it.*

*Constance, 1414 December 31*

1) *As no. 282, but with Fr. Jean Claret, Preceptor of* Tienes, *and Fr. Emanio de Montbrun, Preceptor of Caubin.*

*AOM 338 fol. 162r-v (162r-v), under* prioratus Veneciarum, Lombardie, Vngarie, Vrbis et Pisarum.

Noverint universi et singuli presens procuratorium visuri et audituri, quod nos frater Philibertus etcetera confisi de fidei legalitate et circumspectionis industria venerabilium[a)] virorum Iohannis Auerardi de Medicis et Hylarioni de Bardis, mercatorum Florentinorum, eosdem Iohannem et Hylarionum licet absentes tanquam presentes et eorum quemlibet insolidum ita, quod non sit melior condicio occupantis, sed quod per unum ipsorum ceptum fuerit, per alium resumi valeat, prosequi et finiri, de voluntate, consilio et assensu religiosorum in Christo nobis carissimorum fratrum Galteri Crassi decretorum doctoris prioris ecclesie conventualis Rodi procuratoris nostri Rodi conventus, Iohannis de Porta prioris Capue, Iohannis de Autuno Bellecombe, Iohannis Clareti de Tienes, Emanonis de Montebruno de Caubin, Henrici de Bye hospitalis[b)] sancti Iohannis Parisiensis preceptorum, et aliorum domus nostre fratrum nobis assistentium[c)] citra tamen revocationem aliorum procuratorum nostrorum conventusque nostri Rodi[d)] et dicte sacre domus ubicunque et ad quecunque negocia constitutorum tenore presentium de nostra certa scientia[e)] facimus, creamus, constituimus et sollempniter ordinamus nostros et dicte domus nostre procuratores, actores, factores, sindicos, yconomos negociorumque gestores et nuncios speciales et generales ita, quod specialitas generalitati non deroget nec econtra, ad petendum, recuperandum, levandum, habendum et recipiendum nostro et dicte domus nostre procuratorio nomine atque vice omnes et singulas responsiones, arreragia responsionum omnium et singularum preceptoriarum, baiuliarum et domorum ac aliarum administracionum quarumcunque prioratuum Urbis, Veneciarum, Boemie, Ungarie et Pisarum tam camerarum dictorum prioratuum priorum quam baiuliarum, preceptoriarum, domorum et administracionum aliarum ipsorum prioratuum quarumcunque procrassiave et mortuaria[f)] ac iocalia, res et bona alia, quecunque sint quocunque nomine nuncupata et in quibuscunque consistant, omnium et singulorum fratrum domus eiusdem priorum, preceptorum seu quorumvis aliorum mortuorum iam et inantea moriturorum in dictis prioratibus et eorum singulis ad nos et nostrum Rodi conventum seu communem thesaurum communiter vel divisim spectancia et debencia rationabiliter pervenire. Item ad petendum, recuperandum, levandum, habendum et recipiendum quo supra nomine [162v] procuratorio atque vice omnes et singulas pecuniarum summas ac bona, res et iura alia, quecunque fuerint et quovis nomine nuncupata, nobis et dicto conventui ac communi thesauro communiter vel divisim debitas et debita, debendas et debenda et nobis dictisque conventui et communi thesauro communiter vel divisim pertinencia et debencia rationabiliter pervenire quovis titulo, ratione sive causa tam per domus nostre fratres quam per personas alias ecclesiasticas et mundanas. Item ad faciendum quo supra nomine de recuperatis, levatis, habitis et receptis unacum pacto expresso de aliquid ulterius in futurum non petendo quittancias perpetuo valituras. Procuratores unum vel plures ad predicta et subscripta loco sui semel et pluries substituendum et eum seu eos recovandum et in se procurationis officium reassumendum, et generaliter omnia alia et singula faciendum, dicendum, procurandum, gerendum et exercendum, que in premissis et premissorum quolibet[g)] necessaria fuerint seu eciam opportuna et que veri et legitimi procuratores facere possunt et debent, et que nos ipsi faceremus et facere possemus, si presentes personaliter adessemus, etiam si talia sint, in quibus requiratur mandatum[h)] maius et magis speciale. Promittimus bona fide ratum et gratum habere et perpetuo tenere omne et quid per dictos procuratores et eorum quemlibet ac substituendum vel substituendos ab eis vel eorum altero in premissis et eorum quolibet actum, dictum, petitum[i)], recuperatum, levatum, habitum, receptum[j)], quittatum procuratumve fuerit sive gestum sub ypotheca et obligacione omnium bonorum nostrorum et dicte nostre domus quorumcunque presentium pariter et futurorum. In cuius rei testimonium bulla nostra plumbea in absencia bulle communis plumbee presentibus est appensa. Data Constancie[k)] die[l)] ultima mensis Decembris anno incarnacionis Domini M° CCCC° decimo quarto.

*a)* et circumspectorum *add. ante corr.* *b)* sancti *praem. ante corr.* *c)* de nostra certa scientia *add. ante corr.* *d)* conventus *add. ante corr.* *e)* et speciali gratia *add. ante corr.;* per magistrum Michaelem Paquanti, secretarium domini magistri, cancellario absente *marg.* *f)* morturia *MS* *g)* aliquod *praem. ante corr.* *h)* mai *praem. ante corr.* *i)* s *praem. ante corr.* *j)* q *praem. ante corr.* *k)* Const *praem. ante corr.* *l)* die *dupl. ante corr.*

## 293

*The Master Fr. Philibert de Naillac [and other brethren (as no. 291)] quit Fr. Count Hugo von Montfort, Prior of* Alamania, *for 1,000 ducats of his priory's responsions for the two years of 1413 and 1414. Fr. Hugo has paid 500 and 416 ducats to Giovanni dei Medici of Venice and 100 florins of the Rhine to Fr. Dietrich von Keppenbach. They do this following letters from the Lieutenant Master Fr. Luce de Vallins and the Convent on Rhodes.*

*Constance, 1415 March 23*

*AOM 338 fol. 146r (146r), under* prioratus Alamanie et Boemie.

Noverint universi et singuli presentes recognicionis et quictacionis litteras visuri et audituri, quod nos frater Philibertus de Nailhaco Dei gratia etcetera fatemur, recognoscimus et in verbo veritatis testamur, quoniam de nostri et religiosorum in Christo nobis carissimorum fratrum Galteri Crassi decretorum dottoris prioris ecclesie conventualis Rodi et Iohannis de Maronis preceptoris Vapnicensis, procuratorum nostri Rodi conventus, et aliorum domus eiusdem fratrum nobis assistentium auctoritate, voluntate et consensu[a)] religiosus in Christo nobis carissimus frater Hugo comes[b)] de Montfort prior prioratus nostri Alamanie domus eiusdem in, de et super responsionibus dicti prioratus duorum annorum, videlicet millesimi CCCC XIII et XIIII[ti], finitorum in festo nativitatis sancti Iohannis baptiste proximo preterito tradidit, solvit et realiter consignavit mille ducatos auri in modum inferius declaratum, videlicet venerabilibus viris Iohanni de Medicis et sociis mercatoribus Venetis ducatos auri quingentos in una parte et in alia quatuorcentum sexdecim ducatos auri et religioso in Christo nobis carissimo fratri Theodorico de Kappenbach[c)] prioratus eiusdem vigore quarundam litterarum assignacionis a domus eiusdem fratre Lucio de Vailhins marescallo dicte nostre domus, locum nostrum tenente et nostro Rodi conventu emanatarum[d)] datarum Rodi in prefato conventu die tercia mensis Decembris anno a nativitate Domini millesimo CCCC[mo] duodecimo[1)] et sigillo dicti locum nostrum tenentis sigillatarum ac dicto priori directarum florenos Renenses[e)] centum, in quibus noster communis thesaurus[f)] predicto fratri Theodorico ex[g)] certis racionabilibus causis in dictis litteris lacius expressatis tenebatur. De quibusquidem mille ducatis auri sic, ut premittitur, per dictum priorem solutis de voluntate, consilio et assensu dictorum procuratorum et aliorum domus eiusdem fratrum nobis assistentium predictum priorem eiusque bona et res, et quos tangit et tangere potest et poterit in futurum, quictamus, liberamus et absolvimus per presentes. In cuius rei testimonium bulla nostra plumbea in absencia[h)] bulle communis plumbee presentibus est appensa. Data Constancie die vicesima tercia[i)] mensis Martii anno incarnacionis Domini millesimo quadringentesimo decimo quarto.

*a)* assensu *praem. ante corr.* *b)* com *praem. ante corr.* *c)* cr *praem. ante corr.* *d)* emanatorum *MS* *e)* Remenses *praem. ante corr.* *f)* conventus *praem. ante corr.* *g)* et *MS* *h)* abstencia *MS* *i)* vi *praem. ante corr.*

## 294

*The Master Fr. Philibert [de Naillac] informs Fr. Heinrich von Neuhaus, Prior of Bohemia, that Fr. Vinzenz von Breslau has been absolved by the Conventual prior on Rhodes. Fr. Vinzenz had left the house of Kadaň without licence and ceased to wear his habit publicly. Now he may return to Kadaň or be assigned his maintenance in a more conventient place. His treatment is to follow the usual practices of the Order and is to make sure that he does not have reason to leave again without licence.*

*Constance, 1415 April 2*

*AOM 338 fol. 146r (146v), under* prioratus Alamanie et Boemie.

Frater Philibertus etcetera religioso in Christo nobis carissimo fratri Henrico de Novadomo priori prioratus nostri Boemie domus eiusdem salutem etcetera. Cum domus nostre[a)] frater Vincencius de Wratisslavia conventualis domus in Cadano

*1) 1412 December 3. That document is apparently not included in the extant registers.*

propter nonnulla nobis exposita a dicta conventuali domo recesserit quasi apostatando quamvis habitum[b] religionis absconsum portaret, ad nostram presenciam accesserit, de premissis per priorem ecclesie nostre conventualis Rodi eciam de apostasia et sententia excommunicacionis ac irregularitate, si quam seu quas occasione premissorum vel alterius eorundem incurrerit, absolutum vobis remittentes vos hortamur in Domino ac[c] eciam requirimus, quatenus ipsum benigne recipientes per dicte domus fratrem ·· in Cadano preceptorem, ad quam domum in stagia sua vel alibi, ubi[d] utilior erit pro honore religionis redire volumus fraternaliter et caritative tractari eidem secundum bonos usus et laudabiles consuetudines religionis nostre in suis necessariis provideri faciatis eundem et omnes alios fratres et donatos sic caritative tractantes, quod inantea materiam non habeant in vituperium religionis vagabunde ad nos querelando veniendi. Data Constancie die secunda mensis Aprilis anno incarnationis[e] Domini M° CCCC$^{mo}$ decimo quinto.

*a)* nostri *corr.* *b)* liberum *praem. ante corr.* *c)* et *corr.* *d)* ut *praem. ante corr.* *e)* incarnationis *supra lin.*

## 295

*The Master Fr. Philibert de Naillac receives Henry, Duke of Silesia in Groß-Glogau and Crossen, as a* confrater *of the Order. Duke Henry has sworn an oath to protect and defend the Hospital's brethren and possessions. In case he is informed about dangers or damages he is to send a messenger or letter to the Master or his successor immediately. Duke Henry has promised to pay one pound of wax each year on 24 June.*

*Constance, 1415 April 4*

*AOM 338 fol. 150r (150r), under* prioratus Alamanie et Boemie.

Serenissimo principi et domino domino Henrico alias Rumpoldo, duci Slesie, domino Glogouie maioris et in Crosna, frater Philibertus [a]de Naillaco[a] Dei gracia sacre domus hospitalis sancti Iohannis Iherosolemitani magister humilis et pauperum Christi custos cum omni reverencia salutem in filio Virginis gloriose. Attendentes pie devocionis affectum, quem ad nos et nostrum ordinem habere noscimini et habebitis dante Domino in futurum, inducimur, quantum cum Deo possumus, condescendere votis vestris, ut proinde vestra sublimitas ad religionem eandem tanto fervencius devotionis incrementa suscipiat, quanto salutifera et spiritualia[b] ab eadem rependia reportabitis pociora. Eapropter vos, qui iurastis ad sancta Dei evvangelia corporaliter manu tacta nos et fratres ac bona et iura dicti ordinis ubilibet toto posse deffendere et salvare[c] procurando utilia et inutilia pro viribus[d] evitando et, si per vos evitari non possent, defferri facere vestro posse nuncio vel litteris ad nostram noticiam[e] vel successorum nostrorum dicte sacre domus magistrorum aut alicuius alterius fratris nostri ordinis, qui nos aut dictos nostros successores de eis certos reddant, in confratrem nostrum et dicte nostre religionis recipimus et aliorum confratrum domus eiusdem consortio tenore presencium aggregamus. Facientes vos, qui anno quolibet in festo nativitatis sancti Iohannis baptiste nostre domui libram unam cere dare, ubicunque fueritis, zelo devocionis ductus voluntate spontanea promisistis, ac parentes vestros participes[f)] in omnibus bonis spiritualibus, oracionibus, ieiuniis, missis, elemosinis, suffragiis, vigiliis et quibuscunque aliis piis operibus, que fuerunt in nostro ordine a primeva sui institucione et fient usque in futurum seculi divina gratia suffragante. In cuius rei testimonium bulla nostra plumbea presentibus est appensa. Data[g)] Constancie die quarta mensis Aprilis anno incarnacionis Domini millesimo quadringentesimo decimo quinto.

*a-a) supra lin.* *b)* salubria *praem. ante corr.* *c)* vit *praem. ante corr.* *d)* vicibus *MS* *e)* audienciam *praem. ante corr.* *f)* parent *praem. ante corr.* *g)* Datm *corr.*

*Henry IX (d. 1467) of Glogau, Europäische Stammtafeln 3/1 (1984), no. 13.*

## 296

*The Master Fr. Philibert [de Naillac] receives Nikolaus von Kittlitz as a* confrater *of the Order.*

*[Constance, 1415 April 4]*

*AOM 338 fol. 150r (150r), under* prioratus Alamanie et Boemie.

Frater Philibertus etcetera magnifico et potenti domino domino Nicholao domino de Kittilitz[a)] [b)]salutem in filio Virginis gloriose[b)] etcetera. Attendentes pie devocionis [affectum], quem ad nos et nostrum ordinem habere noscimini et habebitis dante Domino in futurum, inducimur, quantum cum Deo possumus[c)], condescendere votis vestris etcetera omnia ut in littera inmediate suprascripta.

*a)* Kiter *praem. ante corr.* *b-b) dupl.* *c)* etcetera *add. ante corr.*

## 297

*The Master Fr. Philibert de Naillac] receives Kaspar von Dohna, lord, Johann von Berg and Nikolaus von Rechberg, knights, as* confratres *of the Order.*

*[Constance, 1415 April 4]*

*AOM 338 fol. 150r (150r), under* prioratus Alamanie et Boemie.

Sub eisdem tenore et data recepti[a)] fuerunt in confratres magnificus et potens dominus dominus Caspar dominus de Danyn et egregii et strenui milites domini Iohannes de Berge et Nycholaus de Rechemberg.

*a)* retent *praem. ante corr.*

## 298

*[The Lieutenant Master] Fr. Luce de Vallins and the Convent on Rhodes grant to Fr. Friedrich Hubert for ten years the Preceptory of Überlingen (Priory of* Alamania), *which is vacant following the death of Fr. Heinrich Tripscher.*

*Rhodes, 1415 April 5*

*AOM 339 fol. 159r (134r), under* prioratus Almanie et Boemie.

Frater Lucius de Vallinis etcetera et nos conventus Rodi domus prefate religioso in Christo nobis carissimo fratri Frederico Hůbert [a)]dicte domus[a)] prioratus nostri Alamanie salutem et sinceram in Domino caritatis affectum. Religionis decor, morum honestas et alia virtutum dona, quibus vos carismatis gratia insignivit, ad imparciendum vobis nostri favoris gratiam rationabiliter nos moventes, sperantes, quod in comisso vobis regimine effectus administrationis utilis favente Domino vos comendet. Preceptoriam seu baiuliam igitur [b)]de V̊berlinguen[b)] prioratus Alamanie per obitum condam fratris [a)]Henrici Trisper[a)] eiusdem domus presentialiter vacantem et ad nostram dispositionem, collationem et ordinationem propterea rationabiliter devolutam cum omnibus et singulis suis membris, iuribus et pertinenciis ad eam spectantibus et pertinentibus ac spectare et pertinere debentibus, quoquomodo et cum quibus illam habuit, tenuit et possedit dictus condam frater [a)]Henricus[a)], habendam, tenendam, regendam, gubernandam, augmentandam et meliorandam invicem deliberato consilio de nostra certa scientia et speciali gratia ad annos decem incipiendos in festo nativitatis sancti Iohannis baptiste proximo et extunc continuo et integre secuturos vobis auctoritate presencium benefaciendo in eadem conferimus, concedimus et donamus vosque preceptorem et comendatorem in dicta constituimus baiulia hac serie et eciam ordinamus. Comittentes vobis fiducialiter circa etcetera. Quocirca universis et singulis fratribus, sororibus et donatis sub etcetera necnon universis et singulis fratribus domus nostre quacunque auctoritate etcetera ac priori seu presidenti prefato, ut vos vel procuratorem vestrum in corporalem possessionem pacificam et quietam prefate preceptorie inducat et inductum etcetera amoto abinde quolibet alio detentore, si quis sit, quem nos amovemus etcetera. Inhibentes vobis districtius sub virtute sancte obedientie supradicte, ne etcetera. Et si, quod absit, etcetera illud et illa exnunc prout extunc etcetera. In cuius rei testimonium bulla nostra cerea, qua utimur ob defectum bulle communis plumbee dicti nostri conventus, presentibus est appensa. Dat. Rodi in prefato nostro conventu die quinta mensis Aprilis anno a nativitate Domini millesimo quadringentesimo decimo quinto.

*a-a) add. in magna lac. b-b) marg. per manum posteriorem.*

*Fr. Fritz Huber is known as preceptor only in 1429 and 1437, whereas Fr. Ulrich Kubler was Preceptor of Überlingen from 1412 to 1423: Krieger 2 (1905), col. 1220.*

## 299

*The Master Fr. Philibert [de Naillac], two procurators of the Convent, three named and other brethren permit Fr. Count Hugo von Montfort, Prior of* Alamania, *to appoint preceptors for their lifetime, not only for ten years.*

*Constance, 1415 April 11*

*AOM 338 fol. 146v (146v), under* prioratus Alamanie et Boemie.

Frater Philibertus etcetera religioso in Christo nobis carissimo fratri Hugoni comiti de Montfort priori prioratus nostri Alamanie dicte domus salutem etcetera. Supplicatorie peticioni[a] vestre nobis exhibite exprimenti, quod, cum per statuta domus nostre priores domus ipsius preceptorias seu baiulias sive domos spectantes sue donacioni teneantur conferre fratribus domus prestite suorum prioratuum antiquioribus et benemeritis ad annos decem et non ultra salvo semper iure nostri Rodi conventus et communis thesauri et quod nonnulli fratres prioratus predicti timent, ne post dictum tempus decem annorum baiulie, preceptorie sive domus sibi aufferentur et aliis fratribus conferentur, et propter hoc baiulie vel preceptorie sive domus prioratus predicti[b] facilius subiciuntur vastati[c] et ruyne, unde responsiones et alia iura dictorum conventus et communis thesauri diminuuntur[d], preceptorias, baiulias seu domos vaccaturas vestre[e] spectantes donacioni pro commodo et utilitate earundem nostrorumque conventus et communis[f] thesauri predictorum[g] fratribus antiquioribus et benemeritis domus nostre prioratus prelibati[h] ad vitam ipsorum dandi et conferendi quibuscumque statutis seu consuetudinibus ad hec contrariis non obstantibus vobis licentiam et auctoritatem concedere dignaremur, benigne anuentes vestris exigentibus meritis de voluntate, consilio et assensu religiosorum in Christo nobis carissimorum fratrum Galteri Crassi decretorum doctoris, prioris ecclesie conventualis Rodi, Iohannis de Mayronis preceptoris Vapnicensis, procuratorum nostri Rodi conventus, Iohannis de Porta prioris Capue, Iohannis de Autuno Bellecombe, Henrici de Bye hospitalis sancti Iohannis Parisiensis preceptorum[1] et aliorum fratrum nobis assistentium de nostra certa scientia et speciali gracia licentiam et auctoritatem superius postulatam[i] vobis harum serie concedimus et donamus. In cuius rei testimonium bulla nostra plumbea in absencia bulle communis plumbee presentibus est appensa. Data Constancie die[j] undecima mensis Aprilis anno incarnacionis Domini M° quadringentesimo decimo quinto.

*a)* v *praem. ante corr.* *b)* prelibati *praem. ante corr.* *c)* vasatati *MS* *d) marg.;* dimuuntur *in lin.* *e)* vos *corr.* *f)* communis *supra lin.* *g)* eis *praem. ante corr.* *h)* predicti *praem. ante corr.* *i)* postulatas *MS* *j)* de *praem. ante corr.*

1) *The two procurators as no. 293, Fr. Jean de Porta, Prior of Capua, Fr. Jean d'Autun, Preceptor of Bellecombe, and Fr. Henri de Bye, Preceptor of St-Jean in Paris.*

## 300

*The Master Fr. Philibert [de Naillac], two procurators of the Convent, three named and other brethren (as no. 299) declare, at the request of Fr. Count Hugo von Montfort, Prior of* Alamania, *that even with a special licence from the Master no brother shall be received into the Order without notice to the prior, that even with special licence from the Master no brother, except those retained by the Master, is to go to the Convent without the prior's consent, that the prior together with his counsellors can increase or decrease the number of brethren in each house, and that no secular procurator is to be employed in lawsuits between brethren (no. 239).*

*Constance, 1415 April 11*

*AOM 338 fol. 147r-v (147r-v), under* prioratus Alamanie et Boemie. *Cf. Delaville (1913), 332–3 with note 1 (on p. 333).*

Frater Philibertus de Nailhaco etcetera religioso in Christo nobis carissimo fratri Hugoni comiti de Monfort priori prioratus nostri Alamanie dicte domus salutem et sinceram in Domino caritatem. Supplicaciones vestras recepimus continentes, quod, cum nos de gratia speciali alicui fratri seu fratribus prioratus predicti recipiendi viros aliquos[a] in domus nostre fratres licenciam concedimus, ipsi fratres talem gratiam habentes sine aliqua reverencia vobis exhibenda et noticia aliqua recipiendorum viros[b] nonnullos in domus nostre fratres recipiunt, quod facere non possunt nec debent secundum domus nostre statuta, in quibus cavetur, quod non obstantibus quibuscunque litteris per nos sub quocunque verborum tenore concessis frater[c], qui aliquem in domus nostre fratrem sine reverencia suo priori exhibenda nominisque designacione et persone noticia receperit, propter personas inhabiles et minus ydoneas debet amittere habitum et puniri pena in dictis statutis contenta. De voluntate, consilio et assensu religiosorum in Christo nobis carissimorum fratrum Galteri Crassi decretorum doctoris, prioris ecclesie conventualis Rodi, Iohannis de Mayronis preceptoris Vapnicensis, procuratorum nostri Rodi conventus, Iohannis de Porta prioris[d] Capue, Iohannis de Autuno Bellecombe, Henrici de Bie hospitalis sancti Iohannis Parisiensis[e] preceptorum et aliorum domus nostre fratrum nobis assistentium omnibus et singulis fratribus domus nostre prioratus predicti talem gratiam habentibus et habituris sub virtute sancte obediencie et sub penis in dictis statutis contentis prohibemus, ne inantea fratres faciant seu recipiant sine vestri licencia et persone vel personarum noticia vobis facienda et omne, quo contra inhibicionem nostram huiusmodi facere vel attemptare presumpserit, per vos iuxta statutorum predictorum seriem puniri precipimus et mandamus. Item cum alicui dicte domus fratri vel fratribus licenciam eundi ad conventum impartimur, propter hoc, quod nullam personarum habemus noticiam, in litteris nostris semper cavetur, quod dicti fratres ad dictum conventum vadant a suo superiore requisita licentia. Et quod propter tales licentias et fratrum inobedientias in dicto prioratu multa mala et scandala orta fuere, idem prioratus dispendia[f] non modica sustinuit et sustinet[g]. Cupientes talibus obviare de voluntate, consilio et assensu quibus supra volumus et ordinamus, ut decetero quicunque frater ad conventum transfretare volens quacunque licentia a nobis sibi concessa non obstante, nisi tales sint fratres[h)], qui ad manus nostras sint retenti, de dicto prioratu sine licencia a vobis requisita sub penis privacionis baiuliarum[i)] et domorum, quas in dicto prioratu obtinent et inposterum obtinebunt, de dicto prioratu recedere possint nec valeant et qui contra fecerit pena predicta puniatur. Item cum in pluribus baiuliis prioratus predicti sint ultra numerum statutum fratres et donati, propter quorum onus preceptores baiuliarum seu preceptoriarum ipsarum responsiones et alia sibi imposita onera exsolvere non possent nec valent in preiudicium nostri dicti conventus [147v] et in aliis baiuliis seu preceptoriis dicti prioratus quavis redditus habendum nulli sint vel quasi, vobis de consilio et assensu predictis in baiuliis seu preceptoriis dicti prioratus de et [cum] consilio fratrum baillivorum, preceptorum et procerum prioratus ipsius numerum fratrum et donatorum augendi et diminuendi, prout pro comodo et utilitate dictarum baiuliarum vobis videbitur expedire, auctoritatem, licenciam et facultatem harum serie impartimur. Item cum per statuta dicte nostre domus prohibeatur, ne in controversiis de fratre contra fratrem motis et movendis fratrem constituere procuratorem possit nec valeat, nisi fratrem seu fratres domus[j)] eiusdem et nonnulli domus nostre fratres prioratus predicti aliquando personas seculares suos constituerunt procuratores contra dictorum statutorum seriem, unde iurgia et controversie orte fuerint in grande preiudicium dicti prioratus et perniciosum exemplum aliorum, de voluntate, consilio et assensu prescriptis dictos[k)] procuratores seculares, si[l)] qui sunt, de nostra certa scientia revocamus volentes et ordinantes, ne de cetero fratres in controversiis contra fratrem seu fratres motis seu movendis procuratores seculares constituant decernentes exnunc prout extunc et [ex]tunc prout exnunc irritum et inane omne et quicquid per dictos procuratores seculares dictum, actum et procuratum fuerit sive gestum. In cuius rei[m)] testimonium bulla nostra plumbea in absencia bulle communis plumbee presentibus est appensa. Data Constantie die undecima mensis Aprilis anno incarnacionis Domini millesimo quadringentesimo decimo quinto.

*a)* aliquis *corr.* *b)* vros *praem. ante corr.* *c)* fratrem *corr.* *d)* preceptoris *praem. ante corr.* *e)* Ihrlm. *praem. ante corr.* *f)* non modica *praem. ante corr.* *g)* sustinentes *praem. ante corr.* *h)* tm *praem. ante corr.* *i)* seu preceptoriarum ipsarum *add. ante corr.* *j)* eiusdem *praem. ante corr.* *k)* dominos *corr.* *l)* constituant *praem. ante corr.* *m)* res *praem. ante corr.*

## 301

*The Master Fr. Philibert de Naillac, two procurators of the Convent, three named and other brethren (as no. 299) confirm Fr. Count Hugo von Montfort for his lifetime in the Priory of* Alamania *with the prioral chambers of Utrecht, Cologne, Klingnau and Bubikon. He is to rule the priory and its chambers. On 24 June each year he is to pay the responsions of his chambers and of the priory's preceptories to the receptors constituted by the Convent (probably a scribal error, see below note j-j, correct would be "by the Master and Convent") or to others who are ordered to receive them. The prior and the preceptors are also to pay other taxes or dues imposed on them.*

*Constance, 1415 April 11*

*AOM 338 fol. 147v-8r (147v-8r), under* prioratus Alamanie et Boemie. *Partial ed. van Winter (1998), 36–7 no. 17.*

Frater Philibertus de Nailhaco etcetera religioso in Christo nobis carissimo fratri Hugoni comiti de Montfort priori prioratus nostri Alamanie dicte domus salutem etcetera. Digne credimus agere et racionabiliter operari, si quos domus nostre fratres meritorum excellencia ad celsos gradus nostri ordinis evocavit, eos in suis, cum deposcunt[a)], statibus conservamus, ut, dum digni fructus dulcedine se refectos conspiciunt et senciunt honoratos, ad queque[b)] religionis nostre[c)] accomoda[d)] industrie eorum studia iugiter fervencia convertant. Attendentes itaque, quod in administracione prioratus nostri Alamanie predicti estis fructuosus, utiliter comprobatus, prioratum ipsum cum omnibus et singulis suis membris, iuribus et pertinentiis universis ad prioratum ipsum spectantibus et pertinentibus ac spectare et pertinere debentibus quoquomodo cum omni onere, emolumentis et honore et cum preceptoriis [e)]sive baiuliis Traiectensis, Coloniensis, Klingnawie et Bůbikon[e)], cameris suis, pro cameris assignatis cum omnibus et singulis earum et cuiuslibet earum membris, iuribus et pertinenciis habendum, tenendum, regendum, gubernandum, augmentandum et meliorandum in spiritualibus et temporalibus tam in capite quam in membris vobis tamquam digno et benemerito[f)] de voluntate, consilio et assensu religiosorum in Christo nobis carissimorum fratrum Galteri Crassi decretorum doctoris, prioris ecclesie conventualis Rodi, Iohannis de Mayronis preceptoris Vapnicensis, procuratorum nostri Rodi conventus, Iohannis de Porta prioris Capue, Iohannis de Autuno Bellecombe et Henrici de Bye sancti Iohannis Parisiensis preceptorum[1)] et aliorum domus[g)] [148r] nostre fratrum nobis assistencium de nostra certa scientia et speciali gratia auctoritate presencium sub responsione annua ·· florenorum auri de Florencia[h)] et boni ponderis per vos, prout pro cameris vestris vos continget, et per preceptores preceptoriarum dicti prioratus, prout pro preceptoriis suis pro rata eis pertinebit[i)], receptoribus deputatis vel deputandis [j)]per dictum conventum[j)] ad recipiendum responsiones in prioratu prefato aut alii vel aliis, quibus et ubi ordinaverimus et[k)] mandaverimus, in festo nativitatis[l)] beati Iohannis baptiste annis singulis ex pacto expresso infalibiliter exsolvenda et quibuscunque aliis oneribus dicto prioratui qualitercunque et quomodocunque incumbentibus et incumbendis, impositis et imponendis per vos et dictos preceptores, ut predicitur, ex pacto eciam ultra responsionem

1) *As no. 299, but Meyronés now Preceptor of Gap.*

predictam supportandis benefaciendo in eadem ad vitam vestram confirmamus et ad uberiorem vestram cautellam de novo conferimus, concedimus et donamus retento[m)] et specialiter reservato nobis et dicto conventui, quod de[n)] una vel pluribus penis per mortem preceptori etcetera ac eciam retentis nobis ordinationibus omnibus etcetera nichilominus etcetera. Rursum etcetera. Dantes etcetera. Committentes etcetera. Quocirca etcetera. Inhibentes etcetera. In cuius rei testimonium bulla nostra plumbea in absencia bulle communis plumbee presentibus est appensa. Data Constantie die undecima mensis Aprilis anno incarnacionis Domini millesimo CCCC[mo] decimo quinto.

Refecta fuit hec confirmatio de mandato domini propter indesignationem camerarum prius declarari obmissarum per me Michaelem Paquanti etcetera et prima extitit cancellata *marg.* *a)* def *praem. ante corr.* *b)* que *supra lin.* *c) supra lin.* *d)* commode *corr.* *e-e) marg.* *f)* in *praem. ante corr.* *g)* domis *praem. ante corr.* *h)* proitu *praem. ante corr.* *i)* pertinentebat *ante*, pertinentibus *post corr.* *j-j) marg.;* per vos seu fratres *del. in lin.* *k)* in festo sancti Iohannis baptiste *praem. ante corr.* *l)* nativitatis *supra lin.* *m)* rento *MS* *n)* in *praem. ante corr.*

## 302

*The Master Fr. Philibert de Naillac, two procurators of the Convent, three named and other brethren (as no. 301) constitute Fr. Count Hugo von Montfort, Prior of* Alamania, *as receiver and procurator of the Master and the Convent in his priory. He is to collect the responsions and arrears of responsions of preceptories, offices and houses, the pension payments from the Master's present chamber or any other chamber the Master's may obtain, all taxes and other dues which have been imposed or will be imposed, the* procrassia, mortuaria, iocalia *and other dues of dead priors and preceptors and all other dues to the Master and Convent. He is to audit accounts and to enforce payments. Preceptors, vicepreceptors, leaseholders and lieutenants have to be obedient to him; otherwise they are to be deposed or punished according to the statutes of the Hospital. He may issue receipts. With the consent of preceptors and seniors he may unite or divide vacant offices, preceptories or houses to ensure the payment of responsions. He may make legal acts inside and outside law courts. He may constitute and depose one or more Hospitaller brethren as his procurators. What he does and they do is to be valid even if it were momentuous enough to require the Master's special licence; the Master will abide by it. All Hospitallers in the priory are to be obedient to him.*

*Constance, 1415 April 11*

*AOM 338 fol. 148r-9v (148r-9v), under* prioratus Alamanie et Boemie.

Noverint universi et singuli presens procuratorium visuri et audituri, quoniam nos frater Philibertus de Nailhaco, sacre domus etcetera, confisi de fidei legalitate et circumspectionis industria religiosi in Christo nobis carissimi fratris Hugonis comitis de Montfort prioris prioratus nostri Alamanie[a)] domus eiusdem de voluntate, consilio et assensu religiosorum in Christo nobis carissimorum fratrum Galteri Crassi decretorum doctoris, prioris ecclesie conventualis Rodi, Iohannis de Mayronis preceptoris Vapnicensis, procuratorum nostri Rodi conventus, Iohannis de Porta prioris Capue, Iohannis de Autuno Bellecombe, Henrici de Bye sancti Iohannis Parisiensis preceptorum et aliorum domus nostre fratrum nobis assistentium eundem fratrem Hugonem priorem presentem et onus procurationis[b)] huiusmodi in se suscipientem de nostra certa scientia tenore presentium facimus, creamus, constituimus et sollempniter ordinamus nostrum dictique conventus et nostre domus procuratorem, receptorem, sindicum, yconomum et nuncium[c)] specialem et generalem negociorumque gestorem ad petendum et recipiendum, recuperandum, levandum et habendum nostro et dictorum conventus et communis thesauri nomine[d)] atque vice omnes et singulas responsiones et arreragia responsionum omnium et singularum preceptoriarum[e)], baiuliarum et domorum prioratus[f)] nostri predicti pensionesque camere nostre, quam in dicto prioratu obtinemus seu nos contingerit inposterum obtinere. Item ad petendum, recipiendum et habendum quibus supra nominibus tam tailhias et alia onera imposita et imponenda tam de preterito tempore quam presenti et futuro, procrassiave[g)] et mortuaria, iocalia, res et bona et alia, quecunque sint et quocunque nomine [148v] nuncupata et in quibuscunque consistant, omnium et singulorum fratrum domus nostre priorum et preceptorum seu quorumvis[h)] aliorum mortuorum iam et inantea moriturorum[i)] in predicto prioratu ad nos et dictum conventum ac communem thesaurum pertinencia et debencia pervenire[j)] secundum statutum[k)] promulgatum et factum super istis in generali capitulo apud Avinionem de mense Marcii anno incarnacionis Domini millesimo CCC[mo] sexagesimo sexto celebrato, seu quovis alio modo. Item ad petendum et habendum quibus supra nominibus omnes et singulas pecuniarum summas ac bona, res et iura alia, quecunque fuerint et quocunque nomine nuncupata, nobis et dictis conventui et communi thesauro communiter vel divisim[l)] debitas et debita, debendas et debenda et debencia[m)] racionabiliter pervenire quovis titulo, ratione sive causa tam per domus nostre fratres quam personas alias quaslibet aliarum religionum religiosas seu ecclesiasticas et mundanas. Item ad petendum et audiendum quibus supra nominibus compota et raciones de predictis et altero eorundem ab omnibus et singulis, ad quos de premissis compota et rationes ponere spectabit et quomodolibet pertinebit, et ad ponendum dicta compota et raciones eos et eorum quemlibet auctoritate nostra efficaciter compellendum, prout et quociens dicto procuratori et responsionum receptori videbitur expedire, et que nobis et dictis conventui et communi thesauro communiter vel divisim pro dicta composita deberi et pervenire debere competierint. Necnon preceptores, vicepreceptores, firmarios, rendarios et eorum locatenentes ac eorum quemlibet in[n)] dicto prioratu efficaciter compellendum per omnem cohercionis modum racionabilem dicto procuratori et responsionum receptori visum ad solvendum responsiones suas, arreragia responsionum, pensiones camere nostre, procrassiave[o)] et mortuaria et alia per eos quovismodo nobis et[p)] dictis conventui et communi thesauro communiter vel divisim debita et debenda. Eciam eos et eorum quemlibet tam pro deffectu solucionis responsionum suarum quam pro inutili regimine, bonorum[q)] alienacione et dilapidacione baiuliarum, domorum et administracionum suarum, si eorum culpa et contumacia exegerint, a suis administracionibus, eciam si per nos et dictum conventum sibi collate et concesse fuerint, secundum religionis nostre statuta de et [cum] consilio fratrum baillivorum, preceptorum et procerum dicti prioratus destituendum et destitutos seu destituendos huiusmodi ad ipsorum restituendum regimina, si eorum sattisfactio et debita paricio meruerint, rebelles quoque et inobedientes et[r)] per eos debita et debenda solvere recusantes secundum statuta et consuetudines domus nostre, prout demeruerint, puniendum et ducendum per iusticiam dicte nostre[s)] domus seu eum et eos ad nostram presenciam repellendum et transmittendum. Item ad faciendum quibus supra nominibus de receptis compotis et racionibus auditis quittancias perpetuo valituras. Item baiulias, preceptorias sive domos ac membra vaccantes vel vaccancia in et cum aliis baiuliis prioratus predicti, si expediat, [149r] cum consilio[t)] et assensu baillivorum, preceptorum et procerum[u)] dicti prioratus annexandum, uniendum, incorporandum et inserendum et econtra dividendum, segregandum et separandum ipsisque sic annexis, unitis, incorporatis et insertis fratri seu fratribus memorati prioratus sufficienti vel sufficientibus atque ydoneo vel ydoneis et regiminis fructuosi sub annuis responsionibus et aliis oneribus impositis et imponendis racionabiliter[v)] usque ad nostrum beneplacitum secundum statuta domus nostre recommendandum[w)]. Dantes et concedentes predicto nostro procuratori et responsionum receptori licenciam, potestatem et auctoritatem ac mandatum speciale et generale pro omnibus et singulis supra et infra scriptis ac deppendentibus et emergentibus ex eisdem et altero eorundem aut ipsis et eorum cuilibet qualitercunque connexis coram quibuscunque iudicibus et curiis ecclesiasticis et mundanis semel et quociens oporteat et dicto nostro procuratori videbit expedire quibus supra nominibus comparendi, proponendi, agendi et deffendendi, libellum seu libellos et quascunque summarias peticiones dandi et offendi, litem seu lites contestandi, de calumpnia et de veritate dicenda in animas nostras iurandi et subeundi cuiuslibet alterius generis licitum iuramentum, ponendi[x)], proponendi et articulandi posicionibus et articulis[y)] alterius partis respondendi et datis per eum responderi petendi[z)], excipiendi, excepciones dandi, repplicandi, dupplicandi, tripplicandi, testes, instrumenta, litteras et quecunque alia probacionum genera producendi et productis per partem adversam obiciendi, testes iurare videndi et in eos eorunque dicta dicendi crimina et deffectus opponendi, beneficium absolucionis a quacunque sententia excommunicacionis lata vel[aa)] ferenda et restitucionis in integrum semel et pluries simpliciter et ad cautellam[bb)] petendi et obtinendi sententiam seu sententias tam interlocutorias quam diffinitivas ferri, petendi et audiendi et, si opporteat, eas variandi et ab ea vel eis et quocunque alio gravamine illato vel inferendo appellandi, apostolos et litteras dimissorias cum instancia semel et pluries petendi et appellacionum causas prosequendi, expensas et interesse petendi, impetrandi quoque litteras tam simplices quam legendas gratiam seu iusticiam continentes[cc)] et impetratis per partem adversam contradicendi, procuratores unum vel plures domus nostre fratres ad predicta et subscripta et eorum quodlibet loco sui semel vel pluries substituendi et eciam seculares personas ad lites et causas tantummodo et eum[dd)] seu eos revocandi et in se procuracionis officium reassumendi et generaliter omnia alia et singula faciendi, dicendi, procurandi et exercendi, que in premissis et premissorum quolibet necessaria fuerint seu eciam oportuna, et que quilibet verus et legitimus procurator facere potest et debet, et que nos ipsi faceremus et facere possemus, si personaliter adessemus,[ee)] eciam si talia sint, in quibus requiretur mandatum maius et [149v] magis speciale. Et relevantes dictum procuratorem et receptorem et substituendum et substituendos ab eo[ff)] ab omni onere satisdandi, promittimus bona fide ratum, gratum et firmum habere perpetuo et tenere omne et quicquid per dictum procuratorem nostrum[gg)] et substitutum et substitutos ab eo actum, gestum, dictum, petitum, receptum et habitum, quittatum et procuratum fuerit in premissis et quolibet premissorum ac iudicio sisti et iudicatum solvi cum omnibus et singulis suis clausulis oportunis sub ypoteca et obligacione omnium bonorum dicti nostri prioratus presencium pariter et futurorum. Mandantes per presens procuratorium sub virtute sancte obediencie firmiter et districte universis et singulis fratribus domus nostre prioratus predicti et preceptoriarum predictarum, cuiuscunque status, gradus et condicionis existant, et aliis quibuscunque, quibus predicta seu eorum quodlibet pertinebunt et poterunt quomodolibet pertinere, ut premisso procuratori ac deputando vel deputandis ab eo suarum camerarum, domorum et baiuliarum responsiones et arreragia responsionum tam preteriti temporis quam presentis et futuri et omnia alia nobis et dictis conventui et communi thesauro communiter vel divisim spectancia et debencia racionabiliter pervenire, tradant et[hh)] exhibeant contradicione remota. In cuius rei testimonium bulla nostra plumbea in absencia bulle communis plumbee presentibus est appensa. Data Constancie die undecima mensis Aprilis anno incarnacionis Domini millesimo quadringentesimo[ii)] decimo quinto.

*a)* Almanie *corr.* *b)* procuratoris *corr.* *c)* nunciam *praem. ante corr.* *d)* nomine *supra lin.* *e)* responsionum *praem. ante corr.* *f)* prioris *MS* *g)* procurassia[ve] *supra lin.* *h)* quorumvis *dupl. ante corr.* *i)* mortuorum *corr.* *j)* pertinere *corr.* *k)* statum *MS* *l)* divisum *corr.* *m)* et debencia *supra lin.* *n)* cum pro deffectu solucionis responsionum suarum *praem. ante corr.* *o)* procuras *praem. ante corr.* *p)* et *dupl.* *q)* bonorum *dupl. ante corr.* *r)* et *supra lin.* *s)* d *praem. ante corr.* *t)* concilio *MS* *u)* pri *praem. ante corr.* *v)* racionabiliter *supra lin., prius ante imponendis* *w)* recom *dupl. post corr.* *x)* pp *praem. ante corr.vy)* alt *praem. ante corr.* *z)* tenendi *corr.* *aa)* et *corr.* *bb)* cat *praem. ante corr.* *cc)* consequentes *praem. ante corr.* *dd)* enim *corr.* *ee)* adesse *praem. ante corr.* *ff)* ab eo *supra lin.* *gg)* nostrum *supra lin.* *hh)* et *dupl. ante corr.* *ii)* quatercentesimo *corr.*

## 303

*The Master Fr. Philibert de Naillac, two procurators of the Convent, one named and other brethren (as no. 301) confirm Fr. Rupert, son of Henry, Duke of Silesia, for ten years in the Preceptory of Oels (Priory of Bohemia).*

*Constance, 1415 April 18*

*AOM 338 fol. 149v (149v), under* prioratus Alamanie et Boemie.

Frater Philibertus de Nailhaco etcetera religioso in Christo [nobis] carissimo fratri Ruperto filio illustris principis et domini domini Henrici ducis Slesie, preceptori baiulie in Olsna in Wratislaviensi diocesi prioratus nostri Boemie domus eiusdem salutem etcetera. Illustris prosapia, vite ac morum decor aliaque probitatis et virtutum merita, super quibus apud nos fidedigno commendamini testimonio, nos inducunt, ut vobis reddamur in exhibicione gratiarum liberales. Igitur preceptoriam seu baiuliam in Olsna supradictam prioratus nostri predicti cum omnibus et singulis suis membris, pertinenciis et iuribus ad eam spectantibus et pertinentibus ac spectare et pertinere debentibus quoquomodo, prout eam iuste tenetis [a)]presentialiter et habetis[a)], habendam etcetera de voluntate, consilio et assensu religiosorum in Christo nobis carissimorum fratrum Galteri Crassi decretorum doctoris, prioris ecclesie conventualis Rodi et Iohannis de Mayronis preceptoris Vapnicensis, procuratorum nostri Rodi conventus, Iohannis de Porta prioris Capue et aliorum domus nostre fratrum nobis assistencium de nostra certa scientia et speciali gratia ad annos decem continuos et completos vobis auctoritate presentium confirmamus et ad uberiorem vestram cautelam de novo conferimus et donamus benefaciendo in eadem vosque etcetera. Committentes etcetera. Quocirca etcetera necnon etcetera. Inhibentes etcetera. In cuius rei testimonium bulla nostra plumbea in absencia bulle communis plumbee presentibus est appensa. Data Constantie die decimaoctava mensis Aprilis anno incarnacionis Domini millesimo quadringentesimo decimo quinto.

*a-a) supra lin.*

## 304

*[The Lieutenant Master] Fr. Luce [de Vallins] and the Convent quit Fr. Hermann von Ow for all payments due for the lieutenancy on Kos from 1 September 1412 to 31 August 1414 (no. 276).*

*Rhodes, 1415 April 22*

*AOM 339 fol. 192v (no old foliation), under* littere assignationum seu cambiorum.

Frater Lucius etcetera et nos conventus Rodi domus prefate universis et singulis presentes litteras inspecturis notum facimus et attestamur nos a religioso in Christo nobis[a)] carissimo fratre Hermanno de Ow, insule nostre Langonis locumtenente, habuisse realiter atque de facto recepisse bonum ac legale computum, rationem et calculationem et integram satisfactionem de omnibus rebus ac bonis, granis et pecuniis et aliis rebus et bonis quibuscumque, que ad eius manus ratione et nomine dignitatis seu officii locumtenentis de dicta insula Langoni et aliis locis sibi annexis pervenerunt et perventa sunt, et hoc de duobus annis integris, videlicet a primo die mensis Septembris inclusive anni nativitatis Domini M IIII$^{C}$ duodecimi usque per totum mensem Augusti inclusive et usque ad primum diem mensis Septembris exclusive anni nativitatis Domini M IIII$^{C}$ decimiquarti. Et de quibus premissis omnibus et singulis fuimus et sumus contenti et integraliter satisfacti facientes sibi fratri Hermanno per presentes finem, quictationem, remissionem et absolutionem perpetuam de premissis cum pacto perpetuo valituro de aliquid ulterius non petendo seu per aliquem alium peti faciendo. Mandantes universis et singulis fratribus domus nostre, cuiuscunque status, gradus vel conditionis existant, sub virtute sancte obedientie, ne contra presentem nostram confessionem, quitanciam, remissionem et absolutionem aliqualiter venire presumant, quinymo eum fratrem Hermannum locumtenentem prefatum in predicta sua quitantia et absolutione indempnem firmiter et per imperpetuum conservare studeant. In cuius rei etcetera bulla nostra cerea, qua utimur ob defectum bulle communis plumbee dicti nostri conventus, presentibus est appensa. Dat. Rodi in prefato nostro conventu die vigesimasecunda mensis Aprilis anno a nativitate Domini M IIII$^{C}$ decimo quinto.

Pro fratre Hermanno locumtenente Langonis *marg.*  *a)* i *praem. ante corr.*

## 305

*The Master Fr. Philibert [de Naillac], two procurators of the Convent, one named and other brethren (as no. 302) confirm Fr. Nikolaus Lussa for ten years in the Preceptory of Brieg (Priory of Bohemia).*

*Constance, 1415 April 23*

*AOM 338 fol. 150v (150v), under* prioratus Alamanie et Boemie.

Frater Philibertus etcetera religioso in Christo nobis carissimo fratri Nicolao Lussa preceptori in Brega domus eiusdem salutem etcetera. Propter susceptum de vobis testimonium commendandum illa vobis libenter annuimus, que conservacionem vestri status concernere dignoscunter. Eapropter preceptoriam seu baiuliam in Brega supradictam prioratus nostri Bohemie cum omnibus et singulis suis membris, pertinenciis et iuribus ad eam spectantibus et pertinentibus ac spectare et pertinere debentibus quoquomodo, prout illam iuste habetis presencialiter et tenetis, habendam etcetera de voluntate, consilio et assensu religiosorum in Christo nobis carissimorum fratrum Galteri Crassi decretorum doctoris, prioris ecclesie conventualis Rodi, Iohannis de Mayronis preceptoris Vapnicensis, procuratorum nostri Rodi conventus, et aliorum domus nostre fratrum nobis assistencium de nostra certa scientia et speciali gratia ad annos decem continuos et completos vobis auctoritate presencium confirmamus et ad uberiorem vestram cautelam de novo conferimus, concedimus et donamus benefaciendo in eadem vosque etcetera. Committentes etcetera. Quocirca[a] etcetera necnon etcetera. Inhibentes etcetera. In cuius rei testimonium bulla nostra plumbea in absencia bulle communis plumbee presentibus est appensa. Data Constancie die vicesimatercia mensis Aprilis anno incarnacionis Domini millesimo quadringentesimo decimo quinto.

*a)* quo *praem. ante corr.*

## 306

*The Master Fr. Philibert [de Naillac], two procurators of the Convent, three named and other brethren (as no. 301) confirm Fr. Matheus Trente in the church and grange at Maschenholz (Priory of* Alamania), *which have been granted him for his lifetime by Fr. Johann,* prior generalis *of* Dacia, *Sweden and Norway, and the convent at Andvorskov.*

*Constance, 1415 April 24*

*AOM 338 fol. 150v-51r (150v-51r), under* prioratus Alamanie et Boemie. *Cf. Hatt Olsen (1962), 102 no. 8.*

Frater Philibertus etcetera religioso in Christo nobis carissimo fratri Matheo Trente, rectori seu commendatori ecclesie et curie principalis Maskenholte[1] prioratus nostri Alamanie domus eiusdem[a], salutem et sinceram in Domino caritatem. Propter susceptum de vobis testimonium commendandum illa vobis libenter annuimus, per que status vester tranquille pacis munimine[b] fulciatur. Igitur colacionem et donacionem de dictis ecclesia et curia principali de Maskenholte prioratus nostri predicti per domus eiusdem fratrem Iohannem priorem generalem in partibus Dacie, Suecie et Nouergie et conventum[c] domus eiusdem in Andwarchskohon[d] ad vitam vestram factas ratas, gratas et placidas habentes ecclesiam et curiam predictas cum omnibus et singulis pertinentiis et iuribus suis universis de voluntate, consilio et assensu religiosorum in Christo nobis carissimorum fratrum Galteri Crassi decretorum doctoris, prioris ecclesie conventualis Rodi, Iohannis de Mayronis preceptoris Vapnicensis, procuratorum nostri Rodi conventus, Iohannis de Porta prioris Capue, Iohannis de Autuno Bellecombe, Henrici de Bye hospitalis[e] sancti Iohannis Parisiensis preceptorum et aliorum domus eiusdem fratrum nobis assistencium

*1) Mentioned in a list of revenues from the Diocese of Roskilde in about 1380: Büttner (2007), 206–7.*

de nostra certa scientia et speciali gratia vobis ad vitam vestram confirmamus et ad uberiorem vestram cautellam de novo conferimus, concedimus et donamus benefaciendo in eisdem. Quocirca universis et singulis fratribus domus nostre quacunque auctoritate, dignitate vel officio fungentibus, presentibus et futuris sub virtute sancte obedientie precipimus et mandamus, ne [151r] contra presentem nostram confirmacionem, novam[f)] donacionem et gratiam aliquatenus facere vel venire presumant, quinymmo illam servent. Inhibentes vobis districtius[g)] sub virtute sancte obediencie supradicte, ne pretextu confirmacionis, nove donacionis et gratie nostre huiusmodi aliqua de bonis, rebus aut iuribus dictarum ecclesie et curie principalis vendatis, detis, obligetis, inpignoretis, permutetis, alienetis, distrahatis seu in emphiteosim perpetuam concedatis aut quocunque alio colore quesito extra nostram religionem transferatis sine nostra speciali licencia[h)] et mandato. Et si, quod absit, contra inhibicionem nostram huiusmodi aliquid vel aliqua facere vel operari vos contingat, illud et illa exnunc pro[ut ex]tunc et extunc prout exnunc cassamus, annullamus ac decernimus irritum et inane nulliusque existere[i)] penitus efficacie vel valoris[j)]. In cuius rei testimonium bulla nostra plumbea in absentia bulle communis plumbee presentibus est appensa. Data Constancie die vicesima quarta mensis Aprilis anno incarnacionis Domini millesimo quadringentesimo decimo quinto.

*a)* eus *praem. ante corr.* *b)* mune *corr.* *c)* conventus *MS* *d)* Antvaff *praem. ante corr.* *e)* hospitalis *supra lin.* *f)* nos *praem. ante corr.* *g)* ideo *praem. ante corr.* *h)* gratia *praem. ante corr.* *i)* es *praem. ante corr.* *j)* momenti *praem. ante corr.*

## 307

*The Master Fr. Philibert de Naillac appoints Werner von Kilchen to serve as his familiar* commensalis.

*Constance, 1415 May 14*

*AOM 338 fol. 151r (151r), under* prioratus Alamanie et Boemie.

Universis et singulis presentes litteras inspecturis frater Philbertus de Nailhaco Dei gratia sacre domus hospitalis sancti Iohannis Iherosolimitani magister humilis et pauperum Christi custos salutem in Domino sempiternam. Quos experta devotio comprobat et probitas approbata commendat, favoris prerogativa prosequimur. Sane inducentibus nos gratis obsequiorum meritis Wernhero de Kilchen ipsum in familiarem nostrum domesticum continuum et commensalem recipimus et aliorum familiarium[a)] nostrorum domesticorum continuorum et commensalium numero et consortio tenore presentium aggregamus volentes et concedentes eidem Wernhero de Kilchen, ut illis decetero potiatur et gaudeat honoribus, favoribus, privilegiis et graciis, quibus ceteri domestici familiares nostri continui et commensales potiuntur et gaudent ac soliti sunt potiri et gaudere. In cuius rei testimonium bulla nostra plumbea presentibus est appensa. Data Constantie die decimaquarta mensis Maii anno incarnacionis Domini millesimo CCCC° decimo quinto[b].

*a)* familiariorum *praem. ante corr.* *b)* vo *add. ante corr.*

## 308

*[The Master Fr. Philibert de Naillac] appoints Anton Guglar and Ulrich Judicis to serve as his familiars* commensales.

*[Constance, 1415 May 14]*

*AOM 338 fol. 151r (151r), under* prioratus Alamanie et Boemie.

Sub eisdem tenore et data retenti fuerunt in familiares Anthonius Guglar et[a] V̊lricus Iudicis.

*a)* et *supra lin.*

## 309

*[The Lieutenant Master] Fr. Luce de Vallins and the Convent grant for ten years to Fr. Albrecht Böcklin the Preceptory of Villingen (Priory of* Alamania)*, which is vacant following the death of Fr. Hermann von Ow.*

*[Rhodes,] 1415 December 7*

*AOM 339 fol. 159v (134v), under* prioratus Almanie et Boemie.

Frater Lucius de Vallinis etcetera et nos conventus Rhodi religioso nobis in Christo carissimo fratri Auberto Vequelini[a] dicte domus prioratus nostri Alamanie salutem et sinceram in Domino [caritatem]. Dum ad ydoneitatis sufficiencie vestre notam et ali[a] vestra virtuosa merita obsequiave etcetera. Hinc est, quod baiuliam seu preceptoriam de Williguim dicte domus prioratus nostri Alamanie presencialiter per obitum condam fratris Harmant Ow dicte domus vacantem et ad nostram dispositionem etcetera devolutam cum omnibus etcetera – alias secundum continenciam et seriem statuti super deficientibus in responsionum solutione suarum editi in capitulo[1] etcetera – vobis conferimus,

*1) Fr. Albrecht Böcklin was Preceptor of Dätzingen 1428 to 1431: Stälin (1883), 110. As early as 1417 Fr. Johann Söler von Richtenberg was Preceptor of Villingen: Krieger 2 (1905), col. 1280. Fr. Hermann von Ow was granted the Preceptory of Hall by the Convent and confirmed in it by the Master on 11 October 1417, but quarrelled with Fr. Peter Salzfaß: Schön (1910), 98–9. 1367 March 5: Delaville (1913), 161–2.*

concedimus et donamus vosque preceptorem et commandatorem in dicta constituimus baiulia etcetera. Inhibentes vobis districtius et sub virtute sancte obediencie supradicte, ne aliqua de bonis, rebus aut iuribus memorate baiulie vendetis, detis, obligetis, alienetis etcetera prout in forma communi. In cuius rei testimonium bulla nostra cerea, qua utimur ob deffectum bulle communis dicti conventus, presentibus est appensa die septima mensis Decembris anno incarnacionis Domini millesimo quadringentesimo decimo quinto.

Pro fratre Auberto Bequelin *marg.* *a)* q *praem. ante corr.*

## 310

*Licence for Fr. Rupert, Duke of Silesia, Preceptor of Oels, to travel to the Convent and to return.*

*[Rhodes,] 1416 January 21*

*AOM 339 fol. 153v (no old foliation), after* prioratus Anglie.

Die XX[a] I[a] mensis Ianuarii anno incarnacionis Domini millesimo quadringentesimo decimo quinto fuit licencia data fratri duci Ruperto de Slezia preceptori Alussensis prioratus nostri Bohemie veniendi ad nostrum Rhodi conventum et revertendi ad partes cum omnibus fratribus in eius societate venientibus et existentibus, quando sibi placuerit.

## 311

*The Master Fr. Philibert [de Naillac] and other brethren grant for ten years to Fr. Albrecht Böcklin, in virtue of letters from the Lieutenant Master Fr. Luce de Vallins, Marshal, and the Convent dated 7 December 1415 (no. 309), the Preceptory of Villingen (Priory of* Alamania), *which is vacant following the death of Fr. Hermann von Ow.*

*Lyons, 1416 June 10*

*AOM 340 fol. 130r, under* prioratus Almanie et Boemie.

Frater Philibertus etcetera religioso in Christo nobis carissimo fratri Auberto Bequelin domus eiusdem salutem et sinceram in Domino caritatem. Meritorum commendabilium consideratione vestrorum vos specialis favoris gratia prosequentes preceptoriam seu baiuliam de Vilingin prioratus nostri Alamanie per obitum domus predicte fratris Harmant de Ow vacantem presencialiter et ad nostram disposicionem racionabiliter propterea devolutam cum omnibus et singulis suis membris etcetera de voluntate, consilio et assensu religiosorum in Christo nobis carissimorum fratrum domus eiusdem Lucii de Vallinis marescalli nostrique locuntenentis ac nostri Rodi conventus, prout per eorum litteras sigillo eiusdem nostri locumtenentis in cera viridi sigillatas datas Rodi in prefato conventu die septima mensis Decembris anno ab incarnatione Domini M° CCCC^mo^ decimo quinto nobis lacius apparuit, necnon et aliorum fratrum nobis assistencium de nostra certa scientia et speciali gratia ad annos decem continuos et completos salvo iure communis thesauri racione vacancie pro una annuata vobis auctoritate presencium conferimus, concedimus et donamus benefaciendo in eadem vosque etcetera. Committentes etcetera. Quocirca etcetera necnon etcetera. Ac prorsus inhibentes etcetera. In cuius rei testimonium bulla nostra plumbea in absentia bulle communis plumbee[a)] presentibus est appensa. Dat. Lugduni die X^a^ mensis Iunii anno incarnacionis Domini M° CCCC^mo^ decimo sexto.

*a)* plumbe *MS*

## 312

*The Master Fr. Philibert [de Naillac] quits Fr. Heinrich von Neuhaus, Prior of Bohemia, for 500 florins of Hungary from the Priory's responsions in the year ending on 24 June 1415 and 560 florins of Hungary as the* mortuarium *of a deceased brother, all paid in Constance to Giovanni deiAMedici and companions as receivers in Italy,* Alamania *and Bohemia.*

*Constance, 1417 April 15*

*AOM 340 fol. 130r, under* prioratus Almanie et Boemie.

Noverint universi et singuli presentes quictacionis litteras visuri et audituri, quod nos frater Philibertus etcetera fatemur, recognoscimus[a)] et in verbo veritatis testamur, quoniam religiosus in Christo nobis carissimus frater Henricus de Novadomo prior prioratus nostri Boemie solvit, tradidit et realiter consignavit seu solvi, tradi et consignari fecit Iohanni de Medicis et sociis in Constantia per nos et nostri conventus procuratores in partibus[b)] Italie, Almanie et Boemie constitutos ad pecuniarum nostro communi thesauro spectantium recepcionem in, de, pro et super responsionibus predicti prioratus anni Domini M^mi^ CCCC^mi^ XV^ti^ finiti in festo sancti Iohannis baptiste eiusdem anni florenos auri Hungaricales boni et iusti ponderis quingentos et pro mortuario cuiusdam fratris dicti prioratus florenos eciam hungaricales quingentos sexaginta. De quibus florenis Hungaricalibus mille sexaginta sicut prefertur per dictum priorem solutis et per predictos receptis dictum priorem eiusque bona et res et quos tangit et tangere potest et poterit in futurum quittamus, liberamus et absolvimus ac quictos, liberos et absolutos esse volumus et iubemus per presentes. Ceterum propter locorum distanciam et viarum pericula ad uberiorem prenominatorum cautelam presentes litteras sub eisdem tenore et data fecimus duplicari. In cuius rei testimonium bulla nostra plumbea in absentia bulle communis plumbee presentibus est appensa. Dat. Constancie die XV[a] mensis Aprilis anno incarnationis Domini M[mo] CCCC[mo] decimo septimo.

Duplicata, postea triplicata *marg.* *a)* recogniscimus *MS* *b)* procuratores *praem. ante corr.*

Cancellata *AOM 341 fol. 140r under* prioratus Almanie et Boemie: Noverint universi et singuli presentes quictationis litteras visuri et audituri, quod nos frater Philibertus de Nailhaco etcetera fatemur, recognoscimus et in verbo veritatis testamur, quoniam religiosus in Christo nobis carissimus frater Henricus de Novadomo prior prioratus nostri Boemie solvit, tradidit et realiter consignavit seu solvi, tradi et consignari fecit Iohanni de Medicis et sociis in Constantia per nos ac nostri conventus procuratores in partibus Italie, Naciam[a)] et Boemie constitutos ad pecuniarum nostro comuni thesauro spectantium recepcionem in, de, pro et super responsionibus prioratus predicti anni Domini M[mi] CCCC[mi] XV finiti in festo sancti Iohannis baptiste eiusdem anni florenos auri Hungaricales boni et iusti ponderis quingentos et pro mortuario cuiusdem[b)] nostri fratris dicti prioratus florenos eciam Hungaricales quingentos sexaginta. De quibus florenis Hungaricalibus mille sexaginta sic, ut prefertur, per dictum priorem solutis et per predictos receptis dictum priorem eiusque bona et res, et quos tangit, tangere potest et poterit in futurum, quictamus, liberamus et absolvimus ac quictos, liberos et absolutos esse volumus et iubemus per presentes[c)].

*a)* Alamanie *b)* cuius *praem. ante corr.* *c) The text is here incomplete.*

## 313

*The Master Fr. Philibert [de Naillac], two procurators of the Convent, four named and other brethren confirm Fr. Ulrich Kubler in the Preceptory of Überlingen, which has been granted him by the late Prior of* Alamania *Fr. Henman zu Rhein and the prioral chapter when it was vacant following its resignation by Fr. Ulrich Tripscher.*

*Constance, 1417 April 23*

*AOM 340 fol. 130v, under* prioratus Almanie et Boemie.

Frater Philibertus de Nailhaco etcetera religioso in Christo nobis carissimo fratri Vlrico Kuybler prioratus nostri Alamanie domus eiusdem salutem etcetera. Propter susceptum de vobis testimonium commendandum ac sperantes, quod in commisso vobis regimine effectus administrationis utilis dante Domino vos commendet, collacionem, concessionem et donacionem per domus ipsius quondam fratrem Hammannum ze Ryn tunc dicti prioratus priorem in suo provinciali capitulo et de consensu fratrum inibi astantium de preceptoria seu baiulia de Vberlingen ex spontanea resignatione domus prefate fratris Vlrici Tripscher de ea in manibus dicti[a)] quondam prioris facte vacante modo et forma sicut in litteris patentibus sigillo dicti prioratus sigillatis[b)], quibus nostre presentes annectuntur, contentis vobis factas ratas, gratas et placidas habentes collationem, concessionem et donationem huiusmodi ac omnia et singula in eisdem litteris contenta de voluntate, consilio et assensu religiosorum in Christo nobis carissimorum fratrum Galteri Crassi decretorum doctoris, prioris ecclesie nostre conventualis Rodi, Iohannis Griuelli preceptoris Chambarelli, procuratorum nostri Rodi conventus, Galioti Montet Burdegalensis, Guillelmi de Sancto Iuliano de la Marche, Iohannis de Mayronis Vapnicensis, Henrici Stueler de Franquefort preceptorum[1)] pluriumque fratrum aliorum nobis assistentium de nostra certa sciencia et speciali gratia volumus, laudamus, approbamus, ratifficamus, emologamus, confirmamus et ad uberiorem vestri cauthelam, in quantum expedit, dictam preceptoriam de Vberlingen vobis de novo tenore presencium conferimus et donamus. Mandantes et tenore presencium precipientes sub virtute sancte obediencie universis et singulis fratribus domus nostre quacumque auctoritate, dignitate vel officio fungentibus, presentibus et futuris, ne contra premissa in dictis litteris contenta aliquathenus facere vel venire presumant sub penis in huiusmodi contradictoribus per statuta domus eiusdem inflictis, quinymo ea studeant iuxta earum mentem et seriem inviolabiliter observare. In cuius rei testimonium bulla nostra plumbea in absencia bulle communis plumbee presentibus est appensa. Dat. Constancie die XXIII[a] mensis Aprilis anno incarnationis Domini M[mo] CCCC[mo] XVII[o].

*a)* dictis *ante corr.* *b)* sigillatas *MS*

## 314

*The Master Fr. Philibert de Naillac confirms the convocation of a prioral chapter by the Prior of* Alamania *to be held at Straßburg on 8 September 1417 when the Master himself intends to be present.*

*[Constance, 1417] May 10*

*AOM 340 fol. 130v-31r, under* prioratus Almanie et Boemie.

Frater Philibertus de Nailhaco etcetera religioso in Christo nobis carissimo fratri ·· priori prioratus nostri Alamanie domus[a)] eiusdem salutem etcetera. Cum ad promocionem fidei catholice, ad quam nostra professio nos specialiter dedicat et disponit, ac nostre religionis agenda salubriter dirigenda in ultramarinis partibus domus nostre fratribus animositate virili et discretiva naturali virtute

1) *The two procurators as no. 313, Fr. Galliot Montet, Preceptor of Bordeaux, Fr. Guillaume de Saint-Julien, Preceptor of La Marche, Fr. Jean de Meyronés, Preceptor of Gap, Fr. Heinrich Strehler, Preceptor of Frankfurt.*

pollentibus presencialiter indigeat noster Rodi conventus, super quo, prout ex iniuncto nobis incumbit officio, nostra per singulos dicte religionis prioratus mandata direximus[b)] expediatque pro videndis ad huiusmodi servicium nostri iamdicti prioratus fratribus preceptoribus et aliis sufficientibus et ydoneis ac aliis variis prioratus ipsius tractandis negociis vestrum breviter in aliquo congruo loco provinciale capitulum celebrari. Vobis [131r] propterea tenore presencium precipimus et mandamus sub sancte obedientie virtute nichilominus firmiter iniungentes, quatenus vestrum presencialiter dictum provinciale capitulum in Argentina celebrandum in die nativitatis beate Marie virginis proximo futuro per Dei gratiam inhiendum evocetis omnibus et singulis dicti prioratus fratribus preceptoribus et aliis, prout videbitis expedire. Precipientes et mandantes sub dicta sancte obedientie virtute, quatenus eadem die in dicta Argentine civitate coram nobis, qui Deo previo pro nostre religionis utilitate personaliter illuc interesse speramus, vobisque compareant. Quibus eciam sub eadem sancte obedientie virtute precipimus et mandamus, quatenus vestris mandatis huiusmodi, ymo verius nostris obediant, pareant efficaciter et intendant. Quod, si forsitan neglexerint, contra negligentes procedatis rigide secundum statuta domus nostre, super quo plenariam tenore presencium vobis concedimus facultatem. Dat. loco et anno predictis die X[a] mensis Maii.

*a)* d *add. ante corr.* *b)* dixiximus, direximus *praem. ante corr.*

## 315

*The Master Fr. Philibert [de Naillac], two procurators of the Convent (as no. 313) and other brethren grant for ten years to Fr. Albrecht Böcklin the Preceptory of Dätzingen (Priory of* Alamania*), which is vacant following its resignation by Fr. Johann Söler von Richtenberg into the Master's hands. This is made in exchange for the Preceptory of Villingen that Fr. Albrecht resigned in favour of Fr. Johann.*

*Constance, [1417] June 3*

*AOM 340 fol. 134v, under* prioratus Almanie et Boemie.

Frater Philibertus etcetera religioso in Christo nobis carissimo fratri Auberto Bequelin domus eiusdem salutem et sinceram in Domino caritatem. Dum ad laudabilem probitatem vestram consideracionem dirigimus vos dignum favoris nostri gratia cum deposcitis reputantes baiuliam seu preceptoriam de Tetthingen prioratus nostri Alamanie per resignacionem de ea per domus nostre fratrem Iohannem Solren genant Rihtemberg predicti prioratus in manibus nostris sua spontanea voluntate factam et per nos acceptam ex causa tamen permutationis legitime et non alias vobiscum de ea faciende ad preceptoriam seu baiuliam de Vlingen prioratus iamdicti, quam nuper obtinebatis, vacantem presencialiter et ad nostram dispositionem racionabiliter propterea devolutam cum omnibus et singulis suis membris etcetera et cum quibus illam dictus Iohannes habuit, tenuit etcetera de voluntate, consilio et assensu religiosorum in Christo nobis carissimorum fratrum Galteri Crassi decretorum doctoris, prioris ecclesie nostre conventualis Rodi, Iohannis Griuelli preceptoris Chambarelli, procuratorum nostri Rhodi conventus, et aliorum fratrum nostrorum nobis assistentium de nostra certa scientia et speciali gratia ad annos decem continuos et completos vobis[a] auctoritate presentium conferimus, concedimus et donamus benefaciendo in eadem vosque etcetera. Comittentes etcetera. Quocirca etcetera necnon etcetera, quinymo etcetera ac priori etcetera. Inhibentes etcetera. In cuius rei testimonium bulla nostra plumbea in absencia bulle communis plumbee presentibus est appensa. Dat. Constantie die tercia mensis Iunii anno quo supra.

Pro capellanis fratribus *marg. (referring to both Fr. Albrecht and Fr. Johann)* *a)* salvo iure communis *praem. ante corr. In fine marg.:* Hii duo non levarunt bullas usque ad mensem *[*datum *praem. ante corr.]* Septembris. Ideo hic registrantur.

## 316

*The Master Fr. Philibert de Naillac, [two procurators of the Convent and other brethren (as no. 313)] grant for ten years to Fr. Johann Söler von Richtenberg the Preceptory of Villingen (Priory of* Alamania), *which is vacant following its resignation by Fr. Albrecht Böcklin into the Master's hands. This is made in exchange for the Preceptory of Dätzingen that Fr. Johann resigned in favour of Fr. Albrecht.*

*Constance, 1417 June 3*

*AOM 340 fol. 134v, under* prioratus Almanie et Boemie.

Frater Philibertus de Nailhaco etcetera religioso in Christo nobis carissimo fratri Iohanni Solren dicto Rihtemberg domus eiusdem salutem et sinceram in Domino caritatem. Dum ad laudabilem probitatem vestram consideracionem dirigimus vos dignum favoris nostri gratia cum deposcitis reputantes baiuliam seu preceptoriam de Vlingen prioratus nostri Alamanie per resignacionem de ea per domus nostre fratrem Aubertum Bequelin predicti prioratus in manibus nostris sua spontanea voluntate factam et per nos acceptam ex causa tamen permutationis legitime et non alias vobiscum de ea faciende ad preceptoriam seu baiuliam de Tetthingen prioratus iamdicti, quam nuper obtinebatis, vacantem[a] presencialiter et ad nostram propterea disposicionem racionabiliter devolutam cum omnibus et singulis suis membris etcetera et cum quibus illam dictus frater Aubertus habuit etcetera habendam etcetera de voluntate, consilio et assensu religiosorum in Christo nobis carissimorum fratrum ut supra de nostra certa sciencia et speciali gratia ad annos decem continuos et completos vobis auctoritate presencium conferimus, concedimus et donamus benefaciendo in eadem vosque etcetera. Committentes etcetera. Quocirca etcetera necnon etcetera, quinymo etcetera ac priori etcetera. Inhibentes etcetera. In cuius rei testimonium bulla nostra plumbea in absencia bulle communis plumbee presentibus est appensa. Dat. Constancie die III[a] mensis Iunii anno incarnationis Domini M[mo] CCCC[mo] XVII[o].

Pro capellanis fratribus *marg. (referring to both Fr. Albrecht and Fr. Johann)* *a)* vancantem *MS*

## 317

*The Master Fr. Philibert [de Naillac] orders Fr. Heinrich von Neuhaus, Prior of Bohemia, to assign maintenance in the Preceptory of Breslau to Fr. Dietrich Bischoffchen who in virtue of a papal dispensation has been transferred from the Teutonic Order. – Constance, 1417 May 29: Absolution and dispensation by Cardinal-Bishop Giordano [Orsini] of Albano, papal penitentiary, to Fr. Dietrich Bischoffchen, priest of the Teutonic Order in the Preceptory of Rehden (diocese of Kulm), who some time ago left that order but wants to profess in another order.*

*Constance, 1417 June 9*

*AOM 340 fol. 131r-v, under* prioratus Almanie et Boemie.

Frater Philibertus de Nailhaco Dei gratia etcetera religioso in Christo nobis carissimo fratri Henrico de Novadomo priori prioratus nostri Bohemie seu eius locuntenenti domus eiusdem salutem et sinceram in Domino caritatem. Cum et sicuti satis apparentur ac novimus dilectus nobis in Christo frater Theodri-cus Bischoffchen, presbiter professus ordinis fratrum beate Marie Theotonicorum sub regula sancti Augustini degencium[a)] ferventi devocionis zelo ductus[b)] nostram ad hanc sacratissimam religionem transferri peroptet omnipotentique Deo, beate Marie virgini eius genitrici ac beato Iohanni baptiste patrono nostro sub regulari [131v] habitu domus nostre perpetuum impendere famulatum, qua super translacione secum nuper extitit per sedem apostolicam misericorditer dispensatum, prout de huiusmodi dispensatione nobis constitit evidenter. Nos igitur commendabile dicti fratris Theodrici propositum in hac parte favorabiliter prosequentes vobis et vestrum cuilibet tenore presencium committimus et mandamus, quatenus eundem, cuius sufficiencia nobis claruit, in nostre religionis fratrem dicti prioratus nostri Bohemie visa tamen per vos dispensatione pretacta recipiatis ac in domo nostra de Wratislavia suam stagiam assignetis, in qua sibi de neccessariis debite faciatis provideri secundum laudabiles consuetudines prefate domus nostre taliter in premissis vos habentes, quod ipse frater Theodricus, quem eidem nostre religioni fructuosum speramus, hac sua spe votiva qualitercunque non fraudetur. Dat. Constancie die nona mensis Iunii anno incarnationis Domini M[mo] CCCC[mo] XVII[o].

Tenor vero dispensacionis, de qua superius iam est facta mencio, sequitur et est talis: Iordanus miseratione divina episcopus Albanensis dilecto in Christo fratri Theodrico Bischoffchen presbitero professo ordinis fratrum beate Marie Theotonicorum sub regula sancti Augustini degencium domus in Radin Culmensis diocesis salutem in Domino. In nostra proposuisti presencia constitutus, quod tu olim domum et ordinem ipsos, in quibus te voto professionis astrinxeras, habitu et ordine derelictis ex quadam animi levitate illicenciatus exivisti et ad seculum es reversus, in quo sic ligatus tanquam simplex et iuris ignarus et non in contemptum clavium divina celebrasti officia et alias inmiscuisti te eisdem. Cum autem[c)] propter certas et legittimas causas animum tuum ad reditum dicti ordinis non valeas aliqualiter inclinare, cupias tamen ut teneris sub regulari habitu perpetuo Domino famulari, supplicasti humiliter, ut providere tibi super hiis sedes apostolica de opportuno remedio misericorditer dignaretur. Nos igitur, qui tui et singularum animarum salutem ferventi desiderio affectamus, anime tue saluti providere volentes auctoritate sedis apostolice, cuius penitentiarie curam gerimus, te a generali excommunicationis sententia, quam propter premissa incurristi, et excessibus huiusmodi absolvimus in forma ecclesie consueta et iniuncta inde tibi pro modo culpe penitentia salutari, quod petita super hoc per te vel alium tui superioris licentia eciam non obtenta ad aliquem alium ordinem parem vel arctiorem[d)] valeas te transferre et in eo professione facta in dicto primo ordine non obstante gratum Domino reddere famulatum, tibi hac vice tenore presencium licenciam impertimur superiori tuo, qui pro tempore fuerit, dicta auctoritate committentes, quatenus postquam in ordine, ad quem te duxeris transferendum, professus fueris et in eo aliquamdiu laudabiliter conversatus te prius ad tempus, prout eidem expedire videbitur, a tuorum ordinum execucione suspenso demum suffragantibus tibi meritis aliaque canonica non obstante super hoc irregularitate dicto modo contracta tecum misericorditer dispenset, ita tamen, quod infra IIII^or^ mensium spacium a dato presencium[e)] computandum te ad aliquem alium ordinem parem vel arctiorem[f)] ut prefertur transferre nondum negligas[g)] cum effectu. Alioquin legittimo impedimento cessante extunc in statum pristinum relabaris et presentes[h)] littere nullius penitus sint momenti. Dat. Constantie IIII Kalendas Iunii anno nativitatis Domini M^mo^ CCCC^mo^ XVII^o^.

*a)* degenciu *MS* *b) dupl. –* *c)* auctoritate *MS* *d)* alcciorem *ante*, acciorem *post corr.* *e)* presentacionis *corr.* *f)* acciorem *MS* *g)* ne *supra lin.* *h)* presens *MS*

## 318

*The Master Fr. Philibert de Naillac, [two procurators of the Convent and other brethren (as no. 313)] confirm to the Prior of Bohemia and his successors at the request of Bishop Andrew of Posen, present at the general council in Constance, the foundation of the Preceptory of Posen and exempt the* plebanus *of the preceptory as canon of the cathedral from obedience to the preceptor. The document includes copies of two authentications made by the episcopal official of Breslau on 23 June 1417 at the instigation of Fr. Rozdechius, Commander of the hospital of St. Michael outside of Posen, one from Bishop Paul of Posen, the other from Pope Innocent III. On 29 November 1218 Bishop Paul confirmed donations to St. Michael which had been made by Duke Mieszko and three named predecessors of Bishop Paul himself. These donations included St. Michael itself, tithes in named villages and a prebend in the cathedrqal church of Posen. On 2 August 1201 Pope Innocent III confirmed to the Hospitallers in Poland the prebend in the cathedral church of Posen. The Hospitallers had to maintain a vicar there but were permitted to use spare revenues for their own pious purposes.*

*Constance, 1417 September 3*

*AOM 340 fol. 131v-4r, under* prioratus Almanie et Boemie.

Frater Philibertus de Nailhaco etcetera religioso in Christo nobis carissimo fratri priori prioratus nostri Bohemie suisque successoribus in futurum salutem in eo, qui vestrum est vera salus. Ad perpetuam rei memoriam. Votis iusta[a] petencium illis presertim, que divini cultus augmentum Christique fidelium salutem inspiciunt, libenter annuimus et, ut populi devocio magis incalescat, eorum affectum, quantum cum Deo possumus, prosequi nitimur favoribus gratiosis. Nuper siquidem pro parte reverendi in Christo patris domini Andree miseratione divina Poznaniensis episcopi[1] in hoc sacro generali Constanciensi concilio personaliter constituti nobis exhibita peticio continebat gratiosa, quod olim per suos bone memorie predecessores Poznanienses episcopos nostre religioni, quemadmodum et ipse sinceriter afficitur, quamplurimum affectione multe de bonis a Deo sibi collatis religioni prefate dudum extiterunt quantitates elargite utpote parrochialis ecclesia sancti Michaelis prope Poznaniam, que[b] nunc sancti Iohannis ecclesia nuncupatur, ac quoddam hospitale pro Christi pauperum et infirmorum receptione per eos inibi constructum et alias cum suis officinis construendum et reparandum pro eiusdem erectione[c] et pauperum ac infirmorumque affluencium in eodem sustentatione, iidem domini Poznanienses episcopi predecessores nostram religionem eandem in honoribus condignis sublimare cupientes[d] iamdicte parrochialis ecclesie tunc plebanum domus nostre fratrem in sue prescripte Poznaniensis ecclesie canonicum prebendatum receperunt, stallum in choro prout et ceteris eiusdem ecclesie canonicis eidem plebano pro se et suis successoribus assignantes, cui eciam pro ipsius prebende dotacione nonnullas villas, terras et decimas ad[e] mensam episcopalem assignarunt et imperpetuum dimiserunt[f] sub tali tamen condicione, quod fratres in dicta domo nostra Poznaniensi degentes episcopo pro tempore existenti [132r] vicarium unum, qui ecclesie ipsi deserviet in divinis, et dum casus vacacionis occurrerit, presentare tenebuntur. Quiquidem vicarius de dictorum canonicatus[g] et prebende redditibus victum capiat et vestitum, prout ceteri vicarii singulorum canonicorum dicte ecclesie Poznaniensis facere consueverunt. Et residuum vero, quod de dictis redditibus superesse poterit, idem plebanus canonicus in usus dicti hospitalis ad sustentationem pauperum

1) *Andrzej Lascarz Gosławicki (r. 1414–26): Ożóg (2000), pp. 159–86.*

et infirmorum tenebitur applicare legaliter et impendere fideliter, prout hec in litteris superinde confectis, quarum vera transsumpta sub sigillis auctenticis per dicte domus nostre Poznaniensis preceptorem nobis transmissa presentibus sunt inserta, lacius continentur. Tenor vero dictorum transumptorum[h)] de verbo ad verbum sequitur et est talis, [i)]videlicet unius littere:[i)]

In nomine Domini amen. Noverint universi et singuli presens transumptum seu publicum instrumentum inspecturi, quod coram nobis Iohanne Ienkewcz de Namslauia canonico et officiali Wratislauiensi iudicio ad infrascripta pro tribunali sedente, religioso viro fratre Rosdzechio commendatore hospitalis sancti Michaelis extra muros Poznanienses personaliter constituto, idem Rosdzechius commendator quandam patentem litteram reverendi in Christo patris et domini domini Pauli Dei gratia olim episcopi necnon venerabilis capituli ecclesie Poznaniensis in pergameno scriptam sigillis dicti domini episcopi et capituli appendentibus sigillatam, salvam, sanam et integram, non viciatam, non cancellatam nec abolitam, sed omni prorsus vicio et suspicione carentem, cuius tenor de verbo ad verbum inferius est insertus, ibidem coram nobis ad iudicium obtulit originaliter et produxit ibidem ex iustis motivis racionabiliter proponens et asserens, qualiter huiusmodi littere in diversis locis in suis et dicti hospitalis multiplicibus negociis et causis satis arduis agendis et expediendis omnibus modis deferre debent, sed propter ipsius remocioris, ad quem deferenda essent, loci distanciam[j)] et presertim propter viarum intermediarum ac varia, que occurrere possent, periculosa discrimina perdicionem littere prefate et suffocacionem ipsius ex casu fortuitu evenire gravius vereretur. Quare dictus Rosdzechius commendator exhibitam litteram per nos transsumi et transcribi ac[k)] de verbo ad verbum elici et exemplari ac per notarium infrascriptum in formam redigi publici documenti nostraque auctoritate ordinaria cum nostri decreti interposicione roborari et communiri, ut fides ubique locorum in iudiciis et extra eidem transsumpte et transcripte valeat adhiberi, humiliter postulavit. Cuiusquidem littere tenor de verbo ad verbum sequitur per omnia sub hec forma:[2)]

In nomine Patris et Filii et Spiritus Sancti amen. Paulus Dei gratia Poznaniensis episcopus magistro et fratribus Ierosolimitani hospitalis imperpetuum. Quia certum est aliquociens, ymo multociens evenisse, ut res satis bene dispositas et virorum sapientum approbatas examine mater oblivionis reduceret in ambiguum vetustas[l)], unde lites et iurgia, dissensiones et incomoda solent exoriri, ad hec et similia devitanda, ut elemosinarum[m)], orationum, vigiliarum participacionem aliquam valeamus adipisci, ecclesiam beati Michaelis et hospitale[n)] in Poznania, quod Radouarus[o)] predecessor noster bone memorie cum duce Mestone[p3)] noscitur instaurasse et de quibusdam decimis, rebus et

2) *Ed. Codex diplomaticus Poloniae Maioris [= CDPM] 1 (1877), pp. 96–8 no. 104; photo Gąsiorowski (1963), p. 91. Bishop Paweł Grzymała (r. 1211–42).*

3) *Mieszko the Old († 1202), ruler of Greater Poland from 1138 onwards.*

possessionibus ecclesie nostre dotasse, sicut a tempore ipsius ecclesia predicta sive hospitale tenuit et sicut a donacione tempore antecessoris nostri Benedicti quarti ante nos[q] vobis facta usque ad nos pacifice possistis[r], vobis et per vos domui prefato hospitalis Ierosolimitani de consensu tocius capituli ecclesie nostre cum omnibus pertinenciis suis de iamdicta ecclesia nostra[s] precedentibus, videlicet ecclesia beati Michaelis supradicta et hospitali iuxta Poznaniam prenominato cum sanctuariis et servis[t] ascripticiis[u], si qui fuerint ecclesie nostre, et cum decimis in villis nostris, que sunt Milostono,[4] Andreono,[5] Wigiono[6] apud hospitale, Welike,[7] Zuchilez,[8] Obereke,[9] Lipimra[v][10] cum servis ascripticiis et decimis quarundam aliarum villarum, quorum nomina hec sunt: Miteonit,[11] Iagodno,[12] Sannici,[13] Raska,[14] Gorka,[15] Clinka,[16] [132v] Corsucono,[17] Clersono,[18] Cirnelino,[19] Yacognienir[20] et omnibus aliis, si que fuerint. Hiis autem omnibus renunciamus et de omni iure nostro et accione, que[w] vel quam ecclesia nostra contra ecclesiam predictam seu hospitale habuit vel habere potuit, cedimus bona fide. Et prebendam in ecclesia nostra predicta, sicut eam beate memorie antecessor noster Arnoldus secundus ante nos[x] vobis pia liberalitate concessit ita, ut quitquit de expensis vicarii, quem statuetis ibidem, contigerit superesse, per manum vestram in subsidium transeat infirmorum, de pretaxati tocius capituli ecclesie nostre consensu cum omni iure suo et cum omnibus supradictis inviolabili fide donamus et confirmamus et, sicut supra dictum est, de omni cedimus accione. Nomina canonicorum in consensu isto existencium et consencientium hec sunt: Vitorlaus[y] decanus, Gerardus prepositus, Vucus[z] custus[aa], Vicencius cancellarius, Bogsalus[bb] scolasticus, Cabianus[cc], Piziobisla[dd], Robertus, Petreko[ee], Petrus, Egidius, Robertus, Nugo[ff], Nicolaus, Gerassius, Iacobus, Iohannes, Adam, Iohannes, Bokardus[gg],

*4)* Milostovo *CDPM, Miłostowo.*
*5)* Andreovo *CDPM, Jędrzejewo (Czarnków).*
*6)* Wigonovo *CDPM, a deserted settlement.*
*7)* *Wielkie.*
*8)* Zuchiless *CDPM, Suchylas.*
*9)* Obezerrze *CDPM, Objezierze.*
*10)* Lippniza *CDPM, Lipnica.*
*11)* Vriceoviz *CDPM, Wierzyce.*
*12)* *Jagodno.*
*13)* *Sanniki.*
*14)* Ruscha *CDPM, Ruszcza.*
*15)* Gorga *CDPM, Górka.*
*16)* Glinka *CDPM, Glinka;* Costrzen *add. CDPM, Kostrzyn.*
*17)* Cossutovo *CDPM, koszuty.*
*18)* Clessovo *CDPM, Kleszczewo.*
*19)* Cyrnelino *CDPM, Czerlejno.*
*20)* Vargovo *CDPM, Wargovo.*

Nicholaus[hh]. Hec autem omnia, que supra diximus, de nominatorum canonicorum sepedicto consensu vobis et domui vestro iure perpetuo concedimus possedenda[ii]. Et ut hec omnia rata et inconcussa permaneant et confirmacio sive donacio huiusmodi imposterum non valeant[ij] infirmari, presentem paginam[kk] sigillorum nostrorum atestacione dignum duximus roborandam. Quisquis autem hoc immutare vel infringere attemptaverit, anatema sit. Actum anno Dominice[ll] incarnationis M^mo^ CC XVIII, II Kalendas Decembris. Testes autem Albertus sacerdos, Simon, Philippus, Rodgerus[mm], Eusebius[nn], Arnoldus, Stephanus, Blasius, Nicholaus[oo], Fredericus[pp], Ianitus, Degno vicarii, Robertus sacerdos, Garsilius[qq] clericus, Smeragdus[rr], Nicholaus[ss], Iohannes, Florencius, Henricus[tt], Bartholomeus, Irlana[uu], Iohannes capellani, Martinus prepositus de Zedlemin.[21]

Et huic littere duo sigilla ambo oblonge figure tam ab extra quam ad faciem de cera omnino communi sive alba in filis sericiis brunatici coloris erant subappensa, in cuius sigilli videlicet primi medio quedam ymago in sedili sive kathedra sedentis, que propter depressionem cere lucidius videre non poterat, beatum Petrum apostolum representans ab intuentibus sculpta videbatur et apparebant et in ipsius sigilli circunferencia[vv] hec littere capitales pro titulo sculpte legebantur premissa cruce: "Sigillum capituli Poznanien(sis)." In medio vero secundi sigilli quedam ymago directe stans infulata pontificalibus indutta carnacuram[ww] sive baculum pastoralem in sinistra manu tenens, manu dextera quasi ad benedicendum elevata, sculpta[xx] ab intuentibus apparebat. In circumferencia vero prefati sigilli premissa cruce hec littere capitales pro titulo legebantur: "Sigillum Pauli Poznanien(sis) episcopi."

Nos igitur Iohannes Ienkewicz canonicus et officialis visa igitur tam dicta littera quam ipsius sigillis per omnia diligenter ipsisque veris et iustis et absque omni vicio et suspicione penitus reputatis, quapropter ipsam de verbo ad verbum ad peticionem prefati Rosdzechii commendatoris transsumi, transcribi ipsiusque sigilla[yy] per omnia describi per Stephanum Wolff notarium publicum mandavimus diligenter. Qua transsumpta et transcripta invenimus presens transsumptum et transcriptum cum ipsa littera originali tam in tenore quam in ipsa[zz] sigillorum descripcione habita collacione fideli et relacione ad easdem per omnia concordare. Propter quod volentes et auctoritate ordinaria presentibus, quantum in nobis est, decernentes, ut huic presenti transsumpto et transcripto deinceps et inantea hic et ubique locorum tam in iudiciis quam extra tanta fides adhibeatur, quanta adhiberetur littere originali sigillate, si effectualiter per omnia appareret. Quibus omnibus et singulis nostram auctoritatem ordinariam presentibus interponimus pariter et decretum. In cuius rei testimonium et fidem omnium premissorum presens transumptum [133r] et transcriptum sigillo officialatus nostri Wratislaviensis et subscriptione notarii publici infrascripti mandavimus communiri. Actum et datum in summo Wratislauiensi in

*21) Siedlemin, 80 km south-east of Posen.*

domo habitacionis nostre Mercurii die XX[a]III[a] mensis Iunii hora terciarum vel quasi anno Domini millesimo CCCC[mo] decimo septimo indicione decima sede apostolica pastore carente, presentibus ibidem honorabilibus et discretis viris dominis magistro Stephano de Scankaw decano Omnium Sanctorum in castro Pragensi[22)] et canonico Wratislaviensi, Stephano Wolff plebano[aaa)] in Corsluz,[23)] Michaeli signatore[bbb)] sancte Crucis Wratislaviensis et Nicholao Wolff clerico Wratislauiensis diocesis testibus ad premissa vocatis specialiter et rogatis. Et ego Stephanus quondam Theodrici Wolff de Wartinberg clericus W[r]atislauiensis diocesis, publicus auctoritate imperiali notarius, quia prescriptis littere exhibicione, peticione, decreti interposicione omnibusque aliis et singulis premissis, dum sic coram prefato domino Iohanne officiali Wratislaviensi et per eum, ut premittitur, agerentur et fierent, unacum prenominatis testibus presens interfui eaque omnia et singula sic fieri vidi et audivi, ideoque prescriptam litteram dicti reverendi in Christo patris et domini domini Pauli Dei gratia episcopi olim Poznaniensis felicis memorie de mandato pretacti domini Iohannis officialis de verbo ad verbum fideliter transsumpsi et transcripsi et manu mea propria exemplavi nil addens vel minuens, quod sensum aut facti substanciam immutet, viciet aut variet intellectum. Et quia collacione et ascultacione prehabita diligenti presens transsumptum seu publicum instrumentum cum dicta originali littera per omnia concordare inveni, ideoque me hic subscripsi, publicavi et in hanc publicam formam redegi signo et nomine meis solitis unacum appensione sigilli officialatus Wratislauiensis consignando rogatus et requisitus in fidem et testimonium omnium et singulorum premissorum.

Alterius vero littere similiter transsumpte tenor talis est: In nomine Domini amen. Noverint universi et singuli presens transsumptum seu publicum instrumentum inspecturi, quod coram nobis Iohanne de Ienkewricz de Namslauia canonico et officiali Wratislauiensi iudicio ad infrascripta pro tribunali sedente, religioso viro Rosdzechio commendatore hospitalis sancti Michaelis extra muros Poznanienses personaliter constituto, idem Rosdzechius commendator quasdam patentes litteras sanctissimi in Christo patris ac domini domini Innocencii pape tercii sancte memorie eius vera[ccc)] bulla plumbea in filis sericiis glauci et brunatici coloris [iuxta] morem Romane curie impendens bullatas salvas, sanas et integras omnique prorsus vicio et suspicione carentes, quarum litterarum tenor de verbo ad verbum inferius[ddd)] est insertus,[eee)] ibidem coram nobis ad iudicium obtulit originaliter et produxit ibidem ex iustis motivis racionabiliter proponens et asserens, qualiter huiusmodi litterarum apostolicarum in diversis locis in suis et memorati hospitalis multiplicibus negociis et causis satis arduis agendis et expediendis omnibus modis deferre debent, sed [propter] ipsius remocioris, ad quem deferenda[fff)] essent, loci distanciam et presertim propter viarum intermediarum ac varia, que occurrere possent, periculosa

*22) The collegiate church of All Saints in Prague was incorporated into Prague University.*
*23) Korschlitz.*

discrimina perdicionem litterarum apostolicarum prefatarum et suffocacionem earundem ex casu fortuitu evenire gravius vereretur. Quare sepedictus Rosdzechius commendator exhibitas litteras per nos transsumi et transcribi ac[ggg)] de verbo ad verbum elici et exemplari ac per notarium infrascriptum in formam redigi publici documenti nostraque auctoritate ordinaria cum decreti nostri interposicione roborari et [133v] communiri, ut fides ubique locorum in iudiciis et extra eidem transsumpto et transcripto valeat adhiberi, humiliter postulavit. Quarumquidem litterarum apostolicarum tenor de verbo ad verbum sequitur per omnia sub hac forma:[24)]

Innocencius episcopus[hhh)] servus servorum Dei dilectis filiis magistro et fratribus Ierosolimitani hospitalis in Polonia constitutis salutem et apostolicam benedictionem. Venerabilis frater noster A. Postnaniensis[!] episcopus per suas nobis litteras intimavit, quod divine[iii)] pietatis intuitu de canonicorum ecclesie Posnaniensis assensu in eadem ecclesia prebendam vobis pia liberalitate concessit ita, ut quitquid expensis vicarii, quem statuetis ibidem, contigerit superesse, per manum vestram in subsidium transeat infirmorum. Nos igitur prebendam ipsam, sicut eam iuste ac pacifice possidetis, vobis et per vos domui hospitalis auctoritate apostolica confirmamus et[jjj)] presentis scripti patrocinio communimus. Nulli ergo omnino hominum liceat hanc paginam nostre confirmacionis infringere vel ei ausu temerario contraire. Si quis autem hoc attemptare presumpserit, indignacionem omnipotentis Dei et beatorum Petri et Pauli apostolorum eius se noverit incursurum. Dat. Signie[kkk)] IIII nonas Augusti pontificatus nostri anno quarto.

Nos igitur Iohannes Ienkewicz canonicus et officialis Wratislauiensis prefatus visis igitur dictis litteris apostolicis ipsisque veris et iustis et absque omni vicio et suspicione penitus per omnia diligenter reputatis, quapropter ipsas de verbo ad verbum ad peticionem prefati Rosdzechii commendatoris transsumi, transcribi per Stephanum Wolff notarium publicum infrascriptum mandavimus diligenter. Quibus transsumptis et transcriptis invenimus presens transsumptum et transscriptum cum ipsis litteris apostolicis tam in tenore quam eciam in aliis habita collacione fideli et relacione ad easdem per omnia concordare. Propter quod volentes et auctoritate ordinaria presentibus, quantum in nobis est, decernentes, ut huic presenti transsumpto et transcripto deinceps et inantea hic et ubique locorum tam in iudiciis quam extra tanta fides adhibeatur, quanta adhiberetur litteris apostolicis et originalibus, si effectualiter per omnia apparerent. Quibus omnibus et singulis nostram auctoritatem ordinariam presentibus interponimus pariter et decretum. In cuius rei fidem et testimonium omnium premissorum presens transsumptum et transcriptum sigillo nostri officialatus Wratislauiensis et subscripcione notarii publici infrascripti mandavimus communiri. Actum et datum in summo Wratislauiensi in domo habitacionis

24) *Segni, 1201 August 2: Ed. Cart. Hosp. 2 p. 10 no. 1149; CDPM 1 (1877), p. 47 no. 37; photo Gąsiorowski (1963), p. 89.*

nostre Mercurii die vicesima tercia mensis Iunii hora terciarum vel quasi anno Domini $M^{mo}$ $CCCC^{mo}$ $XVII^{o}$ indicione $X^{ma}$ sede apostolica pastore carente, presentibus ibidem honorabilibus et discretis viris dominis magistro Stephano de Stankaw decano Omnium Sanctorum in castro Pragensi et canonico Vratislauiensi, Stephano Wolff plebano[lll)] in Corsluz, Michaele de Strelen signatore sancte Crucis Vratislaviensis et Nicholao Wolff clericis Vratislauiensis diocesis, testibus ad premissa vocatis specialiter et rogatis. Et ego Stephanus quondam Thedrici Wolff de Wartinberg clericus Vratislauiensis diocesis, publicus imperiali auctoritate notarius, quia prescriptarum litterarum apostolicarum exhibicioni, presentacioni, peticioni, decreti interposicioni, omnibus aliis et singulis premissis, dum sic coram prefato domino Iohanne officiali Wratislaviensi et per eum, ut premittitur, agerentur et fierent, unacum prenominatis testibus presens interfui eaque omnia et singula sic fieri vidi et audivi, ideo prescriptas litteras apostolicas de mandato pretacti domini Iohannis officialis de verbo ad verbum fideliter transsumpsi et transcripsi et manu propria exemplavi nil addens vel minuens, quod sensum aut facti substantiam[mmm)] immutet, viciet aut variet intellectum. Et quia auscultacione et collacione[nnn)] prehabita diligenti presens transsumptum seu publicum instrumentum cum dictis litteris originalibus per omnia concordare inveni, [134r] ideoque me hic subscripsi, publicavi et in hanc publicam formam redegi signo et nomine meis solitis unacum appensione sigilli officialatus Wratislaviensis consignando rogatus et requisitus in fidem et testimonium omnium et singulorum premissorum.

Quare pro parte dicti domini Andree Poznaniensis episcopi fuimus in hoc sacro Constanciensi concilio requisiti, ut attentis tam pia fundacione et largiflua donacione predictis a suis predecessoribus religiose factis ad ea manutenenda et efficaciter adimplenda, que preinsertis transsumptis designantur et specificantur, certis temporibus et nunc minus debite completa sunt, quam negligenciam moleste ferimus, dictum plebanum canonicum fratrem nostrum compellere seu compelli facere dignaremur, quodque nequaquam valeat ipse plebanus canonicus causam licitam in contrarium, ut premissa impleat, allegare de preceptoribus[ooo)] illuc pro presenti existentibus suarumque[ppp)] successorum obediencia ipsum eiusque successores imposterum penitus[qqq)] [liberum] sit, quod dumtaxat venerabili fratri nostro priori prioratus nostri Bohemie pro tempore existenti nobisque ac nostris successoribus plebanus ipse canonicus ac eius successores obedientiam prestare tenerentur. Nos igitur pias devotorum Christifidelium fundaciones debite cupientes adimpleri, volentes eciam ipsius domini Andree Poznansis episcopi pro premissis intercedentes contemplationi per nostre plenitudinem potestatis hac in re benigniter extendere, vobis tenore presencium in virtute sancte obedientie precipimus et mandamus, quatenus omnia et singula [in] preinsertis litteris fundatoriis contenta per eundem plebanum canonicum fratrem nostrum presentem et futurum faciatis exequi et ad effectum debitum deduci. Quemquidem plebanum canonicum ex uberiori gratia a predicti preceptoris obedientia per presentes nostras litteras eximimus ac[rrr)] decernimus causis ex predictis perpetuis temporibus eximendum, vobisque et vestris ac nobis et nostris successoribus dumtaxat eum volumus[sss] obedire teneri. Inhibentes harum serie litterarum sub eadem sancte obedientie virtute domus eiusdem Poznaniensis preceptori presenti suisque successoribus in futurum ac omnibus aliis fratribus domus nostre, cuiuscumque preeminencie, gradus aut dignitatis existant, ne contra premissa seu eorum aliquod facere vel venire presumant quoquomodo, quinymo ea studeant iuxta[ttt] earum seriem et tenorem inviolabiliter observare. In cuius rei testimonium bulla nostra plumbea in absencia bulle communis plumbee presentibus est appensa. Datum Constantie die tercia mensis Septembris anno incarnationis Domini M^mo^ CCCC^mo^ XVII^o^ [uuu].

Duplicata P. *marg.* *a)* iuxta *MS* *b)* qui *MS* *c)* tendum eiectione *MS* *d) dupl.* *e) lac. praem.* *f)* assignarunt *corr.* *g)* vicarius *praem. ante corr.* *h)* transuptorum *MS* *i-i) marg.* *j)* distancia *MS* *k)* ad *corr.* *l)* vetustas reduceret in ambiguum *tr. CDPM* *m)* et *add. CDPM* *n)* hospitalie *MS* *o)* Radovanus *CDPM* *p)* Meschone *CDPM* *q)* episcopi Poznaniensis *add. CDPM* *r)* possedistis *CDPM* *s)* nostra ecclesia *tr. CDPM* *t)* suis *male CDPM* *u)* ascriptis *praem. ante corr.*, ascrptis *corr.* *v)* Linp *praem. ante corr.* *w)* quod *CDPM* *x)* episcopus *add. CDPM* *y)* Vitozlaus *CDPM* *z)* Vitus *CDPM* *aa)* custos *CDPM* *bb)* g *supra lin.*, Bogfalus *CDPM* *cc)* Fabianus *CDPM* *dd)* Przibislaus *CDPM* *ee)* Petrcho *CDPM* *ff)* Hugo *CDPM* *gg)* Burgkardus *CDPM* *hh)* Nicolaus *CDPM* *ii)* possidenda *CDPM* *jj)* valeat *CDPM* *kk)* paginem *MS* *ll)* M^mo^ *add. ante corr.* *mm)* Rotgerus *CDPM* *nn)* Cusebius *MS* *oo)* Nicolaus *CDPM* *pp)* Fridricus *CDPM* *qq)* Gars filius *CDPM* *rr)* d *supra lin.;* Smaragdus *CDPM* *ss)* Nicolaus *CDPM* *tt)* Henrichus *CDPM* *uu)* p *praem. ante corr.;* Irlava *CDPM* *vv)* circunstantia *MS* *ww)* corvacuram *forsan* *xx)* l *supra lin.* *yy)* sigillo *MS* *zz)* ipsi *MS* *aaa)* plebanus *MS* *bbb)* signatorum *MS* *ccc)* Innocen. papa III *marg. de manu saec. XVII.* *ddd)* inferiius *corr.* *eee)* intertus *praem. ante corr.* *fff)* defendi *MS* *ggg)* ad *corr.* *hhh)* episcopus *marg. de manu saec. XVII.* *iii)* hospitalis in Polonia *repetit ante corr.* *jjj)* et *supra lin.* *kkk)* Sigrae *MS* *lll)* plebanus *MS* *mmm)* substentiam *MS* *nnn)* collocante *praem. ante corr.* *ooo)* preceptoriis *MS* *ppp)* suarumque *MS* *qqq) signum pro additione* *rrr)* et *corr.* *sss)* valumus *MS* *ttt)* iusta *MS* *uuu)* XVIII^mo^ *praem. ante corr.*

## 319

*Licence for Fr. Richard von Nordheim (Priory of* Alamania) *to travel to the Convent.*
*Straßburg, [1417] September 16*

*AOM 340 fol. 134r, under* prioratus Almanie et Boemie.

Die decimasexta mensis Septembris in Argentina anno quo supra data fuit licencia fratri Richardo de Northeim prioratus Alamanie[a] eundi ad conventum quando voluerit cum equis et armis sufficientibus secundum statuta etcetera.

*a)* nostri *praem. ante corr.*

## 320

*Licence for Fr. Henning Larsen, Bailiff of* Dacia, *to receive six men of legitimate noble birth as knights into the Order, who are to travel to the Convent.*

*[Straßburg, 1417 September 16]*

*AOM 340 fol. 134r, under* prioratus Almanie et Boemie. *Cf. Hatt Olsen (1962), 102 no. 9.*

Eadem die, mense, loco et anno predictis data fuit licencia fratri Hennyngho Laurencii baillivo Dacie prioratus Alamanie recipiendi[a)] sex viros in fratres milites religionis, dum tamen apti sint, sani et integri suis membris ac matrimonio legitimo nati nobiles ex utroque parente. Et eant ad conventum cum equis et armis etcetera.

*a)* Data *praem. ante corr.*

## 321

*Licence for Fr. Johann von Ow, Preceptor of Rottweil, to receive Markward von Ow as a knight brother of legitimate and noble birth into the Order, who is to travel to the Convent.*

*[Straßburg, 1417 September] 17*

*AOM 340 fol. 134r, under* prioratus Almanie et Boemie.

Die decimaseptima dicti mensis, loco et anno predictis data fuit licencia fratri Iohanni de Owe preceptori de Rautwil prioratus Alamanie recipiendi in fratrem militem religionis Margwardum de Owe dicti prioratus, dum tamen nobilis ex utroque parente matrimonio legittimo etcetera sanusque etcetera, ita tamen, quod eat ad conventum cum equis et armis sufficientibus secundum statuta etcetera.

*Cancellatum;* Revocatum fuit *marg.*

## 322

*Licence for Fr. Anton Knoblauch and Fr. Johann Lösel to travel to the Convent.*

*[Straßburg, 1417] September 19*

*AOM 340 fol. 134r, under* prioratus Almanie et Boemie.

Die XIX$^{a}$ dicti mensis Septembris loco et anno predictis data fuit licentia fratribus Anthonio dicto Klobelooch et Iohanni dicto Lôselin prioratus Alamanie eundi ad conventum, quando voluerint, cum equis et armis sufficientibus etcetera secundum statuta etcetera.

## 323

*The Master Fr. Philibert [de Naillac] licenses Fr. Johann Bennefelt, at his own request, to travel to the Convent.*

*Straßburg, 1417 September 20*

*AOM 340 fol. 134v, under* prioratus Almanie et Boemie.

Frater Philibertus etcetera religioso in Christo nobis carissimo fratri Iohanni Bennefelt prioratus nostri Alamanie domus eiusdem salutem et sinceram in Domino caritatem. Cum pro Dei servicio noster presencialiter Rodi conventus fratribus pluribus indigeat vosque, prout ex vestra assercione percepimus, desideretis illuc vestram transferre personam nostram superinde licenciam humiliter implorantes, hinc est, quod nos vestre huiusmodi supplicationi condigne benigniter inclinati eundi ad conventum ipsum in proximo futuro navigio licenciam eandem vobis tenore presencium impertimur. Dat. Argentine die XX$^{a}$ mensis Septembris anno incarnationis Domini M$^{mo}$ CCCC$^{mo}$ XVII$^{o}$.

Pro capellanis fratribus *suprascriptum.*

## 324

*Licence for Fr. Heinrich Walder von Zürich to travel to the Convent.*

*[Straßburg, 1417] September 22*

*AOM 340 fol. 135r, under* prioratus Almanie et Boemie.

Die XXII$^{a}$ mensis Septembris loco et anno predictis data fuit licencia fratri Henrico Walder de Thurego prioratus Alamanie eundi ad conventum cum equis et armis sufficientibus secundum statuta etcetera.

## 325

*The Master Fr. Philibert de Naillac retains Fr. Johann von Monreal, Bailiff of Cologne and Commander of Adenau (Priory of* Alamania).

*Straßburg, 1415 September 25*

*AOM 341 fol. 140r, under* prioratus Almanie et Boemie. *Cf. Delaville (1913), 334 note 4 (from p. 333).*

Frater Philibertus de Nailhaco etcetera religioso in Christo nobis carissimo fratri Iohanni de Monreall, baiulo Coloniensi et commendatori in Adenauwe prioratus nostri Alamanie domus eiusdem, salutem et sinceram in Domino caritatem. Dum laudabilia probitatis vestre merita in considerationis nostre aciem recensemus, digne credimus agere, cum vos inter alios domus nostre proceres attollimus prerogative specialis gratie et honoris. Igitur vestram volentes honorare personam, ut proinde vestre fidei et devocionis zelus ad laudabiliora[a)] inantea ferventius animetur, vos unacum dictis vestris baiuliis et arnesiis solutis per vos integre anuis dictarum baiuliarum responsionibus termino statuto et vobis et dictis baiuliis quibuscunque incumbentibus et incumbendis oneribus supportandis ad manus nostras tenore presencium de speciali gratia retinemus secundum bonos usus et laudabiles consuetudines domus nostre. Mandantes harum serie universis et singulis fratribus domus nostre quacunque auctoritate, dignitate, eminencia vel potestate suffultis, presentibus et futuris in virtute sancte obediencie firmiter et districte, ne contra presentis nostre retencionis gratiam aliquatenus venire presumant, quinymo eam studeant iuxta eius mentem et seriem inconcusse et inviolabiliter[b)] observare. In cuius rei testimonium bulla nostra plumbea presentibus est appensa. Dat. Argentine die vigesima quinta mensis Septembris anno incarnacionis Domini M[mo] CCCC[mo] decimo septimo.

*a)* laudabilia *corr.* *b)* imviolabiliter *MS*

## 326

*The Master Fr. Philibert [de Naillac], two procurators of the Convent, Fr. Gautier le Gras, Prior of the Conventual church, five named and other brethren (as no. 313) confirm the decision these eight brethren made on the same day. Both Fr. Hermann von Ow and Fr. Peter Salzfaß had appealed to the Master in their quarrel about the Preceptory of [Schwäbisch] Hall (Priory of* Alamania). *The Master had commissioned the eight brethren to find a decision. Fr. Gautier le Gras has read the decision in the presence of the legitimate procurators of the two parties. The preceptory belongs to Fr. Hermann von Ow who has been appointed by the Convent, not to Fr. Peter Salzfaß who has been appointed by the Prior. Silence is imposed on Fr. Peter Salzfaß but he shall be repaid all expenses he has spent for the benefit of the preceptory. The Prior of* Alamania *is to induct Fr. Hermann von Ow into possession of the Preceptory of Hall.*

*Straßburg, 1417 September 29*

*AOM 340 fol. 135r [fragm.,* Require ulterius *infrascriptum], fol. (137v-8r) [*Duplicata *marg.], fol. (138v) [fragm. cancellatum], under* prioratus Almanie et Boemie. *Cf. Delaville (1913), 333–4 note 4, with the date 27 September.*

Frater Philibertus etcetera religiosis in Christo nobis carissimis fratribus Hermano de Owe et Petro Saltzfasz prioratus nostri Alamanie domus eiusdem et eorum cuilibet salutem et sinceram in Domino caritatem. Cum certa nuper inter vos controversia coram nobis mota fuerit racione et ad causam baiulie seu preceptorie nostre de Hall dicti prioratus vestrum quolibet ius in eadem pretendente, prout ex vestrum cuiuslibet propositis sane perpendimus, nosque circa alia nostre religionis prepediti negocia rei huius cognicionem, decisionem et omnimodam determinationem religiosis in Christo[a] nobis carissimis fratribus Galtero Crassi decretorum doctori[b] priori ecclesie nostre conventualis Rodi, Iohanni Griuelli preceptori Chambarelli, procuratoribus nostri Rodi conventus, Willo Hulles Anglie, Iohanni de Porta Capue prioribus, Thome Skypuys turcoplerio dicti conventus, Iohanni de Patria ipsius thesaurario, Galioto Montet Burdegalensis et Henrico de[c] Bye sancti Iohannis Parisiensis preceptoribus[1] nobis assistentibus viva voce commiserimus nostram in hac parte plenariam ipsis concedentes auctoritatem, facultatem et potestatem[d], prenominati fratres nostri nostra racionabiliter exequentes mandata vestrum cuiuslibet racionibus et allegacionibus diligenter auditis ac curiose intellectis super hiis inter eos prehabita deliberatione matura ordinaverunt, pronunciaverunt, declaraverunt et sentenciaverunt secundum statuta, stabilimenta ac laudabiles usus et consuetudines nostre religionis, quod equum eis apparuit acque iustum. Quamquidem sententiam palam et publice vestrum de dicta preceptoria concedentes uno alterius vero procuratione legitimo presentibus et audientibus memoratus prior ecclesie nostre conventualis Rodi de prenominatorum collegarum suorum voluntate et assensu ac in vim mandati nostri pretacti alta et intelligibili voce protulit in hunc modum:

Christi nomine invocato nos fratres Galterus Crassi decretorum doctor prior ecclesie conventualis Rodi, Iohannes Griuelli preceptor Chambarelli, procuratores Rodi conventus, Willo Hulles Anglie, Iohannes de Porta Capue priores, Thomas Skypuyt turcoplerius dicti conventus, Iohannes de Patria ipsius thesaurarius, Galiotus Montet Burdegalensis et Henricus de Bye sancti Iohannis Parisiensis preceptores[1] deputati, commissi et ordinati ad infrascripta per reverendissimum in Christo patrem dominum fratrem Philibertum de Nailhaco etcetera visis, auditis et diligenter attentis, que per religiosos viros fratres Hermanum de Owe ex una et Petrum Saltzfasz partibus ex altera super titulo baiulie seu preceptorie de Hall prioratus Alamanie, quam ipsorum quilibet ad se spectare proponebat et asserebat, producta, dicta et allegata extiterunt matura et diligenti discussione et deliberatione prehabitis auctoritate et commissione

1) *The two procurators as no. 313, Fr. William Hulles, Prior of England, Fr. Jean de Porta, Prior of Capua, Fr. Thomas Skipwith, Turcopolier, Fr. Jean de Patria, Preceptor of Thévalles, Fr. Galliot Montet, Preceptor of Bordeaux, Fr. Henri de Bye, Preceptor of St-Jean in Paris.*

dicti reverendissimi in Christo patris domini magistri hospitalis nobis in hac parte factis dicimus, decernimus, pronunciamus, declaramus et sentenciamus dictam preceptoriam et spectasse et spectare debere eidem fratri Hermano de Owe bullas dominorum dicti Rodi conventus super collatione ipsius portanti et nobis eas in iudicio presentanti dictoque fratri Petro Salczfasz in vim collationis de dicta preceptoria per priorem Alamanie sibi facte ius sibi competere pretendenti silencium perpetuum [138r] imponimus et ab ipsius impeticione dictum fratrem Hermanum absolvimus. Item quia dictus frater Petrus in vim dicte collationis per eundem priorem Alamanie sibi facte ius sibi competere in eadem pretendens multas et diversas neccessarias et utiles expensas in dicta preceptoria se fecisse pretendit et asserit dictusque frater Hermanus plura ipsum fratrem Petrum de fructibus dicte preceptorie recepisse quam exposuisse asserit, eisdem commissione et auctoritate dicimus, decernimus, pronunciamus, declaramus et sentenciamus ipsi fratri Petro Saltzfasz debere omnes expensas utiles et neccessarias per ipsum factas per dictum fratrem Hermanum resarciri et refundi et viceversa omnes et singulos fructus, redditus et proventus ipsius preceptorie per dictum fratrem Petrum Saltzfasz perceptos et receptos, et qui per eum percipi et recipi potuerunt, ipsi fratri Hermano primitus debere ex integro restitui et resarciri. Data et pronunciata fuit hec sentencia in domo hospitalis predicti Argentine die penultima mensis Septembris anno Domini M$^{mo}$ CCCC$^{mo}$ XVII$^{o}$.

Nos igitur sententiam huiusmodi iuste facte, sancte et debite nostra auctoritate factam extitisse cognoscentes iuris utriusque vestrum conservacionem, prout ex iniuncto nobis incumbit officio, cupientes vobis et vestrum cuilibet in virtute sancte obedientie precipimus et mandamus, quatenus omnia et singula, que preinserta in sentencia continentur, quemadmodum auctoritate nostra lata sunt pronunciata et declarata, plenarium deducatis ad effectum et efficaciter observetis cautelis et dilacionibus ac aliis obstaculis in contrarium venientibus cessantibus quibuscunque. Mandantes eciam tenore presencium priori prioratus predicti seu et ipsius presidenti, ut vos prefatum fratrem Henricum[!] de Owe vel procuratorem vestrum in corporalem possessionem pacificam et quietam dicte baiulie de Hall inducat et conservet inductum omni contradicione remota amoto abinde quolibet detentore, si quis sit, quem nos amovemus per presentes et decernimus firmiter amovendum. Inhibentes etcetera ut in forma. In quorum omnium testimonium bulla nostra plumbea in absencia bulle communis plumbee presentibus est appensa. Dat. Argentine die predicta penultima mensis Septembris anno incarnationis Domini millesimo CCCC$^{mo}$ decimo septimo.

*a) fine fol. 135r.* *b)* doctoris *corr.* *c)* s *praem. ante corr.* *d) fine fol. 138v.*

## 327

*The Master Fr. Philibert [de Naillac], two procurators of the Convent, one named and other brethren (as no. 326) confirm the grant made by Fr. Hugo von Montfort,*

*Prior of* Alamania, *to Fr. Johann von Masmünster of the Preceptory of Sulz (Priory of* Alamania).

*Straßburg, 1417 October 1*

*AOM 340 fol. 138r-v, under* prioratus Almanie et Boemie.

Frater Philibertus etcetera religioso in Christo nobis carissimo fratri Iohanni de Masemunster prioratus nostri Alamanie domus eiusdem salutem et sinceram in Domino caritatem. Propter susceptum de vobis testimonium commendandum ac sperantes, quod in commisso vobis regimine effectus administrationis utilis dante Domino vos commendet, collacionem, concessionem et donacionem per religiosum in Christo nobis carissimum fratrem Hugonem de Montfort priorem prioratus nostri Alamanie de baiulia seu preceptoria nostra in Sulcz prioratus predicti modo et forma suis in litteris patentibus sigillo dicti prioratus sigillatis, de quibus nobis luculenter apparuit, contentis vobis factas ratas, gratas et placidas habentes collacionem, concessionem et donacionem huiusmodi ac omnia et singula in eisdem litteris collatoriis contenta de voluntate, consilio et assensu religiosorum in Christo nobis carissimorum fratrum Galteri Crassi decretorum doctoris, prioris ecclesie nostre conventualis Rodi, Iohannis Griuelli preceptoris Vallisfranche, procuratorum nostri Rodi conventus, Henrici de Bye preceptoris sancti Iohannis Parisiensis et aliorum fratrum plurium nobis [138v] assistencium de nostra certa sciencia et speciali gratia volumus, laudamus, approbamus, ratifficamus, emologamus ac nostre confirmationis patrocinio tenore presencium roboramus. Mandantes ac earum tenore presencium precipientes sub virtute sancte obedientie universis et singulis fratribus domus nostre quacunque auctoritate, dignitate vel officio fungentibus, presentibus et futuris, ne contra premissa et in dictis litteris contenta aliquathenus facere vel venire etcetera, quinymo etcetera. In cuius rei testimonium bulla nostra plumbea in absencia bulle communis plumbee presentibus est appensa. Dat. Argentine die prima mensis Ottobris anno incarnationis Domini M$^{mo}$ CCCC$^{mo}$ XVII$^{o}$.

## 328

*Licence for the chaplain Fr. Johann Broger (Priory of* Alamania) *to travel to the Convent with the next* passagium (*here* navigium).

*[Straßburg, 1417] October 2*

*AOM 340 fol. 138v, under* prioratus Almanie et Boemie.

Anno et loco predictis die secunda mensis Ottobris data fuit licentia fratri Iohanni Broger capellano[a] prioratus Alamanie eundi ad conventum ipsum[b] in proximo futuro navigio etcetera.

*a) supra lin.* *b)* servituri *add. ante corr.*

## 329

*The Master Fr. Philibert de Naillac orders Fr. Peter Mersner, Preceptor of Reichardsroth, to induct Fr. Hermann von Ow into possession of the Preceptory of [Schwäbisch] Hall (Priory of* Alamania) *in virtue of the sentence (no. 326) against Fr. Peter Salzfaß.*

*Basel, 1417 October 11*

*AOM 340 fol. 138v-9r, under* prioratus Almanie et Boemie. *Cf. Delaville (1913), 333–4 note 4.*

Frater Philibertus de Nailhaco etcetera religioso in Christo nobis carissimo fratri Petro Mersner preceptori de Roden prioratus nostri Alamanie domus eiusdem salutem etcetera. Cum nuper controversia quedam coram nobis inter domus predicte fratres Hermanum de Owe et Petrum Saltzfasz racione preceptorie de Hall predicti prioratus fuerit ipsorum quolibet ius in eadem certis mediantibus titulis sibi vendicante, quorum racionibus et allegacionibus coram nostris commissariis in hac parte propositis hincinde per eosdem commissarios iure cuiuslibet mature discusso sentenciatum extitit, ordinatum et decretum preceptoriam predictam de Hall eidem fratri Hermano spectare debere, alteri vero nullum in eadem fore ius quesitum. Quamquidem sententiam iuste latam extitisse cognoscentes approbavimus, laudavimus et voluimus ad effectum deduci, prout hec in nostra vera bulla plumbea superinde confecta lacius continentur. Volentes igitur, prout racioni congruit, in sententiam huiusmodi execucioni debite indilate deduci vobis tenore presencium in virtute sancte obediencie precipimus [139r] et mandamus, quatenus in vim eiusdem sententie prefatum fratrem Hermanum seu eius procuratorem legitimum in possessionem pacificam et quietam dicte baiulie seu preceptorie de Hall inducatis et conservetis inductum omni contradicione remota, amoto abinde dicto fratre Petro Saltzfasz seu alio quocunque detentore[a] illicito, quos per presentes amovemus et decernimus firmiter amovendum, sic in premissis vos habentes, quod de negligencia qualicunque nequaquam redargui valeatis. In cuius rei testimonium bulla nostra plumbea presentibus est appensa. Dat. Basilie die XI[a] mensis Ottobris anno incarnationis Domini M[mo] quadringentesimo decimo septimo.

Duplicata *marg.* *a)* si quis sit *add. ante corr.*

## 330

*The Master Fr. Philibert de Naillac orders Fr. Peter Mersner, Preceptor of Reichardsroth, to induct Fr. Hermann von Ow into possession of the Preceptory of Hall, since Hermann's claims against Fr. Peter Salzfaß have been accepted by the Master's commissioners.*

*Basel, 1417 October 11*

*AOM 341 fol. 140v, under* prioratus Almanie et Boemie. *Cf. Delaville (1913), 333–4 note 4.*

Frater Philibertus de Nailhaco etcetera religioso in Christo nobis carissimo fratri Petro Mersner preceptori de Roden prioratus nostri Alamanie domus eiusdem salutem etcetera. Cum nuper controversia quedam coram nobis inter domus predicte fratres Hermanum de Owe et Petrum Saltzfasz racione preceptorie de Hallis predicti prioratus fuerit ipsorum quolibet ius in eadem certis mediantibus titulis sibi vendicante, quorum racionibus et allegacionibus coram nostris comissariis in hac parte propositis hincinde per eosdem commissarios iure cuiuslibet mature discusso sentenciatum extitit, ordinatum et decretum preceptoriam predictam de Hallis eidem fratri Hermano spectare debere, alteri vero nullum in eadem fore ius quesitum, quamquidem sententiam iuste latam extitisse cognoscentes approbavimus, laudavimus et voluerimus ad effectum deduci, prout hic in nostra vera bulla plumbea superinde confecta lacius continetur. Volentes igitur, prout racioni congruit, sententiam huiusmodi execucioni debite indilate deduci vobis tenore presencium in virtute sancte obediencie precipimus et mandamus, quatenus in vim eiusdem sentencie prefatum fratrem Hermanum seu eius procuratorem legitimum in possessionem pacificam et quietam dicte baiulie seu preceptorie de Hallis inducatis et conservetis inductum omni contraditione remota, amoto abinde dicto fratre Petro Salczfasz seu alio quocunque detentore illicito, quos per presentes amovemus et decernimus firmiter amovendos[a)], sic in premissis vos habentes, quod de negligencia qualicunque nequaquam redargui valeatis. In cuius rei testimonium bulla nostra plumbea presentibus est appensa. Dat. Basilie die XI[a] mensis Octobris anno incarnacionis Domini M[mo] CCCC[mo] XVII[o].

*a)* ad *praem. ante corr.*

## 331

*The Master Fr. Philibert de Naillac, two procurators of the Convent, two named and other brethren concede that the Preceptory of Straßburg should pay merely 100 florins of the Rhine to the Treasury as* mortuaria *and* vacantia.

*Basel, 1417 October 13*

*AOM 340 fol. 139r, under* prioratus Almanie et Boemie.

Frater Philibertus de Nailhaco etcetera religiosis in Christo nobis carissimis fratribus commendatori et fratribus domus nostre Argentinensis presentibus et futuris prioratus nostri Alamanie domus eiusdem salutem et sinceram in Domino caritatem. Cum ex dicte domus fundacione primeva fuerit in divini cultus augmentacionis favorem per domus ipsius bone memorie fundatorem laudabiliter ordinatum omnes et quoscunque redditus tunc eidem domui datos et dimissos ac imposterum dandos et dimittendos ceteraque bona titulo elemosinario seu alio quovis modo a Christifidelibus collata, donata et conferenda adveniencia seu[a] accrescencia ad Dei servicium penitus applicari sic, quod commendator aut fratres predicti vel eorum aliquis quitquid de bonis huiusmodi sibi minime valeat seu valeant retinere aut in usus suos particulares in vita seu morte convertere quoquomodo. Sintque ad fundacionis eiusdem tuicionem et conservacionem[b] tres iamdicte civitatis cives laici dicte domus protectores, coram quibus et fratribus predictis pro tempore existentibus commendator prefate domus tunc existens tanquam nudus ipsius administrator singulis annis de per eum receptis sufficientem habet reddere racionem ex fundacione iamdicta perpetuo deputati ac eciam ordinati, prout hoc et alias ex predictis dependencia vidimus in fundatione memorata lacius contineri.[1] Quare vestra pro parte nobis humiliter extitit supplicatum, quatenus premissis attentis nostre religionis statutis, stabilimentis, usibus et consuetudinibus, de quibus nostra mediante visitacione maiorem habuistis cognicionem, non obstantibus quibuscunque de mortuario et vacante dicte domus nostro Rodi conventui spectantibus ad certam pecunie quantitatem nostro communi thesauro per vos ac successores vestros, quociens dicte domus casus vacationis evenerit, inantea solvendam graciose componere dignaremur. Nos igitur divini cultus augmentum, vite morumque vestrorum honestatem ac sepedicte fundacionis tenorem attente considerantes vestris in hac parte supplicacionibus favorabiliter inclinati de voluntate, consilio et assensu religiosorum in Christo nobis carissimorum fratrum Galteri Crassi decretorum doctoris, prioris ecclesie nostre conventualis Rodi, Iohannis Griuelli preceptoris Vallisfranche, dicti nostri conventus procuratorum, Iohannis de Porta prioris Capue, Galioti Montet Burdegalensis preceptorum[2] et aliorum fratrum nostrorum plurium nobis assistentium de nostra certa sciencia et speciali gratia volumus, statuimus, decernimus et ordinamus preceptoriam predictam cum suis membris, iuribus et pertinentiis universis exnunc inantea de mortuario et vacante predictis in qualibet vice et quociens eandem per mortem preceptoris pro tempore existentis vacare contigerit [c]pro summa centum florenorum auri Renensis boni et iusti ponderis seu[d] eorum valore receptori responsionum dicti prioratus pro tempore existenti libere solvendorum quictam esse, liberam et immunem. Inhibentes tenore presencium receptori predicto, ne vacantis et mortuarii predictorum occasione, dum eiusdem domus casus vacationis evenerit, quitquam ultra summam petere seu exigere presumat quoquomodo. In cuius rei testimonium bulla nostra plumbea in absencia bulle communis plumbee presentibus est appensa. Dat. Basilie die XIII[a] mensis Ottobris anno incarnationis Domini M[mo] CCCC[mo] decimo septimo.

*a) supra lin.* *b)* pro *add. ante corr.* *c) sublineatum;* Flor. 100 auri pro mortuario et vacante domus Argentinensis solvens receptori communis thesauri *marg. de manu saec. XVII.*

1) *1371 January 5, ed. Buchheit, Commanderies (2014), 281–4.*
2) *The two procurators as no. 313, but Grivel now Vaufranche, Fr. Jean de Porta, Prior of Capua, Fr. Galliot Montet, Preceptor of Bordeaux.*

## 332

*The Master Fr. Philibert [de Naillac], two procurators of the Convent, two named and other brethren (as no. 331) confirm to the Preceptor Fr. Erhard Thome and the brethren of Straßburg the concession made by Fr. Hugo von Montfort, Prior of* Alamania, *that the brethren of Straßburg shall be entitled to elect their preceptor themselves.*

*Basel, 1417 October 13*

*AOM 340 fol. 139v, under* prioratus Almanie et Boemie. *Cf. Delaville (1913), 332 note 2.*

Frater Philibertus etcetera religiosis in Christo nobis carissimis fratribus Erhardo Thome preceptori domus nostre Argentine ceterisque nostris fratribus nunc et imposterum in eadem residentibus salutem et sinceram in Domino caritatis affectum. Religiose vestre vite claritas divina cooperante gratia quamplurimos exemplariter fructus afferens, prout satis novimus apparenter, caritative nos inducit[a)], ut vos ac domum eandem prosequamur favoribus graciosis. Declarationem igitur per religiosum in Christo nobis carissimum fratrem Hugonem de Monteforti priorem prioratus nostri Alamanie in suo provinciali capitulo et de consensu fratrum sibi in eodem assistentium super electione preceptoris dicte domus per fratres ipsius, quociens casus vacationis eiusdem per mortem preceptoris evenerit facienda modo et forma suis in litteris patentibus sigillo communi dicti prioratus sigillatis, quibus nostre presentes annectuntur, lacius contentis factam ac omnes et singulas cautelas dictis in litteris ad opus electionis predicte declaratas ratas, gratas et placidas habentes declarationem huiusmodi ac omnia et singula dictis in litteris contenta de voluntate, consilio et assensu religiosorum in Christo nobis carissimorum fratrum Galteri Crassi decretorum doctoris, prioris ecclesie nostre conventualis Rodi, Iohannis Griuelli preceptoris Vallisfranche, procuratorum nostri Rodi conventus, Iohannis de Porta prioris Capue, Galioti Montet preceptoris Burdegalensis et aliorum fratrum nostrorum plurium nobis assistentium de nostra certa scientia et speciali gratia volumus, laudamus, approbamus, ratifficamus et nostre confirmationis[b)] patrocinio tenore presentium roboramus. Mandantes et tenore presencium precipientes sub virtute sancte obedientie universis et singulis fratribus domus nostre quacunque etcetera, quinymo etcetera. In cuius rei testimonium bulla nostra plumbea in absencia bulle communis plumbee presentibus est appensa. Dat. Basilie die decimatercia[c)] mensis Ottobris anno incarnationis Domini millesimo quadringentesimo decimo septimo.

Bulla confirmationis formam electionis preceptoris domus Argentinens. per fratres illius faciende *marg. de manu saec. XVII.* *a)* inducunt *corr.* *b)* confimationis *MS* *c)* XX *praem. ante corr.*

## 333

*The Master Fr. Philibert de Naillac, two procurators of the Convent, twelve named and other brethren confirm to Fr. Erhard Thome and his Preceptory of Straßburg the incorporation of the house in Schlettstadt made by the late Fr. Hesso Schlegelholz, Prior of* Alamania, *and his prioral chapter.*

*Constance, 1417 November 17*

*AOM 340 fol. 140r, under* prioratus Almanie et Boemie.

Frater Philibertus de Nailhaco etcetera religiosis in Christo nobis carissimis fratribus Erhardo Thome preceptori domus nostre Argentine ceterisque nostris fratribus nunc et imposterum in eadem residentibus prioratus nostri Alamanie domus eiusdem salutem et sinceram in Domino caritatem. Religiose vestre vite mundicia satis nota nostre considerationis in acie odorifera continuatione clarescens vobis ac eidem domui nos favorabiliter promovet inclinatos. Commendacionem igitur, unionem seu adiunccionem de domo nostra in Slezstat prioratus predicti cum iuribus et pertinenciis universis per domus eiusdem quondam fratrem Hessonem Slegelholtz sepedicti prioratus priorem, dum vivebat, in suo provinciali capitulo[1] et de consensu fratrum sibi in eodem assistentium modo et forma suis in litteris superinde confectis, quibus nostre presentes annectuntur, contentis vobis factas ac omnia alia et singula litteris in eisdem specificata et declarata rata, grata et placida habentes commendacionem, unionem seu adiunccionem huiusmodi ceteraque dictis in litteris contenta de voluntate, consilio et assensu religiosorum in Christo nobis carissimorum fratrum Galteri Crassi decretorum doctoris, prioris ecclesie nostre conventualis Rodi, Iohannis Griuelli preceptoris Chambarelli, procuratorum nostri Rodi conventus, Hugonis de Monteforti dicte prioratus Alamanie, Willelmi Hulles Anglie, Iohannis de Porta Capue priorum, Iohannis de Patria thesaurarii dicti conventus, Iohannis de Mayronis preceptoris Vapnicensis et procuratoris nostri generalis in curia Romana, Galioti Montet Burdegalensis, Anthonii de Balardis Florencie, Henrici de Bye sancti Iohannis Parisiensis, Henrici Streler Frankefordie, Petri Salzfasz in Erungen, Henrici Lůfrit in Veltklche, Petri Mersner in Rod, Remboldi[a] de Trůbel in Dorolzhein preceptorum[a][2] et aliorum fratrum nostrorum

1) *Heimbach, 1399: Rödel (1972), 193–4.*

2) *The two procurators as no. 331, Fr. Hugo von Montfort, Prior of* Alamania, *Fr. William Hull, Prior of England, Fr. Jean de Porta, Prior of Capua, Fr. Jean de Patria, Treasurer of the Convent, Fr. Jean de Meyronés, Preceptor of Gap and procruator general at the Roman curia, Fr. Galliot Montet, Preceptor of Bordeaux, Fr. Antonio dei Balardi, Preceptor of Florence, Fr. Henri de Bye, Preceptor of St-Jean in Paris, Fr. Heinrich Strhler, Preceptor of Frankfurt, Fr. Peter Salzfaß, Preceptor in Erdlingen, Fr. Heinrich Leutfrid, Preceptor in Feldkirch, Fr. Peter Mersner, Preceptor in Reichardsroth, Fr. Rembold zum Trübel, Preceptor in Dorlisheim.*

nobis assistentium de nostra certa sciencia et speciali gratia volumus, laudamus, approbamus, ratifficamus, confirmamus ac ex uberiori gratia de voluntate et assensu predictis dictam domum de Slezstat cum suis iuribus et pertinentiis universis eidem domui Argentine tenore presencium perpetuo unimus, adiungimus et annectimus et incorporamus iure tamen nostri conventus quoad responsiones inantea debite solvendas et alia onera racionabiliter incumbencia et incumbenda continue supportanda remanente semper salvo. Mandantes et tenore presencium precipientes universis et singulis fratribus domus nostre quacunque auctoritate, dignitate vel officio fungentibus, presentibus et futuris, ne contra confirmationem, unionem, adiunctionem et annectionem et incorporationem nostras huiusmodi ceterave dictis in litteris contenta aliquathenus facere vel venire presumant, quinymo ea studeant inviolabiliter observare. In cuius rei testimonium bulla nostra plumbea in absencia bulle communis plumbee presentibus est appensa. Dat. Constantie die XVII[tab)] mensis Novembris anno incarnationis Domini M[mo] CCCC[mo] XVII[o].

Confirmatio unionis domus in Sleystat domui Argentinensi *marg. (saec. XVII.)*
*a-a) marg.* *b)* XVI *corr.*

## 334

*The Master Fr. Philibert [de Naillac] confirms a sentence by Fr. Gautier le Gras, Prior of the Conventual church on Rhodes and commissioner of the Master for this case* (noster in hac parte locumtenens), *that Fr. Hugo von Montfort, Prior of* Alamania, *is to permit Fr. Johann von Monreal to remain Bailiff of Cologne. The responsions of the prioral chamber of Cologne are 75 florins, and Fr. Hugo must not permit Fr. Johann to reduce this sum by 25 florins. Fr. Hugo had granted Cologne to Fr. Johann in return for certain annual pension payments.*

*Constance, 1417 November 18*

*AOM 340 fol. 140v-41r, under* prioratus Almanie et Boemie. *Cf. Delaville (1913), 334 note 4 (from p. 333).*

Frater Philibertus etcetera. Cum questio quedam seu controversia mota coram nobis nuper extiterit inter religiosos in Christo nobis carissimos fratres Hugonem de Monteforti priorem prioratus nostri Alamanie parte ex una et Iohannem de Montreal baillivum Colonie parte ex altera in, de et super dicta Colonie baiulia priorali camera, quam prior ipse, licet eidem baillivo ad terminum vite sue in arrendamentum seu annuam pensionem certis sub pactis et convencionibus tradiderit, ut ex suis superinde confectis patentibus litteris liquet satis plane, tamen cuiusdam verbalis renunciationis per dictum baillivum, ut asserit idem prior, de arrendamento huiusmodi suis in manibus facte occasione dictam baiuliam seu cameram suam prioralem arrendamento predicto non obstante reassumere poterat et in effectu suis in manibus tenere volebat dicti baillivi renunciacionem acceptans. Ipse vero baillivus Colonie per organum domus eiusdem fratris Hermani commendatoris in Cronenberg procuratoris sui ad hec legitime constituti, ut ex instrumento procurationis sufficienter apparuit, multis mediis iamdicti prioris assercioni prefate respondendo dictam baiuliam dimittere non debere, sed eam pocius ad tempus vite sue sub pactis et conventionibus predictis regere et tenere allegabat petens insuper iuxta dicti prioris promissum viginti quinque florenos per eum super dicte baiulie responsione annua sibi data annuatim de responsione predicta singulis annis defalcari seu per dictum priorem sibi solvi. Dictis siquidem partibus, ipso videlicet priore personaliter, alterius vero baillivi prenominati procuratore predicto coram religioso in Christo nobis carissimo fratre Galtero Crassi decretorum doctore priore ecclesie nostre conventualis Rhodi, nostro in hac parte locumtenente, hodie comparentibus ac instantissime iusticiam super premissis sibi ministrari petentibus iuxta et secundum stabilimenta, statuta ususque et[a] laudabiles consuetudines domus nostre memoratus prior, noster in hac parte locuntenens, visis, auditis et diligenter inspectis allegatis, dictis et obiectis hincinde matura deliberatione prehabita cum religiosis in Christo nobis carissimis fratribus Iohanne de Porta Capue, Michaele Ferrandi Hungarie prioribus, Iohanne Griuelli Vallisfrance, Iohanne de Maronis Vapnicensis, Iohanne de Patria de Theualle nostri conventus thesaurario, Galioto Montet Burdegalensis, Anthonio de Balardis Florencie, Henrico de Bye sancti Iohannis Parisiensis preceptoribus et aliis fratribus nostris pluribus sibi assistentibus auctoritate nostra Christi nomine invocato dixit, pronunciavit, declaravit, decernit et sentenciando diffinivit dictam baiuliam Coloniensem cameram prioralem eis modo et forma, quibus eam dictus prior ipsi baillivo tradidit seu arrendavit, sibi remanere debere pensione tamen arrendamenti dicto priori iuxta tenorem instrumenti super hec confecti, ut pax inter eos servetur et pacta custodiantur, continue per eundem baillivum soluta. Quantum vero ad dictos viginti quinque florenos super responsione annua dicte baiulie eidem baillivo per dictum priorem remissos dixit, pronunciavit, declaravit, decernit et sentenciando diffinivit, ut supradictum priorem ipsos remittere [141r] nec quittare potuisse, cum responsio annua ad conventum spectet non ad ipsos dictum baillivum ad totalem responsionem dicte baiulie, que ad summam septuaginta quinque florenorum ascendit, singulis annis teneri dictum priorem a dictorum XXV florenorum ulteriori solucione[b] penitus absolvendo. Decernens insuper noster[c] in hac parte locuntenens sepedictus omnes et singulos baillivos et preceptores pretacti prioratus Alamanie ad integras soluciones responsionum suarum baiuliarum et preceptoriarum singulis annis teneri pactis, conventionibus seu remissionibus de quascunque quota seu parte per dictum priorem aliquibus preceptoribus seu baillivis hactenus factis et imposterum faciendis non obstantibus quibuscunque pacta, conventiones seu remissiones huiusmodi, si que forsitan facta fuerint, annullando et revocando ipsumque priorem penitus ab hiis absolvendo. Que supradicta omnia et singula per eundem nostrum locuntenentem dicta, pronunciata, declarata, decerta et sentenciando diffinita tanquam rationabilia rata et grata habentes laudamus, approbamus et ratifficamus nostrum in eisdem interponentes decretum pariter et assensum. Mandantes eisdem priori et baillivo et in virtute sancte obedientie tenore presencium precipientes, quatenus hanc nostri locuntenentis sententiam inviolabiliter observent. In cuius rei testimonium bulla nostra plumbea presentibus est appensa. Dat. Constantie die XVIII$^{a}$ mensis Novembris anno incarnationis Domini M$^{mo}$ CCCC$^{mo}$ XVII$^{o}$.

Duplicata *marg.* *a)* et c *praem. ante corr.* *b)* solucone *MS* *c)* nostri *corr.*

## 335

*The Master Fr. Philibert [de Naillac], two procurators of the Convent, five named and other brethren confirm to Fr. Rembold zum Trübel, Preceptor of Dorlisheim, 13 pounds 4 ounces of pennies of Straßburg as the annual revenues donated by the Hospitaller* soror *Anna, widow of the knight Wilhelm Knoblauch, in Dorlisheim and Hermolsheim on property of the squire Cunemar von Udenheim.*

*Constance, 1417 November 22*

*AOM 340 fol. 141r-v, under* prioratus Almanie et Boemie.

Frater Philibertus etcetera religioso in Christo nobis carissimo fratri Reimboldo in Trubel preceptori in Dorolzheim prioratus nostri Alamanie salutem et sinceram in Domino caritatem. Racioni congruit et condecens arbitramur laudabiles defunctorum intenciones extremasque voluntates, presertim cum a racionis tramite non deviant, efficaciter adimpleri. Cum igitur, sicuti vestra relatione accepimus, religiosa[a)] condam domus nostre soror Anna Kelobelochin defuncti domini Willelmi Kelobeches militis, dum viverit, a nobili Cůnemerario de V̊temhein armigero tridecim libras et quatuor uncias Argentinensium denariorum super redditibus et annuis censibus, bonis ceteris dicti nobilis in districtu Dorolzheim et Hermoltzheim existentibus annuatim capiendas pro se vobisque ac alio quod suo consanguineo vita exeunte vestrum cuiuslibet evicerit dictas tridecimas libras et quatuor uncias Argentinensium denariorum annui et perpetui redditus domui prefate in Dorelzheim post suum ac vestrum cuiuslibet decessum pro sue anime salute dimittens, prout hec eciam in litteris superinde confectis, quibus nostre presentes annectuntur, lacius continentur, dimissionem, voluntatem et ordinationem predictas ac cetera dictis in litteris contenta rata, grata et placida habentes de voluntate, de consilio et assensu religiosorum in Christo nobis carissimorum fratrum Galteri Crassi decretorum doctoris, prioris ecclesie nostre conventualis Rodi, Iohannis Griuelli preceptoris Vallisfranche, procuratorum nostri Rodi conventus, Iohannis de Porta prioris Capue, Iohannis de Patria thesaurarii dicti conventus, Iohanis de Mayronis procuratoris nostri generalis in curia Romana, Galioti Montet Burdegalensis et Henrici de Bye sancti Iohannis Parisiensis [preceptorum][1)] et aliorum fratrum plurium [141r] nobis assistentium de nostra certa sciencia et speciali gratia volumus, laudamus, approbamus, ratifficamus et nostre confirmationis patrocinio tenore presencium roboramus. Mandantes universis et singulis fratribus etcetera, ne contra dimissionem, voluntatem et ordinacionem predictas aliquathenus facere vel venire presumant, quinymo etcetera. In cuius rei testimonium bulla nostra plumbea in absencia bulle communis plumbee presentibus est appensa. Dat. Constancie die XXII[a] mensis Novembris anno incarnationis Domini M[mo] CCCC[mo] decimo septimo.

*a)* religioso *MS*

## 336

*Order to Fr. Peter Salzfaß, Preceptor of Erdlingen, Rexingen, Rothenburg and Regensburg, to travel to the Convent within nine months from presentation of the present letter. He has to obtain his superior's licence and is permitted to rent out his preceptories for three years.*

*[Constance, 1417] December 10*

*AOM 340 fol. 141v, under* prioratus Almanie et Boemie.

Die X[a] mensis Decembris loco et anno predictis mandatum fuit in virtute santte obedientie venerabili fratri Petro Saltzfasz commandatori Erlimgen, Rexsingen, Rotebourg, Regelspurg prioratus Alamanie, quod eat ad conventum infra novem menses a data presentacionis presencium computandos unacum licencia arrendandi dictas suas preceptorias et[a)] membra ipsarum ad tres annos ut in forma mandati super hoc confecti fratri Iohanni Bertier preceptori de Carguanilla prioratus Francie folio XXIII[o] ad longum continetur etcetera.

*a)* vel *corr.*

## 337

*The Master Fr. Philibert [de Naillac] orders the Preceptor of Zittau (Priory of Bohemia) to receive Peter le Bissig as sergeant-at-office into the Order and to maintain him in his preceptory.*

*Constance, [1417] December 10*

*AOM 340 fol. 141v, under* prioratus Almanie et Boemie.

1) *The two usual procurators, Porta, Patria, Mayronés, Montet and Bye.*

Frater Philibertus etcetera religioso in Christo nobis carissimo fratri commendatori in Ditaw prioratus nostri Boemie domus eiusdem salutem et sinceram in Domino caritatem. Votis dilecti nobis in Christo honesti viri Petri le Bissig desiderantis sub regulari habitu nostre religionis mundane conversacionis reiectis illecebris ferventi affeccione Deo omnipotenti, beate Marie virgini ac sancto Iohanni baptiste patrono nostro Christique pauperibus perpetuum impendere famulatum benigniter annuentes vobis tenore presencium committimus, precipimus et mandamus sub virtute sancte obediencie nichilominus firmiter iniungentes, quatenus eundem Petrum ad eius requisitionem, si opus fuerit, dum tamen ydoneus existat, recipiatis in nostre religionis fratrem servientem officii solenniter, ut moris est, sibique sic in fratrem recepto in dicta vestra commendaria stagiam seu residentiam assignetis, in qua ei provideatis seu provideri faciatis de suis neccessariis secundum bonos usus et laudabiles [consuetudines] sepedicte domus nostre, ad quod pariter vestri successores seu prefate commendarie regimini quovis titulo nunc vel imposterum presidentes teneantur. Dat. Constantie die decima mensis Decembris anno ut supra.

Ibi debet esse *[*propter *dupl. ante corr.]* propter datam *marg.*

## 338

*The Master Fr. Philibert [de Naillac] confirms a sentence by the Prior of the Convent Fr. Gautier le Gras who acted as the Master's commissioner and consulted four named and other experienced brethren. The parties involved had had to produce their proofs until 13 December. Following this sentence the Preceptory of Rothenburg (Priory of* Alamania*) belongs to Fr. Peter Mersner by reason of his appointment by Master and Convent (no. 213) and not to Fr. Peter Salzfaß and Fr. Johann Jagstheimer by reason of their appointment by the Prior of* Alamania.

*Constance, 1417 December 17*

*AOM 340 fol. 142r-v, under* prioratus Almanie et Boemie.

Frater Philibertus etcetera. Cum lis seu controversia quedam mota coram nobis nuper extiterit inter religiosos in Christo nobis carissimos fratres Petrum Merschmer agentem ex una[a)] et Petrum Saltzfasz ac Iohannem Iacsmer reos seu deffensores partibus ex altera super facto preceptorie de Rothembourg an der Duber, quam quelibet dictarum parcium, dictus videlicet Petrus Merschmer agens virtute collationis de eadem per nos et nostrum Rodi conventum sub bulla nostra[b)] communi et dicti conventus sibi facte, alii vero rei seu deffensores cuiusdam alterius collationis per religiosum in Christo nobis carissimum fratrem priorem prioratus nostri Almanie etcetera eis facte virtute sibi spectare, vendicabat, proponebat et allegabat, ipsisque partibus pro iusticia unicuique facienda terminum peremptorium assignaverimus ad comparendum coram nobis in die beate Lucie proxime lapsa et ad producendum hincinde bullas, litteras, cartas, instrumenta ac alia quecumque probacionum genera ius utriusque partis continencia procedendumque[c] in causa usque ad sententiam diffinitivam inclusive. Ad quem terminum prefate[d] partes cum omnibus et singulis suis iuribus coram religioso [142v] in Christo nobis carissimo fratre Galtero Crassi decretorum doctore priore ecclesie nostre conventualis Rodi, nostro in hac parte locumtenente, personaliter comparuerunt renunciato per dictas partes in causa et concluso. Memoratus prior, noster ut prefertur in hac parte locumtenens, visis, auditis et diligenter inspectis allegatis, dictis et obiectis hincinde matura deliberacione prehabita cum religiosis in Christo nobis carissimis fratribus Iohanne de Porta priore Capue, Iohanne Griuelli Vallisfranche, Michaele Ferrandi Verone, Henrico de Bie sancti Iohannis Parisiensis preceptoribus[1] et aliis quamplurimis fratribus nostris et iurisperitis sibi de nostro mandato assistentibus solum Deum habens pre oculis auctoritate nostra Christi nomine invocato dixit, pronunciavit, declaravit, decrevit et sentenciando diffinivit dictam baiulliam de Rothembourg ex causis dictis in bullis nostris eadem communi bulla communitum contentis et alias ad collationem nostram et dicti nostri conventus spectasse et pertinuisse nullumque ius ad eam conferendam dicto priori competiisse et sic consequenter collationem per eum de dicta preceptoria iamdictis fratribus Petro Saltzfasz et Iohanni Iacsmer contra nostrarum bullarum predictarum tenorem[e] factam nullam fuisse et esse quamquidem prefati prioris collationem seu donacionem sic ut premititur inaniter factam. Quatenus de facto processit, idem noster locumtenens auctoritate nostra cassavit, irritavit, revocavit et penitus adnullavit dictamque preceptoriam prenominato fratri Petro Merschmer in vim nostre sepedicte collationis adiudicandam fore decernit et adiudicavit ac ipsum in corporalem possessionem realem et liberam dicte preceptorie inducendum fore decernit et induxit sillencium perpetuum dictis reis seu deffensoribus super premissis imponendo ipsosque reos seu deffensores in fructibus dicte preceptorie, membrorum[f] et pertinenciarum eiusdem per eos aut suis nominibus perceptis[g] et qui percipi[h]potuerint restituendo dicto fratri Petro Merschmer in vim dictarum nostrarum bullarum et alias necnon in expensis per eum in hac causa factas condempnavit taxacione tamen ipsarum expensarum nobis reservata. Que supradicta omnia et singula per eundem nostrum locumtenentem dicta, pronunciata, declarata, decerta et sentenciando diffinita tanquam racionabilia et nostris statutis, stabilimentis, usibus et consuetudinibus laudabilibus consona rata et[i] grata habentes laudamus, approbamus et ratifficamus nostrum in eisdem decretum pariter et assensum. Mandantes eciam tenore presencium eidem priori in virtute sancte obedientie, ut prefatum fratrem Petrum Merschmer vel procuratorem suum in[j] corporalem possessionem pacificam et quietam dicte baiullie de Richembourg inducat et conservet inductum[k] omni contradicione remota amotis abinde dictis fratribus Petro Saltzfasz et Iohanni Iacsmer et aliis

1) *Fr. Jean de Porta, Prior of Capua, Fr. Jean Grivel, Preceptor of Vaufranche, Fr. Michele Ferrandi, Preceptor of Verona, Fr. Henri de Bye, Preceptor of St-Jean in Paris.*

detentoribus[l)] seu alio detentore, si qui sint, quos nos amovemus per presentes et decernimus firmiter amovendos ac dictis partibus sub eadem sancte obedientie virtute, quatenus prescriptam nostri eiusdem locumtenentis sentenciam inviolabiliter observent. In cuius rei testimonium bulla nostra plumbea presentibus est appensa. Datum Constantie die XVII[a] mensis Decembris anno incarnationis Domini millesimo[m)] CCCC[mo] decimo septimo.

*a)* partem *add. ante corr.* *b)* nostri *MS* *c)* procendum *MS* *d)* perfate *MS* *e)* teno *praem. ante corr.* *f)* memborum *MS* *g)* preceptis *MS* *h)* precipi *MS* *i) supra lin.* *j)* in p *praem. ante corr.* *k)* indutum *MS* *l)* detten *praem. ante corr.* *m)* M *praem. ante corr.*

## 339

*The Master Fr. Philibert de Naillac, two procurators of the Convent, Fr. Ulrich Kubler, Preceptor of Überlingen, and other brethren permit Fr. Heinrich Leutfrid, Preceptor of Feldkirch (Priory of* Alamania), *to leave his preceptory, where wars threaten his safety, and to reside in the Preceptory of Überlingen, whose Preceptor Fr. Ulrich Kubler agrees to provide him with the usual maintenance.*

*Constance, 1417 December 22*

*AOM 340 fol. 141v-2r, under* prioratus Almanie et Boemie.

Frater Philibertus de Nailhaco etcetera religioso in Christo nobis carissimo fratri Henrico Lůtfrid preceptori domus nostre in Veltkilch prioratus nostri Alamanie salutem et sinceram in Domino caritatem. Odor religiose vestre vite cum aliorum suffragancia meritorum nostram adusque noticiam fidedignorum relatione perductus nos inducit, ut vobis reddamur ad gratiam liberales. Cum itaque, prout vestra pro parte nobis fuit expositum, de vestre preceptorie residencia causantibus guerris inibi vigentibus diversis et variis speccibus vestre sit persone periculosa desideretisque omnipotenti Deo et nostre religioni secundum professionem per vos emissam acetero pacifice famulari residenciam [142r] vestram seu stagiam hiis de causis in domo nostra de V̊berlingen predicti prioratus, quoad vixeritis, humiliter implorantes. Hinc est, quod nos vestrum huiusmodi laudabile propositum considerantes de voluntate, consilio et assensu religiosorum in Christo nobis carissimorum fratrum Galteri Crassi decretorum doctoris, prioris ecclesie nostre conventualis Rodi et Iohannis Griuelli preceptoris Chambarelli, procuratorum nostri Rodi conventus, Vlrici Cubler dicte domus nostre de V̊berlingen preceptoris et aliorum fratrum nostrorum nobis assistencium de nostra certa scientia et speciali gratia vobis auctoritate presencium in preceptoria predicta de V̊berlingen ad vitam vestram stagiam assignamus. Mandantes sub virtute sancte obedientie preceptori predicto et suis successoribus aut quovis alio titulo prefate preceptorie regimini presidentibus nunc vel imposterum, ut vos ad eandem moraturum venientem pro stagia ad stagiam ipsam benigne admittat et caritative pertractet vobisque, quamdiu vixeritis, in preceptoria ipsa de vestris neccessariis provideat secundum usus bonos et consuetudines laudabiles domus nostre dicta preceptoria de Veltkilch, quam obtinetis, non obstante. Volumus tamen, quod[a)], quamdiu stagiam in eadem preceptoria de V̊berlingen vos habere contigerit, eidem preceptori suisque successoribus reverenciam exhibeatis ac sub eius obediencia persistatis. Quocirca universis et singulis fratribus domus nostre presentibus et futuris, cuiuscunque status, gradus vel condicionis existant, sub virtute sancte obedientie supradicta districte[b)] mandantes precipimus, ne contra predictam nostram assignationem stagie nullathenus venire presumant, quinymo efficaciter illam servent. In cuius rei testimonium bulla nostra plumbea in absencia bulle communis plumbee presentibus est appensa. Dat. Constantie die vigesima II$^{a}$ mensis Decembris anno incarnationis Domini M$^{mo}$ CCCC$^{mo}$ XVII$^{o}$.

*a)* quam *MS* *b)* virtute *praem. ante corr.*

## 340

*The Master Fr. Philibert [de Naillac] retains Fr. Nikolaus Weisly, Preceptor of Freiburg and Neuenburg (Priory of* Alamania), *with his preceptories.*

*Constance, 1418 January 3*

*AOM 341 fol. 140v-41r, under* prioratus Almanie et Boemie.

Frater Philibertus etcetera religioso in Christo nobis carissimo fratri Nicholao[a)] Weisly commandatori de Friburg ac de Novo Castro prioratus nostri Alamanie domus eiusdem salutem et sinceram in Domino caritatem. Dum laudabilia probitatis vestre merita in considerationis nostre aciem recensemus, digne credimus agere, cum vos inter alios domus nostre proceres attollimus prerogativa specialis gratie et honoris. Igitur vestram volentes honorare personam, ut proinde vestre fidei et devotionis zelus ad laudabiliora[b)] inantea fervencius animetur, vos unacum dictis vestris baiuliis membrisque ipsarum ac arnesiis solutis per vos integre anuis dictarum baiuliarum responsionibus termino statuto et vobis et dictis baiuliis quibuscunque incumbentibus et incumbendis oneribus supportandis ad manus nostras tenore presencium de speciali gratia retinemus secundum bonos usus et laudabiles consuetudines domus nostre. Mandantes harum serie universis et singulis fratribus domus nostre quacumque auctoritate, dignitate, eminencia vel potestate suffultis, presentibus et futuris [141r] in virtute sancte obediencie firmiter et districte, ne contra presentis nostre retentionis gratiam aliquathenus venire presumant, quinymo eam studeant iuxta[c)] eius mentem et seriem inconcusse et inviolabiliter observare. In cuius rei testimonium bulla nostra plumbea presentibus est appensa. Data Constancie die tercia mensis Ianuarii anno incarnationis Domini millesimo CCCC$^{mo}$ decimo septimo.

*a)* Nicholaus *corr.* *b)* laudabilia *corr.* *c)* inviolabiliter *praem. ante corr.*

## 341

*The Master Fr. Philibert [de Naillac] orders the Preceptors of Villingen Fr. Johann [Söler von] Richtenberg and of Mergentheim Fr. Wilhelm von Hailfingen to induct Fr. Peter Mersner according to a sentence (no. 338) in his favour against Fr. Peter Salzfaß and Fr. Johann Jagstheimer into possession of the preceptory of Rothenburg (Priory of* Alamania).

*Constance, 1418 January 5*

*AOM 340 fol. 143r, under* prioratus Almanie et Boemie. *Cf. Delaville (1913), 334 note 4 (from p. 333).*

Frater Philibertus etcetera religiosis in Christo nobis carissimis fratribus Iohanni[a] Richttemberg commendatori de Filingen et Willelmo de Halfingen commendatori de Mergelhaym et eorum cuilibet prioratus nostri Almanie domus eiusdem salutem et sinceram in Domino caritatem. Cum nuper controversia quedam coram nobis inter religiosos in Christo nobis carissimos fratres Petrum Merschner[b] agentem ex una[c] et Petrum Saltzfasz ac Iohannem Iacsmer reos seu deffensores partibus ex altera super facto preceptorie de Rothembourg an der Duber dicti prioratus mota fuerit ipsorum quolibet ius in eadem certis mediantibus titulis sibi vendicante, quorum rationibus et allegationibus coram nostris commissariis in hac parte propositis hincinde per eosdem commissarios iure cuiuslibet mature discusso sentenciatum extitit ordinatum et decretum preceptoriam predictam de Rotthembourg eidem fratri Petro Merschmer spectare debere, alteri vero Petri nullum in eadem fore ius quesitum, quamquidem sententiam iuste latam extitisse cognoscentes approbavimus, laudavimus et voluimus ad effectum deduci, prout hec in nostra vera bulla plumbea superinde confecta lacius continentur. Volentes igitur, prout rationi congruit, sententiam huiusmodi execucioni debite indilate deduci vobis et vestrum cuilibet tenore[d] presencium in virtute sancte obedientie precipimus et mandamus, quatenus in vim eiusdem sentencie prefatum fratrem Petrum Merschmer seu eius procuratorem[e] legitimum in possessionem[f] pacificam dicte baiullie seu preceptorie de Rotthembourg inducatis et conservetis inductum omni contradictione remota amotis abinde dictis fratribus Petro Saltzfasz et Iohanni Iacsmer seu aliis quibuscumque detentoribus illicitis, quos per presentes amovemus et decernimus firmiter amovendum sic in premissis vos habentes, quod de negligentia qualicumque nequaquam redargui valeatis. In cuius rei testimonium bulla nostra plumbea presentibus est appensa. Datum Constantie die quinta mensis Ianuarii anno incarnationis Domini millesimo quadringentesimo decimoseptimo.

*a)* Ri *praem. ante corr.* *b)* Mes *praem. ante corr.* *c)* vana *MS* *d)* tonere *MS* *e)* procurem *praem. ante corr.* *f)* ppo *praem.*, passificam, pacis *add. ante corr.*

## 342

*The Master Fr. Philibert [de Naillac] licenses Fr. Heinrich Schildknecht (Priory of* Alamania) *to travel to the Convent with the next* navigium.

*Constance, 1418 January 10*

*AOM 340 fol. 143r, under* prioratus Almanie et Boemie.

Frater Philibertus etcetera religioso in Christo nobis carissimo fratri Henrico Schiltkneht prioratus nostri Alamanie domus eiusdem salutem etcetera. Cum pro Dei servicio noster presencialiter Rodi conventus fratribus pluribus indigeat vosque, prout ex vestra assercione percepimus, desideretis illuc vestram personam transferre nostram superinde licenciam humiliter implorantes, hinc est, quod nos vestre huiusmodi supplicationi condigne benigniter inclinati eundi ad conventum ipsum in proximo futuro navigio licenciam eandem vobis tenore presencium impertimur. Dat. Constantie die decima mensis Ianuarii anno incarnationis Domini M$^{mo}$ CCCC$^{mo}$ XVII$^{o}$.

## 343

*The Master Fr. Philibert [de Naillac], two procurators of the Convent, three named and other brethren confirm Fr. Konrad von Burgel in the house of Bruchsal, which has been granted him by Fr. Konrad von Biblis, Preceptor of Heimbach, with the consent of Fr. Hugo von Montfort, Prior of* Alamania, *and his prioral chapter.*

*Constance, 1418 January 14*

*AOM 340 fol. 143v, under* prioratus Almanie et Boemie.

Frater Philibertus etcetera religioso in Christo nobis carissimo fratri Cůnrado de Burgel prioratus nostri Alamanie domus eiusdem salutem et sinceram in Domino caritatem. Propter susceptum de vobis testimonium commendandum ac sperantes, quod in commisso vobis regimine effectus administrationis utilis dante Domino vos commendet, collationem, concessionem, tradicionem et donacionem per domus eiusdem fratrem Cůnradum de Bybellosz preceptorem in Heimbach de voluntate, consilio et assensu religiosi in Christo nobis carissimi fratris Hugonis de Montfort dicti prioratus[a] prioris et aliorum fratrum sibi in suo provinciali capitulo assistentium de domo nostra de Brůszel a dicta preceptoria in Heimbach dependente modo et forma suis in litteris patentibus sigillo dictorum prioratus et preceptoris sigillatis, quibus nostre presentes annectuntur, contentis vobis factas ratas et gratas et placidas habentes collationem, concessionem, tradicionem et donacionem huiusmodi ac omnia et singula in eisdem litteris contenta de voluntate, consilio et assensu religiosorum in Christo nobis carissimorum fratrum Galteri Crassi decretorum doctoris prioris ecclesie nostre conventualis Rodi, Iohannis Griuelli preceptoris Chambarelli, procuratorum nostri Rodi conventus, Iohannis de Porta prioris Capue, Michaelis Ferrandi Verone et Henrici de Bye Parisiensis preceptorum[1] pluriumque fratrum nostrorum aliorum nobis assistentium de nostra certa scientia et speciali gratia volumus, laudamus, approbamus, ratifficamus, emologamus ac nostre confirmationis patrocinio tenore presencium roboramus. Mandantes et tenore presencium precipientes sub virtute sancte obedientie universis et singulis fratribus domus nostre quacumque auctoritate, dignitate vel officio fungentibus, presentibus et futuris, ne contra premissa et in dictis litteris contenta aliquathenus facere vel venire presumant, quinymo ea studeant iuxta eorum mentem et seriem inviolabiliter observare. In cuius rei testimonium bulla nostra plumbea in absentia bulle communis plumbee presentibus est appensa. Dat. Constantie die XIIII[ta] mensis Ianuarii anno incarnationis Domini M[mo] quadringentesimo decimoseptimo.

*a) dupl.*

## 344

*The Master Fr. Philibert de Naillac, two procurators of the Convent, four named and other brethren constitute the Preceptors of Frankfurt Fr. Heinrich Streler and of Straßburg Fr. Erhard Thome as receivers in the Priory of* Alamania. *The two receivers have exactly the same powers. What one of them begins can be continued and finished by the other. They are to collect the responsions and arrears of responsions of all preceptories, offices and houses in the Priory of* Alamania *and of all chambers, the* procrassia, mortuaria, iocalia *and other dues of dead brethren and all other dues to the Treasury according to the statute of 1367. They are to audit accounts and to issue receipts.*

*Constance, 1418 January 15*

*AOM 340 fol. 143v-4r, under* prioratus Almanie et Boemie.

Noverint universi et singuli visuri et audituri presentem constitucionem procuratorum et receptorum responsionum et aliorum in presenti constitucione contentorum et expressorum, quoniam nos frater Philibertus de Nailhaco etcetera confisi de fidei legalitate et circunspeccionis industria religiosorum in Christo nobis carissimorum fratrum Henrici Streler Frankefordie et Erhardi Thome Argentine preceptorum[a] domus eiusdem eosdem fratres Henricum Streler et Erhardum Thome licet absentes[b] tanquam presentes et eorum quemlibet insolidum ita, quod non sit melior condicio primitus occupantis, sed quod per unum ipsorum inceptum[c] fuerit, per eum resumi valeat, prosequi et finiri, tenore presencium de voluntate, consilio et assensu religiosorum in Christo nobis carissimorum fratrum Galteri Crassi decretorum doctoris prioris ecclesie nostre

1) *The two procurators as no. 313, Fr. Jean de Porta, Prior of Capua, Fr. Michele Ferrandi, Preceptor of Verona, Fr. Henri de Bye, Preceptor of St-Jean in Paris.*

conventualis Rodi, Iohannis Griuelli[d] preceptoris Vallisfranche, procuratorum nostri Rodi conventus, Iohannis de Porta Capue prioris, Iohannis de Mayronis Vapnicensis, procuratoris nostri generalis in curia Romana, Michaelis Ferrandi Verone, [144r] Henrici de Bie sancti Iohannis Parisiensis preceptorum[1] et aliorum nostrorum fratrum plurium domus nostre nobis assistentium de nostra certa scientia facimus, creamus et solenniter ordinamus nostros ac dicti conventus et dicte domus nostre procuratores, receptores, actores, sindicos, yconomos et nuncios speciales et generales negociorumque gestores ad petendum, recipiendum, recuperandum et habendum nostri ac dicti conventus et domus nostre predicte procuratorio[e] nomine atque vice omnes et singulas responsiones, arreragia responcionum omnium et singularum preceptoriarum, baiuliarum et domorum prioratus nostri Alamanie tam camerarum dicti prioratus quam omnium et singularum baiuliarum et domorum aliarum quarumcumque prioratus eiusdem. Item ad petendum, recuperandum et habendum quo supra nomine tam de preterito tempore quam presenti et futuro omnia procrassia[f] et mortuaria ac iocalia, res et bona alia, quecumque sint et quovis nomine nuncupata et in quibuscumque consistant, omnium et singulorum fratrum domus nostre, prioris et preceptorum seu quorumvis aliorum mortuorum iam inantea moriturorum, in predicto prioratu ad nos et dictum conventum ac communem thesaurum debencia pervenire secundum statutum promulgatum[g] et factum super hoc in generali capitulo[h] apud Avinionem de mense Marcii anno incarnationis Domini M° CCC$^{mo}$ sexagesimo sexto celebrato[2] seu quovis alio modo. Item ad petendum, recuperandum, recipiendum et habendum quo supra nomine omnes et singulas pecuniarum summas ac bona, res et iura alia, quecumque fuerint et quovis nomine nuncupata, nobis et dicto conventui ac communi thesauro debitas et debita, debendas et debenda et nobis et dicto conventui et communi thesauro pertinentes et debencia pervenire quovis titulo, racione vel causa tam per domus nostre quam per personas alias quaslibet aliarum religionum religiosas seu ecclesiasticas et mundanas[i]. Item ad petendum et audiendum raciones, compota quo supra nomine de predictis et altero eorundem ab omnibus et singulis, ad quos de premissis compota, raciones ponere[j] spectabit et quomodolibet pertinebit, et ad ponendum dicta compota et raciones eos et eorum quemlibet auctoritate nostra dictorumque conventus et communis thesauri efficaciter compellendum ipsaque compota et raciones examinandum, allocandum, approbandum et reprobandum in toto vel in parte ipsaque concludendum et diffiniendum, prout dictis procuratoribus aut eorum alteri videbitur expedire et que nobis predictisque conventui et communi thesauro predicta compota deberi et provenire debere compecierint petendum, recipiendum et habendum. Item ad faciendum quo supra nomine de receptis quittantias perpetuo valituras. Dantes etcetera et generaliter etcetera. Mandantes etcetera. In cuius rei testimonium bulla nostra

1) *As no. 343, and Fr. Jean de Meyronés, Preceptor of Gap.*

2) *March 1367: Delaville (1913), 162.*

plumbea in absencia bulle communis plumbee presentibus est appensa. Datum Constantie die decimaquinta mensis Ianuarii anno incarnacionis Domini millesimo quadringentesimo decimoseptimo.

*a)* sancti Iohannis Iherosolim. *praem. ante corr.* *b)* abstentes *MS* *c)* in *praem. ante corr.* *d)* Griuelli *praem. ante corr.* *e)* procurato *MS* *f)* procra *praem. ante corr.* *g)* premulgatum *MS* *h)* consilio *praem. ante corr.* *i)* mundanas *praem. ante corr.* *j)* spectare *praem. ante corr.*

## 345

*The Master Fr. Philibert [de Naillac] appoints Fr. Johann [Söler] von Richtenberg, Preceptor of Villingen (priory of* Alamania), *to be his* socius *and familiar.*

*Constance, [1418] January 22*

*AOM 341 fol. 141r, under* prioratus Almanie et Boemie.

Frater Philibertus etcetera religioso in Christo nobis carissimo fratri Iohanni de Richemberg preceptori de Vilingen prioratus nostri Alamanie domus eiusdem salutem et sinceram in Domino caritatem. Probitatis merita, morum decor et religionis honestas, quibus personam vestram illarum largitor Dominus multipliciter insignivit, necnon fervens ac fidelis devotio, quam ad nos et religionem nostram vos exibere dignoscimus, mentem nostram hortantur et pulsant, ut personam vestram eandem congruis, quibus possimus[a)], honoribus decoremus. Hinc est, quod premissorum meritorum vestrorum intuitu vos exnunc in socium et familiarem nostrum de speciali benivolencia admittentes aliorum sociorum et familiarium nostrorum consortio tenore presencium aggregamus, ut tanto libencius de cetero cultui bonitatis intendere conemini, quanto exhibitus vobis honor pocioris vel onus maturitatis importat, quantoque facilius pro hoc ad maiora poteritis dante Domino promoveri, volentes, ut, ubicunque deinceps fueritis, tanquam nostrum et inter nostros socios et familiares ascriptum vos nostre protectionis et tuicionis presidio confoveri ac pro vestris agendis, cum expedierit, ubicunque fuerimus, ad nostram presenciam cum fiducia accessum liberum vos habere. In cuius rei testimonium bulla nostra plumbea presentibus est appensa. Dat. Constancie die XXII[a] mensis Ianuarii anno quo supra.

*a)* possemus *corr.*

## 346

*The Master Fr. Philibert de Naillac confirms a sentence by Fr. Gautier le Gras, Prior of the Conventual church, his commissioner for this case, and three named brethren that the brethren of the Mark of Brandenburg and of Lower* Alamania, *represented by their procurator Fr. Heinrich Streler, Preceptor of Frankfurt, shall continue to support the usual expenses for running the priory.*

*Constance, 1418 January 28*

*AOM 340 fol. 144r-v, under* prioratus Almanie et Boemie.

Frater Philibertus de Nailhaco etcetera. Cum lis seu controversia quedam mota racione et ad causam nostre baiullie de Marchia nuper extiterit inter religiosos in Christo nobis carissimos fratres superioris Almanie ex una et alios inferioris Almanie partibus ex altera super contributacionibus[!], nusiis[a] et expensis interdum pro negociis in nostro prioratu Almanie supportari neccessariis ipsisque partibus pro bono pacis [144v] et iusticia cuilibet ipsarum ministranda terminum peremptorium assignaverimus ad comparendum coram nobis ad diem undecimam mensis Novembris ultimo preteriti et ad producendum hincinde quecumque sua iura ceteraque probacionum[b] genera ius utriuslibet ipsarum partium concernencia[c] procedendumque in causa usque ad sentenciam diffinitivam inclusive, ad quem terminum comparente religioso viro fratre Henrico Streler preceptore[d] de Frankafordia[e], procuratore fratrum[f] de bassa Almania tam nomine proprio quam procuratorio, de quo fidem fecit, parte ex una, aliis vero nomine comparentibus in ipsorum contumaciam Dei presentia repletam cum omnibus et singulis suis iuribus coram religioso in Christo nobis carissimo fratre Galtero Crassi decretorum doctore, priore ecclesie nostre conventualis Rodi, nostro[g] in hac parte locumtenente coram quo per ipsum procuratorem comparentem renunciato et concluso sentenciam ferri petentem memoratus prior noster ut prefertur in hac parte locumtenens visis, auditis et diligenter inspectis dictis, allegatis et obiectis hincinde matura deliberacione prehabita cum religiosis in Christo nobis carissimis fratribus Iohanne de Porta priore Capue, Iohanne Griuelli Valisfranche, Henrico de Bye sancti Iohannis Parisiensis preceptoribus[1] et aliis quamplurimis fratribus nostris sibi de mandato nostro assistentibus solum Deum habens pre oculis auctoritate nostra Christi nomine invocato dixit, pronunciavit, declaravit, decernit et sentenciando diffinivit pacem inter dictas partes inantea servari ac consueta iuxta pacta hactenus inter eas super contributacionibus[!] huiusmodi facta custodiri secundum tenorem instrumenti super hoc confecti, nostro tamen ac Rodi nostri conventus iure in omnibus semper salvo. Que supradicta omnia[h] et singula per eundem nostrum locumtenentem dicta, pronunciata, declarata, decerta et sentenciando diffinita tamquam racionabilia et nostris statutis, stabilimentis, usibus et consuetudinibus laudabilibus consona rata et grata habentes laudamus, approbamus et ratifficamus nostrum in eisdem interponentes decretum pariter et assensum. Mandantes in virtute sancte obedientie[i] tenore presencium partibus predictis, quatenus nostri

1) *Fr. Jean de Porta, Prior of Capua, Fr. Jean Grivel, Preceptor of Vaufranche, Fr. Henri de Bye, Preceptor of St-Jean in Paris.*

prefati locumtenentis huiusmodi sentenciam studeant inviolabiliter observare. In cuius rei testimonium bulla nostra plumbea in absencia bulle communis plumbee presentibus est appensa. Datum Constantie die XXVIII[a] mensis Ianuarii anno incarnacionis Domini millesimo quadringentesimo decimoseptimo.

*a) forsan* noxiis. *b)* probaconum *MS* *c)* concernenciam *MS* *d)* preceptor *MS* *e)* Frank *praem. ante corr.* *f)* de *praem. ante corr.* *g) supra lin.* *h) praem. corr.* *i)* obdientie *MS*

## 347

*The Master Fr. Philibert [de Naillac] quits Fr. Johann von Ow, Preceptor of Rottweil, for 30 florins of the Rhine or 24 ducats of Venice received through Fr. Johann von Monreal, Preceptor of Cologne. The Master promises to pay this sum which is for one year's* pitancia *to the Tongue of* Alamania *in the Convent.*

*Constance, 1418 February 10*

*AOM 341 fol. 141r, under* prioratus Almanie et Boemie.

Noverint universi et singuli presentes recognitionis litteras inspecturi[a)], quod nos frater Philibertus de Nailhaco etcetera fatemur, recognoscimus et in verbo veritatis testamur habuisse et recepisse[b)] a religioso in Christo nobis carissimo fratre Iohanne de Auwe, commendatore de Rotwyl, per manus domus eiusdem fratris Iohannis de Monreal[c)], commendatori[s] Coloniensis, pro pitanciis unius anni fratrum lingue Alamanie in nostro Rodi conventu degencium summam triginta florenorum auri Renenis viginti quatuor ducatorum Venetorum auri valentium, de quaquidem summa per nos quo supra nomine recepta dictos fratres Iohannem de Rotwyl et Iohannem de Monreal et alios, quos tangit et tangere potest aut poterit in futurum, quittamus, liberamus et absolvimus per presentes ac erga dictos fratres eiusdem lingue Alamanie quittos reddere promittimus et immunes. In cuius rei testimonium nostrum presentibus fecimus apponi sigillum. Dat. Constancie d[i]e[d)] X[a] mensis Februarii anno incarnationis Domini M[mo] CCCC[mo] XVII[o].

*a)* visuri *add. ante corr.* *b)* relig *praem. ante corr.* *c)* Montebel *praem. ante corr.*

## 348

*The Master Fr. Philibert [de Naillac] orders Fr. Hugo von Montfort, Prior of* Alamania, *to expend 2,000 florins and other goods of the* mortuarium *of Fr. Hesso Schlegelholz on the ruined Preceptory of Freiburg, as had been previously ordered (no. 272).*

*Constance, 1418 February 10*

*AOM 340 fol. 169v-70r, after* prioratus Baroli, Capue et Messane et alie partes regni. *Cf. Delaville (1913), 333 note 2, with the date 18 February.*

Frater Philibertus etcetera religioso in Christo nobis carissimo fratri Hugoni de Monfort priori prioratus nostri Alamanie domus eiusdem salutem et sinceram in Domino caritatem. Cum dudum per has partes anno videlicet Domini millesimo CCCC^mo^ XIII° transitum faciendo post habitam per vos et alios fratres nostros quamplures fidedignos de nostre domus Friburgensis desolacione, ruina et quasi totali detrimento noticiam, duo mille florenos ex mortuario domus eiusdem quondam fratris Hessonis Selegelholz provenientibus et nostro comuni thesauro spectantes ac omnia quecunque alia bona dicti defuncti, ubicunque reperiri possent, ad reedificationem, reparationem et manutenenciam prefate domus nostre Friburgensis ordinaverimus[a] et expresse converti voluerimus ac domus eiusdem fratri Erhardo Thome preceptori Argentine dictorum duorum milium florenorum custodi mandaverimus ipsa duo milia et alia quecunque dicti defuncti bona in usus predictos nec alibi quomodolibet applicanda vestris in manibus deponi vobis tunc nobis personaliter assistenti et omne huiusmodi liberaliter assumenti nostrarum ordinacionis et voluntatis predictarum execucionem committentes, prout hec et alia nostris in litteris superinde confectis lacius continentur desideremusque summopere dicta duo milia florenorum et alia bona de mortuario dicti fratris Hessonis recuperata [170r] et recuperanda, que nondum[b] ut asseritur fuerunt ad id applicata, ad usus predictos infallibiliter applicari iuxta dictarum nostrarum litterarum seriem et tenorem. Vobis in virtute sancte obediencie precipimus et mandamus, quatenus omnia per vos recepta tam a dicto preceptore Argentine quam aliis quibuscumque de dicto mortuario pertinencia ad usus dicte preceptorie Friburgensis applicetis indilate. Omnes et quoscunque nobis et nostre religioni subditos bonorum predictorum dententores seu occupatores ad restitucionem debitam faciendam auctoritate nostra viis omnibus et modis, quibus melius videbitis expedire, compellendo, quibus eciam tenore presencium sub eadem sancte obediencie virtute ac sub penis contra rebelles et inobedientes per statuta domus nostre inflictis precipimus et mandamus, quatenus de bonis huiusmodi, cuiuscunque speciei existant, plenariam et integram vobis faciant restitucionem. Dat. Constancie die decima mensis Februarii anno incarnationis Domini M^mo^ CCCC^mo^ XVII°.

In prioratu Alamanie debet poni, sed non erat spacium. *marg.* *a)* ordiaverimus *MS* *b)* nundum *MS*

*AOM 340 fol. 144v:* Quere quoddam mandatum priori Alamanie factum super restitucione duorum milium florenorum mortuarii domus istius sancti Iohannis fratris Hessonis etcetera in prioratibus[a] Baroly, Capue et Messane in folio VIII^XXIX^.

*a)* seque *praem. ante corr.*

## 349

*Licence for Fr. Johann Brun (Priory of* Alamania) *to travel to the Convent.*

*Zwingen, 1418 February 27*

*AOM 340 fol. 144v, under* prioratus Almanie et Boemie.

Die penultima mensis Februarii in Zwinguen[1] anno incarnationis Domini millesimo CCCC^mo XVII^o data fuit licencia fratri Iohanni Brun prioratus Alamanie eundi ad conventum etcetera[a].

*a)* quando voluerit *praem. ante corr.*

## 350

*The Master Fr. Philibert [de Naillac] constitutes Fr. Ulrich Kubler, Preceptor in Überlingen, and Fr. Johann Staler, Preceptor in Hohenrain, as administrators of the Master's chamber of Buchsee (Priory of* Alamania). *Both have exactly the same powers. What one of them begins may be continued and finished by the other. They rule Buchsee in both spiritual and temporal affairs. They collect present and futures revenues and dues. They can constitute one or more Hospitaller brethren as their substitutes. They can audit accounts and issue receipts.*

*Bern, 1418 March 3*

*AOM 341 fol. 141v, under* prioratus Almanie et Boemie.

Noverint universi et singuli presens procuratorium visuri et audituri, quod nos frater Philibertus etcetera confisi de fidei legalitate et circumspeccionis industria religiosorum in Christo nobis carissimorum fratrum Vlrici Kubler in Vberlinguen et Iohannis Staler in Hohenrein preceptorum domus eiusdem eosdem fratres licet absentes tamquam presentes et eorum quemlibet insolidum ita, quod non sit melior condicio primitus occupantis, sed quod per unum eorum inceptum fuerit, per alium resumi valeat, prosequi, mediari et finiri melioribus via, modo et forma, quibus melius et utilius fieri potest et debet, facimus, creamus, constituimus et solenniter ordinamus nostros veros et[a] indubitatos procuratores, actores, factores, sindicos, yconomos et nuncios speciales et generales negociorumque gestores ita tamen, quod specialitas generalitati non deroget nec econtra, videlicet ad regendum, gubernandum, administrandum, visitandum, meliorandum et augmentandum nomine nostro et pro nobis domum seu baiuliam nostram in Buchsz, quam in prioratu nostro Alamanie pro camera nostra obtinemus, in spiritualibus et temporalibus tam in capite quam in membris necnon ad petendum, exigendum, recipiendum et

1) *20 km south of Basel.*

recuperandum omnes et singulos fructus, redditus et debita quecunque, que nobis racione dicte camere nostre debentur et debebuntur quacunque racione, titulo sive causa tam pro preterito et presenti quam futuro tempore a quibuscunque personis tam religiosis domus nostre fratribus seu aliis quam clericis et laycis cuiuscunque status et condicionis existant. Item ad ponendum[b)], instituendum et inducendum ad regimen et gubernacionem dicte camere nostre unum vel plures domus nostre fratres puta sufficientes et ydoneos et eos seu eorum alterum destituendum ac loco destituti seu destitutorum alium seu alios reponendum, reinstituendum et reinducendum usque ad nostre beneplacitum voluntatis, prout eisdem procuratoribus nostris et eorum cuilibet videbitur expedire. Item ad petendum et audiendum raciones et compota quo supra nomine de predictis et eorum altero ab omnibus et singulis, ad quos de premissis compota et raciones ponere spectabit et quomodolibet pertinebit, et ad ponendum dicta compota et raciones eos et eorum quemlibet auctoritate nostra efficaciter compellendum ipsaque compota et raciones examinandum, allocandum, approbandum et reprobandum in toto vel in parte ipsaque concludendum et diffiniendum, prout eisdem nostris procuratoribus et eorum cuilibet videbitur expedire, et que per dicta compota nobis deberi et pervenire debere reperientur et compecierint petendum, recuperandum, recipiendum et habendum. Item ad faciendum quo supra nomine de receptis quictancias perpetuo valituras. Dantes et concedentes eisdem procuratoribus nostris et eorum cuilibet insolidum plenam et liberam potestatem, licenciam et auctoritatem cum plena, libera et generali administratione pro omnibus et singulis supra et infrascriptis etcetera et generaliter etcetera. Et relevantes etcetera. Quocirca etcetera. In cuius rei testimonium bulla nostra plumbea presentibus est appensa. Dat. Berne die III$^{a}$ mensis Marcii anno incarnationis Domini M$^{mo}$ CCCC$^{mo}$ XVII$^{o}$.

*a) supra lin.* *b)* ponendun *MS*

## 351

*Assignation of maintenance for his lifetime to Fr. Konrad von Gengenbach (Priory of* Alamania) *in the house of Buchsee.*

*Bern, 1418 March 3*

*AOM 340 fol. 144v, under* prioratus Almanie et Boemie.

Die tercia mensis Marcii in Berna anno incarnationis Domini millesimo quadringentesimo decimoseptimo fratri Cůnrado de Gengenbach prioratus[a)] Alamanie assignata fuit stagia in domo de Buchsz ad vitam suam ut in forma etcetera.

*a)* ass *praem. ante corr.*

## 352

*The Master Fr. Philibert [de Naillac] confirms Fr. Johann Staler und Fr. Nikolaus Staler for their lifetime in the Preceptory of Hohenrain, which Fr. Hugo von Montfort, Prior of* Alamania, *and the prioral chapter at Basel had granted them.*

*Bern, 1418 March 3*

*AOM 340 fol. 144v and 170v, after* prioratus Baroli, Capue et Messane et alie partes regni.

[144v] Quere quendam confirmatoriam fratribus Iohanni Staler et Nicolao Staler prioratus Alamanie factam de domo in Hohenrein etcetera in prioratibus Baroli, Capue et Messane in folio VIII$^{\mathrm{XXIX}}$.

[170v] Frater Philibertus etcetera religiosis in Christo nobis carissimis fratribus Iohanni Staler et Nicolao Staler fratribus prioratus nostri Alamanie domus eiusdem salutem et sinceram in Domino caritatem. Propter susceptum de vobis testimonium commendendum ac sperantes, quod in commisso vobis regimine effectus administrationis utilis dante Domino vos commendet, collacionem, concessionem, commendacionem et donacionem per religiosum in Christo nobis carissimum fratrem Hugonem de Montfort predicti prioratus priorem in suo provinciali capitulo Basilee celebrato et de consensu, voluntate et consilio fratrum inibi assistentium de domo nostra in Hohenrein dicti prioratus modo et forma suis in litteris patentibus sigillo prioratus ipsius sigillatis, quibus nomine presentes annectuntur, contentis ad vitam vestram et superviventis vestrum vobis factis ratas, gratas et placidas habentes, collacionem, commissionem, commendacionem et donacionem huiusmodi ac omnia et singula in eisdem litteris contenta de voluntate, consilio et assensu fratrum plurium nostrorum nobis assistentium de nostra certa scientia et speciali gratia volumus, laudamus, approbamus, ratifficamus, emologamus ac nostre confirmationis patrocinio tenore presencium roboramus. Mandantes et tenore presencium precipientes sub virtute sancte obediencie universis et singulis fratribus domus nostre quacunque auctoritate, dignitate vel officio fungentibus, presentibus et futuris, ne contra premissa et in dictis litteris contenta aliquatenus facere vel venire presumant, quinymo ea studeant iuxta eorum mentem et seriem inviolabiliter observare. In cuius rei testimonium bulla nostra plumbea in absencia bulle communis plumbee presentibus est appensa. Dat. Berne die III$^{a}$ mensis Marcii anno incarnacionis Domini millesimo CCCC$^{mo}$ XVII$^{o}$.

## 353

*The Master Fr. Philibert [de Naillac] asks the local judge, council and community of Bern not to permit any sale, pledge or other alienation of Hospitaller properties in the Priory of* Alamania *by Hospitaller officers without the Master's special licence. The Master had recently renewed his prohibition of any such action in a prioral chapter at Straßburg.*

*Bern, 1418 March 4*

*AOM 340 fol. 144v, under* prioratus Almanie et Boemie, *and 170v-71r, under* prioratus Baroli, Capue et Messane et alie partes regni. *Cf. Delaville (1913), 333 note 3.*

[144v] Quere consequenter in eodem folio et in prioratibus predictis quendam litteram communitati Bernensi factam etcetera.

[170v] Frater Philibertus etcetera magnificis et spectabilibus viris sculteto, consulibus et communitati ville Bernensis salutem et sincere dilectionis affectum. Ex suscepto servitutis officio vigiliis angimur assiduis et meditacione pulsamur continua, ut sacre huius religionis, catholice fidei deffensatricis, pauperum Christi et peregrinorum nutricis ac divino cultui[a] iugiter obsequentis, quantum cum Deo possumus, obviemus[b] detrimentis. Cum itaque pro dicte religionis perpetua sustentacione fuerit ab ipsius fundacionis inicio bonorum eiusdem mobilium quorumcumque nobis omnibus religionis eiusdem fratribus alienacio penitus et imperpetuum inhibita, prout semper inhibetur tam per religionis ipsius statuta quam apostolica mandata continue renovata, de cuius contrario nullus prefate religionis domorum administrator quamquam potest ignoranciam allegare, fueritque[c] nichilominus certis in partibus huius nostri prioratus Alamanie nonnulli preceptoriarum aliquarum sepedicte religionis administratores, preceptores et gubernatores, qui plura huiusmodi bona immobilia, census, redditus et proventus domorum pretacte religionis de facto, licet ad hoc minimam haberent potestatem, vendiderunt, alienarunt, distraxerunt et impignorarunt in ipsorum ac bona, redditus et proventus huiusmodi recipiencium et emencium animarum periculum dicteque [171r] religionis et nichilominus fidei catholice pauperumque Christi et divini cultus predictorum preiudicium maximum et gravamen, prout hec nuper fratribus dicti prioratus in capitulo per nos Argentine celebrato reseravimus, exposuimus et declaravimus manifeste tunc eis et eorum cuilibet in virtute sancte obediencie et sub penis per eiusdem religionis statuta contra tales inflictis et infligendis precipientes et in vim dictorum statutorum et apostolicorum mandatorum inhibentes, ne decetero qualiacunque domorum baiuliarum seu preceptoriarum eis in administracione commissarum et committendarum bona immobilia, censusve redditus aut proventus qualescunque vendere, alienare, permutare, distrahere seu quovis alio modo impignorare presumerent ac decernentes, prout alias decretum est, nullum, irritum et inane, quicquit per eos seu eorum alterum in contrarium hacthenus fuit et inantea foret actum. Expediatque pro remedio super premissis apponendo, presertim ne bona predicta quocunque titulo detinentes ignorancie sentenciarum excommunicationis in eos auctoritate apostolica latarum sub umbra in bonorum predictorum perceptione ulterius se immisceant dominiis, in quibus talia perpetrantur, hec indicare. Nos igitur magnum devocionis zelum, quem vestrorum universitas nostram ad prelibatam religionem habere dignoscitur, attendentes sperantesque vestram huiusmodi devotionem ad hec et alia religionem sepedictam tangencia favorabilem existere propiciam et et benignam premissa veritate intencia, vobis fideliter significamus universitatis

vestre sinceritatem deprecantes ac benigniter hortantes in Domino, quatenus imposterum domorum, baiuliarum et preceptoriarum nostrarum quarumcunque in vestro dominio degencium[c] bona immobilia, censusve redditus aut proventus nequaquam ab eisdem alienari, vendi, distrahi seu impignorari per quosvis domus nostre fratres[d] seu alios permittat[e] sine nostra speciali licencia et mandato, circa iam in contrarium factorum reparacionem laborando, super quibus tenore presencium auctoritatem vobis damus. In cuius rei testimonium nostrum presentibus fecimus imprimi sigillum. Dat. Berne die IIII[ta] mensis Marcii anno incarnacionis Domini M[mo] CCCC[mo] XVII[o].

*a) dupl.* *b)* obtinemus *corr.* *c)* mo *add. ante corr.* *d) dupl. ante corr.* *e)* per quovis domus *add. ante corr.*

## 354

*Licence for the sergeant Fr. Nikolaus Staler, Preceptor of Hohenrain (Priory of* Alamania), *to travel to the Convent with his horses and armour.*

*[Bern, 1418 March 4]*

*AOM 340 fol. 171r, after* prioratus Baroli, Capue et Messane et alie partes regni.

Eadem die, loco, mense et anno predictis data fuit licencia fratri Nicolao Staler fratri servienti[a], preceptori de Honrein prioratus Alamanie eundi ad conventum cum equis et armis secundum statuta etcetera.

*a)* fratri servienti *in marg. altera manu.*

## 355

*The Master Fr. Philibert [de Naillac] orders Fr. Henri de Bye, Preceptor of St-Jean in Paris, to receive Johann Magnus und Emmerich Graf, two men who may be ordained as priests, into the Order in the Priory of* Alamania *with maintenance in the house of Buchsee (Priory of* Alamania).

*Bern, 1418 March 4*

*AOM 340 fol. 171r, after* prioratus Baroli, Capue et Messane et alia partes regni.

Frater Philibertus etcetera religio in Christo nobis carissimo fratri Henrico de Bye preceptor sancti Iohannis Parisiensis domus eiusdem salutem et sinceram in Domino caritatem. Votis dilectorum nobis in Christo Iohannis Magni et Ymerii Comitis prioratus nostri Alamanie Deo et beato Iohanni baptiste patrono nostro sub nostre religionis habitu desiderancium perpetuum impendere famulatum benigniter annuentes, vobis tenore presencium committimus et mandamus, quatenus dictos Iohannem et Ymerium, dum tamen ydonei existant, et quam cito etatem legitimam attingerint, ad sacrum presbiteratus ordinem se faciant promoveri, in nostre religionis fratres recipiatis ipsisque stagiam in domo nostra in Buchsz dicti prioratus assignetis ac de suis neccessariis eisdem provideri faciatis secundum[a)] bonos usus et consuetudines domus nostre. Quocirca plenam et liberam vobis tenore presencium concedimus facultatem. Dat. Berne die quarta mensis Marcii anno incarnacionis Domini millesimo quadringentesimo decimo VII°.

*a)* sd *praem. ante corr.*

## 356

*Licence for Fr. Konrad von Gengenbach [of the Preceptory of Buchsee] to receive Rudolf Brevis as brother into the Order with maintenance in the Preceptory of Buchsee.*

*[Bern, 1418 March 4]*

*AOM 340 fol. 171r, after* prioratus Baroli, Capue et Messane et alie partes regni.

Eadem die, mense, loco et anno predictis et sub predicta forma data fuit licencia fratri Cunrado de Gengenbach recipiendi in fratrem religionis Radulfum Breuis et dare stagiam in dicta preceptoria de Buchsz etcetera.

## 357

*The Master Fr. Philibert [de Naillac] retains Fr. Wilhelm Velga, Preceptor of Freiburg im Üchtland (Priory of* Alamania), *with his preceptory and harness.*

*Freiburg im Üchtland, 1418 March 6*

*AOM 341 fol. 142r, under* prioratus Almanie et Boemie.

Frater Philibertus etcetera religioso in Christo nobis carissimo fratri Willelmo Velgen preceptori seu commendatori domus nostre Friburgensis in Oecland prioratus nostri Alamanie domus eiusdem salutem et sinceram in Domino caritatem. Dum laudabilia probitatis vestre merita in considerationis nostre aciem recensemus, digne credimus agere, cum vos inter alios domus nostre proceres attollimus prerogativa specialis gratie et honoris. Igitur vestram volentes honorare personam, ut proinde vestre fidei et devocionis zelus ad laudabiliora inantea fervencius animetur, vos unacum dicta vestra baiulia et arnesiis solutis per vos integre annuis dicte baiulie responsionibus termino statuto et vobis et dicte baiulie quibuscunque incumbentibus[a)] et incombendis oneribus supportandis ad manus nostras tenore presencium de speciali gratia retinemus secundum bonos usus et laudabiles consuetudines domus nostre. Mandantes harum serie universis et singulis fratribus domus nostre quacunque auctoritate, dignitate, eminencia vel potestate suffultis, presentibus et futuris in virtute sancte obedientie firmiter et districte, ne contra presentis nostre retentionis graciam aliquathenus venire[b)] presumant, quinymo eam studeant iuxta eius mentem et seriem inconcusse[c)] [et] inviolabiliter observare. In cuius rei testimonium bulla nostra plumbea presentibus est appensa. Dat. Friburgi die VI[a] mensis Marcii anno incarnationis Domini M[mo] CCCC[mo] XVII[o].

*a)* incumbendibus *corr.* *b)* facere *praem. ante corr.* *c) supra lin.*

## 358

*The Master Fr. Philibert de Naillac, two named procurators of the Convent and 30 named brethren, acting in chapter general, order the Priors of* Alamania *and Bohemia to attend the chapter general in Rhodes on 1 November 1419, each with the receiver of responsions and with two brethren elected by their next prioral chapter. – By the devil's instigation the church has suffered from the schism. After consultation with the above mentioned brethren the Master convokes a chapter general on Rhodes in fifteen months. All priors are to come in person and to report about the status of their priories. They are to have written authorisations. They are to provide detailed written information about their prioral chambers and the priory's preceptories, especially about their old responsions.*

*Avignon, 1418 August 10*

*AOM 342 fol. 141r (141r), under* Alamanie et Boemie.

Die X[a] mensis Augusti in Avinione anno incarnationis Domini millesimo CCCC[mo] XVIII[o] sub forma simili contenta de verbo ad verbum in prioratu Francie foliis XVII[o] et XVIII[o] mandatum fuit prioribus Almanie et Boemie, quod irent ad capitulum generale in Rodi celebraturum etcetera.

*AOM 342 fol. 17v-8r (17v-8r), under* prioratus Francie, *letter to the prior of* Francia*:*

Frater Philibertus de Nailhaco etcetera religioso in Christo nobis carissimo fratri priori prioratus nostri Francie[a)] domus eiusdem salutem et sinceram in Domino caritatem. Clamat ecclesia Christi fidelium pia mater, que dampnati scismatis eius inimici diutius temporibus regnante – proch dolor! – sevicia causantibus hominum perfidus[b)] suo viduata sponso remansit nunc divina ministrante gracia suam erigens cervicem et gremium universis apperiens nostrisque mesticiis[c)] compaciens conatur et instat benigniter, ut nos, qui suorum dolorum amaritudinem velut alterum ipsius membrum gustavimus, dultorem eciam mellifluum[d] in sue felicitatis eventu cum ea participando senciamus. Ut igitur tam salubres tamquam pios et fructuosos monitus nostre matris huius sacre religionis bonum concernentes universum, prout ex iniuntto nobis incumbunt officio, ceteris abiettis meditationibus ad effectum deducere valeamus et quociens vocati fuerimus coram Deo et hominibus tam in sacro generali proxime futuro ecclesie concilio quam alibi, quo expedierit, de preffate nostre religionis dicto causante scismate quam plurimum subverse statu et regimine debitam reddere rationem, habita super hiis cum religiosis in Christo nobis carissimis fratribus Galtero Crassi decretorum doctore priore ecclesie nostre conventualis Roddi et Iohanne Griuelli preceptore Vallisfranche, procuratoribus nostri Roddi conventus, Iohanne Flote [18r] Sancti Egidii, Gaufrido de Canadal Catalonie, Petro Pignatelli Messane prioribus, Anthonio de Verneto Forensis, Iohenne[!] de Patria dicti conventus thesaurario de Theuale, Petro de Gualberto Arelatensis, Iohanne de Autuno baillivo nostre insule Rodi de Bellacomba, Guillelmo de Sancto Iuliano Marchie, Philiberto de Aqua de Maloleone, Anthonio de Sancto Amendo de Bugues, Georgio de Criuellis Avinionensis, Michaele Ferrandi de Verona, Petro de Lynyan de Torrente de Cinqua, Paschali Martini de Morraille priore Montissoni, Ludouico de Galbis Barchinonensis, Dalmacio Ycitmar de Marllorqua, Iohanne de Villagut de Greynen, Garsie de Turribus legum doctore de Villafrancha de Penedes, Gabrielle de Galbes de Aquaviua, Bertrando de Cosqueri de Saluera, Michaele de Pegna de Nonasp, Gabriele de Asmeriis Montiscalerii, Iohanne Goyrandi Sancti Petri Auesii preceptoribus, Petro Medici, Iohanne de Villafrancha, Raymondo de Linas, Freschina de Pereyra, Aymaro de Sessello, Clemente de Tretis et Reginaldo Paruiclerici[1] ac pluribus aliis diversorum domus eiusdem prioratuum et linguarum nostris fratribus in nostra presenti assembleya nobis assistentibus in multitudine copiosa deliberatione matura conclusimus nostrum generale capitulum Rodi divina favente clemencia infra tempus quindecim mensium a data presencium proximo futurorum infallibiliter celebrare universis et singulis fratribus prioribus domus nostre nostra presentibus mandata similia, ut inibi pro dicti celebratione capituli et religionis eiusdem salubri reformatione et ad statum debitum reductione personaliter compareant, presencialiter dirigentes. Vestram itaque fraternitatem exortamur in Domino vobis nichilominus sub virtute sancte obedientie precipiendo mandantes, quatenus dicto tempore, videlicet infra annum a die festi Omnium Sanctorum proxime venturi computandum, in nostro Rodi conventu receptore responsionum necnon duobus domus eiusdem fratribus preceptoribus vestri prioratus prudentibus et in eadem religione antiquis, sufficientem pro toto prioratu in eodem capitulo comparendi ac omnia et singula faciendi, tractandi, paciscendi, concordandi et concludendi, que totus idem prioratus facere, tractare, pacisci, concordare et concludere posset, si presens interesset, potestatem habentibus sociatus ac

1) *For the 30 brethren see the index.*

de camerarum vestrarum prioralium necnon singularum preceptoriarum vobis subdictarum[!] statu et valore ac earum antiqua responsione particulariter et ad plenum instructus fidedignis cartularium et scripturarum mediantibus documentis compareatis personaliter coram nobis omni excusatione cessante. Quibus duobus fratribus in vestro provinciali capitulo primo celebrando per vos et idem vestrum capitulum eligendis ac eidem responsionum receptori sub simili sancte obedientie virtute tenore presencium precipimus et mandamus, quatenus ad nostrum generale capitulum vobiscum accedant de factis vestri prioratus pariter eruditi super vestra et ipsorum veridica relatione mediantes super necessariis prioratus ipsius negociis ad nostre religionis utilitatem possimus quam cicius providere. In cuius [rei] testimonium bulla nostra plumbea presentibus est appenssa. Dat. Avinione in prefata nostra assembleya die decima mensis Augusti anno incarnationis Domini millesimo quadringentesimo decimo octavo.

*a)* Urbis *praem. ante corr.* *b)* prefici *praem. ante corr.* *c) primo* mencus, *postea* menticus *praem. ante corr.* *d)* melliflum *MS*

## 359

*The Master Fr. Philibert [de Naillac, two procurators of the Convent and other brethren] quit Fr. Heinrich von Neuhaus, Prior of Bohemia, for 490 florins of Hungary for the responsions of the year ending on 24 June 1418. The Master has received this sum from Giovanni dei Medici in Constance and issues two duplicate receipts.*

*Avignon, 1418 September 6*

*AOM 342 fol. 141r (141r), under* Alamanie et Boemie.

Noverint universi et singuli presentes quittationis litteras visuri et audituri, quod nos frater Philibertus etcetera fatemur, recognoscimus et in verbo veritatis testamur, quoniam religiosus in Christo nobis carissimus frater Henricus de Novadomo prior prioratus[a] nostri Boemie solvit, tradidit et realiter consignavit seu solvi, tradi et consignari fecit Iohanni de Medicis et sociis in Constantia per nos ac nostri conventus procuratores in partibus Italie, Alamanie et Boemie constitutis ad pecuniarum nostro comuni thesauro spectantium recepcionem in, de, pro et super responsionibus predicti prioratus anni Domini M[mi] CCCC[mi] decimiseptimi finiti in festo beati Iohannis baptiste ultimo preteriti florenos auri Hungaricales boni et iusti ponderis quadringentos nonaginta, de quibus florenis Hungaricalibus quadringentis nonaginta sic, ut prefertur, per dictum priorem solutis et per predictos receptis dictum priorem eiusque bona et res et quos tangit et tangere potest et poterit in futurum quictamus, liberamus et absolvimus ac quittos, liberos et absolutos esse volumus et iubemus per presentes. Ceterum propter locorum distanciam et viarum pericula ad uberiorem prenominatorum cautelam presentes litteras sub eisdem tenore et data fecimus duplicari. In cuius rei testimonium bulla nostra plumbea in absencia bulle communis plumbee presentibus est appensa. Dat. Avinioni die sexta mensis Septembris anno incarnationis Domini M^mo CCCC^mo XVIII°.

Duplicata *marg.* *a)* proratus *ante corr.*

## 360

*The Master Fr. Philibert de Naillac constitutes, with consent of two named and other brethren, the Preceptors Fr. Erhard Thome of Straßburg, Fr. Heinrich Streler of Frankfurt and Fr. Nikolaus Weisly of Freiburg to collect subsidies for repairs in the Preceptory of Freiburg.*

*Avignon, 1419 April 20*

*AOM 342 fol. 141r-v (141r-v), under* Alamanie et Boemie.

Noverint universi et singuli presentem procuracionem visuri et audituri, quoniam nos frater Philibertus de Nailhaco etcetera confisi de fidei legalitate et circumspeccionis industria religiosorum in Christo[a)] nobis carissimorum fratrum Erhardi Thome Argentine, Henrici Streler Frankefordie et Nicholai Weisly Friburgi preceptorum prioratus Alamanie domus eiusdem eosdem fratres et eorum quemlibet insolidum ita, quod non sit melior condicio occupantis, sed quod per unum eorum inceptum fuerit, per alium seu alios resumi valeat, prosequi, mediari et finiri, licet absentes tanquam presentes citra tamen revocacionem omnium et singulorum procuratorum nostrorum ubicunque et ad quecunque nostra et dicte nostre domus negocia constitutorum de voluntate, consilio et assensu religiosorum in Christo nobis carissimorum fratrum Galteri Crassi decretorum doctoris prioris ecclesie nostre conventualis Rodi et Iohannis de Porta prioris Capue[1)] ac aliorum fratrum nostrorum plurium nobis assistentium facimus, creamus, constituimus et sollenniter ordinamus nostros et dicte domus nostre procuratores[b)], actores, sindicos, yconomos et nuncios speciales et generales negociorumque gestores videlicet ad petendum, requirendum, exigendum, recipiendum et habendum nostro et dicte domus nomine et ad opus et utilitatem domus nostre Friburgensis a quibuscunque viris ecclesiasticis et secularibus domus eiusdem hospitalis fratribus et aliis religiosis, cuiuscunque gradus, preeminencie seu dignitatis [141v] existant, omnes[c)] et singulas pecunias ac alia bona, in quibuscunque consistant, que per nos et dicti conventus procuratores ad usus et reparaciones dicte domus Friburgensis dudum fuerunt specialiter ordinata. Item ad petendum et audiendum computa et raciones de

*1) Fr. Gautier le Gras, Prior of the Conventual church, Fr. Jean de Porta, Prior of Capua.*

pecuniis et bonis huiusmodi ab omnibus et singulis, ad quos de premissis computa et raciones ponere spectabit et quomodolibet pertinebit, et ad ponendum dicta computa et raciones eos et eorum quemlibet auctoritate predicta efficaciter compellendum, prout dictis nostris procuratoribus videbitur expedire, necnon dictas pecunias atque bona sic recuperata et recepta in reparacionem et reedifficacionem dicte domus Friburgensis convertendum. Item ad faciendum quo supra nomine de receptis quictancias perpetuo valituras. Dantes et concedentes etcetera procuratores unum vel plures domus nostre fratres ad predicta et subscripta [d)]et eorum quelibet[d)] loco sui semel et pluries substituendi etcetera et generaliter etcetera. In cuius rei testimonium bulla nostra plumbea in absencia bulle communis plumbee presentibus est appensa. Dat. Avinioni die vicesima mensis Aprilis anno incarnationis Domini M$^{mo}$ CCCC$^{mo}$ XIX$^{o}$.

*a)* nostro *MS* *b)* procuratorum *MS* *c)* quibus *praem. ante corr.*, a *supra lin.* *d-d) marg.*

## 361

*Licence for Fr. Nikolaus Weisly, Preceptor of Freiburg (Priory of* Alamania), *to travel to the Convent.*

*[Avignon, 1419] April 22*

*AOM 342 fol. 141v (141v), under* Alamanie et Boemie.

Die vicesimasecunda mensis Aprilis loco et anno predictis data fuit licentia fratri Nicholao Weisly preceptori Friburg. prioratus Alamanie eundi ad conventum Rodi, quando voluerit, etcetera.

## 362

*Licence for Fr. Peter Mersner, Preceptor of Rothenburg [and Reichardsroth] (Priory of* Alamania), *to rent out these preceptories for three years.*

*Les Échelles, [1419] June 4*

*AOM 342 fol. 141v (141v), under* Alamanie et Boemie.

Die IIII$^{ta}$ mensis Iunii anno quo supra in Scalis data fuit licentia fratri Petro Merschner preceptori de Rothemburg an der Duber prioratus Alamanie arrendandi dictas preceptorias cum earum membris ad annos tres incipiendos ad festum beati Iohannis baptiste proxime tamen futuri etcetera solutis primitus annuis dictarum baiuliarum responsionibus et aliis oneribus supportatis etcetera ut in forma.

## 363

*Licence for the same Fr. Peter to travel to the Convent on Rhodes.*
*[Les Échelles, 1419 June 4]*

*AOM 342 fol. 141v (141v), under* Alamanie et Boemie.

Item eadem die eidem fratri Petro data fuit licencia eundi ad conventum Rodi.

## 364

*The Master Fr. Philibert [de Naillac] orders the two Preceptors of Straßburg and Heimbach to ensure that Fr. Peter Mersner obtains possession of the Preceptory of Rothenburg with the deduction, however, of the expenses that Fr. Peter Salzfaß and Fr. Johann Jagstheimer allegedly spent on repairs of that preceptory; Fr. Peter Mersner is also to recover his expenses in obtaining the Master's sentence against his two opponents.*
*Les Échelles, 1419 June 4*

*AOM 342 fol. 141v-2r (141v-2r), under* Alamanie et Boemie.

Frater Philibertus etcetera religiosis in Christo nobis carissimis fratribus ·· preceptori Argentinensi et preceptori de Hånbach[a] prioratus nostri Alamanie domus eiusdem salutem et sinceram in Domino caritatem. Pro parte domus eiusdem fratris Petri Merschner preceptoris de Rotthembourg an der Duber dicti prioratus nobis fuit expositum cum querela, quod licet per sentenciam nostram dudum pro eo contra domus ipsius fratres Petrum Saltzfasz ac Iohannem Iacsmer super facto dicte preceptorie latam et pronunciatam diffiniverimus et sentenciaverimus seu per solennem locumnostrumtenentem priorem ecclesie nostre conventualis Rodi per nos ad hoc cum quibusdam suis in hac parte collegis commissum et deputatum diffiniri et sententiari fecerimus dictos fratres Petrum [142r] Saltzfasz et Iohannem Iacsmer in fructibus dicte preceptorie membrorumque et pertinenciarum eiusdem per eos aut suis nominibus perceptis et qui percepi potuerunt eidem fratri Petro Merschner restituendis in vim collationis per nos et nostrum Rodi conventum de eadem preceptoria sibi facte teneri ac eciam eosdem fratres in expensis per dictum fratrem Petrum Merschner factis in hac causa condempnaverimus seu per dictum locumtenentem nostrum fecerimus condempnari, prout hec et alia lacius in sententia nostra huiusmodi continentur. Ipsi nichilominus fratres Petrus Salczfasz et Iohannes Iacsmer nostram prefatam contempnentes sentenciam nec fructus predictos eidem fratri Petro Merschner restituerunt seu de eisdem compotum vel racionem reddere voluerunt, sed se asserunt plures in reparationibus dicte preceptorie pecunias exposuisse, quam ascendant fructus per eos percepti de eadem, quod in presentis fratris exponentis preiudicium cedit non modicum et gravamen. Volentes igitur super premissis debite provideri vobis et vestrum cuilibet committimus et mandamus sub sancte obediencie virtute nichilominus precipientes, quatenus de et super expensis, quas dicti fratres Petrus Salczfasz et Iohannes Iacsmer in reparacione dicte preceptorie fecerunt seu fecisse asserunt, diligenter et omni cessante favore vos informetis et, si per informacionem debitam dictos fratres Petrum Salczfasz et Iohannem Iacsmer plures fructus de eadem preceptoria, quam ascendant dictarum reparacionum expense per eos facte, reperitis recepisse seu eorum nominibus et per eis receptos extitisse, quod supererit eidem fratri Petro Merschner per eosdem fratres Petrum et Iohannem solvi et restitui faciatis. Si vero plures[b] fuerint dictarum reparacionum expense quam fructus per eos ab eadem preceptoria percepti, dictum fratrem Petrum Merschner ad condignam satisfactionem viceversa compellatis. Preterea vos informantes de expensis per dictum fratrem Petrum Merschner factis in hac causa, quarum taxacionem alias per nostram sententiam nobis retentam vobis omnino remittimus terminandam. Et pro omnibus hiis et singulis execucioni plenarie demandandis vobis[c] et vestrum cuilibet committimus vices nostras. Mandantes insuper harum serie sub simili sancte obediencie virtute religioso in Christo nobis carissimo fratri priori prioratus nostri Alamanie, quatenus ad premissorum execucionem vobis et vestrum cuilibet auxilium prestet et favorem et que per vos super hiis ordinata fuerint teneri faciat et inviolabiliter observari dictos fratres et eorum quemlibet, prout casus exegerit, compellendo sic, quod alias dictus frater Petrus Merschner propter iusticie defectum ad nos redeundi causam non habeat cum conquestu. In cuius rei testimonium bulla nostra plumbea presentibus est appensa. Dat. Scalis die quarta mensis Iunii anno incarnationis Domini M$^{mo}$ CCCC$^{mo}$ X$^{o}$ nono.

*a)* Waͤnbach *male post corr.* *b)* plr *add. ante corr.* *c)* vestrum *MS*

## 365

*The Master Fr. Philibert de Naillac retains Fr. Peter Mersner, Preceptor of Rothenburg ob der Tauber (Priory of* Alamania), *with his preceptories and harness.*

*Les Échelles, 1419 June 4*

*AOM 343 fol. 158r (141r), under Alamanie et Boemie.*

Frater Philibertus de Nailhaco etcetera religioso in Christo nobis carissimo fratri Petro Merschner preceptori de Rothembourg an der Duber prioratus nostri Alamanie domus eiusdem salutem et sinceram in Domino caritatem. Dum laudabilia probitatis vestre merita in considerationis nostre aciem recensemus, digne credimus agere, cum vos inter alios domus nostre proceres prerogativa specialis gratie et honoris [attolimus]. Igitur vestram volentes honorare personam, ut proinde vestre fidei et devotionis zelus ad laudabiliora inantea fervencius animetur, vos unacum dictis vestris baiuliis et arnesiis solutis per vos integre annuis dictarum baiuliarum responsionibus termino statuto et vobis et dictis baiuliis quibuscunque incumbentibus et incumbendis oneribus supportandis ad manus nostras tenore presencium de speciali gratia retinemus secundum bonos usus et laudabiles consuetudines domus nostre. Mandantes harum serie universis et singulis fratribus domus nostre quacunque auctoritate, eminencia vel potestate suffultis, presentibus et futuris in virtute sancte obediencie firmiter et districte, ne contra presentis nostre retencionis gratiam aliquathenus venire presumant, quinymmo eam studeant iuxta eius mentem et seriem inviolabiliter [a)]et inconcusse[a)] observare. In cuius rei testimonium bulla nostra plumbea presentibus est appensa. Dat. Scalis die quarta mensis Iunii anno incarnationis Domini millesimo CCCC$^{mo}$ XIX$^{o}$.

*a-a) supra lin.*

## 366

*The Master Fr. Philibert [de Naillac] orders Fr. Erhard Thome, Preceptor of Straßburg (Priory of* Alamania), *to collect the* mortuarium *and the* vacantia *after the death of Fr. Heinrich Streler, Preceptor of Frankfurt.*

*Chambery, 1419 August 15*

*AOM 342 fol. 142v (142v), under* Alamanie et Boemie.

Frater Philibertus etcetera religioso in Christo nobis carissimo fratri Erhardo Thome preceptori Argentine prioratus nostri Alamanie domus eiusdem salutem et sinceram in Domino caritatem. Quoniam fidedigno relatu comperimus religiosum in Christo nobis carissimum fratrem Henricum Streler preceptorem Frankefordie diem suum clausisse extremum, super cuius mortuarii et vacantie recuperacione, etsi alias vobis ex vestre procurationis officio sit iniunctum facultas et mandatum, vobis tamen ad premissorum vigorem ampliorem ex speciali mandato committimus et in virtute sancte obediencie mandamus, quatenus pro recuperatione mortuarii et vacantie predictorum nostro communi thesauro spectantium diligenciam adhibeatis omnimodam contra premissorum illicitos detentores, [a)]quantum poteritis iuxta statuta et viriliter procedentes[a)]. Mandantes insuper tenore presencium sub dicta sancte obediencie virtute universis et singulis fratribus preceptoribus et aliis quibuscunque in dicto nostro prioratu existentibus ac sub penis contra rebelles et inobedientes secundum statuta nostre religionis editis, quatenus tam in dictorum mortuarii et vacantie recuperatione quam omnibus aliis nobis et nostro predicto communi thesauro spectantibus vobis tociens, quociens per vos ipsi aut eorum alter et uniusquisque fuerint requisiti, [a)]auxilium, consilium et favorem concedant[a)], nam in hoc vobis potestatem[b)] plenariam concedimus et donamus. Dat. in Chambariaco die XV$^{a}$ Augusti anno incarnationis Domini millesimo CCCC$^{mo}$ XIX$^{o}$.

*a-a) supra lin.* *b)* pot *add. ante corr.*

## 367

*Licence for Fr. Johann von Monreal, Preceptor of Cologne (Priory* Alamania), *to travel to the Convent with the next sailing* (passagium, *here* navigium).

*[Chambery, 1419 August 15]*

*AOM 342 fol. 142v (142v), under* Alamanie et Boemie.

Loco, anno et die predictis data fuit licentia fratri Iohanni de Monreall preceptori Colonie prioratus Alamanie eundi ad conventum Rodi in proximo futuro navigio.

## 368

*Fr. Konrad von Gengenbach is licensed to receive a chaplain into the Order and to maintain him in the Master's chamber of Buchsee.*

*Les Échelles, [1419] August 30*

*AOM 342 fol. 142v (142v), under* Alamanie et Boemie.

Die penultima Augusti in Scalis anno quo supra data fuit licentia fratri Conrado de Gengenbach recipiendi in fratrem capellanum religionis stagiamque sibi assignet in camera nostra de Buch, in qua ei provideat in suis neccessariis etcetera secundum bonos usus etcetera.

*Fr. Konrad von Gengenbach was the prior of the house and the steward in Buchsee: Helvetia Sacra 4/7/1 (2006), 399. The Preceptor or Chamberlain was apparently absent.*

## 369

*The Master Fr. Philibert [de Naillac] quits Count Konrad von Freiburg for 575 écus he had held as guarantor for the Duke of Brieg and annuls the Duke's promissory note held by the Medici company at the Roman curia.*

*Avignon, 1419 November 16*

*AOM 343 fol. 158r (141r), under* Alamanie et Boemie.

Noverint universi et singuli presentes quittacionis litteras visuri et audituri, quod nos frater Philibertus de Nailhaco etcetera fatemur, recognoscimus et in verbo veritatis testamur habuisse et recepisse ab illustri principe domino Conrando comite Friburgi et domino Novicastri[1] sommam quadringentorum

1) *Count Konrad von Freiburg, who died in 1422, was through his mother since 1395 Lord of Neuenburg.*

septuaginta quinque scutorum auri, de quibus apud nos pro duce de Briga[2)] dudum remanserat fideiussor et se pro eodem constituerat debitorem. De quaquidem somma prefatum dominum comitem suique causam habentes ac eundem dominum ducem et quos tangit et tangere potest et poterit quomodolibet in futurum quittamus, liberamus et absolvimus per presentes litterasque quadringentorum septuaginta quinque scutorum auri predictorum obligatorias per dictum dominum comitem nobis factas, que in manibus mercatorum de Medicis in Romana curia remanserunt, tenore presencium annullamus et eas eidem domino comiti restitui volumus et mandamus cedentes eidem domino comiti omnes et singulas acciones nobis propterea competentes contra prefatum ducem principalem debitorem. In cuius rei testimonium bulla nostra plumbea presentibus est appensa. Dat. Avinioni die XVI[a] mensis Novembris anno incarnacionis Domini M[mo] CCCC[mo] XVIII[o].[3)]

## 370

*The Master Fr. Philibert [de Naillac] orders Fr. Peter Salzfaß, Preceptor of Erdlingen, and Fr. Johann Jagstheimer finally to cede the Preceptory of Rothenburg ob der Tauber (Priory of* Alamania*) to Fr. Peter Mersner. They owe him 333 florins from which according to the commissioners' report 329 florins are to be deducted.*

*Florence, 1419 December 2*

*AOM 342 fol. 142v-3r (142v-3r), under* Alamanie et Boemie.

Frater Philibertus etcetera religiosis in Christo nobis carissimis fratribus Petro Salczuasz preceptori de Erlingen et Iohanni Iachzsmer prioratus nostri Alamanie domus eiusdem salutem et[a)] nostris firmiter obedire mandatis. Cum ad execucionem sentencie dudum in Argentina per nos late vobis et vestrum cuilibet iam vicibus iteratis in virtute sancte obediencie et sub formidabilibus penis contra rebelles et inobedientes per statuta nostre religionis inflictis mandaverimus, quatenus preceptoriam de Rotthemburg en der Duber dicti prioratus, quam [143r] magno tempore detinuistis et adhuc contra nostram nostreque religionis voluntatem detinetis occupatam, religioso in Christo nobis carissimo fratri Petro Mersner dicti prioratus vero dicte preceptorie preceptori pacificam expediretis indilate visis presentibus liberam et quietam sibique de fructibus eiusdem per vos hactenus perceptis responderetis plenarie[b)] iuxta sententie nostre seriem et tenorem nostraque mandata huiusmodi, sicuti pro parte dicti

2) *Perhaps Louis II, Duke of Brieg in Silesia from 1399 to his death in 1436. Louis was present at the Council of Constance: Augenzeuge (2014), 188–9.*

3) *Delaville (1913), 386: According to the Master's itinerary, the date is clearly 1419, not 1418.*

fratris Petri nobis cum querela fuit lacrimabiliter et dolenter expositum, contempseritis hucusque, prout debebatis, adimplere penas incurrendo supradictas. Vobis igitur et vestrum cuilibet iterato precipimus et mandamus sub eadem sancte obedientie virtute et sub penis predictis contra rebelles et inobedientes inflictis, quas tenore presencium contra vos ferimus, nisi compleveritis hac vice indilate, que mandamus, quatenus iuxta dicte sentencie tenorem preceptoriam eandem de Rotthemburg ac ipsius fructus per vos et vestrum quemlibet hactenus perceptos eidem fratri Petro Mersner tradatis et expediatis integre, pacifice et libere et quiete. Quoniam vero nobis constitit vos eidem fratri Petro Mersner in somma trecentorum triginta trium florenorum auri teneri, volumus, ut racionis est, summam trecentorum viginti novem florenorum auri per commissarios super hoc deputatos adiudicatorum[c)] per eum vobis debitorum de summa predicta trecentorum triginta trium florenorum auri refalcari et deduci. Scituri attente, quod casu, quo in predictis vel aliquo premissorum defeceritis, omni via iuridica possibili contra vos procedemus. Dat. Florencie die II[a] mensis Decembris anno incarnationis Domini M[mo] CCCC[mo] XIX[o].

*a)* sinceram in Domino caritatem *del.* *b)* indilate *praem. ante corr.* *c)* adiucatorum *MS*

## 371

*The Master Fr. Philibert de Naillac orders Fr. Erhard Thome, Preceptor of Straßburg, Fr. Konrad von Biblis, Preceptor of Heimbach, and Fr. Johann von Ow, Preceptor of Rottweil, to calculate the expenses incurred by Fr. Peter Mersner in obtaining the Preceptory of Rothenburg ob der Tauber and to have these expenses paid by his opponents Fr. Peter Salzfaß and Fr. Johann Jagstheimer.*

*Florence, 1419 December 2*

*AOM 342 fol. 143r-v (143r-v), under* Alamanie et Boemie.

Frater Philibertus de Nailhaco etcetera religiosis in Christo nobis carissimis fratribus Erhardo Thome, Argentine, Conrado de Bibellos, in Haymbach, et Iohanni von Owe, in Rotwil [preceptoribus] prioratus nostri Alamanie domus eiusdem, et eorum cuilibet salutem et sinceram in Domino caritatem. Quoniam in prosecucione execucionis cuiusdam sentencie nostre in Argentina dudum late pro et ad utilitatem religiosi in Christo nobis carissimi fratris Petri Mersner super facto preceptorie de Rotthemburg en der Duber contra domus eiusdem fratres Petrum Saltuasz et Iohannem Iaczmer, dicte preceptorie detentores et occupatores, idem frater Petrus Mersner magna sustinuit dampna et expensas, que racionabiliter per eosdem occupatores et illicitos detentores sibi debent compensari, vobis et vestrum cuilibet committimus et mandamus, quatenus expensas huiusmodi, prout racionis fuerit, taxetis et ad solucionem plenariamque satisfactionem earundem prenominatos fratres Petrum Saltzuasz et Iohannem Iaczsmer efficaciter [143v] compellatis auctoritate nostra sic, quod iamdictus frater Petrus Mersner amodo causam non habeat hac occasione nostram ad presenciam redeundi cum querela. Super hiis autem vobis et vestrum cuilibet committimus plenarie vices nostras. Dat. Florencie die secunda mensis Decembris anno incarnationis Domini millesimo quadringentesimo decimonono.

## 372

*The Master Fr. Philibert de Naillac orders Fr. Johann Reichenberg, Fr. Johann von Ow or Fr. Johann von Masmünster to incarcerate Fr. Peter Salzfaß, Fr. Johann Jagstheimer and Fr. Eberhard Romrod if they continue to disobey the Master's commands concerning Fr. Peter Mersner, Preceptor of Rothenburg ob der Tauber.*

*Florence, 1419 December 2*

*AOM 342 fol. 143v (143v), under* Alamanie et Boemie.

Frater Philibertus de Nailhaco etcetera religiosis in Christo nobis carissimis fratribus Iohanni[a] Rychemberg, Iohanni de Owe et Iohanni de Masmeyster prioratus nostri Alamanie et eorum cuilibet insolidum salutem et sinceram in Domino caritatis affectum. Quia domus nostre fratres Petrus Saltfasz, Iohannes Iaczmer et Eberhardus Růmrot pluribus mandatis nostris patentibus per religiosum in Christo nobis carissimum fratrem Petrum Mersner preceptorem de Rothemburg en der Duber contra eos a nobis racionabiliter obtentis parere neglexerunt hucusque penas per statuta domus nostre religionis contra rebelles et inobedientes suo dampnabili more solito cetera mandata nostra, que presencialiter ad instanciam dicti fratris Petri Mersner eis et eorum cuilibet dirigimus, contempnere non cessabunt, eapropter ipsorum temere presumpcioni providere volentes, ut eidem fratri Petro Mersner dimittatur, quod suum est, et restituatur ablatum, dictorum rebellium punicio, si perseverare studeant in exemplum[b] ceteris transeat, vobis et vestrum cuilibet tenore presencium committimus et mandamus[c] sub eadem sancte obedientie virtute ac sub penis eisdem nichilominus precipientes districte, quatenus prefatos fratres rebelles et inobedientes, nisi mandatis nostris de dicta presencium confectis et per vos seu vestrum alterum, qui super hoc primo fuerit requisitus, vel dictum fratrem Petrum Mersner aut alium ab eo constitutum eis et eorum cuilibet presentandis reverenter, ut decuerit, paruerint et inobediverint cum effectu capiatis et tutis nostre religionis carceribus mancipetis sub fideli custodia, quousque per nos de ipsorum punicione secundum eadem statuta fuerit ordinatum, invocato ad hoc eciam, si opus extiterit, auxilio brachii secularis, quod in vestri subsidium benigniter imploramus, committentes in hac parte vobis et vestrum cuilibet plenarie vices nostras. Dat. Florencie die IIª mensis Decembris anno incarnationis Domini M$^{mo}$ CCCC$^{mo}$ XIX$^{o}$.

*a)* Iohamni *MS* *b)* in exemplum *add. duo cruces* *c)* quatenus *add. ante corr.*

## 373

*The Master Fr. Philibert [de Naillac], two procurators of the Convent, six named and other brethren confirm Fr. Johann Cruze for his lifetime in the Bailiwick of Westphalia (Priory of* Alamania).

*Florence, 1419 December 10*

*AOM 342 fol. 144r (144r), under* Alamanie et Boemie. *Cf. van Winter (1998), 37 no. 18.*

Frater Philibertus etcetera religioso in Christo nobis carissimo fratri Iohanni Cruze, baiulo seu preceptori baiulie seu preceptorie Westphalie domus eiusdem, salutem et sinceram in Domino caritatem. Vestrorum commendabilium etcetera. Idcirco baiuliam seu preceptoriam supradictam prioratus nostri Alamanie cum omnibus et singulis suis membris, iuribus et pertinenciis universis ad eam spectantibus et pertinentibus ac spectare et pertinere debentibus quoquomodo, prout eam tenetis presencialiter et habetis, habendam, tenendam, regendam, gubernandam, augmentandam et meliorandam in spiritualibus et temporalibus etcetera usque precipimus provideri confirmacione et nova donacione huiusmodi de dicta baiulia vobis facta in aliquo non obstante – de voluntate, consilio et assensu religiosorum in Christo nobis carissimorum fratrum Galteri [Crassi] decretorum doctoris prioris ecclesie nostre conventualis Rodi, Iohannis Griuelli preceptoris Chambarelli, procuratorum nostri Rodi conventus, Iohannis de Venteuolio Manoasce, Iohannis de Autuno de Bellacumba, baillivi nostre insule Rodi, Guillelmi de Sancto Iuliano Marchie, Anthonii de Sancto Amado de Bugnois, Petri de Liniano de Casp et Georgii de Criuellis Avinionensis preceptorum[1)] pluriumque fratrum nostrorum aliorum nobis assistencium de nostra certa sciencia et speciali gratia ad vitam vestram vobis auctoritate presencium confirmamus et ad uberiorem vestri cautelam de novo conferimus et donamus vosque baiulum seu preceptorem in dicta constituimus baiulia etcetera. Committentes etcetera. Quocirca etcetera necnon etcetera, quinymo etcetera. Inhibentes etcetera. In cuius rei testimonium bulla nostra plumbea in absencia bulle communis plumbee presentibus est appensa. Dat. Florencie die decima mensis Decembris anno incarnationis Domini M$^{mo}$ CCCC$^{mo}$ XIX$^{o}$.

1) *The procurators as no. 331, but Grivel now Preceptor of Chamberaud; Fr. Johannes Ventevolio, Preceptor of Manosque, Fr. Jean de Autuno, Preceptor of Bellecombe, Fr. Guillaume de Saint-Julien, Preceptor of La Marche, Fr. Antoine de Saint-Amand, Preceptor of Bugnais, Fr. Pedro de Linyan, Preceptor of Caspe, Fr. Georges de Crivelli, Preceptor of Avignon.*

## 374

*The Master Fr. Philibert de Naillac, [two procurators of the Convent an other brethren] confirm to Fr. Johann Cruze, Bailiff of Westphalia, an annual pension payment of 70 florins granted him by the former Priors of* Alamania *Fr. Hugo Schlegelholz and Fr. Henman zu Rhein at their prioral chapters (here* capitula generalia) *in Heimbach, because he defended the Order at great risk to himself, his family and friends.*

*Florence, 1419 December 16*

*AOM 342 fol. 144r-v (144r-v), under* Alamanie et Boemie.

Frater Philibertus de Nailhaco etcetera religioso in Christo nobis carissimo fratri Iohanni Cruze baiulo seu preceptori balie seu preceptorie Westphalie domus eiusdem salutem et sinceram in Domino caritatem. Vestrorum commendabilium gratia meritorum et ob administrationem accommodam per vos habitam in commisso vobis regimine in nostra religione, maxime propter vestros claros labores et assiduos ac expensas graves guerrarumque turbaciones, que unacum[a)] consanguineis vestris et amicis non sine magno corporis vestri periculo pro defensione honoris et iurium ordinis eiusdem in Alamania contra nonnullos eiusdem ordinis bonorum et iurium invasores tam animose quam eciam utiliter intrepide subiistis, illa libenter vobis annuimus, que conservacionem status vestri quomodolibet concernere dignoscuntur. Idcirco responsionem et concessionem septuaginta florenorum Renensium vobis annuatim in aliqualem satisfaccionem et recompensam ipsorum laborum et expensarum de domibus eiusdem hospitalis in Westphalia ad vitam vestram alias nondum in ecclesia Dei unione habita in capitulo generali in Hymbach Spirensis diocesis per religiosos in Christo nobis carissimos fratres Hugonem Slegelholtz et Hermanum zo Rijn successive prioratus nostri Alamanie quondam priores[b)] de voluntate, approbatione[c)] et consensu in ipso capitulo tunc eisdem prioribus assistencium, prout in litteris vobis super hoc concessis latius continetur, vobis factam et concessam, dummodo [144v] preceptorie iamdicta annua responsio nostro communi thesauro pertinens per hoc minime diminuta existat, sed pocius integra remaneat, prout in ceteris est hacthenus consuetum, auctoritate presencium ad vitam vestram confirmamus inhibentes expresse universis et singulis fratribus domus nostre, ne contra presentem confirmationem aliquathenus facere vel venire presumant, inhibentes eciam vobis nichilominus expresse, ne pretextu huiusmodi confirmationis aliqua de bonis, rebus aut iuribus ad vos et bailliam predictam spectantibus detis, obligetis, impignoretis, alienetis aut quomodolibet distrahatis. Et si, quod absit, contra inhibicionem nostram huiusmodi quicquid forsan feceritis aut attemptaveritis[d)], illud[e)] exnunc prout extunc annullamus et cassamus ac decernimus nullius roboris, efficacie vel momenti. In cuius rei testimonium bulla nostra plumbea in absencia bulle communis plumbee presentibus est appensa. Dat. Florencie die decimasexta mensis Decembris anno incarnationis Domini M$^{mo}$ CCCC$^{mo}$ quadringentesimo decimonono.

*a)* cum *add. MS* *b)* fratres *MS* *c)* approbate *praem. ante corr.* *d)* attemptari *corr.* *e)* illuc *MS*

## 375

*The Master Fr. Philibert [de Naillac, two procurators of the Convent and other brethren] grant for ten years to Fr. Johann Harder von Gertringen the Preceptory of Frankfurt (Priory of* Alamania), *which is vacant following the death of Fr. Heinrich Streler. To this grant the Drapier and Lieutenant Master Fr. Antoni de Fluvià and the Convent gave their consent on 2 December 1419.*

*Ancona, 1420 May 20*

*AOM 344 fol. 141r, under* prioratus Alamanie et Boemie.

Frater Philibertus etcetera religioso in Christo nobis carissimo fratri Iohanni Harder de Gertringen prioratus nostri Alamanie domus eiusdem salutem et sinceram in Domino caritatem. Religionis decor, morum honestas aliaque virtutum dona, quibus vos carismatis gratia insignivit[a], ad impartiendum vobis nostri favoris gratiam racionabiliter nos moventes, sperantes, quod in comisso vobis regimine effectus administracionis utilis favente Domino vos commendet. Preceptoriam igitur seu baiuliam de Franckenfort dicti prioratus per obitum quondam fratris Henrici Streler predicte domus vacantem presencialiter et ad nostram dispositionem et collacionem et ordinacionem racionabiliter propterea devolutam cum omnibus et singulis suis membris, iuribus et pertinenciis universis ad eam spettantibus et pertinentibus ac spettare et pertinere debentibus, quoquomodo et cum quibus illam habuit, tenuit et possedit dictus quondam frater Henricus, habendam etcetera de voluntate, consilio et assensu religiosorum in Christo nobis carissimorum fratrum domus eiusdem Anthonii Fluvian, nostre dicte domus hospitalis draperii nostrique locumtenentis, ac nostri Rodi conventus, prout per ipsorum litteras sigillo eiusdem nostri locumtenentis in cera viridi sigillatas, dattas Rodi in prefato nostro conventu die secunda mensis Decembris anno incarnacionis Domini millesimo CCCC$^{mo}$ decimonono nobis lacius apparuit, necnon et aliorum fratrum nostrorum plurium nobis assistencium de nostra certa scientia et speciali gratia ad annos decem continuos et completos salvo iure communis thesauri racione vacantie pro una annata vobis auctoritate presencium conferimus, concedimus et donamus benefaciendo in eadem vosque etcetera. Committentes etcetera. Quocirca etcetera necnon etcetera, quinymmo etcetera ac priori etcetera. Inhibentes etcetera[b]. In cuius rei testimonium bulla nostra plumbea in absencia bulle communis plumbee presentibus est appensa. Datum Ancone die vicesima Maii anno incarnationis Domini millesimo quadringentesimo vicesimo.

*a)* insig *praem. ante corr.* *b)* inhibentes etcetera ac priori etcetera *corr.*

## 376

*The Master Fr. Philibert [de Naillac, two procurators of the Convent and other brethren] grant for ten years to Fr. Johann Schlegelholz, who has resigned the Preceptory of Mergentheim to the Drapier and Lieutenant Master Fr. Antoni de Fluvià and the Convent on 24 May 1419, the Preceptory of Rheinfelden (Priory of* Alamania), *which is vacant following the death of Fr. Johann von Munzingen.*

*Ancona, 1420 May 22*

*AOM 344 fol. 141v, under* prioratus Alamanie et Boemie.

Frater Philibertus etcetera religioso in Christo nobis carissimo fratri Iohanni Schlegelholtz prioratus nostri Alamanie domus eiusdem salutem et sinceram in Domino caritatem. Religionis decor, morum honestas et alia virtutum dona, quibus vos carismatis gratia insignivit, ad impartiendum vobis nostri favoris gratiam racionabiliter nos moventes, sperantes, quod in commisso vobis regimine effectus administracionis utilis favente Domino vos commendet, resignata prius per vos vestra spontanea voluntate preceptoria Marguetensi in manibus religiosorum in Christo nobis carissimorum fratrum Anthonii Fluvian, nostre dicte domus draperii et nostri locumtenentis, ac nostri Rodi conventus, prout per ipsorum litteras sigillo eiusdem nostri locumtenentis in cera viridi sigillatas datas Rodi in prefato nostro conventu die vicesimaquarta mensis Maii anno incarnationis Domini millesimo CCCC$^{mo}$ decimonono nobis lacius apparuit, ac resignacione per eos recepta et admissa preceptoriam seu baiuliam de Rinuelden dicti prioratus per obitum domus eiusdem quondam fratris Iohannis de Montzinguen presencialiter vacantem et ad nostram disposicionem et ordinacionem racionabiliter propterea devolutam cum omnibus et singulis suis membris, iuribus et pertinenciis universis ad eam spettantibus et pertinentibus ac spettare et pertinere debentibus, quoquomodo et cum quibus illam habuit, tenuit et possedit dictus quondam frater Iohannes, habendam etcetera de voluntate, consilio et assensu predictorum[a)] nostri locuntenentis et nostri Rodi conventus et aliorum fratrum nostrorum plurium nobis assistentium de nostra certa scientia et speciali gratia ad annos decem continuos et completos salvo iure communis thesauri racione vacantie pro una annata vobis auctoritate presencium conferimus etcetera vosque etcetera. Committentes etcetera. Quocirca etcetera necnon etcetera, quinymmo etcetera ac priori etcetera. Inhibentes etcetera. In cuius rei testimonium bulla nostra plumbea in absencia bulle communis plumbee presentibus est appensa. Datum Ancone die vicesimasecunda mensis Maii anno incarnationis Domini millesimo CCCC$^{mo}$ XX$^{mo}$.

*a)* religioso *praem. ante corr.*

## 377

*The Master Fr. Philibert [de Naillac] and the Convent, acting in chapter general, confirm Fr. Konrad Guntfrid for ten years in the Preceptory of Hagenau (Priory of* Alamania), *which has been granted him by the Prior Fr. Hugo von Montfort.*

*Rhodes, 1420 September 19*

*AOM 345 fol. 139r (140r), under* prioratus Alamanie et Boemie. *Cf. van Winter (1998), 37 no. 19.*

Frater Philibertus etcetera et nos conventus Rhodi domus eiusdem capitulum generale celebrantes religioso in Christo nobis carissimo fratri Conrado Guntfrid dicte domus prioratus nostri Alamanie salutem et sinceram in Domino caritatem. Propter susceptum de vobis testimonium commendandum ac sperantes, quod in commisso vobis regimine effectus administracionis utilis dante Domino vos commendet, collacionem, concessionem et donacionem de domo nostra seu baiulia in Hagnouo dicti prioratus per religiosum in Christo nobis carissimum fratrem[a)] Hugonem Montisfort., prefati prioratus priorem, ad annos decem sub modo, forma et modifficacionibus in litteris, quibus nostre presentes annectentur, contentis vobis factas ratas et gratas habentes predictas collacionem, concessionem et donacionem ac omnia et singula in dictis litteris contenta invicem deliberato consilio de nostra certa scientia et speciali gratia auctoritate presencium et nostri presentis generalis capituli volumus, laudamus, approbamus, rattifficamus ac nostre confirmacionis patrocinio roboramus. Mandantes et tenore presencium precipientes sub virtute sancte obediencie universis etcetera, quinymo etcetera. In cuius rei testimonium bulla nostra communis plumbea presentibus est appensa. Dat. Rhodi durante nostro prefato generali capitulo die decimanona mensis Septembris anno incarnationis Domini millesimo CCCC$^{mo}$ XX$^{mo}$.

Dominus magister frater Anthonius Fluuian et domini de conventu revocaverunt istam bullam, quia tacita veritate fuit ab ipso fratre Conrado impetrata, de qua revocatione vide in registro prefati domini MCCCCXXIII. *marg.;* vacat *supra- et infrascript.* *a)* fratris *MS*

## 378

*Fr. Henri de Bye and Fr. Johann von Monreal are constituted as visitors in the Priory of* Alamania.

*Rhodes, [1420 September] 19*

*AOM 345 fol. 139r (140r), under* prioratus Alamanie et Boemie. *Partial ed. van Winter (1998), 37–8 no. 20.*

Die XIX[a] fuerunt constituti ad visitandum in prioratu Alamanie fratres Henricus de Bye et Iohannes de Monreall., prout in prioratu Urbis continent mutatis mutandis folio CLXV°.

## 379

*Constitution of Fr. Jean de Patria and Fr. Johann [Söler] von Richenberg, Preceptor of Villingen, as visitors in the Priories of* Alamania, *Bohemia and Hungary. – They are to go to the priories in person. They are to visit, correct and reform and meliorate the priors and preceptors, the chambers, preceptories and houses, the Hospital's brethren, sisters, donats and subjects in spiritual and temporal affairs. They have to ensure that the responsions and arrears of responsion and the pension payments of the Master's chambers in these priories and all other dues imposed on the priories, the* procrassia, mortuaria, vacantia *and other dues of dead brethren that belong to the Master and Convent are paid. They are to audit accounts and issue receipts. In case of default they may depose, punish or reinstate officers. They may convoke assemblies of senior brethren. They may redeem estates and goods. They can make legal acts inside and outside law courts. What they do is to be valid as if the Master himself were present. Following a decision of the general council and an order of Pope Martin V one half of all revenues has been imposed on all Hospitallers as a tax for two years and is due to the Treasury for a period that commenced on 24 June 1420. So they are to obtain all the necessary information on the value of the incomes of the Master's chambers, the prioral chambers, the preceptories, offices and houses and to decide about the amount of the tax. They are to enforce its payment, and if necesary they may appeal to secular powers. In case of default they may depose, punish or reinstate officers. What they do is valid as if the Master himself were present, even if it were momentuous enough to require the Master's special licence; and the Master will abide by it. The preceptors, officers and rulers of the Master's chambers and the Hospital's subjects are to be obedient to them, notwithstanding any retentions by the Master. However, without the Master's special licence they are not permitted to alienate estates, revenues and goods.*

*[Rhodes, 1420] September 19*

*AOM 345 fol. 143v (144v), under* prioratus Alamanie et Boemie.

Item in prioratibus Alamanie, Boemie et Hungarie fuit ordinatus et constitutus visitator frater Iohannes de Patria ex parte magistri et conventus [a)]unacum fratre Iohanne de Richembergh preceptore de Willinghen[a)], ut continetur de verbo ad verbum in prioratu Urbis folio CLXV mutatis mutandis. Dat. die XIX[a] Septembris durante generali capitulo anno quo supra.

*a-a) marg.*

*AOM 345 fol. 164v-7v (165v-8v), under* prioratus Veneciarum, Lombardie, Vrbis et Pisarum*:*

Frater Philibertus etcetera et nos conventus Rodi domus eiusdem capitulum generale celebrantes religioso in Christo nobis carissimo fratri Iohanni de Patria nostri dicti conventus thesaurario salutem et sinceram in Domino caritatem. Inter solicitudines alias mentis nostre illa quadam indesinenti meditatione solicita[a] nostrum pulsat animum, ut prioratibus, baiuliis et domibus nostre dicte domus visitatione, correctione et reformatione indigentibus de salubri celeri remedio ocurratur, antequam dilatione illius gravibus dispendiis exponatur. Fidedigna itaque relatione noviter intellecto, quod prioratus nostri Urbis et Pisarum causa presertim inveterati dampnabilis scismate nunc per Dei gratiam extirpati, cum nondum sufficienter visitati fuerint, visitatione, correctione et reformatione predictis adhuc noscuntur indigere, de fidei vestri legalitate et mature circumspectionis industria speciali fiducia confidentes ac pariter sperantes, quod studiosa vestra providencia et natura discretiva virtute, quibus gratiarum largitor vos dotavit, premissi prioratus corrigentur et formabuntur[b] spiritualiter et temporaliter ad honorem et[c] commodum ipsius nostre domus vos invicem deliberato consilio de nostra certa scientia auctoritate presencium et nostri dicti generalis capituli facimus, creamus, constituimus et solemniter ordinamus nostrum ac domus eiusdem procuratorem, commissarium, visitatorem, correctorem et reformatorem in prioratibus predictis in spiritualibus et temporalibus tam in capite quam in membris. Dantes et concedentes vobis auctoritatem, potestatem et licenciam vos ad dictos prioratus et eorum quemlibet personaliter transferendi, ipsorumque prioratuum priores ac preceptores eorumque cameras, preceptorias sive domus ac fratres, sorores et donatos, homines et vassallos visitandi, reformandi, [165r] corrigendi et meliorendi[!] in spiritualibus et temporalibus tam in capite quam in membris necnon ipsorum prioratuum priores et preceptores ac firmarios seu rendarios et eorum quemlibet compellandi efficaciter per omnem cohercionis modum racionabilem vobis visum ad solvendum responsiones suas, arreragia[d] responsionum pensionesque camerarum nostri dicti magistri, quas in dictis prioratibus obtinemus, ac earum responsiones et alia onera imposita et imponenda procrassiave et mortuaria atque vacantia et quevis alia bona fratrum domus nostre deffunttorum seu moriturorum in prioratibus prefatis vel eorum altero, quorum bona, res et iura in toto vel in parte ad nos communiter vel divisim pertineant et debeant racionabiliter pervenire, ac eciam omnia et singula alia quacunque racione, titulo sive causa nobis communiter vel divisim pertinentia et ad recipiendum illa de per nos deputatis seu inantea deputandis responsionum receptoribus seu aliis quibuscunque, de receptisque et habitis quittancias dandi perpetuo valituras, eciam destituendi dictos preceptores et responsionum receptores seu eorum alterum ab administracionibus et officiis sic destitutorum seu destituendorum loco eorum[e] alios domus nostre fratres puta sufficientes et ydoneos usque ad nostrum beneplacitum surrogandi, baiulias[f], preceptorias sive domus, si que in dictis prioratibus vacent de presenti aut[g] in futurum vacaverint seu a dittis prioribus vel eorum altero aut aliis fratribus indebita detineantur occupate, arrendandi et affittandi seu arrendandum[h] et administrandum tradendi nostro nomine, donec et quousque alias duxerimus providendum, fratresque huiusmodi destitutos ad sua restituendi regimina et officia, si ipsorum sattisfacio et debita paritio meruerint, rebelles quoque et inobedientes et solvere per eos debita et debenda recusantes ad vestram presentiam evocandi et eos secundum statuta et consuetudines nostre dicte domus, prout demeruerint, puniendi et ducendi per iusticiam domus ipsius seu eum et eos ad nostram citra mare presenciam repellandi et transmittendi, inter fratres, sorores, donatos, homines et vassallos et nostre dicte domus prioratuum predictorum super quibuscunque causis et casibus iusticiam ministrandi, culpabiles puniendi[i] et ducendi per iusticiam nostre dicte domus, [165v] plantam et plantas faciendi, fratrum esgardia petendi et tenendi et mandare teneri, raciones et compota seu raciocinia ab omnibus et singulis, quorum interest seu interesse potest et poterit, audiendi et ad ponendum dicta compota et raciones seu raciocinia eos et eorum quemlibet auctoritate nostra efficaciter compellendi, ipsaque compota et raciones examinandi, allocandi, approbandi et reprobandi in toto vel in parte, ipsaque concludendi et diffiniendi, prout vobis pro utilitate nostri communis thesauri videbitur expedire, et que reperientur nobis communiter vel divisim deberi dari restitui faciendi, receptoribus[j], procuratoribus nostris aut aliis per nos communiter vel divisim ad talia constitutis in prioratibus prefatis seu eorum altero, prout ad ipsorum quemlibet pertinebit iuxta commissionem et commissiones nostras eis factas[k], capitulum et capitula, assembleyam et assembleyas et congregationes fratrum in prioratibus ipsis et eorum quolibet mandandi et tenendi super quibuscunque negociis, quocienscunque vobis visum fuerit expedire, et in illis disponendi et ordinandi cum consilio fratrum et procerum prioratuum eorumdem omnia et singula concernencia utilitatem nostre dicte domus, castra, loca, bona, domus, possessiones, iura et quasvis res alias prioratuum predictorum alienatas et alienata et per quascunque personas ecclesiasticas vel mundanas iniuste occupatas et occupata, detentas et detenta petendi et recuperandi et ad ius et proprietatem nostre domus revocandi et reducendi pro nobis quoque et nostra dicta domo communiter vel divisim quibuscunque dominis ecclesiasticis[l] et secularibus, eciam si pontificali, regia, ducali vel alia quacunque prefulgeant dignitate, supplicandi et ab eis et eorum quolibet litteras gratie et simplicis iusticie petendi et obtinendi et impetratis et impetrandis contra nos et nostram dictam domum communiter vel divisim et personas ipsius et loca obiciendi et contradicendi, homagia et fidelitatis sacramenta ab hominibus et vassallis dictorum prioratuum, si expediat, petendi et recipiendi necnon terras, loca, dominia, castra, domus, possessiones, iura et quevis alia bona mobilia vel immobilia, quecunque et qualiacunque fuerint seu quovis nomine nuncupata, per quoscunque dominos spirituales vel temporales, eciam si pontificali, regali, ducali vel alia [166r] quacunque prefulgeant dignitate, cives, mercatores, rurales vel alios cuiuscunque status nobis et nostre religioni communiter vel divisim in ultima eorum voluntate vel alias inter vivos quovismodo dimissas et dimissa seu dimittendas et dimittenda petendi, requirendi, recipiendi et ad nos et prefatam religionem trahendi et, si neccesse fuerit, homagia et fidelitatis iuramenta proinde faciendi, litterasque quittacionis vel alias ad hoc neccessarias passandi et concedendi nostro et dicte domus nostre nomine atque vice perpetuo valituras ac eciam fratrem unum dicte domus per vos in dictis prioratibus vel eorum altero capiendi, eligendi et vobiscum assumendi, qui in predictis et subscriptis consimilem habeat potestatem[m)] et sibi tributa per presentes et omnia et singula alia et insuper dependencia, incidencia et emergencia ex predictis et eorum altero ac ipsis et eorum cuilibet quoquomodo connexis, prout vobis melius et utilius videbitur, exercendi, excequendi, faciendi, disponendi et ordinandi cum consilio fratrum et procerum dictorum prioratuum et eorum cuiuslibet, que nos ipsi visitare, reformare, corrigere, exercere et facere possemus, si in dictis prioratibus personaliter adessemus, et insuper predictorum prioratuum et ipsorum cuiuslibet negocia qualiacunque ad honorem et utilitatem ipsorum et nostre dicte domus in quibuscunque curiis et partibus proponendi, promovendi et exequendi et proponi, promoveri et exequi faciendi per alium seu alios, quos ad singula vobis visa pro nostra et dicte domus utilitate procurens constituere possitis, super quo facultatem vobis tenore presencium concedimus, quotiens vobis expedire videbitur et fuerit oportunum. Dantes insuper vobis auctoritatem, potestatem atque speciale mandatum iuxta determinationem, ordinationem et decretum nostri presentis generalis capituli necnon reformationis sanctissimi in Christo patris et domini nostri domini Martini divina providentia pape quinti moderni, in qua cavetur specialiter et expresse, quod medietatem omnium et singulorum fruttu[u]m, reddituum et proventuum ex magisterio, prioratibus, castellaniis, preceptoriis[n)], bailliviis, domibus et aliis quibuscunque[o)] locis nostre religionis ubicunque consistentibus et quolibet eorum per biennium ab ultimo lapso festivitate nativitatis beati Iohannis baptiste inante proventurorum annis singulis dicti biennii per magistrum, priores, castellanos, preceptores, baillivos et rectores magisterii, prioratuum, castellaniarum, preceptoriarum, bailliviarum, domorum et locorum huiusmodi illis, qui ad id in nostro prefato generali capitulo constituti et deputati fuerint, integre fore solvendam[p)], assignandam et exhibendam pro nostro communi thesauro predicto et ipsi thesauro pro fidei catholice tutella et augmento manutencioneque et sustentacione nostra et nostri ordinis fratrumque nostrorum et personarum aliarum ad has ultramarinas partes confluencium applicandam, prout hec et alia in reservacione apostolica huiusmodi, cuius processum apostolicum dictorum Urbis et Pisarum nostrorum prioratuum prioribus et preceptoribus in eorum capitula [!] assembleiis vel congregacionibus et alibi, quibus et quo vobis expedire videbitur, mandamus et volumus exhiberi, plenius et seriosius continentur seriem expressionem et tenorem habita prius per vos informatione sufficienti de valore communi camerarum magistralium et[q)] prioralium ac preceptoriarum, baiulliarum et domorum aliarum prioratuum predictorum in dictis prioratibus valorem medietatis fruttuum, reddituum et proventuum ex cameris magistralibus et prioralibus ac preceptoriis, bailiviis et aliis domibus prioratuum huiusmodi per dictum biennium proventurorum extimandi et inponendi secundum Deum et conscientiam vestram, quam super hoc[r)] oneramus, et preterea cum dictis prioribus, preceptoribus et baiulis ac camerarum magistralium rettoribus seu eas quovis titulo tenentibus, si ad racionabilem fruttuum, reddituum et proventuum huiusmodi composicionem condescendere voluerint, trattandi, componendi et concludendi omnemque finalem determinacionem faciendi, prout melius ad utilitatem prefati communis thesauri, prioratuum[s)], camerarum magistralium, preceptoriarum, baiuliarum et domorum predictorum vobis videbitur expedire, peccunias quoque taxacionis vel composicionis fruttuum, reddituum et[q)] proventuum huiusmodi seu alia quecunque prefato nostro communi thesauro debencia his vel aliis de causis racionabiliter pervenire nostro et ditti communis thesauri nomine petendi, exigendi, recipiendi, levandi et habendi et ad ipsorum solucionem et exactionem priores, preceptores et baiulios ac camerarum magistralium rettores supradictos compellendi per captionem et vendicionem bonorum suorum mobilium quorumcunque ac reddituum, fruttuum et proventuum prioratuum, magistralium camerarum, preceptoriarum et baiuliarum huiusmodi et omnem alium cohercionis[t)] modum vobis visum invocatus ad hoc, si opus fuerit, preter sententias apostolicas contra rebelles et inobedientes ac solvere recusantes latas et ferendas auxilio brachii secularis, quod tenore [167r] presentium in vestri et substituendorum a vobis subsidium evocamus, ac de receptis et habitis nostro et dicte domus ac communis thesauri nomine quittancias dandi perpetuo valituras et nichilominus ad receptionem, levacionem, exattionem et recuperacionem reddituum, proventuum et fruttuum predictorum sive pecuniarum proventiarum ex eisdem procurens unum vel plures[u)] domus nostre fratres, qui de receptis similes quittancias dare valeant ac eosdem priores, preceptores et baiulos ac camerarum magistralium rettores similiter compellere, loco vestri semel et pluries substituendi et ad lites et causas, que forsitan hac de causa possent ex aliquorum inobediencium et rebellium protervia suboriri, seculares per suae et eum seu eos recovandi et in vobis procuracionis officium reassumendi et generaliter omnia alia et singula faciendi, dicendi, procurendi et exercendi, que in premissis et premissorum quolibet neccessaria fuerint seu etiam oportuna et que quilibet verus et legitimus procurator, negociorum gestorum potitor et receptor facere potest et debet et que nos ipsi faceremus, si presentes[v)] personaliter adessemus, eciam si talia fuerint, que mandatum exigant maius et magis speciale. Mandantes dictis prioribus et eorum cuilibet ac universis et singulis fratribus preceptoribus, baiulis, camerarum magistralium rettoribus et aliis quibuscunque dictorum prioratuum presentibus et futuris, cuiuscunque status, gradus vel condicionis existant, sub virtute sancte obediencie firmiter et districte ac hominibus et vassallis nobis et nostre domui subdictis in ipsis prioratibus et ipsorum quolibet constitutis sub sacramento fidelitatis et homagii, quo nobis et nostre domui sunt astritti, expresse precipimus et mandamus, ut in premissis et quolibet premissorum vobis tamquam nostro et dicte domus vero procuratori et visitatori et reformatori pareant, obediant et intendant reverenter tamquam nobis, imparciendo vobis auxilium, consilium et favorem, quociens eos et eorum singulos duxeritis requirendos, veritati eciam, super quibus eos et eorum alterum interrogaveritis aut interrogari feceritis, testimonium perhibendo[w], non obstante, quod, si aliqui [167v] ex dictis fratribus ad manus nostras sunt retenti aliasve exempti per nos sub quacunque forma verborum, quibus exemptiones suas in executione eorum, que vos atturus fueritis in dictis prioratibus et eorum quolibet, nolumus de certa scientia in aliquo suffragare, quinimo[x] prorsus ut fratres ceteri non exempti in omnibus vestre obediencie subsint necnon ad mandatum vestrum et vocacionem ad locum et loca, quem et que[y] ipsos aut aliquem seu aliquos ex eis semel aut pluries vocaveritis, veniant[z] contradictione et excusacione remotis. Super quibus omnibus et singulis vobis tamquam nostro procuratori et visitatori committimus harum serie vices nostras, inhibentes vobis sub dicta virtute sancte obedientie firmiter et districte, ne pretextu visitacionis predicte aut alias aliqua de bonis, rebus aut iuribus dictorum prioratuum aut eorum cuiuslibet vendatis, detis, obligetis, impignoretis, permutetis, alienetis, distrahatis seu in emphiteosim perpetuam concedatis aut quocunque alio colore quesito extra nostram religionem transferatis sine nostra speciali licencia et mandato. Et si, quod absit, contra inhibicionem nostram huiusmodi aliquid vel aliqua operari vel facere vos contingat, illud et illa exnunc prout extunc et extunc prout exnunc cassamus, annullamus et decernimus irritum et inane nulliusque penitus existere efficacie vel valoris. In cuius rei testimonium bulla nostra communis plumbea presentibus est appensa. Dat. Rodi durante nostro prefato generali capitulo die decimanona mensis Septembris anno incarnacionis Domini M° CCCC° XX$^{mo}$.

*a)* solita *praem. ante corr.* *b)* formantur *ante corr.* *c)* et *dupl.* *d)* arreragias *ante corr.* *e) supra lin.* *f)* seu *add. ante corr.* *g) supra lin.*, ac *in lin. ante corr.* *h)* adrendendi *add. ante corr.*, arrendendum *post corr.* *i)* per *add. ante corr.* *j)* receptori *ante corr.* *k)* Registratum *marg.* *l) dupl.* *m)* presentatem *MS* *n)* preceptoris *MS* *o)* nostre *add. ante corr.* *p)* solvendi *ante corr.* *q) om. MS* *r) supra lin.*, fide *in lin. et add. lac.* *s)* magistralium *add. ante corr.* *t)* v *add. ante corr.* *u)* pluries *MS* *v)* et *add. ante corr.* *w)* prohibendo *MS* *x)* quim *MS* *y) add. post corr.* *z)* ex *add. ante corr.*

## 380

*The Master Fr. Philibert [de Naillac] and the Convent, acting in chapter general, confirm Fr. Johann Söler von Richtenberg, Preceptor of Villingen, for ten years in the Preceptory of Rohrdorf (Priory of* Alamania), *which had been granted him by the Prior Fr. Hugo von Montfort.*

*Rhodes, 1420 September 19*

*AOM 345 fol. 139v-40r (140v-41r), under* prioratus Alamanie et Boemie.

Frater Philibertus etcetera et nos conventus Rhodi domus eiusdem capitulum generale celebrantes religioso in Christo nobis carissimo fratri Iohanni Soler dicto Richemberch, dicte domus preceptori in Vilingen et Rorderf prioratus nostri Alamanie, salutem et sinceram in Domino caritatem. Exigunt vestra commendabilia merita, ut tam in conservacione vestri status quam aliis nobis decenter possibilibus vos in vestris desideriis graciosis favoribus prosequamur. Prelibatam igitur preceptoriam in Rorderf vestris meritis exigentibus vobis dudum per religiosum in Christo nobis carissimum fratrem Hugonem Montisfortis, predicti prioratus priorem, collatam et deinde per nos dictum conventum cum omnibus et singulis suis membris, iuribus et pertinenciis universis ad eam spectantibus [140r] et pertinentibus ac spectare et pertinere debentibus, quoquomodo et cum quibus illam habetis, presencialiter tenetis et possidetis, vobis per nostras litteras confirmatam habendam, tenendam etcetera invicem deliberato consilio auctoritate presencium et nostri presentis generalis capituli de nostra certa scientia et speciali gratia ad annos decem continuos et completos iterum confirmamus, ratifficamus, roboramus et emologamus et ad uberiorem vestram cautelam de novo benefaciendo in eadem conferimus, concedimus et donamus vosque etcetera. Committentes etcetera. Quocirca etcetera necnon etcetera, quinymmo etcetera. Inhibentes etcetera. In cuius rei testimonium bulla nostra communis plumbea presentibus est appensa. Dat. Rhodi durante nostro predicto generali capitulo die decimanona mensis Septembris anno incarnacionis Domini millesimo quadringentesimo vicesimo.

## 381

*The Master Fr. Philibert [de Naillac] and the Convent, acting in chapter general, declare that the house in Hagenau is to be a separate preceptory, as the Prior of* Alamania *Fr. Hugo von Montfort and his prioral chapter had declared in order to save more than 20,000 florins for the Order and also as following a decision of the chapter general held at Aix; Hagenau is not to be a member of the Preceptory of Dorlisheim, as Fr. Rembold zum Trübel, Preceptor of Dorlisheim, had asserted according to a donation made by the father of the Emperor [Sigismund].*

*Rhodes, 1420 September 24*

*AOM 345 fol. 141v-2r (142v-3r), under* prioratus Alamanie et Boemie.

Frater Philibertus etcetera et nos conventus Rodi domus eiusdem capitulum generale celebrantes ad futuram rei memoriam. Cum discordia sive questionis[a)] materia in nostro generali capitulo mota fuerit coram nobis inter religiosos in Christo[b)] nobis carissimos fratres Reymboldum Zumtrubel preceptorem de Dorelczhem prioratus nostri Alamanie ex una et Hugonem de Montfort priorem dicti prioratus partibus ex altera super eo, quod dictus frater Raymboldus[c)] pretendebat et asserebat domum de Hagenow per progenitorem imperatoris moderni religioni nostre collatam et eidem sue preceptorie coniunctam et unitam tamquam dicte sue preceptorie membrum ab antiquo ad se spettare et pertinere debere et ideo non obstante collatione de eadem domo de Hagenow duobus fratribus successive per dictum priorem in sui preiudicium fatta ad eandem preceptoriam de Dorelczhem tamquam ad suum caput semota difficultate fore reducendam; dicto priore in contrarium dicente, quod, licet domus ipsa de Hagenow membrum fuerit certis temporibus preceptorie memorate, tamen ad evitanda scandala dampnosaque discrimina, que nostre religioni secutura videbantur, prout hactenus visa sunt, usque ad perditionem viginti milium florenorum et ultra propter defectum capitis in eadem domo de Hagenow pridem pro parte religionis predicte non constituti, quod notorium erat[d)] et est inter fratres predicti prioratus, prior ipse de consensu et determinacione sui provincialis [142r] capituli dudum post obitum sui predecessoris, cui fuerat in capitulo generali Aquis celebrato faciendi de dicta domo de Hagenow pridem membro preceptoriam per se ad dictam preceptoriam de Dorelczhem[e)] disgregatam, ut ferebatur, data et commissa potestas pro bono et utilitate religionis nostre sepedicte, prout in eodem suo provinciali capitulo cognitum fuerat et conclusum, quod mortis impedimento facere non potuerat eius predecessor antedictus, curaverat fideliter adimplere preceptoriam de dicta domo de Hagenow faciendo et de eadem tamquam de[f)] vacante preceptoria tunc providendo etiam antequam dicto fratri Raymboldo de dicta preceptoria de Dorelczhem provisum extitisse aliis pluribus hincinde dictis prepositis ac eciam allegatis. Tandem dictis partibus in eodem nostro generali capitulo comparentibus coram nobis visis, auditis, consideratis et attentis hincinde prepositis, dictis, allegatis et probatis invicem deliberato consilio reductionem dicte domus de Hagenow de membro ad preceptoriam per dictum priorem factam gratam habentes et placidam pronunciavimus, declaravimus, sentenciavimus et adiudicavimus ac tenore presencium et auctoritate predicti nostri generalis capituli pronunciamus, declaramus, sentenciamus et adiudicamus fuisse, fore et[g)] esse iustam ac nostre religioni futuro tempore fructuosam dictamque domum de Hagenow preceptoriam per se inantea permansuram[h)] eidem fratri Raymboldo suisque successoribus in futurum dicte preceptorie de Dorelczhem preceptoribus perpetuum super impeticione huiusmodi silentium imponentes ac tenore presencium in virtute sancte obedientie universis et singulis domus nostre fratribus quacumque dignitate vel officio fungentibus, presentibus et futuris precipiendo mandantes, ne contra sententiam nostram huiusmodi ac alia superius contenta aliquatenus facere vel venire presumant, quinymo ea studeant iuxta eorum mentem et seriem inviolabiliter observare. In cuius rei testimonium bulla nostra communis plumbea presentibus est [appensa]. Dat. Rodi durante nostro prefato generali capitulo die vicesimaquarta mensis Septembris anno incarnacionis Domini millesimo quadringentesimo vicesimo.

Vacat retentionibus superius expresatis in prima bulla huius registri. *marg.* *a)* questiones *MS* *b)* Christos *MS* *c)* Raymboldum *MS* *d)* est *supra lin. ante corr.;* erat inter fratres *add. ante corr.* *e)* de Dolrel *praem. ante corr.* *f) supra lin.* *g)* et i *praem. ante corr.* *h)* permensuram *MS*

*The* imperator modernus *was Sigismund. Under his father Charles IV the Hospitallers had finally got the parish church of St. Georges at Hagenau which they had been donated already in 1262. Later in the fifteenth and sixteenth centuries Hagenau was still regarded as a member of Dorlisheim: Rödel (1972), 221–2.*

## 382

*The Master Fr. Philibert [de Naillac] and the Convent, acting in chapter general, confirm Fr. Rembold zum Trübel, Preceptor of Dorlisheim, for ten years in the Preceptory of Rottweil (Priory of* Alamania), *which had been granted him by the Prior Fr. Hugo von Montfort.*

*Rhodes, 1420 September 27*

*AOM 345 fol. 139r-v (140r-v), under* prioratus Alamanie et Boemie.

Frater Philibertus etcetera et nos conventus Rhodi domus eiusdem capitulum generale celebrantes religioso in Christo nobis carissimo fratri Reinboldo Zoumtrubel preceptori domus in Doroltzheim prioratus nostri Alamanie domus eiusdem salutem et sinceram in Domino caritatem. Propter susceptum de vobis testimonium commendandum ac sperantes, quod in commisso vobis regimine effectus [139v] administracionis utilis dante Domino vos commendet, collacionem, concessionem et donacionem de domo nostra seu preceptoria de Rotwilr dicti prioratus per religiosum in Christo nobis carissimum fratrem Hugonem Montisfortis, prefati prioratus priorem, ad annos decem sub modo, forma et modifficacionibus in litteris, quibus nostre presentes annectuntur, contentis vobis factas ratas et gratas habentes predictas collacionem, concessionem et donacionem ac omnia et singula in dictis litteris contenta invicem deliberato consilio de nostra certa scientia et speciali gratia auctoritate presencium et nostri presentis generalis capituli volumus, laudamus, approbamus, ratifficamus, emologamus ac nostre confirmacionis[a)] patrocinio roboramus. Mandantes et tenore presencium precipientes sub virtute sancte obediencie universis etcetera, quinymmo etcetera. In cuius rei testimonium bulla nostra communis plunbea presentibus est appensa. Dat. Rhodi durante prefato nostro generali capitulo die vicesimaseptima mensis Septembris anno incarnacionis Domini millesimo CCCC[mo] XX[mo].

*a)* certifficacionis *praem. ante corr.*

## 383

*The Master Fr. Philibert [de Naillac] licenses Fr. Hugo von Montfort, Prior of* Alamania, *to leave the Convent for his priory.*

*Rhodes, 1420 September 27*

*AOM 345 fol. 140r (141r), under* prioratus Alamanie et Boemie. *Partial ed. van Winter (1998), 38 no. 21.*

Frater Philibertus etcetera religioso in Christo nobis carissimo fratri Hugoni de Monteforti priori nostri prioratus Alamanie domus eiusdem salutem et sinceram in Domino caritatem. Ex certis causis per vos nobis expositis peticiones vestras benigne admittentes de nostro Rhodi conventu recedendi et vos transferendi ad partes vestras visitaturus et gubernaturus dictum vestrum prioratum, ne in ruina, quod absit, deveniat, et deinde ad dictum conventum redeundi vobis tenore presencium impertimur. Data Rhodi in prefato nostro conventu die vicesimaseptima Septembris anno incarnacionis Domini millesimo CCCC$^{mo}$ XX$^{mo}$.

## 384

*Licence for Fr. Konrad Guntfrid, Preceptor of Hagenau (Priory of* Alamania), *to leave the Convent.*

*[Rhodes, 1420 September 27]*

*AOM 345 fol. 140r (141r), under* prioratus Alamanie et Boemie.

Sub forma prescripta dieque, loco et anno prescriptis fuit data licentia recedendi de conventu et deinde redeundi a suo superiori prius requisita licencia fratri Conrado Guntfrit preceptori in Hagueno prioratus Alamanie.

## 385

*Licence for Fr. Johann Söler von Richtenberg, Preceptor of Villingen and Rohrdorf (Priory of* Alamania), *to leave the Convent and return, with licence of the Prior [of* Alamania*].*

*[Rhodes, 1420] September 27*

*AOM 345 fol. 141v (142v), under* prioratus Alamanie et Boemie.

Die XXVII[a] mensis Septembris anno et loco predictis data fuit licencia fratri Iohanni Soler dicto Richemberch preceptori in Willingen et Rorderf prioratus Alamanie recedendi et deinde redeundi prius licencia requisita suo priori etcetera.

## 386

*Licence for Fr. Heinrich Weife, Preceptor of Weisel (Priory of* Alamania), *to leave the Convent.*

*[Rhodes, 1420] October 4*

*AOM 345 fol. 141v (142v), under* prioratus Alamanie et Boemie.

Item fratri Henrico Weife preceptori de Wiessell. prioratus Alamanie fuit data licentia recedendi a conventu et deinde ut supra etcetera die IIII[ta] Ottobris anno quo supra.

## 387

*The Master Fr. Philibert [de Naillac] and the Convent, acting in chapter general, confirm to the Preceptory of Straßburg the concession that in future it pays only 100 florins of the Rhine for the* mortuarium *and the* vacantia. *They also confirm the incorporation of the house of Schlettstadt by the former Prior of* Alamania *Fr. Hesso Schlegelholz and by the Master himself.*

*Rhodes, 1420 October 4*

*AOM 345 fol. 140v-41r (141v-2r), under* prioratus Alamanie et Boemie.

Frater Philibertus etcetera et nos conventus Rodi domus eiusdem celebrantes capitulum generale religiosis in Christo nobis carissimis fratribus commendatori et ceteris domus nostre Argentinensis presentibus et futuris. Religiose vite vestre claritas divina cooperante gratia, qua plurimos exemplariter fructus afferetis, prout veridice intelleximus, caritative nos inducit, ut vos ad domum eandem favoribus prosequamur propiciis. Declaracionem igitur et ordinacionem per nos prelibatum magistrum de consensu nonnullorum fratrum tunc nobis assistencium vobis factam super solucione mortuorum et vacantiarum dicte preceptorie seu domus, quociens ipsa vacare contingerit, de solvendo pro dictis mortuariis et vacantiis summam florenorum auri Renensis boni et iusti ponderis centum seu eorum valorem receptori responsionum dicti prioratus, qui [pro] tempore fuerit, prout in litteris nostris inde confectis lacius continetur, necnon annexionem, unionem, adiunctionem et incorporacionem domus de Scleczstat ad pretactam preceptoriam Argentinensem dudum per quondam fratrem Hessonem Slegelholcz, dicti prioratus priorem, in suo provinciali, dum vivebat, et de consensu fratrum sibi in eodem assistentium factam per suas patentes litteras inde confectas et subsequenter per[a)] nos dictum magistrum cum consilio fratrum tunc nobis assistentium confirmatas per nostras patentes litteras, prout in eisdem lacius continetur, habentes ratas et gratas et firmas ac prefatas litteras, quarum omnium tenores in quodam transumpto, transcripto[b)] et instrumento publico, cui presentes nostre littere annectuntur, sunt inserti, et omnia contenta in eisdem invicem deliberato consilio de nostra [certa] scientia et speciali gratia auctoritate capituli nostri generalis et presentis scripti patrocinio et comunimus[c)], emologamus, ratificamus[d)], laudamus atque approbamus. Mandantes universis et singulis fratribus domus nostre quacumque auctoritate, dignitate vel officio fungentibus, presentibus et futuris sub virtute sancte [141r] obediencie, ne contra premissa vel eorum aliqua in dictis litteris et tenoribus earundem contenta aliquatenus facere vel venire presumant, quinymmo ea studeant inviolabiliter observare. In cuius rei testimonium bulla nostra communis plumbea presentibus est appensa. Data Rodi nostro generali capitulo durante die quarta mensis Ottobris anno incarnationis Domini M° CCCC° XX°.

*a)* d *praem. ante corr.* *b)* inst *praem. ante corr.* *c)* committimus *praem. ante corr.* *d)* ratisfacamus *MS*

## 388

*The Master Fr. Philibert [de Naillac] and the Convent, acting in chapter general, confirm to the Preceptor Fr. Erhard Thome and the house of Straßburg (Priory of* Alamania) *the concession made by the Prior Fr. Hugo von Montfort and by the Master himself that a new preceptor for Straßburg is to be appointed by the prior together with the brethren of the house in Straßburg.*

*Rhodes, 1420 October 4*

*AOM 345 fol. 141r (142r), under* prioratus Alamanie et Boemie.

Frater Philibertus etcetera et nos conventus Rodi domus eiusdem capitulum generale celebrantes religiosis in Christo nobis carissimis fratribus Erhardo Thome preceptori domus Argentinensis prioratus Alamanie ceterisque fratribus domus nostre nunc et inposterum in eadem residentibus salutem et sinceram in Domino caritatem. Odor religiose vite vestre et fame cum aliorum suffragancia laudabilium meritorum usque ad nos fidedignorum relacione[a)] perducto nos inducit, ut vos aut domum eandem favoribus prosequamur gratiosis. Cum igitur dudum religiosus in Christo nobis carissimus frater Hugo de Montfort prioratus predicti prior in suo provinciali capitulo cum consilio et consensu fratrum dicti prioratus sibi in eodem assistentium per suas patentes litteras declaraverit, quod[b)], cum quociens casus vacacionis dicte domus per mortem preceptoris seu alias evenerit, quod ipse prior et successores sui cum consilio et eleccione fratrum eiusdem domus alteri commitere debuerit, prout hec et alia in dictis litteris inde confectis lacius continentur, et qua declaracio et omnia contenta in dictis litteris subsequenter per nos dictum magistrum confirmata fuere per nostras patentes litteras nostra bulla plumbea munitas, quarum litterarum tenores in sumpto, transcripto et instrumento publico, cui presentes nostre littere[c)] annectuntur, sunt inserti. Unde prefatas litteras et omnia contenta in eisdem de nostra certa scientia atque speciali gratia invicem deliberato consilio auttoritate capituli nostri generalis et presentis etcetera. In cuius rei testimonium bulla nostra communis plumbea presentibus[b)] est appensa. Dat. Rodi nostro generali capitulo durante die quarta mensis Ottobris anno incarnationis Domini M° CCCC° XX°.

*a)* relax *praem. ante corr.* *b) supra lin.* *c)* litteres *MS*

## 389

*The Master Fr. Philibert [de Naillac] and the Convent, acting in chapter general, order the Bailiff of Westphalia to attend the prioral chapter (here* capitulum provinciale) *of the Prior of* Alamania *on 24 June [1421] with all his preceptors and to produce all papal privileges for the Order which they may have.*

*Rhodes, [1420] October 4*

*AOM 345 fol. 143r-v (144r-v), under* prioratus Alamanie et Boemie. *Cf. van Winter (1998), 38 no. 22.*

Frater Philibertus etcetera et nos conventus Rodi dicte domus religioso in Christo nobis carissimo fratri baillivio Westfalie salutem in Domino et nostris firmiter obedire mandatis[a]. Quia ad vestram pervenisse noticiam credimus, qualiter ex apostolico mandato pro reparacione et confirmacione nostre religionis presenti anno capitulum generale in nostro conventu Rodi cum magna baillivorum[b], priorum, preceptorum et procerum comitiva extitit celebratum, in quo quidem inter alios interfuit religiosus in Christo nobis carissimus prior nostri prioratus Alamanie, qui ex parte nostra et totius capituli vobis referre debet aliqua sibi imposita specialiter et eciam per nos mandata religioni spectanti et cum effectu pertinenti, ideoque vobis ballivio sub virtute sancte obedientie, qua nobis et domui nostre estis astrictus, precipiendo mandamus, quatenus in capitulo provinciali, quod prior prioratus[c] Alamanie citra in festo sancti Iohannis baptiste proximo celebraturus ad ipsum capitulum personaliter debeatis accedere cum omnibus et singulis preceptoribus in vestra baiulia commorantibus. Et si forsan aliqua privilegia apostolica, bullas, litteras et scripturas quocumque modo habita et obtenta a predecessoribus fratribus nostris pretacte religionis mencionem faciencia ad dictum capitulum[d] portare minime et postponatis. Et ulterius quisquid predictus prior vobis et ceteris fratribus in ipso provinciali capitulo exponere, narrare vel dicere voluerit ex[e] nostra tociusque generalis capituli de omnibus hic conclusis, finitis et determinatis, sub eadem virtute [143v] mandamus districtius precipiendo, quatenus eidem plenariam fidem debeatis adhibere taliter nichilominus circa premissa vos et ceteros alios nostros fratres habentes, ut de vera obediencia apud nos merito commendari valeatis. Scripta Rodi in prefati nostri capituli conclusione die quarta mensis Ottobris.

*a) supra lin.* *b)* baiulliorum *MS* *c)* prefattus *MS* *d)* pri *praem. ante corr.* *e)* ex tocius *praem. ante corr.*

## 390

*The same to the two Bailiffs of Brandenburg and of Denmark.*

*[Rhodes, 1420 October 4]*

*AOM 345 fol. 143v (144v), under* prioratus Alamanie et Boemie. *Cf. Hatt Olsen (1962), 102 no. 10.*

Item eadem die, loco et anno predictis sub eadem forma prescripta mandatum fuit fratribus baillivo de Brandeburgh ac baillivo de Donnamarche et cuilibet eorum etcetera prioratus Alamania.

## 391

*Licence for Fr. Rembold zum Trübel, Preceptor of Dorlisheim and Rottweil (Priory of* Alamania), *to leave the Convent for the West and return.*

*[Rhodes, 1420] October 15*

*AOM 345 fol. 144v (145v), under* prioratus Alamanie et Boemie.

Die XV$^{a}$ mensis Octobris anno quo supra data fuit licencia fratri Remboldo Zoumtrubel preceptori Dorolzhein et Rotwil prioratus Alamanie recedendi a conventu et se transferendi ad partes ponentis et deinde revertendi a suo superiore prius requisita licencia ad dictum conventum.

## 392

*Licence for Fr. Johann von Monreal, Bailiff of Cologne (Priory of* Alamania), *to leave the Convent.*

*[Rhodes, 1420 October 15]*

*AOM 345 fol. 144v (145v), under* prioratus Alamanie et Boemie.

Item eadem die, modo et forma quibus supra data fuit licencia fratri Iohanni de Monreall, baiulo Coloniensi dicti prioratus, recedendi etcetera.

## 393

*Licence for Fr. Johann Lösel (Priory of* Alamania) *to leave the Convent where he has long been sick.*

*[Rhodes, 1420 October 15]*

*AOM 345 fol. 144v (145v), under* prioratus Alamanie et Boemie.

Item ut supra fratri Iohanni Loͤslin dicti prioratus licencia recedendi etcetera propter infirmitatem nimiam, quam hic paciebatur a longo tempore.

## 394

*The Master Fr. Philibert [de Naillac] and the Convent constitute Fr. Johann von Monreal, Preceptor of Cologne, and Fr. Erhard Thome, Preceptor of Straßburg, as their receivers in the Priory of* Alamania. *They have exactly the same powers. What one of them begins can be continued and finished by the other. They are to collect the responsions and arrears of responsions of the preceptories, offices and houses of the priory and of its chambers, the* procrassia, mortuaria, iocalia *and other dues of dead brethren according to the statute of 1367 and all other dues to the Master and Convent. They are to audit accounts and to issue receipts.*

*Rhodes, 1420 October 21*

*AOM 345 fol. 143v-4r (144v-5r), under* prioratus Alamanie et Boemie. *Cf. Hatt Olsen (1962), 102 no. 10a.*

Noverint universi et singuli visuri et audituri presentem constitucionem procuratorum[a)], receptorum responsionum et aliorum in presenti constitucione contentorum et expressorum, quod nos frater Philibertus etcetera et nos conventus Rodi domus eiusdem, nos videlicet dictus magister de voluntate, consilio et assensu fratrum baillivorum et aliorum fratrum et procerum dicti conventus et[b)] nos fratres baillivi et alii nominati conventus de licencia, consilio et assensu dicti domus magistri[c)] superioris, confisi de fidei legalitate et circumspectionis industria religiosorum in Christo nobis carissimorum fratrum Iohannis de Monreal, Colonie, et Erhardi Thome, Argentine preceptorum domus eiusdem, eosdem fratres Iohannem de Monreal et Erhardum Thome licet absentes tamquam presentes et eorum quemlibet insolidum ita, quod[d)] non sit melior condicio primitus occupantis, sed quod per unum ipsorum inceptum fuerit, per alium[e)] resumi valeat, prosequi et finiri, tenore presentium de nostra certa scientia facimus, creamus et solenniter ordinamus nostros ac dicte domus nostre procuratores, receptores, actores, syndicos, yconomos et nuncios speciales et generales negociorumque gestores ad petendum, recipiendum, recuperandum et habendum nostro ac dicte domus nostre predicte procurationis nomine atque vice omnes et singulas responsiones, arreragia [144r] responsionum omnium et singularum preceptoriarum, baiuliarum et domorum prioratus nostri Alamanie tam camerarum prioris dicti prioratus quam omnium et singularum baiuliarum ac domorum aliarum quarumcumque prioratus eiusdem. Item ad petendum, recuperandum, recipiendum et habendum quo supra nomine tam de preterito tempore quam presenti et futuro omnia procrassia et mortuaria ac iocalia, res et bona alia, quocumque sint et quovis nomine nuncupata et in quibuscumque consistant, omnium et singulorum fratrum domus nostre priorum et preceptorum seu quorumvis aliorum mortuorum[f)] iam et inantea moriturorum in predicto prioratu ad nos et dictum conventum ac communem thesaurum debentia pervenire secundum statutum promulgatum et factum super hoc in generali capitulo apud Avinionem de mense Marcii anno incarnacionis Domini millesimo $CCC^{mo}$ sexagesimo sexto celebrato[1)] seu quovis aliorum. Item ad petendum, recuperandum, recipiendum et habendum quo supra nomine omnes et singulas pecuniarum summas ac bona, res et iura alia, quecumque fuerint et quovis nomine nuncupatas, nobis communiter vel divisim debitas et debita, debendas et debenda et nobis pertinencia et debencia pervenire quovis titulo, ratione vel causa tam per domus nostre fratres quam per personas alias quaslibet aliarum religionum religiosas seu ecclesiasticas et mundanas. Item ad petendum et audiendum raciones et compota quo supra nomine de predictis et altero eorundem ab omnibus et singulis, ad quos de premissis compota et raciones ponere spectabit et quomodolibet pertinebit, et ad ponendum dicta compota et raciones eos et eorum quemlibet auctoritate nostra efficaciter compellendum ipsaque compota et raciones examinandum, allocandum, approbandum et reprobandum in toto vel in parte ipsasque concludendum et diffiniendum, prout dictis procuratoribus aut eorum alteri videbitur expedire, et que nobis per compota supradicta deberi et pervenire debere competierantis petendum, recipiendum et habendum. Item ad faciendum quo supra nomine de receptis quittantias perpetuo valituras. Dantes etcetera procuratores unum vel plures etcetera. Mandantes etcetera. In cuius rei testimonium bulla nostra communis plumbea presentibus est appensa. Dat. Rodi in prefato nostro conventu die $XXI^{a}$ mensis Octobris anno incarnacionis Domini millesimo $CCCC^{mo}$ $XX^{o}$.

*a)* procurationem *corr.* *b)* nos vid *praem. ante corr.* *c)* eiusdem *praem. ante corr.* *d)* itaque *MS* *e)* eum *MS* *f) corr.*

## 395

*The Master Fr. Philibert [de Naillac] and the Convent order the receivers of responsions in the Priory of* Alamania *to pay 100 ducats owed by the Treasury to Fr. Johann [Söler] von Richtenberg.*

*Rhodes, 1420 October 24*

*AOM 345 fol. 142v-3r (143v-4r), under* prioratus Alamanie et Boemie.

Frater Philibertus etcetera et nos conventus Rodi domus eiusdem religiosis in Christo nobis carissimis fratribus responsionum receptoribus prioratus nostri Alamanie salutem in Domino et nostris firmiter obedire mandatis. Noveritis nostrum communem thesaurum teneri dare et restare debere religioso in Christo nobis carissimo fratri Iohanni de Richtenbergh facto finali computo cum eodem nostro communi thesauro sui parte ducatos aureos boni et legalis ponderis centum, quosquidem ducatos C seu eorum valorem in pecunia

1) *1367 March 5: Delaville (1913), 162.*

numerata promisimus per vos prefato fratri Iohanni de Richtenbergh debite persolvi. Volentes igitur pollicita adimplere, ut tenemur, vobis et vestrum cuilibet districte precipiendo mandamus, quatenus visis presentibus de pecuniis eidem communi thesauro pertinentibus per vos receptis [143r] et recipiendis detis, tradatis et consignetis eidem fratri Iohanni seu eius procuratori legitimum mandatum habenti dictos ducatos centum, quibus solutis [re]cognicionem recipiatis, que nobis et vobis sufficiat ad cautelam, presentesque retineatis apud vos incisas. In cuius rei testimonium bulla nostra communis plumbea presentibus est appensa. Dat. Rodi in prefato conventu die vicesimaquarta mensis Ottobris anno incarnacionis Domini millesimo CCCC$^{mo}$ XX$^{mo}$.

## 396

*The Master Fr. Philibert [de Naillac] and the Convent order the receivers of responsions in the Priory of* Alamania *to pay 64 florins 18 aspers of Rhodes or 36 ducats 2 aspers of Venice to Fr. Hugo von Montfort, Prior of* Alamania, *to whom the Treasury owes this.*

*Rhodes, 1420 October 25*

*AOM 345 fol. 142v (143v), under* prioratus Alamanie et Boemie.

Frater Philibertus etcetera et nos conventus Rodi domus eiusdem religiosis in Christo nobis carissimis fratribus responsionum receptoribus prioratus nostri Alamanie salutem in Domino et nostris firmiter obedire mandatis. Noveritis nostrum[a] communem thesaurum teneri dare et restare debere religioso in Christo nobis carissimo fratri Hugoni de Montford, dicti prioratus priori, facto finali computo cum eodem nostro communi thesauro sui parte florenorum currentium Rodi sexaginta quatuor aspera XVIII valentium ducatorum Venetorum triginta sex aspera II, quosquidem ducatos auri Venetos XXXVI aspera II seu eorum valorem in pecunia numerata promisimus per vos prefato priori debite persolvi. Volentes igitur pollicita adimplere, ut tenemur, vobis et vestrum cuilibet districte precipiendo mandamus, quatenus visis presentibus de pecuniis eidem communi thesauro pertinentibus per vos receptis et recipiendis detis, tradatis et consignetis eidem priori seu eius procuratori legitimum mandatum habenti dictos ducatos XXXVI aspera II, quibus solutis recognicionem [recipiatis], que nobis et vobis sufficiat ad cautelam, presentesque apud vos retineatis incisas. In cuius rei testimonium bulla nostra communis plumbea presentibus est appensa. Dat. Rodi in nostro prefato conventu die vicesimaquinta mensis Octobris anno incarnacionis Domini M$^{o}$ CCCC$^{o}$ XX$^{o}$.

*a)* co *praem. ante corr.*

## 397

*The Tongue of* Alamania*, meeting with the Master's licence, grants Fr. Johann von Monreal, Preceptor of Cologne and Adenau, the seniority enjoyed by other officers serving the Master and Convent within the Bailiwicks of Cologne, Utrecht and Westphalia.*
*[Rhodes], 1420 October 25*

*AOM 345 fol. 144v (145v), under* prioratus Alamanie et Boemie. *Ed. van Winter (1998), 38 no. 23.*

Anno Domini millesimo CCCC° XX° die XXV[a] mensis Octobris ipso die cum licencia reverendissimi domini magistri congregata et in unum convocata extitit lingua Alamanie, in qua quidem convocacione una voce nemine discrepante concessa extitit venerabili fratri Iohanni de Monreal, Colonie et Denhune preceptori, sua ancianitas sive antiquitas ad petendum, postulandum commendarias, beneficia, officia et per sua[m] dictam ancianitatem in baiulis[i]s scilicet Colonie, Traiectensis et Westfalie ipso exeunte[a)] in legacione, servicio et ambassorie ex magistri et conventus in modo et forma, quibus aliis ambassiatoribus est concessum, quod eciam domino nostro recitavimus more solito conventus,[b)] qui suam voluntatem et consensum omnibus supradictis exhibuit. Dat.

*a)* eunte *praem. ante corr.* *b)* concessum *praem. ante corr.*

## 398

*On behalf of the Master and the Convent Fr. Eberhard Thome, receiver of responsions in the Priory of* Alamania*, is ordered to pay 24.5 ducats plus one third of a ducat to Fr. Johann von Monreal; this sum is to be deducted from the responsions Fr. Johann owed.*
*[Rhodes, 1420] October 31*

*AOM 345 fol. 145v (144v), under.*

Die ultima mensis Octobris anno quo supra et loco mandatum fuit ex parte magistri et conventus fratri Eberhardo Thome receptori responsionum Alamanie, quatenus sommam viginti IIII[or] ducatorum cum dimidio et terciam partem unius ducati defalcari[a)] debeat fratri Iohanni de Monreal super suis responsionibus etcetera.

*a)* in communis sue *praem. ante corr.*

## 399

*The Master Fr. Philibert de Naillac and the Convent constitute for two years Giovanni Averardi dei Medici and Ilarione dei Bardi and their company as receivers of responsions and other incomes in the seven Priories of Venice, Rome, Pisa, Lombardy,* Alamania, *Hungary and Bohemia. They have exactly the same powers. What one of them begins can be continued and finished by the other. They are to collect one half of all revenues of the priories, preceptories, offices and houses, the Master's chambers, the prioral chambers and other offices that the chapter general has imposed on the Hospital's possessions for two years. These and all other dues to the Master and Treasury they are to receive, and they may issue receipts for it. They may constitute and depose procurators. What they do is valid as if the Master himself were present and the Master will abide by it.*

*Rhodes, [1420] October 31*

*AOM 345 fol. 223r (226r), under* assignationes pecuniarum.

Die ultima mensis Octobris[a] in Rodo anno quo supra et ordinati et constituti fuerunt ex parte magistri et conventus nobiles viri Iohannes Auerardi de Medicis et Hylarioni de Bardi mercatores Florentinorum et consociorum adinvicem ad recipiendum in prioratibus Veneciarum, Vrbis, Pisarum, Lombardie, Alamanie, Vngarie et Boemie omnes et singulas responsiones etcetera prout de verbo ad verbum mutatis mutandis in alia constitucione eadem die facta in prioratu[c] sancti Egidii folio LVI venerabilibus viris Francisco [et] Bernardo de Riccis et Iacobo Serrat continetur.

*a)* Novembris *corr.* *b)* et consociorum adinvicem *in marg.* *c)* prioratus *corr.*

*AOM 345 fol. 57r-v, 183r (57r-v, 185r), both under* prioratus sancti Egidii, *the second time after* prioratus Baroli et Capue*:*

Noverint universi et singuli presens procuratorium visuri et audituri, quod nos frater Philibertus etcetera et nos conventus Rodi, nos videlicet dictus magister de consilio et assensu dicti conventus et nos conventus de voluntate et assensu dicti domini magistri superioris nostri ad sonum campane, ut moris est, in nostra sancto Iohannis Colocensi ecclesia congregati de fide, legalitate et circumspectionis industria venerabilium virorum Francisci et Bernardi de Riccis et Iacobi Sarrat mercatorum et sociorum adinvicem plenam in Domino fiduciam obtinemus eosdem Franciscum, Bernardum et Iacobum licet absentes tanquam presentes et eorum quemlibet insolidum ita, quod non sit melior[a] condicio occupantis, sed quod per usum ipsorum ceptum fuerit, per alium resumi valeat, prosequi et finiri, citra tamen revocationem aliorum procuratorum nostrorum ubicunque et ad quecunque negotia constitutorum tenore presencium de nostra certa scientia facimus, creamus, constituimus et solenniter ordinamus nostros et dicte domus nostre procuratores, actores, factores, sindicos, yconomos negociorumque gestores et nuncios speciales et generales ita, quod specialitas generalitati non[b] deroget nec econtra, ad petendum, recuperandum, levandum, habendum et recipiendum nostro et dicte domus nostre procuratorio nomine atque vice omnes et singulas responsiones ac arreragia responsionum omnium et singulorum preceptoriarum, baiuliarum et domorum, cameralium prioralium et aliarum administrationum quarumcunque prioratuum nostrorum Francie, Acquitanie, Campanie, Aluernie, sancti Egidii, Tholose et Nauarre procrassia[57v]ve et mortuaria ac iocalia, res et bona alia quecunque nomine sint quocunque nuncupata et in quibuscunque consistant, omnium et singulorum fratrum domus eiusdem priorum, preceptorum seu aliorum, quorum mortuorum iam et inantea moriturorum in dictis prioratibus et eorum singulis ad nos seu nostrum communem thesaurum communiter vel divisim spectantia et debencia racionabiliter pervenire. Item ad petendum, recuperandum, recipiendum, levandum et habendum quo supra nostro procuratorio nomine atque vice a quibuscunque per nos deputatis seu per visitatores nostros auctoritate nostra deputandis in dictis prioratibus et eorum quolibet ad receptionem, levacionem, exactionem et recuperacionem medietatis omnium et singulorum fructuum, reddituum et proventuum prioratuum predictorum ac preceptioriarum, baiuliarum et domorum, camerarum magistralium et prioralium ac administracionum aliarum quarumcunque in ipsis prioratibus constitutarum per biennium nostro communi thesauro tam per nostrum generale capitulum quam certam reservacionem apostolicam pro sustentacione nostri conventus ac ceteris aliis de causis vigentibus et necessariis in litteris apostolicis reservacionis huiusmodi latius declaratis aplicatorum, prout de magisterio ceterisque prioratibus, castellaniis, preceptoriis et domibus ac aliis administracionibus nostre religionis quibuscunque per universorum consistentibus in prefato capitulo liciter est conclusum, omnes et singulas pecuniarum summas, que de subsidio, reservacione et aplicacione huiusmodi nobis et prefato communi thesauro de dictis septem prioratibus et ipsorum preceptoriis, baiuliis et domibus ac cameris magistralibus et prioralibus seu aliis administracionibus quibuscunque debuerint prout debent racionabiliter pervenire necnon omnes et singulas alias pecuniarum summas ac bona, res et iura alia, quecunque fuerint et quovis nomine nuncupata nobis et dicto communi thesauro communiter vel divisim debitas et debita, debencia et debendas et nobis ac eidem communi thesauro communiter vel divisim pertinencia et debencia racionabiliter pervenire titulo, racione sive causa tam per domus nostre fratres quam per personas[c)] [183r] alias ecclesiasticas vel mundanas. Item ad faciendum quo supra nomine de recuperatis, levatis, habitis et receptis una cum pacto expresso de aliquid in futurum ulterius pettando, quittancias perpetuo valituras. Dantes et concedentes eisdem nostris procuratoribus et eorum cuilibet insolidum potestatem, auctoritatem et licentiam ad omnia et singula[d)] infrascripta unum vel plures procuratores loco sui semel et pluries substituendi et eum seu eos revocandi ac in se procuracionis officium reassumendi et generaliter omnia alia et singula faciendi, dicendi, procurandi[e)], gerendi et exercendi, que in premissis et premissorum quolibet neccessaria fuerint seu eciam oportuna et que veri et legitimi procuratores facere possunt et debent et que nos ipsi faceremus et facere possemus, si presentes personaliter adessemus, eciam si talia sint, in quibus requiratur mandatum maius et magis speciale. Promittimus bona fide ratum, gratum habere et perpetuo tenere omne id et quitquit per dictos procuratores et eorum quemlibet ac substituendum[f] seu substituendos ab eis vel eorum altero in premissis eorum quolibet actum, dictum, petitum, recuperatum, levatum, habitum, receptum, quittatum procuratumve fuerit seu gestum sub ypotheca et obligatione omnium bonorum nostrorum et dicte nostre domus quorumcunque presencium pariter et futurorum. In cuius rei testimonium bulla nostra communis plumbea presentibus est appensa. Dat. Rodi die ultima mensis Ottobris anno incarnacionis Domini millesimo CCCC° XX°.

*a)* d *add. ante corr.* *b) dupl.* *c) add.* Quere residuum in prioratibus Baroli et Capue CLXXXV *d)* singulia *MS* *e)* procurendi *MS* *f)* fratres v *add. ante corr.*

## 400

*Fr. Gautier le Gras, Prior of the Conventual church at Rhodes and Lieutenant of the vacant Master's office, and the Convent grant to Fr. Johann Pragher, chaplain of the Priory of* Alamania, *the Preceptory of Colmar (Priory of* Alamania), *which is vacant because Fr. Hugo von Montfort, Prior of* Alamania, *has deposed Fr. Berthold von Hohencastell on account of his mismanagement.*

*Rhodes, 1421 June 9*

*AOM 346 fol. 122r, under* prioratus Alamanie.

Frater Gualterus Crassy decretorum doctor, prior ecclesie sancti Iohannis Colaci Rodi conventus ac locumtenens humilis magisterii nuper vacantis, sacerdos hospitalis sancti Iohannis Iherosolimitani et nos conventus Rodi domus eiusdem religioso in Christo nobis carissimo fratri Iohanni Pragher dicte domus capellano prioratus nostri Alamanie salutem et sinceram in Domino caritatem. Religionis decor, morum honestas et alia virtutum dona, quibus vos carismatis gratia insignivit, ad imparciendum favoris nostri gratiam rationabiliter nos moventes, sperantesque in comisso vobis regimine effectus administrationis utilis favente Domino vos commendet. Preceptoriam igitur seu baiuliam de Colmar dicti prioratus vacantem per remocionem seu destitucionem fratris Bertholdi de Alteri Castel ob eius malam gubernationem et indebitam per venerabilem fratrem nostrum Hugonem de Montfort dicti prioratus priorem presencialiter vacantem seu quocunque alio modo vacantem et ad nostram disposicionem, collacionem et ordinacionem propterea rationabiliter devolutam cum omnibus et singulis suis membris, iuribus et pertinenciis ad dictam preceptoriam spectantibus et pertinentibus seu spectare et pertinere debentibus, quoquomodo et cum quibus illam habuit, tenuit et possedit dictus frater Bertholdus, habendam, tenendam etcetera invicem etcetera ad annos decem etcetera. Comittentes etcetera. Quocirca etcetera ac priori etcetera amoto etcetera. Inhibentes etcetera. In cuius rei testimonium bulla nostra cerea ob defectum bulle communis plumbee vacante dicto magisterio presentibus est appensa. Data Rodi die IX mensis Iunii anno incarnacionis Domini M IIII[C] XXI.

## 401

*Quittance issued by the Lieutenant [of the vacant Master's office] Fr. Gautier le Gras and twelve brethren of four tongues,* Alamania, *Saint-Gilles, Spain, and Lesser Provence, about passage payments and seniority for twelve named brethren in the same way as the earlier receipt issued by Fr. Luce [de Vallins].*

*Rhodes, 1421 June 10*

*AOM 346 fol. 162r-v, under* partes citramarine. *Cf. Sarnowsky, Macht (2001), 220 note 54.*

Die decima mensis Iunii anno incarnacionis Domini in presencia domini locumtenentis[1)] fratris Galteri Crassi decretorum doctoris et aliorum dominorum comparuerunt fratres diversarum linguarum et rogaverunt predictos dominos, qualiter placeret eis quittare passagium ipsorum, prout iam a domino locumtenente fratre Lucio[2)] et eius consilio fuit scriptum in partibus ponentis fratribus volentibus venire ad conventum ad serviendum Deo et religioni ipsorum passagium esse quittum domini locumtenentis et consilium auditis racionibus et iuribus dictorum fratrum quittaverunt passagium et quod thesauro nichil solvere debeant et quod ipsorum anchienitas[a)] cur[r]ere debeat [162v] a die prima, qua venerunt ad conventum, uniusquisque ipsorum vero dictorum fratrum debeat cur[r]ere a dicta die superius denotata. Et ipsorum fratrum nomina sunt hec: frater Bertrandus de Cradies lingue Spanie, frater Hugo de Melquinghem lingua Alamanie, frater[b)] Brocardus Hant dicte lingue, frater Anthonius Nablo dicte lingue, frater Iohannes Lossel dicte lingue, frater Iohannes de Biting dicte lingue, frater Iohannes Bnin dicte lingue, Iohannes Chuicus dicte lingue, frater Iohannes de Cabelut prioratus sancti Egidii, frater Mercus de Rostuel dicte lingue Almanie, frater Anthonius Bal lingue parve Provincie, frater Raymundus Richardi prioratus sancti Egidii.

*a)* anchienttas *MS* *b)* C *add. ante corr.*

## 402

*The Master Fr. Antoni de Fluvià and the Convent grant for ten years to the chaplain Fr. Simon Bracht the Preceptory of Arnheim (Priory of* Alamania), *which is vacant following the death of Fr. Arnold von Groenheim.*

*Rhodes, 1421 July 4*

1) *Fr. Gautier had been Lieutenant of the vacant Mastership in 1421 (no. 400) and acted now as Lieutenant of the absent Master. Cf. Countryside (2019), 275–8.*

2) *Fr. Luce de Vallins was Lieutenant Master on Rhodes from 1412 to 1419.*

*AOM 346 fol. 122r-2v, under* prioratus Alamanie. *Ed. van Winter (1998), 39 no. 24.*

Frater Anthonius Fluuian Dei gratia sacre domus hospitalis sancti Iohannis Iherosolimitani magister humilis et pauperum Christi custos et nos conventus Rodi domus eiusdem religioso in Christo nobis carissimo fratri Simoni de Bracht cappellano prioratus nostri Almanie dicte domus salutem et sinceram in Domino caritatem. Vestris exposcentibus meritis paterna benevolentia prosequentes baiuliam sive preceptoriam de Arnheym dicti prioratus vacantem per mortem dicte domus quondam fratris Arnoldi de Groenhem[1] dicti prioratus ultimi eiusdem preceptoris et propterea ad nostram collacionem et disposicionem racionabiliter devolutuam cum omnibus et singulis suis membris, iuribus et pertinenciis universis ad eam spectantibus et pertinentibus ac spectare [122v] et pertinere debentibus, quoquomodo et cum quibus illam habuit, tenuit et possedit dictus quondam frater[a] Arnoldus, habendam, tenendam, regendam etcetera invicem etcetera ad X annos etcetera. Committentes etcetera. Quocirca etcetera ac priori etcetera amoto etcetera. Inhibentes etcetera. In cuius rei testimonium[b] bulla nostra[c] plumbea presentibus est appensa. Dat. Rodi in nostro conventu die quarta mensis Iulii anno incarnacionis Domini millesimo quadringentesimo vicesimo primo.

*a)* fratri *MS* *b)* p *add. ante corr.* *c)* pl *add. ante corr.*, cerea *add. ante corr.*

## 403

*Licence for Fr. Simon von Bracht, Preceptor of Arnheim, to leave the Convent and return with his superior's permission.*

*Rhodes, 1421 July 10*

*AOM 346 fol. 122v, under* prioratus Alamanie. *Ed. van Winter (1998), 39 no. 25.*

Data fuit licencia fratri Symoni de Bracht preceptori de Arnheym recedendi a conventu et iterum redeundi ad dictum conventum, prius tamen habita licencia a suo superiori, die decima mensis Iulii anno incarnacionis Domini M° CCCC° vigesimo primo.

## 404

*Assignation of 104.5 florins of the Rhine to Fr. Simon [von Bracht] in the Priory of* Alamania.

*[Rhodes], 1421 July 12*

1) *Correct would be Grünwald, Groenewoud.*

*AOM 346 fol. 122v, under* prioratus Alamanie. *Ed. van Winter (1998), 39 no. 26.*

Die duodecima mensis Iulii anno ut supra fuit facta dicto fratri Simoni assignacio centum quatuor et cum dimidio florenorum Renensium in prioratu Almanie.

## 405

*Licence for Fr. Simon [von Bracht], Preceptor of Arnheim, to receive two chaplains and one sergeant into the Order.*

*[Rhodes], 1421 July 13*

*AOM 346 fol. 122v, under* prioratus Alamanie. *Ed. van Winter (1998), 40 no. 27.*

Die XIII[a] mensis Iulii anno ut supra data fuit licencia fratri Simoni preceptori de Arnheyn prioratus Alamanie faciendi duos fratres cappellanos et unum servientem, ut moris est.

## 406

*The Master Fr. Antoni de Fluvià and the Convent grant to Fr. Johann von Monreal, Bailiff of Cologne, Preceptor of Cologne and Adenau (Priory of* Alamania*), the Preceptory of Breisig, which is vacant following the death of Fr. Nikolaus von Adenau.*

*Rhodes, 1422 May 6*

*AOM 346 fol. 122v-3r, under* prioratus Alamanie.

Frater Anthonius Fluuiani Dei gratia sacre domus hospitalis sancti Iohannis Iherosolimitani magister humilis et pauperum Christi custos et nos conventus Rodi domus eiusdem religioso in Christo nobis carissimo fratri Iohanni de Montreall baillivo baiulie Coloniensis ac preceptori domorum in Colonia et in Adenauwe prioratus nostri Alamanie dicte domus salutem et sinceram in Domino caritatem. Propter probitatis vite merita et administrationem accomodam, quam in comissis vobis regiminibus in nostro ordine, sicut fidedigno testimonio accepimus, habuistis, illa vobis libenter annuimus, que conservationem vestri status concernere dignoscuntur. Hinc est, quod non obstante, quod dictam baiuliam et domos supradictas noscamini presentialiter obtinere, preceptoriam de Bisge vacantem presentialiter per mortem quo[n]dam dicte domus fratris Nicolay de Adenawe ultimi eiusdem preceptoris et propterea ad nostram collationem et dispositionem rationabiliter devolutam cum omnibus et singulis suis membris, iuribus [123r] et pertinenciis universis ad eam spectantibus et pertinentibus ac spectare et pertinere debentibus, quoquomodo et cum quibus illam habuit, tenuit et possedit dictus quondam frater Nicolaus, habendam, tenendam, regendam, gubernandam, augmentandam et meliorandam in spiritualibus et temporalibus tam in capite quam in membris etcetera invicem etcetera. Quocirca etcetera quinymo etcetera necnon etcetera. Inhibentes etcetera. In cuius rei testimonium bulla nostra communis plumbea presentibus est appensa. Data Rodi in nostro conventu die VI[ta] mensis Maii.

## 407

*The Master Fr. Antoni de Fluvià and the Convent have been informed by Fr. Johann von Monreal, visitor and receiver of responsions in the Priory of* Alamania, *by Fr. Rembold zum Trübel, also receiver of responsions in the Priory of* Alamania, *and by Fr. Johann Cruze, Bailiff of Westphalia, the Master's chaplain and familiar, that after the death of Fr. Arnold van Groenwald, Preceptor of Arnheim, three officers, Fr. Henri de Bye, Preceptor of Paris, the said Fr. Johann von Monreal, Preceptor of Cologne, and the said Fr. Johann Cruze, Bailiff of Westphalia and Preceptor of Steinfurt, Lage and Wesel (all in the Priory of* Alamania), *tried to collect the* mortuarium *due to the Convent on Rhodes. But this was thwarted by Fr. Arnold Zeuwelkin and his supporters, who excused themselves from obedience to the Master with reference to Fr. Hugo von Montfort, Prior of* Alamania. *Together with Fr. Karl von Bingen, Preceptor of Mainz, they also refused to accept Fr. Simon von Bracht as the new preceptor of Arnheim. If Fr. Hugo, Fr. Arnold and Fr. Karl persist in this, they are to be summoned to Rhodes to stand trial.*

*Rhodes, 1422 May 26*

*AOM 346 fol. 123r-4r, under* prioratus Alamanie. *On fol. 123v-4r no. 408.*

Frater Anthonius Fluuiani sacre domus hospitalis sancti Iohannis Iherosolimitani magister humilis et pauperum Christi custos et nos conventus Rodi domus eiusdem religioso in Christo nobis carissimis fratribus Iohanni de Monreal procuratori, visitatori, correctori et reformatori ac responsionum nostrarum in prioratu nostro Alamanie receptori, Rembaldo Zemtrubel responsionum earundem in prelibato nostro prioratu receptori et Iohanni Cruze baillivo Wesualie capellano et familiari nostro domestico salutem in Domino et nostris firmiter obedire mandatis. Tenore presentium vobis et cuilibet vestrum duximus fore notificandum, quod ad nostram presentiam ex veridicis documentis, lettris[a)] et relationibus supervenit, quod post mortem fratris Arnoldi de Groenwald olim preceptoris preceptorie nostre de Arnhem iamdicto prioratu nostro ad dictum locum religiosi in Christo nobis carissimi fratres Heinricus de Bie Parisiensis, Iohannis de Monreal Coloniensis una cum supradicto baillivo Westfalie preceptorie domorum nostrarum Steynfordie, Lage, Wesalie preceptores pre[de]cessores prenominati asserunt tamquam procuratores, visitatores, correctores et reformatores et responsionum nostrarum aliarumque iurium conventus nostri receptores pro recuperando, exigendo et levando mortuaria, vacantia et certa alia bona ipsius fratris olim preceptoris secundum nostre religionis stabilimenta et consuetudines laudabiles nostro[b)] communi tesauro pro sustentatione nostri conventus Rodi fideique chatolice defensione spectantia. Qui supradicti maliciis, dolo et fraude dicti fratris Arnoldi Zewelquin aliorumque sibi adherentium conventualium non potuerunt exigere nec mortuaria supradicta et bona nostro comuni tesauro[c)] spectantia et pertinentia recuperare quibusdam opinionibusque, contradictionibusque frivolis adherendo sub umbra[d)] nichilominus et protectione, ut dicitur, venerabili fratris Hugonis de Montfort nostri prioratus Alamanie prioris se excusantes nec fratrem Simonem de Bracht preceptorem de Arnheim non obstantibus colatione et mandata ipsi priori per nos factis dictus frater Arnoldus Zewelquin et ipsius coadherentes tamquam inobedientes nec se visitare permittentes et nostris mandatis omnino reluctantes in pacificam possessionem supradictam admittere voluerunt. Nos vero volentes unicuique racionem eius, prout tenemur, ministrare nec oculis coniunctibus iniuste facta scilentio[e)] pertransire, mandamus vobis supradictis procuratoribus, visitatoribus, correctoribus, reformatoribus et responsionum nostrarum receptoribus et quibuscumque nostre religionis subditis, qui primitus requisitus vel requisiti fuerint, contra prefatos priorem et fratrem Arnoldum et quoscumque alios inobedientes auxilium, consilium et favorem tam circa recuperationem omnium bonorum mortuariorum, vacantium et responsionum[f)] nostro communi tesauro spectantium et pertinentium, [123v] ut est premissum, quam ad ponendum et introducendum prefatum fratrem Simonem preceptorem in possessionem corporalem, pacificam et quietam dicte preceptorie impendere necnon eciam [etcetera]. Mandantes sub eadem virtute precipiendo districtius iuxta illud, quod nemo suo dolo, fraude et violentia gaudere debeat, quatinus omnibus exceptionibus et cavillationibus quibuscumque postpositis facitis[g)] Simoni supradicto preceptori omnia dampna et itinerum ipsius dispensa resarcare plenarie et restituere ab eodem fratre Arnaldo vel ab ipso priore alias quis eorum primitus ad vestras manus prevenerit, cohartetur. Et quoniam informati veris et certis relationibus dictum priorem baillivo et capellano ac familiari[h)] et domestico nostro Westfalie in capitulo Spirensi dudum in prioratu celebrato magnam intulisse et inmanem ex[s]poliationem de quibusdam litteris obligatoriis datis et ratifficatis ab eodem[i)] priore, cum quodam subscripto fratre Karolo Bing nunc Ma[g]untin. ut dicitur preceptore quequidem littere tenorem centum florenorum Renensium camil.[?] ipsi baillivo iamdicto nimirum[j)] anuatim debere, insuper dictum nostrum baillivum et domesticum capellanum ac familiarem ab ipso iamdicto priore expoliatum in dicto capitulo fuisse [k)]intelleximus, unde vobis et cuilibet vestrum sub eadem virtute precipiendo mandamus, quatenus dicto ballivo iusticie complementum, auditus et examinatus utrisque partibus administrari faciatis et quod iura disponunt, quos ecclesiastica corrigere discrimina non potest principum mundanorum potentia, subsidium debet prestare et cum effectu favorabiliter subvenire. Rogamus igitur pro premissorum adimplendorum executioni et effectu, quatenus in iuris subsidium et nostre religionis contemplacione et amore, cum a nostris supradictis procuratoribus, visitatoribus, correctoribus et reformatoribus fueritis requisiti, contra tales inobedientes[l] et vere [124r] excommunicatos ac secundum nostre religionis stabilimenta laudabilia eorum preceptoriis et dignitatibus privatos auxilium, consilium et favorem prestare et impendere dignentur. Circa premissa taliter [se] habentes, ut eisdem dominis ecclesiasticis et temporalibus teneamur ad similia et maiora cum gratiarum actionibus. Et si omnino dicti[m] prior[n], frater Arnoldus dictusque Karolus de Binge Maguntinensis preceptor obedire recusaverint in sua pertinacia persistentes, omnes et singulos huiusmodi ex parte nostra citetis, quos[o] eciam presentium tenore citamus, quatenus coram nobis in conventu nostro Rodi infra terminum iuris per se vel[p] per procuratores religiosos sufficienter instructos compareant. Protestantes siquidem, quod, si in termino prefixo comparere non curaverint, contra ipsos ipsorumque contumacia non obstante procedemus, prout statuta religionis exigunt. In cuius rei testimonium bulla nostra communis plumbea presentibus est appensa. Dat. in nostro Rodi conventu die XXVI mensis Maii anno incarnacionis Domini M° IIII$^{C}$ XXII.

*a)* litteris *recte* *b)* convenerit *add. ante corr.* *c)* tangentia *add. ante corr.* *d)* subra *corr.* *e)* silentio *recte* *f)* si *add. ante corr.* *g)* fratris *MS* *h)* familiati *MS* *i)* eadem *MS* *j)* mime *praem. ante corr.* *k) hincinde script. nova manu* *l)* inobedientis *MS m)* p *praem. ante corr.* *n)* priores *MS o)* h *praem. ante corr.* *p)* vel *praem. ante corr.*

## 408

*The Master Fr. Antoni de Fluvià retains Fr. Johann Cruze, Bailiff of Westphalia, with his Preceptories of Steinfurt, Lage and Wesel, provided that the usual responsions and other dues are paid to the Order.*

*Rhodes, 1422 May 31*

*AOM 346 fol. 123v-4r, under* prioratus Alamanie.

Frater Anthonius Fluuiani sacre domus hospitalis etcetera religioso in Christo nobis carissimo fratri Iohanni Cruse ballivo nostre baiulie Westphalie prioratus nostri Almanie dicte domus salutem et sinceram in Domino caritatem. Dum laudabilia probitatis vestre merita in considerationis nostre aciem recensemus, digne credimus agere, cum vos inter alios domus nostre proceres attollimus prerogativa specialis gratie et honoris. Igitur vestram volentes honorare personam, ut proinde vestre fidei et devocionis zelus ad laudabiliora inantea ferventius animetur, vos unacum dicta vestra baiulia et preceptoriis vestris Steynfordie, Lage et Wesalie solutis per vos integre annuis eiusdem baiulie responsionibus termino statuto et vobis et dicte baiulie incumbentibus et incumbendis oneribus supportandis ad manus nostras tenore presentium de speciali gratia retinemus ab omni alia superioritate exemptum secundum bonos usus et laudabiles consuetudines domus nostre. [124r] Mandantes harum serie universis et singulis fratribus preceptoribus domus nostre quacumque auctoritate, eminentia vel potestate suffultis, presentibus et futuris sub virtute sancte obediencie firmiter et districte, ne contra presentis nostre retentionis gratiam aliquatenus venire presumant, quinymmo eam studeant iuxta eius mentem et seriem inconcusse et inviolabiliter observare. In cuius rei testimonium bulla nostra plumbea presentibus est appensa. Dat. Rodi in nostro conventu die ultima Maii anno incarnacionis Domini M° CCCC° XXII°.

## 409

*The Master Fr. Antoni de Fluvià orders Fr. Sander von Hellbick, Bailiff of Utrecht, Fr. Arnold Zeuwelkin, Preceptor of Arnheim, and the prior [of the house of Arnheim] to permit the payment of the usual* mortuarium *and* vacantia, *which they refused to do because they claimed without sufficient proof that Arnheim was not an independent commandery but only a member.*

*Rhodes, 1422 May 31*

*AOM 346 fol. 124v, under* prioratus Alamanie. *Ed. van Winter (1998), 40–1 no. 28.*

Frater Anthonius Fluuiani sacre domus hospitalis sancti Iohannis Iherosolimitani humilis magister et pauperum Christi custos religiosis in Christo nobis carissimis fratribus Zandro de Hellbick ballivo domus nostre Traiecti, Arnaldo Zeuwelkin ac priori conventus dicte domus necnon fratribus conventualibus domus eiusdem salutem in Domino et nostris firmiter obedire mandatis. Ad nostram presentiam olim ex veris et manifestis litterarum nostrorum procuratorum relacionibus pervenit, quod dudum nostros responsionum receptores mortuaria, vacantia et alia iura nostro communi thesauro pro defensione catholice fidei spectantia et pertinentia exhigentes repulistis sub umbra cuiusdam frivole[a)] excusacionis dictam domum membrem[!] Traiectensem camere asserentes, super quo nullam fidedignam probacionem non obstant. termino ab ipsis receptoribus dato in capitulo provinciali demonstratis, insuper vos novissime visitari a nostris procuratoribus, visitatoribus et correctoribus quibusdam interpositis reprobandis allegacionibus minime permisistis secularesque personas contra nostre religionis statuta et consuetudines laudabiles procuratoribus nostris iamdictis minas et terrores incucien. introduxistis. Et quia nemo suo dolo et fraude debet gaudere, vobis et unicuique vestrum in virtute sancte obediencie districte precipiendo mandamus, quatenus emendacionis spiritum resumpti procuratoribus nostris predictis dicta iura nostro dicto thesauro pertinencia et possessionem dicte domus omni contradictione postposita assignetis. Taliter vos in predictis exhibentes, ut de vestra obediencia apud nos recommendari valeatis. Valete in Christo. Dat. in nostro Rodi conventu die ultima mensis Maii M° CCCC° XXII°.

*a)* responsionis *add. ante corr.*

## 410

*Licence for Fr. Rembold zum Trübel, receiver of responsions in the Priory of* Alamania *and Preceptor of Dorlisheim and Rottweil, to come to the Convent and to rent out his preceptories for three years.*

*[Rhodes, 1422] June 3*

*AOM 346 fol. 124v, under* prioratus Alamanie.

Die III[a] mensis Iunii anno ut supra data fuit licentia fratri Ramboldo Zemtrubel receptori responsionum in prioratu Allamanie et preceptori de Dorenzel[!] et de Rotwil veniendi ad conventum et arrendandi pro tres annos predictas preceptorias.

## 411

*Protest by the procurators of the Tongue of* Alamania *that the appointment of Fr. Rupert, Duke of Silesia, to the Priory of Bohemia should not be to the future detriment of this tongue. Any future prior of Bohemia may come from either of the two priories, Bohemia or* Alamania.

*Rhodes, 1422 June 25*

*AOM 346 fol. 125r, under* prioratus Alamanie.

Protestatum est a procuratoribus lingue Alamanie ex parte fratrum dicte lingue in conventu commorantium, quod collacio facta fratri Roberto duci Slezie de prioratu Boemie[a)] non debeat futuri[b)] temporis ipsis fratribus dicte lingue Almanie a quo modo cedere in preiudicium, quinymo dicti fratres de cetero debeant et possunt dictum prioratum inter se una cum consensu magistri et consilii, quando casus evenerit, iuxta consuetudines laudabiles et statuta probata ipsius religionis conferre cuiquam[c)] fratri benemerito utriusque prioratus sive Boemie[a)] sive Almanie. Scripta XX[ma] quinta die mensis Iunii. Dat. M° CCCC et XXII.

*a)* Boemine *MS* *b)* futuris *corr.* *c)* cuiusquam *MS*

## 412

*The Master Fr. Antoni de Fluvià and the Convent grant to Fr. Rupert, Duke of Silesia, the Priory of Bohemia, which is vacant following the death of Fr. Heinrich von Neuhaus. He is to govern the priory, it preceptories and chambers. He is to pay the responsions of his chambers and of the priory's preceptories each year on 24 june and all other dues. The Master reserves for himself the right to grant one or more offices which are vacant following the death of the officer, according to the statute of 1367. In case of default and with the counsel of senior brethren the Master also reserves the right to grant the priory to another officer, following a statute of the same chapter general. As before that chapter general the brethren in the priory had had a right to certain death duties which were then reserved to the Treasury, the prior is permitted to choose an additional chamber from offices which fall vacant and which he may grant to the new officer. Fr. Rupert is to rule the priory in spiritual and temporal affairs and to dispense justice. Following another statute of 1367 he is to grant certain offices, castellanies and houses which fall vacant, without violating the Master's rights.*

*Rhodes, [1422] June 26*

*AOM 346 fol. 125r-v, under* prioratus Alamanie.

Frater Anthonius Fluuiani Dei gratia sacre domus hospitalis sancti Iohannis Iherosolimitani magister humilis et pauperum Christi custos et nos conventus Rhodi domus eiusdem venerabili ac religioso in Christo nobis carissimo fratri Rupperto duci Slezie prioratus nostri Bohemie dicte domus salutem et sinceram in Domino caritatem. Digne credimus agere et racionabiliter operari, si, quos domus nostre fratres excellentia meritorum extollit, ad celsiores gradu[s] nostri ordinis evocamus. Et cum, dum digni fructus dulcedine se refectos conspiciunt et secum honoratos, ad queque nostre religionis accommodo industrie eorum studia iugiter fervenciora convertant. Attendentes itaque proceritatis vestre notam et alia virtutum dona multimoda, quibus multipliciter prefulgetis, necnon quod sub vestro fructuoso regimine vestra industri soli[ci]tudine operante prioratus noster Boemie procurabitur accomode in spiritualibus et temporalibus quamplurima suscipiet incrementa, horum consideracione suasi prioratum ipsum per mortem quondam dicte domus fratris Henrici de Novadomo ultimi eiusdem prioris vacantem presencialiter et ad nostram collationem et dispositionem racionabiliter devolutam cum omnibus et singulis suis membris, iuribus et pertinenciis universis ad prioratum ipsum spectantibus et pertinentibus ac spectare et pertinere debentibus quoquomodo cum omni onere, emolumentis et honere et cum preceptoriis et cameris suis, et quas vobis pro cameris assi[g]namus, cum omnibus et singulis earum et cuiuslibet earum membris, iuribus et pertinenciis universis habendum, tenendum, regendum, gubernandum, augmentandum et meliorandum in spiritualibus et temporalibus tam in capite quam in membris vobis tamquam digno et benemerito invicem deliberato consilio, auctoritate presencium sub responsione annua consueta per vos, prout pro cameris vestris vos continget, et per preceptores preceptoriarum dicti prioratus, prout pro preceptoriis suis pro rata eis pertinebit, receptoribus deputatis vel deputandis per nos ad recipiendum responsiones in prioratu prefato aut alii vel aliis, quibus et ubi ordinaverimus et mandaverimus, in festo sancti Iohannis baptiste annis singulis ex pacto expresso infallibiliter exsolvanda et quibuscumque aliis oneribus dicto prioratui qualitercumque et quomodocunque incumbentibus et incumbendis, impositis et imponendis per vos et dictos preceptores, ut predicitur, ex pacto eciam ultra responsionem predictam supportandi de nostra certa scientia et speciali gratia benefaciendo in eadem ad[a] conferimus, concedimus et donamus. Retento nobis et specialiter reservato, quod de una vel pluribus, prout per mortem preceptoris evenire contingerit, vacantibus vel vacaturis baiulia vel baiuliis in dicto prioratu possumus anno quolibet providere secundum continenciam et seriem statuti, ac eciam retentis et reservatis nobis dicto magistro ordinacionibus omnibus pro bono memorie dominum fratrem Ra[i]mundum Berengarii dicte sacre domus magistrum predecessorem nostri prelibati magistri factis et sibi reservatis in generali capitulo per eum anno sexagesimo sexto in Avinione celebrato.[1] Nichilominus nobis dicto magistro[b] retento et eciam reservato, ut, si, quod absit, [125v] in solucione per vos statuto termino facienda annuarum vestrarum camerarum et baiuliarum responsionum, quas ad manus vestras habetis vel habebitis in premisso prioratu, defficere vos contingat, quod nos cum[c] consilio fratrum et procerum dicte domus possumus disponere et ordinare de premisso prioratu secundum continenciam statuti editi in generali capitulo prelibato. Rursum cum ante celebracionem dicti capituli priores domus nostre supra bona et arnesia preceptorum moriencium haberent et reciperent certa iura et iura huiusmodi fuerunt ex statuto[d] et ordinacione in iamdicto capitulo promulgatis urgenti necessitate applicata et reservata communi thesauro dicte nostre domus et propterea ex dictis ordinacione et statuto fuerit concessum et promissum prioribus, ut in recompens[a]tione iurium premissorum eorum cuilibet ultra suas ordinarias cameras haberet et habere posset in suo prioratu unam aliam baiuliam, cum vacabit, in vestro prioratu vestre collacioni pertinentem potestatem et licenciam indulgemus. Dantes vobis et concedentes auctoritatem et potestatem plenariam regendi, gubernandi et administrandi prioratum prefatum tam in capite quam in membris, in spiritualibus et temporalibus et quecumque alia celebrandi, agendi et exercendi, que ad prioris spectant officium et que pro utili regimine prioratus ipsius necessaria fuerint et eciam opportuna. Insuper dandi et conferendi cum consilio et assensu fratrum et procerum dicti prioratus baiulias, castellanias atque domos vacaturas in iamdicto prioratu vestre spectantes donacioni secundum statutum nostre dicte domus editum super istis fratribus ydoneis et benemeritis domus nostre prioratus prefati per dictum tempus[a], prout melius et ultimis vobis videbitur expedire, nostris tamen predictis retencionibus in omnibus semper salvis. Committentes etcetera. Invicem etcetera ad[e] decem annos etcetera comminantes etcetera. Quocirca etcetera necnon etcetera ac priori etcetera. Inhibentes etcetera. In cuius rei testimonium bulla nostra communis plumbea presentibus est apensa. Data Rhodi [in] nostro conventu die XXVI mensis Iunii anno incarnacionis ut supra.

1) *March 1367: Delaville (1913), 162.*

*marg. manu recentiori* collatio prioratus Boemie *a) add. lac.* *b)* ordinacionibus *add. ante corr.* *c)* in *corr.* *d)* fuerit concessum et permissum prioribus, ut in recompensationem et ordinacionem *add. ante corr.* *e)* a *MS*

## 413

*The Master Fr. Antoni de Fluvià informs Fr. Wilhelm Hartung that Fr. Johann Prager, Preceptor of Colmar (Priory of* Alamania), *has complained against him and that he is to give that preceptory to Fr. Johann. If he thinks he has claims to the Preceptory of Colmar, he is to come to Rhodes within nine months either in person or by sending a procurator in order to face trial. Otherwise his disobedience will be punished.*

*Rhodes, 1422 August 10*

*AOM 346 fol. 125v-6r, under* prioratus Alamanie.

Frater Anthonius Fluuiani Dei gratia sacre domus hospitalis sancti Iohannis Iherosolimitani magister humilis et pauperum Christi custos religioso in Christo nobis carissimo fratri Guillermo Harttung dicte domus salutem in Domino et nostris firmiter obedire mandatis[a)]. Tenore presencium vobis denotamus, quod ad nostram presenciam his diebus elapsis comparuit religiosus in Christo nobis carissimus frater Iohannes Proger eiusdem domus preceptor baiulie Columbarie nostri prioratus Alamanie et querellando nobis exposuit, quod possessiones dicte preceptorie suis procuratoribus restituere minime voluistis, imo violenter et sine aliquo iusto titulo prefatam preceptoriam detinetis. Ideoque vobis districtius sub virtute sancte obediencie precipiendo [126r] mandamus, quatenus visis presentibus omni excepcione et cavillacione remota preceptoriam iamdictam dicto fratri Iohanni vel eius procuratoribus restituatis iuxta tenorem bullarum nostrarum ipsi preceptori concessarum. Et si forsan in ipsa preceptoria aliquod ius habere pretenditis, quod nos penitus ignoramus, vobis terminum iuris assignamus, videlicet novem mensium, ad comparendum coram nobis personaliter vel per procuratorem fratrem nostre religionis sufficiens mandatum habentem ad allegandum et preponendum omnia iura vobis competencia, offerentes nos, ut ex debito tenemur, vobis et unicuique vestrum iusticie complementum administrare. Et si comparere coram nobis, ut superius est denotatum, neglexeritis, quod tamen non credimus, procedemus contra vos et personam vestram tamquam contra inobedientem secundum nostre religionis stabilimenta et consuetudines antiquas [h]actenus approbatas. Datum in nostro conventu Rhodi die decima mensis Augusti millesimo quadringentesimo vicesimo secundo sub impressione sigilli nostri, quo utimur in cera nigra.

*a)* mandamus *corr.*

## 414

*Licence for Fr. Johann Schwalbach to leave the Convent, to go to the West and return.*
*Rhodes, 1422 October 15*

*AOM 346 fol. 125v, under* prioratus Alamanie.

Fuit data licentia fratri Iohanni Suvalbach recedendi de conventu et eundi ad partes ponentis et redeundi, ut in forma. Dat. Rodi die XV[a] mensis Octobris millesimo quadringentesimo vigesimo secundo.

## 415

*Declaration by the Master and the Convent that the Tongue of* Alamania *is to be respected as one of the seven tongues with all honours and duties, including the captaincy of the castle of St. Peter [at Bodrum] in its turn.*
*Rhodes, 1422 November 9*

*AOM 346 fol. 126r, under* prioratus Alamanie. *Ed. Roger (2010), 101.*

Die nona mensis Novembris anno incarnacionis Domini M° IIII[Co] XXII° inter dominos magistrum, baiulos, priores et proceres in conventu Rodi[a)] commorantes fuit obtentum, quod fratres lingue Alamanie ipsorum lingua debeat una de septem linguis reputari in omnibus honoribus et oneribus in conventu Rodi et in capitaneatu castri sancti Petri secundum cursum aliorum linguarum.

*a)* et in capitaneatu *add. ante corr.*

## 416

*The Master Fr. Antoni de Fluvià and the Convent grant to Fr. Johann Lösel for his lifetime the Preceptory of Rheinfelden (Priory of* Alamania*), which is vacant following its resignation by Fr. Johann Schlegelholz into the Master's hands.*
*Rhodes, 1427 March 20*

*AOM 347 fol. 134r (122r), under* prioratus Alamanie, Boemie.

Frater Anthonius Fluuian etcetera et nos conventus Rhodi domus eiusdem religioso in Christo nobis carissimo fratri Iohanni Lo̊sel dicte domus prioratus Alamanie salutem et sincere dilectionis affectum. Religionis decor, morum honestas et alia virtutum dona, quibus vos carismatis gratia insignivit ad impartiendum vobis nostri favoris gratiam racionabiliter nos moventes, sperantesque in commisso vobis regimine effectus administracionis utilis favente Domino vos fructus uberes alaturum, preceptoriam de Rinfelden dicti prioratus vacantem presencialiter per ressignacionem fratris Iohannis Schlegelholtz dicte domus de sua spontanea voluntate factam in manibus nostri prelibati magistri et per nos dictum magistrum susceptum et propterea ad nostram dispositionem devolutam cum omnibus et singulis suis membris, iuribus et pertinenciis universis etcetera et cum quibus illam dictus frater Iohannes vel quicumque alius frater ultimus legitimus eiusdem possessor habuit etcetera invicem deliberato consilio de nostra certa scientia et speciali gratia ad vitam vestram vobis auctoritate presentium conferimus, concedimus et donamus etcetera. Committentes vobis fiducialiter etcetera. Quocirca universis et singulis etcetera necnon universis etcetera ac priori seu presidenti prefato etcetera. Inhibentes vobis districtius etcetera. Et si, quod absit, contra inhibitionem nostram huiusmodi etcetera. In cuius rei testimonium bulla nostra communis plumbea presentibus est impensa. Dat. Rhodi in nostro conventu die vicesima mensis Marcii anno incarnationis Domini millesimo CCCC XXVII.

*According to the Hospitaller style the date should be 1428 March 20, but the entry here starts the year from 1427 March 25 to 1428 March 24; so 1427 March 20 is the probable date.*

## 417

*The Master Fr. Antoni de Fluvià and the Convent grant for ten years to Fr. Peter Mersner, who has resigned the Preceptories of Reichardsroth and Rothenburg ob der Tauber (Priory of* Alamania) *into the Master's hands, the Preceptories of Erdlingen and Hemmendorf (Priory of* Alamania), *which are vacant following the death of Fr. Peter Salzfaß.*

*Rhodes, [1427] May 20*

*AOM 347 fol. 134r (122r), under* prioratus Alamanie, Boemie.

Frater Anthonius Fluuian etcetera et nos conventus Rhodi domus eiusdem religioso in Christo nobis carissimo fratri Petro Merschner dicte domus prioratus nostri Alamanie salutem in Domino sempiternam. Experto in regimine fructuosos, ut eorum virtus in amplioribus cura regiminis in ipsorum laudis preconium famosius divulgetur, rationabiliter eorum status de bono in melius commutamus. Sane cum baiulie seu preceptorie Richartzrod et Rottemburg voff der Tuber dicti prioratus vestre dudum administrationi commisse sub industri vestra gubernatione varia susceperint prosperitatis augmenta, perinde[a] spes certa resiliet, quod in nunc collatis baiuliis sive preceptoriis accomoda procurare studebitis gra[n]diora, resignatis per vos prius in manibus dicti nostri magistri de vestra spontanea voluntate baiuliis sive preceptoriis predictis et per nos dictum magistrum ipsa resignatione recepta, baiulias sive preceptorias de Erling et de Hemmendorff dicti nostri prioratus per mortem quondam fratris Petri Salczefas vacantes presentialiter et ad nostram donationem et collationem propterea devolutas, cum omnibus et singulis suis membris, iuribus etcetera et cum quibus illas habuit et tenuit dictus frater Petrus Salczefas, habendas etcetera – alias secundum continentiam et seriem statutorum etcetera invicem deliberato [consilio] de nostra certa scientia et speciali gratia ad annos decem incipiendos in festo sancti Iohannis baptiste proximo extunc continuo etcetera. Committentes vobis etcetera. Quocirca universis etcetera necnon universis etcetera ac priori seu presidenti etcetera. Inhibentes vobis districtius etcetera. Et si, quod absit, etcetera. In cuius rei testimonium bulla nostra communis plumbea presentibus est appensa. Dat. Rhodi in nostro conventu die XX mensis Maii anno incarnationis Domini ut supra.

*a)* proinde *recte*

## 418

*The Master Fr. Antoni de Fluvià and the Convent grant for ten years to Fr. Johann Schlegelholz the Preceptories of Reichardsroth and Rothenburg (Priory of* Alamania), *which are vacant following their resignation into the Master's hands by Fr. Peter Merschner.*

*Rhodes, [1427] May 20*

*AOM 347 fol. 134r (122r), under* prioratus Alamanie, Boemie.

Frater Anthonius Fluuian etcetera et nos conventus Rhodi domus eiusdem religioso in Christo nobis carissimo fratri Iohanni Schlegelhoz dicte domus prioratus nostri Alamanie [salutem] et sincere dilectionis affectum. Ad illos libenter gratiosum favorem nostrum extendimus, quos benemeritos reputamus, ut reffecti ex gratia et exhilarati ex honore suscepto ad providenda nostre religionis comoda libentius invigilent et ad virtutum studia ferventius eveniatur. Grata igitur fidedigna relatione percepto, quod gratiarum largitor Dominus vos morum compositione, vite munditia et naturali discretiva virtutum dotavit, sperantes in commissio vobis regimine favente Domino vos fructus uberes alaturum, baiulias seu preceptorias de Richartezrod [et] Rotemburg dicti prioratus vacantes per resignationem per fratrem Petrum Merschner dicte domus de sua spontanea voluntate factam in manibus nostri prelibati magistri et per nos dictum magistrum susceptas[a] et propterea ad nostram dispositionem devolutas, cum omnibus et singulis suis membris et iuribus universis etcetera habendas, tenendas etcetera invicem deliberato consilio etcetera de nostra certa scientia et speciali gratia ad annos decem etcetera. Committentes vobis etcetera. Quocirca etcetera nec[non] universis et singulis etcetera [b]ac priori etcetera[b]. Inhibentes vobis etcetera. In cuius rei testimonium bulla nostra communis plumbea presentibus est appensa. Dat. Rhodi in nostro conventu die XX mensis Maii anno quo supra.

*a)* susceptam *MS* *b-b) marg.*

## 419

*The Master Fr. Antoni [de Fluvià] informs the brethren of the Priory of* Alamania *that Fr. Peter Merschner, Preceptor of Erdlingen and Hemmendorf (Priory of* Alamania), *has borrowed a sum of money from Fr. Fritz Huber, Preceptor of Überlingen. Fr. Peter's preceptories serve as a surety.*

*Rhodes, 1428 September 10*

*AOM 347 fol. 136r (134r), under* prioratus Alamanie, Boemie.

Frater Anthonius etcetera universis et singulis fratribus religionis nostre presentibus et futuris prioratus nostri Alamanie, ad quos presentes nostre[a)] littere pervenerint, salutem in Domino sempiternam. Tenore presentium vobis notificamus, quod, cum religiosus in Christo nobis carissimus frater Petrus Merschner dicte domus preceptor in Erlingen et Hemmendorff dicti prioratus certa[m] quantitatem pecuniarum pro magnis suis necessitatibus indiguerit et frater Fritz Huober dicte domus preceptor in Wberlingen certam quantitatem inter ipsos conventam gratis et amore prefato fratri Petro nostri magistri voluntate interveniente mutuavit, ut inter prefatos contrahentes nostra etiam voluntate interveniente prefatus preceptor frater Petrus allegavit dictas suas preceptorias dicto fratri Fritz et que fructus illarum et emolumenta debeat percipere, donec et quousque erit sibi integraliter satisfactum. In cuius rei testimonium bulla nostra, qua utimur in cira nigra, presentibus est impensa. Dat. Rhodi in nostro conventu die X mensis Septembris M CCCC° XXVII.

*a)* p *add. ante corr.*

## 420

*Licence for Fr. Peter Merschner, Preceptor of Erdlingen and Hemmendorf, to leave the Convent.*

*Rhodes, 1427 September 23*

*AOM 347 fol. 134v (132v), under* prioratus Alamanie, Boemie.

Fuit data licentia fratri Petro Merschner preceptori in Erlyngen et Emendorff recedendi de conventu ut in forma. Dat. Rhodi die XXIII mensis Septembris anno incarnationis Domini M CCCC$^{mo}$ XXVII.

## 421

*The Master Fr. Antoni de Fluvià and the Convent grant for ten years to Fr. Anton Knoblauch the Preceptory of Regensburg (Priory of* Alamania), *which is vacant following the death of Fr. Peter Salzfaß.*

*Rhodes, [1427] September 25*

*AOM 347 fol. 136r (134r), under* prioratus Alamanie, Boemie.

Frater Anthonius Fluuian etcetera et nos conventus Rhodi domus eiusdem religioso in Christo nobis carissimo fratri Anthonio Klobeloch[e]ri[a] dicte domus prioratus nostri Alamanie salutem et sinceram in Domino caritatem. Ad illos libenter gratiosum nostrum favorem extendimus, quos benemeritos reputamus, ut refecti ex gratia et exhilarati ex honore suscepto ad promovenda nostre religionis comoda libentius invigilent et ad nutum studia libentius animentur. Grata igitur fidedigna relatione percepta, quod gratiarum largitor Dominus vos morum compositione, vite mundicia et naturali discretiva virtutum dotavit, sperantes in comisso vobis regimine favente Domino vos fructus uberes alaturis, preceptoriam seu baiuliam Regelspurg prioratus prefati per mortem quondam dicte domus fratris Petri Saltzfas ultimi eiusdem preceptoris vacantem seu alio quovis modo aut ex alterius cuiuscumque persone vacet, ad nostram collationem [et] dispositionem favorabiliter devolutam cum omnibus et singulis suis membris etcetera habendam, tenendam etcetera invicem deliberato consilio de nostra certa scientia et speciali gratia ad annos X etcetera. Comittentes vobis fiducialiter etcetera. Quocirca universis et singulis fratribus etcetera, quinimo etcetera ac priori seu presidenti prefato etcetera amoto abinde etcetera. Inhibentes etcetera. In cuius rei testimonium bulla nostra communis plumbea est appensa. Dat. Rhodi in nostro conventu die XXV mensis Se[p]tembris anno quo supra[b].

*a)* ri *supra lin.* *b) add.* Ista preceptoria fuit collata de gratia speciali prefato fratri Anthonio etcetera, quod non possit sibi obstare talis collatio, quod non possit ad aliam collationem vel alterius preceptorie collationem promoveri pro suo cabimento.

## 422

*The Master Fr. Antoni de Fluvià and the Convent grant for ten years to Fr. Emmerich Otrat von Bacharach (Priory of* Alamania) *the Preceptory of Freiburg im Üchtland (Priory of* Alamania), *which is vacant following the death of Fr. Marcellus de Clarmont.*

*Rhodes, 1427 October 8*

*AOM 347 fol. 135v (133v), under* prioratus Alamanie, Boemie.

Frater Anthonius Fluuian etcetera et nos conventus Rhodi domus eiusdem religiosos in Christo nobis carissimo fratri Emenricho Otrat de Bacherch prioratus nostri Alamanie dicte domus salutem et sinceram in Domino caritatem. Vestris exposcentibus meritis probitatis vos specialis favoris gratia prosequentes preceptoriam seu baiuliam de Friburg in Ohtlant prioratus nostri Alamanie prefati per mortem quondam dicte domus fratris Marcelli de Claramont ultimi eiusdem preceptoris vacantem seu alio quovis modo aut ex alterius cuiuscumque persone vacet, ad nostram collationem et dispositionem rationabiliter devolutam cum omnibus et singulis suis membris etcetera habendam, tenendam etcetera invicem deliberato consilio de nostra certa scientia et speciali gratia ad annos X continuos et completos vobis auctoritate presentium conferimus, concedimus et donamus benefaciendo in eadem etcetera. Committentes vobis fiducialiter etcetera. Quocirca universis et singulis fratribus, sororibus etcetera necnon universis et singulis etcetera ac priori seu presidenti prefato etcetera. Inhibentes vobis districtius etcetera. Et si, quod absit, etcetera. In cuius rei testimonium bulla nostra communis plumbea presentibus est appensa. Dat. Rhodi in nostro conventu die VIII mensis Octobris anno incarnationis Domini[a)] M CCCC XXVII.

*a)* dn *cum abbreviatione corr.*

## 423

*The Master Fr. Antoni de Fluvià and the Convent, acting in chapter general, constitute Fr. Pierre Lamand, Preceptor of [Saint-]Vaubourg and lieutenant of the Treasurer General, as their procurator to proceed against two persons, one falsely claiming to be a Hospitaller, the other falsely claiming to be a Franciscan, who collected money on behalf of the King of Cyprus and of the Order in certain regions of Germany, especially in Lübeck and [Stral]Sund.*

*Rhodes, 1428 May 20*

*AOM 348 fol. 124v-5r (122v-3r), under* prioratus Alamanie, Boemie. *Ed. Documents concerning Cyprus (2011), 100–1 no. 87.*

Noverint universi et singuli has presentes litteras inspecturi, quod nos frater Anthonius Fluuiani Dei gratia etcetera et nos conventus Rodi capitulum generale celebrantes, anima[d]vertentes ad nostram nuper pervenisse noticiam duos viros pseudones, quorum unus sub habitu dis[s]imulato[a)] nostre religionis se faciens fratrem militem religionis nostre, alter vero in habitu fratrum minorum ad partes Alamanie et precipue ad Lubeque, Zon et alias civitates et opida maris transeuntes subsidia pro serenissimo rege Cippri et religione nostra petentes, quodque plures peccunias cum falsis bullis et litteris a fidelibus personis recolligerunt et, antequam eorum perversam[b)] et sinistram poterint adimplere intentionem et dictas peccunias in eorum convertere usus, viri sagaces atque prudentes ipsorum locorum[c)], sicut Deo placuit, eorum perversitatem[d)] atque nequiciam opinantes dictas pecunias arestari ad opus ipsius domini regis et religionis nostre fecerunt. Unde pro recuperacione ipsarum pecuniarum religioni nostre tantum dumtaxat datarum ex nostra certa sciencia omnibus melioribus via, modo et forma, quibus melius et aptius valemus, nostrum facimus, constituimus, creamus et solempniter ordinamus procuratorem, actorem, factorem, sindicum et yconpremum ac negociorum nostrorum infrascriptorum[e)] gestorem et nuncium specialem et generalem, ita tamen quod specialitas [generalitati] non deroget [aut] econverso, videlicet religiosum in Christo nobis carissimum fratrem Petrum Lamandi preceptorem Vallisburgi et locumtenentem thesaurarii[f)] generalis religionis, presentem et onus huiusmodi procurationis in se reverenter suscipientem. Videlicet specialiter et expresse ad prefactas pecunias religioni nostre datas a quibuscumque personis ecclesiasticis vel mundanis habentibus et tenentibus in sequestro, custodia vel acomanda seu quocunque alio titulo, occasione seu causa habendum, petendum, levandum et recipiendum quascunque res et pecuniarum summas[g)] [125r] religioni nostre in partibus illis spectantes et pertinentes seu spectare et pertinere debentes quocunque titulo, occasione seu causa a quibuscunque personis ecclesiasticis vel mundanis ipsas res et pecunias habentibus seu debentibus. Et de habitis seu receptis, habendis et recipiendis quictanciam et quictancias vallidas et solempnes faciendum cum obligationibus, penis, iuramento et ad hec necessariis et opportunis. Et, si expedit, requirendum, protestandum, penas et deffenssas inponendum et, si opus et necesse fuerit, pro predictis comparandum usque ad litis finem, unumque et plures procuratorem seu procuratores loco sui cum simili potestate substituendum et eum ac eos revocandum, quociens opus fuerit et dicto procuratori videbitur expedire. Dantes et concedentes dicto nostro procuratori plenam et liberam potestatem ac mandatum speciale et generale predicta omnia et singula faciendum et generaliter omnia alia et singula agendum, dicendum et procurandum, que nosmet ipsi faceremus et facere possemus, si premissis omnibus et singulis personaliter interessemus, etiam si talia essent, que mandatum propterea exigerent magis speciale. Promittentes nos bona fide ratum et firmum omne id et quitquid per dictum nostrum procuratorem et substituendum actum, factum fuerit in premissis seu quolibet premissorum procuratum. Relevantes exnunc dictum nostrum procuratorem et substituendum ab omni onere satisdandi, de iudicio scisti[h)] et exnunc iudichatum solvi cum omnibus suis clausulis necessariis et opportunis, cum omni iuris et facti renunciatione ad hec necessaria pariter et cauthella sub ypotheca et obligatione omnium bonorum nostrorum et dicte domus nostre mobilium et immobilium presencium et futurorum. In quorum omnium testimonium bulla nostra communis plumbea presentibus est appenssa. Data in prefacto Rodi conventu durante nostro [generali] capitulo die vicessima mensis Maii anno incarnationis Domini millesimo quadringentesimo vicesimo octavo.

*a)* disimilato *MS* *b)* preversam *MS* *c)* licorum *MS* *d)* preversitatem *MS* *e)* infrascrip *praem. ante corr.* *f)* thesauriis *MS* *g)* res et pecunias *add. ante corr.* *h)* sisti *recte*

*According to Hatt Olsen (1962), 102 no. 13, AOM 348 fol. 195r Fr. Pierre Lamandi was visitor in* Dacia.

## 424

*The Master Fr. Antoni de Fluvià grants, with consent of the Convent, for ten years to Fr. Johann Schlegelholz, Preceptor of Rheinfelden, the Bailiwick of Hohenrain (Priory of* Alamania), *which is vacant following the death of Fr. Nikolaus Staler. The grant belongs to the Master following the statute issued in February 1379 during a chapter general on Rhodes which declared that every ten years the Master may grant one or two preceptories in each priory.*

*Rhodes, 1428 May 26*

*AOM 348 fol. 124r (122r), under* prioratus Alamanie, Boemie.

Frater Anthonius Fluuiani etcetera religioso in Christo nobis carissimo fratri Iohanni Schlegelholtz dicte domus preceptori domus nostre ad Rinuuelden prioratus nostri Alamanie salutem et sinceram in Domino caritatem. Ad illos libenter gratiosum nostrum favorem extendimus, quos benemeritos reputamus, ut refecti ex gratia ex exhilerati[!] ex honore suscepto ad promovenda nostre religionis commoda libentius invigilent et ad virtutum studia ferventius comminentur. Grata igitur fidedigna relatione percepto, sperantes in commisso vobis regimine favente Domino vos fructus uberes alaturum, non obstante igitur, quod dictam baiuliam noscamini presentialiter obtinere, domum seu baiuliam de Hohenrein dicte prioratus vacantem presentialiter per mortem fratris Nicholay Stoler dicte domus ultimi eiusdem preceptoris seu alio quovis modo vacet, et ad nostram col[l]ationem, ordinationem et dispositionem secundum seriem et continentiam statuti editi in generali capitulo Rodi de mense Februarii anni incarnationis Domini M[i] trecentesimi septuagesimi octavi celebrato[1] specialiter et expresse caventis, quod de una vel duabus vacante vel vacantibus preceptoria vel preceptoriis in quolibet prioratu de decennio in decennium[a] domus eiusdem fratribus benemeritis in nostro conventu Rodi residentibus providere et disponere possimus, rationabiliter propterea devolutam cum omnibus et singulis suis membris, iuribus et pertinentiis universis ad eam spectantibus et pertinentibus ac spectare et pertinere debentibus quoquomodo, et cum quibus illam habuit, tenuit et possedit dictus quondam frater Nicholaus vel quicumque alter ultimus eiusdem possessor, habendam, tenendam, regendam etcetera de voluntate et consensu balliviorum, priorum et procerum nostri Rodi conventus de nostra certa scientia et speciali gratia ad annos decem continuos et completos vobis auctoritate presentium conferimus, concedimus et donamus benefaciendo in eadem, vosque preceptorem et commendatorem[b] in dicta constituimus domo seu baiulia hac serie et eciam ordinamus. Committentes vobis etcetera. Quocirca universis et singulis fratribus etcetera necnon universis etcetera ac priori etcetera. Inhibentes vobis districtius etcetera. Et si,

1) *1379 February: Delaville (1913), 206–7.*

quod etcetera. In cuius rei testimonium bulla nostra plumbea presentibus est appensa. Datum Rodi in nostro conventu durante nostro capitulo generali die XXVI[a] mensis Maii anno incarnationis Domino M° CCCC° XXVIII°.

*marg.* duplicata  *a)* decennio in decennium *scriptura elargita*  *b)* cammendatorem *MS*

## 425

*The Master Fr. Antoni de Fluvià and the Convent loaned 2,000 gold ducats to King Eric of Denmark, Sweden and Norway, when he was on his pilgrimage to the Holy Sepulchre; acting in chapter general they instruct Fr. Pierre Lamand, Preceptor of Sainte-Vaubourg and lieutenant of the Treasurer General, to collect this money either by himself or through sub-procurators.*

*Rhodes, 1428 May 26*

*AOM 348 fol. 125v-6r (123v-4r), under* prioratus Alamanie, Boemie. *Cf. Hatt Olsen (1962), 102 no. 11.*

Noverint universi et singuli has presentes litteras procurationis, quod nos frater Anthonius Fluuiani Dei gratia etcetera et nos conventus Rodi domus eiusdem capitulum generale celebrantes, reminiscentes nos dudum serenissimo ac excellentissimo principi et domino domino Erico Dei gratia Suecie et Norwergie ac regnorum Gotorum et Slavorum rege duceque Promeranie[!] dudum, dum peregre visitaverit Dominicum sanctum sepulcrum,[1)] hic in Rhodo ad eius requisicionem summam duorum millium ducatorum auri graciose mutuas[s]e, ad quorum recuperacionem, cum idem dominus rex non solverit, necessarium nobis existat aliquem domus nostre fratrem ad conspectum ipsius domini regis transmittere pro recuperatione ipsorum ducatorum duorum millium. Unde confidentes de legallitate, industria ac probitate religiosi in Christo nobis carissimi fratris Petri Lamandi preceptoris sancte Valli Burgis et locumtenentis thesaurarii generalis nostre religionis, ex nostra certa scientia omnibus melioribus via, modo et forma, quibus melius et aptius valemus et scimus, de iure facimus[a)], constituimus, creamus et sollempniter ordinamus nostrum et dicte domus nostre procuratorem, actorem, factorem, sindicum et yconomum ac negociorum nostrorum infrascriptorum gestorem et nuncium specialem et generalem, ita tamen, quod specialitas generalitati non deroget aut econverso, videlicet eundem fratrem Petrum locumtenentem thesaurii[!] presentem et onus procurationis huiusmodi in se reverenter recipientem, videlicet specialiter et expresse ad petendum, exigendum, recipiendum, recuperandum et obtinendum nomine

*1) King Eric was on pilgrimage from 1423 until May 1425, whilst his wife Philippa served as regent.*

nostro et pro nobis a dicto domino rege et aliis, quorum interest, dictos ducatos duo mille et de habitis et receptis seu habendis et recipiendis quictantiam et quictancias vallidas et sollempnes cum obligationibus, penis, iuramento ad hec necessariis et oportunis, et si expedit, requirendum et protestandum et pro premissis comparendum coram quibuscumque principibus, dominationibus, communitatibus de iusticiarum rectoribus et in quibuscumque curiis ecclesiasticis et mundanis et communi ipsis proponendum, agendum et deffendendum usque ad litis finem, unumque et plures procuratorem seu procuratores loco sui substituendum et eum ac eos revocandum, quociens opus fuerit et dicto procuratori videbitur expedire. Dantes et concedentes dicto nostro procuratori plenam et liberam potestatem predicta omnia et singula faciendi et generaliter omnia et singula agendi, dicendi et procurandi, que nosmet ipsi faceremus et facere possemus, si premissis omnibus et singulis personaliter interessemus, eciam si talia essent, que mandatum proprium exigerent magis speciale[b)]. Promittentes nos bona fide habere ratum, gratum et firmum omne id et quitquid per dictum nostrum procuratorem et substituendum actum, factumve fuerit in premissis seu quolibet premissorum procuratum. Relevans exnunc eundem procuratorem ab omni onere satisdandi, de iudicio scisti et exnunc iudicatum solvi cum omnibus suis clausulis necessariis et oportunis, cum omni iuris et facti renunciatione ad hec necessaria pariter et cauthela[c)] sub ypotheca et obligatione omnium bonorum nostrorum et dicte domus nostre mobilium et immobilium, presencium [126r] futurorum. In quorum omnium testimonium bulla nostra communis plumbea presentibus est appenssa. Dat. Rodi in nostro conventu durante prefacto nostro generali capitulo die vicessimo sexta mensis Maii anno incarnacionis Domini millesimo quadringentesimo vicesimo octavo.

*a)* constitui mmiur *add. ante corr.* *b)* speciali *MS* *c)* ch *praem. ante corr.*

## 426

*The Master Fr. Antoni [de Fluvià] and the Convent quit King Eric of Denmark, Sweden and Norway for 2,000 gold ducats of Venice to whom they had lent this money in 1424, while he was on Rhodes on pilgrimage to the Holy Sepulchre.*

*Rhodes, 1428 May 26*

*AOM 348 fol. 127v (125v), under* prioratus Alamanie, Boemie. *Cf. Hatt Olsen (1962), 102 no. 12.*

Noverint universi et singuli hanc presentem quictanciam et liberationem inspecturi, lecturi eciam et audituri, quod nos frater Anthonius etcetera et nos conventus Rodi domus eiusdem capitulum generale celebrantes tenore presentium confitemur et in verbo veritatis palam et publice recognoscimus nos integraliter fuisse solutos et satisfactos atque contentos de serenissimo principe et domino domino Erico Dei gratia Dacie, Suecie et Nowergie ac regnorum

Gotorum Slavorum rege duxque Pomeranie de ducatis auri Venetis duobus milibus sibi per nos dudum de anno millesimo quadringentesimo vicesimo quarto, dum peregre veniret de Dominico sepulcro, gratiose mutuatis, facientes per nos et successores nostros eidem domino regi et suis per presentes finem, quictationem, remissionem, absolutionem de predictis[a] ducatis duobus millibus ac pactum expressum perpetuo valiturum ad aliquid ulterius non petendo seu per alium peti faciendo, cassantes, irritantes et annullantes obligationem per dictum dominum regem nobis de dictis ducatis duobus millibus factam ita, quod de cetero sic[b] inesse debeat nullius valloris in iudicio et extra. Promittentes nos bona fide contra presentem nostram confessionem et quictanciam ullo tempore non obicere vel venire per nos vel alios de iure vel de facto sub pena duplici ducatorum duorum millium applicandorum dicto domino rege, qua pena soluta vel non aut gratis remissa predicta omnia et singula firma perdurent, item reficere[c] et restituere eidem domino regi omnia et singula dampna, expensa et interesse[d] litis et extra, que propterea fierent. Pro quibus omnibus et singulis firmiter attendentis et observandis obligamus omnia nostra et dicte domus nostre religionis bona mobilia et immobilia presentia et futura cum omni iuris et facti renunciatione ad hec necessaria pariter et cauthella. In cuius rei[e] testimonium bulla nostra communis plumbea presentibus est appenssa. Dat. Rodi in nostro conventu die vicesima sexta mensis Maii anno incarnacionis Domini millesimo quadringentesimo vicesimo octavo.

*a)* absolutionem de predictis *alia manu script. in lac.* *b)* sit *MS* *c)* restituere *praem. ante corr.* *d)* inters *praem. ante corr.*

*AOM 349 fol. 195r, Hatt Olsen (1962), 102–3 no. 14, 1428 May 28, order for Silvestro Mauroceno to pay 2,000 ducats to Fr. Pierre Lamandi, lieutenant of the Treasurer, on account of King Erik's debt.*

## 427

*The Master Fr. Antoni de Fluvià and the Convent, acting in chapter general, constitute Fr. Roberto di Diana, Prior of Messina, as visitor, corrector and reformer the Priories of* Alamania, *Bohemia and Hungary. He is to go there in person and to visit, reform, correct and meliorate the priors, officers and preceptors, the convents, preceptories, offices and houses, the Hospital's brethren, sisters, donats and subjects in spiritual and temporal affairs. He is to ensure that the priors, officers, preceptors and leaseholders pay the responsions and arrears of responsions, the pension payments of the Master's chambers and other dues imposed on them, the* procrassia, mortuaria *and other dues from dead brethren which are due to the Master and Convent. He is to receive them from the receivers of responsions and from others who collect them. He may issue receipts of perpetual validity. In case of default he may depose, punish and reinstate preceptors and receivers of responsions. Vacant offices, preceptories and house he may lease out until the Master decides their case in Rhodes. He may dispense justice among brethren, sisters, donats and subjects of the Hospital. He may audit accounts. He may convoke assemlies of senior brethren. He may redeem estates, revenues and goods of the Hospital. He may make legal acts even in front of bishops, kings and dukes. He may demand oaths and issue receipts of perpetual validity. What he does is to be valid as if the Master himself were present. He may constitute procurators. He is to calculate the tax rates of the priors, preceptors, officers and rulers of the Master's chambers. In case of default he may enforce payment, if necessary with the help of secular powers. He may issue receipts, even those with perpetual validity. He may constitute one or more procurators with the same powers. What he does and they do is to be valid as if the Master himself were present, even if it were momentuous enough to require the Master's special licence. The priors, preceptors, officers, rulers of the Master's chambers and other brethren and subjects of the Hospital are to be obedient to him and to support him, even if some of them are exempt. However, he may not alienate revenues and goods without the Master's special licence.*

*Rhodes, 1428 May 28*

*AOM 348 fol. 126v-8v (124v-6v), under* prioratus Alamanie, Boemie. *On fol. 127v nos. 426, 436.*

Frater Anthonius Fluuiani etcetera et nos conventus Rodi domus eiusdem generale capitulum celebrantes venerabili ac religioso in Christo nobis carissimo fratri Roberto de Diana priori nostri prioratus Messane dicte domus salutem in Domino. Inter solicitudines alias mentis nostre studio inherentes illa quadam indesinenti meditacione solicita animum nostrum pulsat, ut prioratibus et baiuliis ac[a)] domibus nostre dicte domus visitacione, correctione et reformatione indigentibus de salubri celerique remedio occurratur, antequam dilatione illius gravibus dispendiis exponantur. Fidedigna relacione itaque intellecto noviter, quod prioratus nostri Almanie, Bohemie et Hongarie visitatione, correctione et reformatione noscuntur indigere, de fidei vestre legalitate et mature circumspectionis industria speciali fiducia confidentes et pariter sperantes, quod[b)] studiosa vestra providentia et vestra discretiva virtute, quibus vos dotavit graciarum largitor Dominus, prioratus predicti consolidabuntur, corrigentur et reformabuntur[c)] spiritualiter et temporaliter ad honorem et comodum ipsius domus nostre, nos invicem deliberato consilio ex nostra certa scientia[d)] auctoritate presencium et nostri dicti generalis capituli facimus, creamus et solempniter ordinamus nostrum ac domus nostre procuratorem, commissarium, visitatorem, correctorem et reformatorem in prioratibus predictis et eorum quolibet in spiritualibus et temporalibus tam in capitibus quam in membris. Dantes et concedentes vobis auctoritatem, potestatem et licentiam vos ad dictos prioratus et eorum quemlibet personaliter transferendi, ipsorum prioratuum priores, baiulos ac preceptores eorumque conventus, preceptorias, baiulias, domus, fratres, sorores, donatos, homines, vassalos visitandi et reformandi, corrigendi et meliorandi in spiritualibus et temporalibus, in capitibus et membris necnon ipsorum prioratuum priores, baiulos, preceptores, firmarios et arrendarios et eorum quemlibet compellendi efficaciter per omnem cohersionis modum rationabilem, prout vobis visum erit, ad solvendum responsiones suas, arreragia responsionum, pensiones camerarum nostri prelibati magistri, quas in dictis prioratibus obtinemus, ac earum responsiones et alia onera inposita et inponenda, procrassiave et mortuaria et quevis alia bona et iura fratrum domus nostre deffunctorum et inantea moriendorum in prioratibus prefatis vel eorum altero, quorum res, bona et iura in toto vel in parte ad nos communiter vel divisim pertineant et debeant racionabiliter pervenire, ac etiam omnia alia et singula quacumque racione nobis communiter vel divisim pertinentia, ad recipiendum illa de per nos deputatis vel inantea deputandis responsionum receptoribus seu aliis quibuscumque de receptis et habitis quictancias dandi perpetuo vallituras, eciam destituendi dictos preceptores et responsionum receptores seu eorum alterum ab administrationibus et aliis officiis, si opporteat et si[e] ipsorum exigerit contumatia vel defectus et pro nostre religionis utilitate visum fuerit expedire, et in huiusmodi administrationibus et officiis sic destitutorum vel destituendorum locorum alios domus nostre fratres puta sufficientes et ydoneos usque ad nostrum beneplacitum subrogandi, baiulias, preceptorias sive domus, si que in dictis prioratibus vacent de presenti aut in futurum vacaverint seu a dictis prioribus vel eorum altero aut aliis fratribus indebite detineantur [127r] occupate, arrendandi et affictandi seu arrendandum et administrandum tradendi nostro nomine, donec et quousque alias duxerimus providendum, fratresque huiusmodi destitutos ad sua restituendi regimina et officia, si ipsorum satisfacio et debita peticio meruerint, rebelles quoque[f] et inobedientes et solvere per eos debita et debenda recusantes ad vestram evocandi presenciam et eos secundum statuta et consuetudines nostre dicte domus, prout demeruerint, puniendi et ducendi per iusticiam domus ipsius seu eum et eos ad nostram citra mare presenciam repellendi et transmittendi, inter fratres, sorores, donatos, homines, vassallos nostre dicte domus prioratuum predictorum super quibuscumque causis et casibus iusticiam ministrandi, culpabiles puniendi et ducendi per iusticiam nostre dicte domus, planctam[g] et planctas faciendi, fratrum esgardia petendi et tenendi et mandare teneri, raciones et conputa seu raciocinia ob omnibus et singulis, quorum interest seu interesse potest et poterit, audiendi et ad petendum dicta computa et raciones sive[h] raciocinia eos et eorum quemlibet auctoritate nostra efficaciter compellendi, ipsaque computa et raciones examinandi, allocandi, approbandi et reprobandi in toto vel in parte et ea[i] concludendi et diffiniendi, prout vobis pro utilitate nostri communis thesauri videbitur expedire, et que reperierunt vobis communiter vel divisim deberi, dari, restitui, facientes receptoribus procurationibus nostris aut alias communiter vel divisim ad talia constitutis in prioratibus prefatis seu eorum altero, prout ad ipsorum quemlibet pertinebit iuxta commissionem et commissiones nostras eis factas capitulum et capitula, assambleiam et assambleias et congregationes fratrum in prioratibus ipsis et eorum quolibet mandandi et tenendi super quibuscumque[j] negotiis, quocienscumque vobis visum fuerit expedire, et in aliis disponendi et ordinandi cum consilio fratrum et procerum prioratuum eorundem omnia et singula concernentia utilitatem nostre dicte domus castra, loca, bona, domus, possessiones, iura et quasvis res alias prioratuum predictorum alienatas et alienata et per quoscumque personas ecclesiasticas vel mundanas iniuste occupatas et occupata, detentas et detenta petendi et recuperandi et ad ius et proprietatem nostre domus recovandi et reducendi pro nobis quoque et nostra dicta domo communiter vel divisim a quibuscumque dominis ecclesiasticis et secularibus, etiam si pontificali, regia vel ducali vel alia quacumque prefulgeant[k)] dignitate, supplicandi et ab eis et eorum quolibet litteras gratie et simplicis iusticie petendi et obtinendi et impetratis et impetrandis contra nos et nostram dictam domum communiter vel divisim et personas ipsius et loca obiciendi et contradicendi homagia et fidelitatis sacramenta ab hominibus et vassalis dictorum prioratuum, si expediat, petendi et recipiendi, necnon terras, loca, dominia, castra, domus, possessiones, iura et quevis bona alia mobilia et immobilia, quecumque et qualiacumque fuerunt seu quovis nomine nuncupata per quoscumque dominos spirituales et temporales eciam si pontificali, regali, ducali vel alia quacumque prefulgeant dignitate, cives, mercatores, rurales vel alias cuiuscumque status nobis et nostre domui communiter vel divisim in ultima[l)] eorum voluntate vel alias inter vivos quovismodo[m)] [127v] dimissas et dimissa seu dimittendas et dimittenda petendi et requirendi, recipiendi et ad nostram prefatam religionem trahendi et, si necesse[n)] fuerit, homagia fidelitatis iuramenta proinde faciendi litterasque quictationis vel alias ad hec necessarias passandi et concedendi nostro et dicte domus nostre nomine atque vice perpetuo valituras ac eciam fratrem unum dicte domus per vos in dictis prioratibus vel eorum altero recipiendi, eligendi et vobiscum assumendi, qui in predictis et subscriptis consilium habeant, potestatem et sibi traditam per presentes ad omnia alia et singula alia et insuper dependentibus, incidentibus et emergentibus ex predictis et eorum altero [128r] ac ipsis et eorum cuilibet quoquomodo connexis, prout melius vobis et utilius videbitur exercendi, exequendi, faciendi, disponendi et ordinandi, que nos ipsi visitare, reformare, corrigere, exercere et facere possemus, si in dictis prioratibus personaliter adessemus et insuper ad dictorum prioratuum et ipsorum cuiuslibet negocia qualiacumque ad honorem et utilitatem ipsorum et nostre dicte domus in quibuscumque curiis[o)] et partibus proponendi, promovendi et exequendi et proponi, promoveri et exequi faciendi per alium seu alios, quos ad singula vel visa pro nostra et dicte domus utilitate procuratores constituere possitis, super que facultatem vobis tenore presencium[p)] concedimus, quociens vobis expedire videbitur et fuerit opportunum, insuper ad annatam pro sustentacione nostri communis thesauri inpositam in ipsis prioratibus et preceptoriis, in quibus non fuerint per nostros deputatos taxata extimandi, inponendi et taxandi secundum Deum et conscientiam vestram, quam super hec oneramus, et preterea cum dictis prioribus, preceptoribus, baiuliis ac camerarum magistralium rectoribus seu eas quovis titulo tenentibus, si ad racionabilem fructuum, reddituum huiusmodi composicionem condescendere voluerint taxandi, concludi et componendi omnemque finalem determinationem faciendi, prout melius ad utilitatem prefati communis thesauri prioratuum camerarum magistralium, baiuliarum, preceptoriarum et domorum predictarum vobis videbitur expedire, in illis vero in quibus per nostros deputatos fuerint taxata et extimationes extimare et taxare[q)] una cum extima et taxa per vos, ut prefertur, fiende executioni demandendi, peccunias quoque taxationis vel composicionis fructuum, reddituum et proventuum huiusmodi seu alia quecumque prefato nostro communi thesauro deben(tia) hiis vel aliis de causis rationabiliter pervenerint[r)] nostro et nostri communis thesauri nomine petendi, exigendi, recipiendi, levandi et habendi et ad ipsorum solucionem et executionem priores, proceres, preceptores et ballivos ac camerarum magistralium rectores supradictos compellendi per captionem et venditionem bonorum suorum mobilium quorumcumque ad reddituum, fructuum[s)], proventuum prioratuum, magistralium camerarum, preceptoriarum et baiuliarum huiusmodi et omnem cohercionis modum vobis visum invocato ad hec[t)], si opus fuerit, preter sententias apostolicas contra rebelles et inobedientes ac solvere recusentes latas et ferendas auxilio brachii secularis, quod tenore presencium in vestri et substituendorum a vobis subsidium evocamus ac de receptis et habitis nostro et dicte domus ac communis thesauri nomine quictantias dandi perpetuo vallituras et nichillominus ad receptionem, levationem, exactionem et recuperationem reddituum, proventuum et fructuum predictorum sive peccuniarum proventurarum ex eisdem, procuratores unum vel plures domus nostre fratres, qui de receptis similes quictancias dare valeant ac eosdem priores, preceptores et ballivos ac camerarum magistralium rectores similiter compellere loco vestri semel vel pluries substituendi et ad lites et causas, que forsitan hac de causa possent ex aliquorum inobedientium et rebellium protervia suboriri, seculares personas et eum[u)] seu eos revocandi et in vobis procurationis officium reassumendi et generaliter omnia alia et singula faciendi, dicendi, procurandi et exercendi, qui in premissis et premissorum quolibet necessaria fuerint seu[v)] opportuna et que quilibet verus[w)] et legitimus procurator, negotiorum[x)] gestor, petitor et receptor facere posset et deberet et que nos ipsis faceremus, si presentes personaliter adessemus, eciam si talia fuerint, que mandatum exigant maius et magis speciale. Mandantes dictis prioribus et eorum quilibet ac universis et singulis fratribus, preceptoribus, baillivis, camerarum magistralium rectoribus et aliis quibuscumque dictorum prioratuum presentibus et futuris, cuiuscumque status, gradus vel condisionis[y)] existant, sub virtute sancte obedientie firmiter et districte ac hominibus et vassallis nobis et nostre domui subditis expresse precipimus et mandamus, ut in premissis et quolibet premissorum vobis[z)] tamquam nostro et dicte domus vero procuratori et reformatori pareant, obediant et intendant reverenter, quod tamquam nobis inparticiendo [128v] vobis auxilium, consilium et favorem, quociens eos et eorum singulos duxeritis requirendos, veritati eciam super quibus eos[aa)] et eorum alterum interrogaveritis aut interrogari feceritis testimonium perhibere non obstante, quod, si aliqui[bb)] ex dictis fratribus ad manus nostras sint retenti aliasve exempti per nos sub quacumque forma verborum quibus exemptiones suas in[x)] exequcione eorum, que vos acturus fueritis in dictis prioratibus et eorum quolibet, volumus de certa scientia in aliquo suffragare, quinimo prorsus ut fratres ceteri non exempti in omnibus vestre obedientie subsint, necnon ad mandatum vestrum et advocationem[cc] ad locum et loca, quem et que ipsos aut aliquem seu aliquos ex eis semel aut pluries vocaveritis[dd], veniant contradictione[ee] et excusatione remotis. Super quibus omnibus et singulis vobis tamquam nostro procuratori et visitatori committimus harum serie vices nostras, inhibentes vobis sub virtute sancte obedientie, ne pretextu visitacionis predicte aut alias aliqua de bonis, rebus aut iuribus predictorum prioratuum aut eorum cuiuslibet vendatis, detis, obligetis, impignoretis, permutetis, alienetis, distrahatis seu in emphiteosim[ff] perpetuam concedatis ac quocumque alio colore quesito extra nostram religionem transferatis sine nostra speciali licentia et mandato. Et si, quod absit, contra inhibicionem nostram huiusmodi aliquid vel aliqua operari vel facere vos contingat, illud et illa exnunc prout extunc et extunc prout exnunc cassamus, anullamus ac decernimus iritum et inane nulliusque existere efficacie vel valloris. In cuius rei testimonium bulla nostra communis plumbea presentibus est appenssa. Dat. Rodi in nostro conventu durante nostro prefato capitulo die vigesima[gg] octava mensis Maii anno incarnacionis Domini millesimo quadringentesimo vigesimo octavo.

*a)* ad *corr.* *b)* sperantesque *MS* *c)* int *add. supra lin.* *d)* et speciali *add. ante corr.* *e)* is *MS* *f)* quoq(ue)ie *MS* *g)* plantat *praem. ante corr.* *h)* sues ratino *corr.* *i)* et ea] ipsaque conputa *corr.* *j)* p *add. ante corr.* *k)* profulgeant *MS* *l)* utilitate *add. ante corr.* *m)* disi *add. ante corr.* *n)* neccem *praem. ante corr.* *o)* cure *corr.* *p)* eos *add. ante corr.* *q)* extimam *praem. ante corr.* *r)* pervenerinto *MS* *s)* fuc *praem. ante corr.* *t)* v *add. ante corr.* *u)* omni *corr.* *v)* vel *add. ante corr.* *w)* vera *MS* *x)* *supra lin.* *y)* conditionis *recte* *z)* universis vobis *add. ante corr.* *aa)* anno *corr.* *bb)* aliquem *corr.* *cc)* ad *del.* *dd)* veneritis *corr.* *ee)* cond *praem. ante corr.* *ff)* in emphiteosim] imemphiteosim *MS* *gg)* me *add. ante corr.*

## 428

*The Master Fr. Antoni de Fluvià and the Convent, acting in chapter general, declare, that the Preceptory of Rottweil was so far granted by the Prior of* Alamania *to a brother of his choice who agreed to pay a moderate pension to the Tongue of* Alamania. *In other priories there were also preceptories which promised similar pension payments as a* pitancia *to their tongue. But this caused shortages and damages when the pension was not paid. Following a petition by the brethren of the Tongue of* Alamania, *they now declare that when Fr. Rembold zum Trübel is no longer Preceptor of Rottweil, the Preceptory is to be granted in future to a brother of Tongue of Alamania on Rhodes who agrees to pay the pension.*

*Rhodes, [1428] May 31*

*AOM 348 fol. 124r-v (122r-v), under* prioratus Alamanie, Boemie.

Frater Antonius Fluuian etcetera et nos conventus Rhodi domus eiusdem capitulum generale celebrantes universis et singulis fratribus presentibus et futuris nostri prioratus Alamanie et quibusvis aliis, ad quos presentes nostre littere pervenerint, salutem in Domino sempiternam. Cum verum sit, quod preceptoria in Rotwil dicti prioratus a longo tempore fuerit ordinata pro pitantiis fratrum dicti prioratus in conventu Rhodi degentium, prout in aliis prioratibus similes preceptorie ordinate existunt, et dicta preceptoria conferatur a priore ipsius prioratus sub parva pensione in maximum da[m]num et detrimentum dictorum fratrum et contra bonos usus et laudabiles consuetudines conventus nostri, ob cuius rei causam procuratores lingue dicti prioratus in nostra comparuerunt presentia supplicando, quatenus dignaremur et vellemus, quod ipsius preceptorie collatio deberet spectare et solummodo pertinere et dumtaxat ipsis fratribus de eligendo preceptorem ipsius preceptorie sub certa pensione pro eis melius et utilius videbitur pro bono et utilitati [124v] dictorum fratrum et electione ipsius fratris facta per nos seu successores nostri magistri et conventum bulle exinde debeant fieri, prout est consuetum. Nos vero magister et capitulum generale conventus Rhodi celebrantes iuxta regulam, quod iuste deprecantibus non est denegandus as[s]ensus, decernimus et exnunc per presentes ordinamus, quod decedente seu mortuo fratre Remboldo Zůmnold ipsius preceptorie preceptore dictam preceptoriam de Rotwil exnunc et inantea et quotienscumque eam vacare contingerit, conferri, donari et dari debere per fratres conventuales Rhodi ipsius lingue alicui fratri ipsius lingue ad pensionem annalem, prout eis melius et utilius videbitur, pro comodo et bono ipsorum fratrum secundum bonos usus nostre religionis. Mandantes sub virtute sancte obedientie universis et singulis fratribus predictis, ne contra presentem nostram ordinationem aliquatenus venire, facere aut contradicere presumant, quinimo eam iuxta eius mentem et seriem studeant inviolabiliter observare. In cuius rei testimonium bulla nostra plumbea presentibus est appensa. Dat. in dicto nostro conventu durante nostro dicto capitulo generali prefato die ultima mensis Maii anno quo supra.

## 429

*The Master Fr. Antoni de Fluvià and the Convent grant to Fr. Richard von Nordheim the house or Bailiwick and Preceptory of Steinfurt in Westphalia (Priory of* Alamania), *which is vacant following the death of Fr. Nikolaus Staler.*

*Rhodes, [1428] June 1*

*AOM 348 fol. 128v (126v), under* prioratus Alamanie, Boemie. *Cf. van Winter (1998), 41 no. 29.*

Frater Anthonius Fluuiani etcetera religioso in Christo nobis carissimo [fratri] Ricardo de Norchei dicte domus prioratus nostri Alamanie salutem et sinceram in Domino caritatem. Ad illos libenter nostrum favorem extendimus[a], quod benemeritos reputamus. Preceptoriam domum seu baiuliam Steinfort situatam in Westualia dicti prioratus vacantem presentialiter per mortem quondam fratris Nicholai Stoler dicte domus ultimi eiusdem preceptoris cum omnibus et singulis suis membris etcetera habendam, tenendam etcetera. Committentes vobis etcetera. Quocirca universis etcetera necnon universis etcetera. Inhibentes vobis etcetera quinymo etcetera. In cuius rei testimonium bulla nostra communis plumbea presentibus est appensa[b]. Dat. Rhodi in nostro conventu die prima mensis Iunii anno ut supra.

*a)* exetendimus *MS* *b)* a *praem. ante corr.*

## 430

*The Master Fr. Antoni [de Fluvià] and the Convent, acting in chapter general, inform Fr. Hugo von Montfort, Prior of* Alamania, *and the brethren of his priory that Fr. Johann Lösel has received the above mentioned letter.*

*Rhodes, 1428 June 1*

*AOM 348 fol. 129r (127r), under* prioratus Alamanie, Boemie.

Frater Anthonius etcetera et nos conventus Rodi capitulum generale celebrantes venerabili ac religioso in Christo nobis carissimo fratri Hugoni de Montfort priori prioratus nostri Alamanie ac preceptoribus dicti prioratus, ad quos presentes nostre littere patentes pervenerint, quatenus fratri Iohanni Loͤsel data est talis executoria littera die prima mensis Iunii durante capitulo generali anno M° CCCC° XXVIII°.

## 431

*The Master Fr. Antoni de Fluvià and the Convent, acting in chapter general, confirm Fr. Johann Vetscholt for ten years in the Preceptory zu Horst (Priory of* Alamania).

*Rhodes, 1428 June 2*

*AOM 348 fol. 126r (124r), under* prioratus Alamanie, Boemie.

Frater Anthonius Fluuiani etcetera et nos conventus Rodi domus eiusdem capitulum generale celebrantes religioso in Christo nobis carissimo fratri Iohanni Vetscholt preceptori zů der Hurst[a] prioratus nostri Alamanie salutem et sinceram in Domino caritatem. Propter probitatis merita, vite mundiciam et religiositatis decorem, que secundum fidedigno testimonio accepimus habuistis, illa vobis libenter annuimus, que conservacionem vestri status cernere dinoscuntur. Hinc est, quod preceptoriam predictam seu baiuliam prioratus nostri prelibati cum omnibus et singulis suis membris, iuribus et pertinenciis universis ad eam spectantibus et pertinentibus ac spectare et pertinere debentis, et cum quibus illam presencialiter habetis ac tenere et possidere et habere debetis, habendam, tenendam etcetera sub annua responsione etcetera confirmationem huiusmodi de dicta baiulia etcetera invicem deliberato consilio de nostra certa scientia et speciali gratia ad annos decem continuos et completos vobis auctoritate presencium ac huiusmodi nostri presentis capituli generalis confirmamus et ad uberiorem vestri cautelam de novo conferimus, concedimus et donamus benefaciendo in eadem, vosque preceptorem etcetera. Committentes etcetera. Quocirca etcetera quinymo etcetera. Inhibentes etcetera. In cuius rei[b] testimonium bulla nostra plumbea presentibus est appenssa[c]. Dat. Rodi in nostro conventu die secunda mensis Iunii anno incarnacionis Domino millesimo[d] quadringentesimo vigesimo octavo.

*a)* zů der Hurst *supra lin., desupter* Nota, quod in secunda linea prescripte bulle fuit error in nomine preceptorie. *b) supra lin.* *c)* appenssat *MS* *d)* miss *praem. ante corr.*

## 432

*Confirmation of Fr. Markus Helfant as Preceptor of Heimbach, issued during the chapter general.*

*Rhodes, 1428 June 2*

*AOM 348 fol. 129r (127r), under* prioratus Alamanie, Boemie.

Anno M° CCCC° XXVIII° die secunda mensis Iunii durante capitulo generali data est confirmatio fratri Marco Helfant de preceptoria de Heymbach ut in forma.

## 433

*Following a petition from Fr. Rupert [of Silesia], Prior of Bohemia, who received five named men as knights into the Order, these receptions are confirmed as if Fr. Rupert had had the necessary licence.*

*Rhodes, [1428] June 10*

*AOM 348 fol. 125r (123r), under* prioratus Alamanie, Boemie.

Cum ex parte venerabilis fratris Ruperti comitis[a] [1] prioris Boemie fuerit notificatum domino nostro magistro, quod sua auctoritate propria fecerit quosdam fratres milites, quorum nomina sunt inferius descripta, ut dictus magister suam[b] confirmationem faceret et imponeret, qui dominus dicti prioris confirmavit et

1) ducis Slesie *recte*.

ratifficavit receptionem ipsorum fratrum perinde, acsi de sua licentia in religione fuissent as[s]umpti. Nomina vero ipsorum fratrum[c] sunt hec, videlicet fratres Conradus Nymaz, Iacobus Korncheyn, Georgius Falkenhayn, Nicholaus Valde et Octo Predil. Dat. Rhodi die X mensis Iunii anno quo supra.

*a)* fratris Ruperti comitis *supra lin. post* prioris *b)* suum *MS.* *c)* sunt hec *praem. ante corr.*

## 434

*Licence for [Fr. Rupert], Prior [of Bohemia], to receive 20 men as knights and 5 men as chaplains and sergeants into the Order.*

*[Rhodes, 1428 June 10]*

*AOM 348 fol. 125r (123r), under* prioratus Alamanie, Boemie.

Fuit data licentia fratri venerabili priori prefato faciendi fratres milites XX et V inter fratres capellanos et servientes ut in forma. Dat. die, mense et anno quo supra.

## 435

*The Master Fr. Antoni de Fluvià and the Convent, acting in chapter general, decide, following a complaint from the brethren of the Tongue of* Alamania, *that this tongue is to have the same honours and duties as the other tongues in the Convent. Given that they aim at peace in the Convent and want to encourage brethren from* Alamania *to come to the Convent, they creat the Grand Bailiff as a Conventual officer for this tongue similar to the other seven Conventual officers including the Prior of the Conventual church. He is to receive the same salary of 225 florins each year from the Treasury as does the Admiral. The Grand Bailiff is to visit at least once a year the Castle of St. Peter [at Bodrum] with all its mercenaries, weapons, missiles and artillery and to report about his findings to the Master.*

*Rhodes, 1428 June 10*

*AOM 348 fol. 130r (128r), under* prioratus Alamanie, Boemie.

Frater Anthonius Fluuiani etcetera et nos conventus Rhodi domus eiusdem capitulum generale celebrantes universis et singulis presentibus et futuris nostre religionis fratribus, ad quos presentes nostre patentes littere pervenerint, salutem in eo, in quo est vera salus et gaudium. Dignum existimamus huius thematis presentis materiam preponere et inscientibus ad eternam rei memoriam dilucidare. Ideoque in hiis prorumpere sermonibus et sub breviloquio illam progrediendo declaramus reserantes, quod longissimis temporibus iam transactis a fratribus lingue Alamanie in nostro conventu Rhodi commorantibus querelosa insinuatio sepenumero porrecta fuit, quod, cum ipsa lingua Alamanorum inter Christianos in potentia[a] et amplitudine dominii teneat principatum, erant intentionis et voluntatis in hoc generali capitulo aliquod officium baiuliatus cum stipendio debito in conventu nostro prefato habere et obtinere, prout fratres aliarum nationum hactenus in ipso conventu habebant et obtinebant, alias si ad huiusmodi requisitionem et petitionem per nos consensus sive assensus minime tribueretur, petitionem et requisitionem eorum indiscussam novi relinquere labores et expensas in ipsorum ius prosequendo eciam pariere nequaquam formidabunt. Nos vero prefati magister, baillivi, prior[b] et priores volentes iuridicis petitionibus et requisitionibus nostrorum fratrum, ut tenemur, adherere et illud benignis auribus exaudiri, iuxta regulam iuris communis dictantis: "Iuste deprecantibus non est denegandus assensus"[1], premissorum igitur occasione, ut fruamus pace et concordia in nostro dicto conventu, et quod iuris est semper nostris subditis administrare, ac ut ipsi fratres lingue predicte ferventiori amore nostro conventui servire teneantur, et ut ardentius ad conventum accedendi ad serviendum Deo et nostre religioni animentur, et ut materiam expensarum et laborum amputemus, auctoritate huiusmodi nostri capituli generalis fratribus lingue Alamanie baiuliatum nuncupatum magnum concedimus et donamus. Et quod dictus baiulus magnus per nos nuper creatus in nostro conventu Rhodi de numero septem baiuliorum ultra priorem ecclesie, qui spiritualibus preest, imposterum haberi, revereri et reputari debeat cum stipendiis florenorum ducentorum et XXV, prout admiratus nostri dicti conventus est assuetus et consuetus, annuatim percipere et habere a nostro communi thesauro. Et quod quolibet anno saltem semel, vel prout necessitate casuum venire contingerit, de licentia et voluntate nostri dicti magistri visitare debeat stipendiarios, munitiones, arma, missilia sive artellariam nostri castri sanctorum Petri et Pauli in acie Turcorum et infidelium situati[c] et conservati. Et in ipsius baiulii reversione a dicto castro nobis magistro et successoribus nostris, quicumque in ipso officio erit succesurus[d], relationem de omnibus repertis et inventis facere ad plenum[e] teneatur et debeat. In cuius rei testimonium bulla nostra communis plumbea presentibus est appensa. Dat. Rhodi in nostro conventu prefato nostro generali capitulo durante die decima mensis Iunii anno incarnationis Domini millesimo quadringentesimo XX° VIII°.

*a)* pontentia *MS* *b)* priore *MS* *c)* scituati *MS* *d)* sus- *praem. ante corr.* *e)* plenus *corr.*

## 436

*Licence for Fr. Johann Lösel to rent out his Preceptories of Mainz and Rheinfelden.*
*Rhodes, 1428 June 28*

1) *See Corpus Iuris Civilis, Institutiones 1.8.21.*

*AOM 348 fol. 127v (125v), under* prioratus Alamanie, Boemie.

Die XXVIII[a] mensis Iunii anno M° CCCC° XXVIII° datum fuit fratri Iohanni Lősel arrendamentum super preceptorias suas Mentz et Rinfelden.

## 437

*Licence [for Fr. Johann Lösel] to deduct 180 florins and 7 aspers from his responsions, because the Treasury owes him that sum for his salary.*

*[Rhodes, 1428] June 30*

*AOM 348 fol. 129r (127r), under* prioratus Alamanie, Boemie.

Item eodem die ultima mensis Iunii anno quo supra data est littera resecandi[a)] de responsionibus suis CLXXX[b)] florenos aspera VII, quos communis thesaurus sibi debebat pro soldeo suo.

*a)* recip *praem. ante corr.* *b)* CLXVIII *corr.*

## 438

*Licences for Fr. Johann Lösel, Preceptor of Mainz and Rheinfelden, to be retained, to receive two men as knight brethren into the Order, to leave the Convent and return.*

*[Rhodes], 1428 July 1*

*AOM 348 fol. 129r (127r), under* prioratus Alamanie, Boemie.

Die prima mensis Iulii anno M° CCCC° XXVIII° [a)] data est littera receptoria fratri Iohanni Lősel preceptori de Maguncia et de Rinfelden sub bulla plumbea magistri ipsum recipientis ad manus proprias cum preceptoriis suis ut in forma.

Item eodem die, mense, anno quo supra data est licentia faciendi duos fratres milites ut in forma.

Item eodem die, mense, anno quo supra data est licentia recedendi de conventu et reveniendi ut in forma.

*a)* anno M° CCCC° XXVIII° *supra lin.*

## 439

*Retention by the Master for [Fr. Markus Helfant, Preceptor of Heimbach].*

*[Rhodes, 1428] July 1*

*AOM 348 fol. 129r (127r), under* prioratus Alamanie, Boemie.

Die prima mensis Iulii anno quo supra data est eodem retentio ad manus magistri ut in forma.

## 440

*Licences for Fr. Markus Helfant to leave the Convent and to receive two men as brethren into the Order.*

*[Rhodes, 1428] July 1*

*AOM 348 fol. 129r (127r), under* prioratus Alamanie, Boemie.

Data est licentia fratri Marco Helfant recedendi de conventu et duos fratres faciendi[a] die prima mensis Iulii anno quo supra.

*a)* et duos fratres faciendi *supra lin.*, et domus suas arrendandi *corr.*

## 441

*Licence for Fr. Anton Knoblauch, Preceptor of Regensburg, to rent out his preceptory.*

*Rhodes, [1428] July 10*

*AOM 348 fol. 129r (127r), under* prioratus Alamanie, Boemie.

Fuit data licentia fratri Anthonio Knoploch preceptori Regelspurg suam preceptoriam arrendandi ut in forma. Dat. Rhodi X Iulii anno quo supra.

## 442

*Licence for the Grand Bailiff Fr. Johann Schlegelholz to rent out his houses.*

*[Rhodes], 1428 July 10*

*AOM 348 fol. 129r (127r), under* prioratus Alamanie, Boemie.

Data est licentia fratri Iohanni Slegelholtz magno balivo arrendandi domus suas die X mensis Iulii anno Domini M° CCCC° XXVIII°.

## 443

*The Master Fr. Antoni de Fluvià and the Convent license Fr. Anton Knoblauch, Preceptor of Regensburg (Priory of* Alamania*), to travel to the West in order to claim his paternal inheritance. As this inheritance includes fiefs, he may swear oaths of homage and fidelity.*

*Rhodes, [1428] July 10*

*AOM 348 fol. 129v (127v), under* prioratus Alamanie, Boemie.

Frater Anthonius Fluuiani Dei gratia sacre domus hospitalis etcetera et nos conventus Rodi religioso in Christo nobis carissimo fratri Anthonio Knobeloch preceptori de Regelspurg dicte domus prioratus nostri Almanie salutem in Domino sempiternam. Vestre supplicacioni continenti, ut ad petendum et recuperandum hereditatem paternam vobis contingentem et quecumque alia bona vobis debita et debenda in partibus ponentis licentiam concedendi[!] inpartiri dignaremur, premissorum occasione damus vobis licentiam et congetum ipsam hereditatem et patrimonium ac veoda quondam genitoris vestri a quibuscumque personis recuperandi et habendi, in quibuscumque rebus dictas hereditas et patrimonium ac veoda consistunt, et illa regendi et gubernandi prout genitor vester, dum vitam agebat in humanis, vos eadem forma agere et facere possitis ac homagia prestare et quecumque sacramenta fidelitatis auctoritate presencium damus licentiam, potestatem et iurisdictionem. In cuius rei testimonium bulla nostra communis plumbea presentibus est appenssa. Dat. Rodi in nostro conventu die Xª mensis Iullii anno ut supra.

## 444

*Licence [for Fr. Markus Helfant] to rent out his houses.*

*[Rhodes, 1428] July 12*

*AOM 348 fol. 129r (127r), under* prioratus Alamanie, Boemie.

Anno quo supra die XII mensis Iulii data est eodem licentia arrendandi domus suas.

## 445

*Constitution of Fr. Johann Lösel as receiver of responsions in the upper bailiwick and of Fr. Johann Schwalbach as receiver of responsions in the lower bailiwick of the Priory of* Alamania.

*[Rhodes], 1428 July 20*

*AOM 348 fol. 129r (127r), under* prioratus Alamanie, Boemie.

Anno M° CCCC° XXVIII° die vigesima Iulii data est bulla procuratoria fratri Iohanni Loͤsel essendi receptor responsionum in prioratu Alamanie in baiulia superiori ut in forma.

Item anno, die quo supra data est talis bulla fratri Iohanni Swalbach in prioratu predicto in baiulia inferiori.

## 446

*The Master Fr. Antoni [de Fluvià] and the Convent inform Fr. Johann von Monreal, Commander of Adenau and Breisig, and Fr. Eberhard von Url about a complaint by Fr. Simon von Bracht, Commander of Arnheim and Mecheln. Simon was granted Mecheln, but favouring Simon's opponent, the late Fr. Basilius von Hall, Johann and Eberhard refused to induct Simon into actual possession. When Basilius died, Johann and Eberhard, who now claim Mecheln, again refused to obey orders issued by Fr. Emondus de Armecione and to induct Simon into its actual possession. Johann and Eberhard are now ordered to be obedient, as is Fr. Hugo von Montfort, Prior of* Alamania. *Otherwise they will all be punished. The* spolium *of Fr. Basilius is to be ascertained and listed in an inventory by the visitor of the Master and Convent.*

*Rhodes, 1428 August 10*

*AOM 348 fol. 130r-v (128r-v), under* prioratus Alamanie, Boemie.

Frater Anthonius etcetera et nos conventus Rhodi domus eiusdem religiosis in Christo nobis carissimis fratribus Iohanni de Monreal commendatori domorum nostrorum in Adenaw, Brisig etcetera ac Euerardo de Vrl salutem et nostris firmiter inherere mandatis. Coram nobis comparuit dilectus in Christo nobis carissimus frater Symon de Bracht commendator in Arnheim et Mechelin querelose exponens[a], qualiter, cum iam dudum per nos de dicta domo Mechelin legitime sibi fuerit provisum iuxta tenorem litterarum executorialium sibi super hoc concessarum, quasquedam litteras presentibus volumus haberi pro expressis, quibus eciam litteris tam in capitulo provinciali quam[b] assemblea per eundem fratrem Symonem ostensis inter alios vos fratrem Iohannem supradictum tanquam ballivum et procuratorem conventus ac proximiorem et utiliorem executorem requisivit, quatenus huiusmodi nostro executoriali mandato parere velletis, dictum fratrem Symonem ad pocessionem prefate domus de Mechelin inducendo, quod tamen non ut executor, sed potius ut alterius partis fautor omnino adimplere renuistis, prout in quodam publico instrumento super hoc confecto nobis constat magnifeste, sicque nostra mandata differendo et quendam fratrem Basilius de Hal, dum viveret, contra ipsum fratrem Symonem ac nostrarum bullarum tenorem manutenendo. Non obstante eciam, ut accepimus[c], quod post obitum dicti fratris Basilii detentoris eiusdem venerabilis in Christo nobis carissimus frater Emondus de Armecione tamquam obediencie filius iamdicto fratri Symoni vice nostra piettate[!] domus pocessionem assignasse et vobis super hoc in nostrarum bullarum ac ipsius fratris Symonis favorem necnon cuiusdam fratris Euerardi de Vrl ammocionem graciose scripsisset, pocius induratus ac sub quodam velamine et nomine thesauri dictam pocessionem occupatam hucusque tenetis et ab eodem fratre Everardo intruso detineri procuratis. Hiis itaque per nos mature discussis et intellectis, et quia unicuique absque ulla acceptione personarum iusticiam administrare tenemur, vobis predictis fratribus Iohanni necnon Everardo coniunctim et divisim in virtute sancte obedientie ac sub penis contra rebelles et inobedientes per nostra statua promulgatis districtius precipiendo mandamus, quatenus post decem dierum spacium a die presentacionis presencium eidem fratri Symoni seu eius legittimo procuratori sepedicte domus pocessionem liberam et expeditam, corporalem[d] et realem cum omnibus et singulis eius membris ac pertinentiis fructibus, redditibus et proventibus perceptis et percipiendis assignetis omni contradictione seu excusatione remotis [130v], amoventes ac penitus detrahentes manus vestras ab eadem, amoto abinde alio quocumque detentore, sicut sit, quem nos eciam vigore presencium amovemus ac decernimus amovendum. Spolium tamen dicti fratris Banilii[!] defuncti, cuius de iure debeat esse, visitatori[e] nostro ad determinandum atque discuciandum relaxamus. Mandantes nichilominus sub eadem virtute venerabili in Christo nobis carissimo fratri Hugoni de Montfort priori prioratus nostri Almanie ceterisque baiulis, preceptoribus, vicepreceptoribus et aliis quibuscumque nostris subditis communiter et divisim, ut, si quis vestrum ab eodem fratre Symone commendatore aut eius procuratore simul vel insolidum primitus fuerit requisitus, presens nostrum mandatum infra terminum prefixum absque ulla dilacione vel excusacione fideliter et efficaciter exequi debeat, contradicentes vero per sensuras ecclesiasticas aut per brachium seculare, si oportunum fuerit, compescendo. In hiis itaque tam religiose quam solerter vos exhibentes, ut apud nos de vera obediencia merito valeatis commendari. In cuius rei testimonium bulla nostra communis plumbea presentibus est appensa. Data in nostro Rhodi conventu anno Domini M° quadringentesimo XX° VIII° die decima mensis Augusti.

*a)* exponans *MS* *b)* in *add. ante corr.* *c)* aperimus *MS* *d)* quam pluralem *MS* *e)* visitari *MS*

## 447

*Declaration that the Grand Bailiff [Fr. Johann Schlegelholz], the Preceptor of Cyprus [Fr. Hermann von Ow] and the other brethren of the Tongue of* Alamania *should cease dividing their* pitancie *among themselves but use these incomes for repairs to their auberge and other concerns of their tongue.*

*Rhodes, 1428 August 12*

*AOM 348 fol. 129v (127v), under* prioratus Alamanie, Boemie. *Ed. Roger (2010), 102*

Magnus balivius, preceptor Cipri[1] et alii quam plures fratres lingue Alamanie iverunt ad presentiam reverendissimi domini magistri et sui venerabilis consilii

*1) Fr. Hermann von Ow: Hartmann (1981), 108.*

et dixerunt, quod inter ipsos fuit concordatum et conventum, quod pitancie fratrum, que de prioratu Alamanie ad conventum transmittuntur, non debeant de cetero inter fratres dividi, sed in thesauro fratrum lingue debeant deponi pro reparatione albergie et aliarum rerum spectantium ad honorem lingue. Dat. Rhodi die XII mensis Augusti anno M CCCC$^{mo}$ XXVIII.

## 448

*The Master Fr. Antoni [de Fluvià] and the Convent inform the brethren of the Priory of* Alamania *that the Prior Fr. Hugo von Montfort and Fr. Johann von Monreal have been quarrelling for a long time about the house and prioral chamber of Cologne. In order to avoid further damages, the Master and Convent sequester the goods and commission Fr. Karl von Bingen, leaseholder of the house of Mainz, with their administration until the case is decided. Fr. Karl may name a sub-adminstrator. Moreover, he is to pay all necessary expenses for those who live in the house of Cologne not only from now on but from the time the dispute commenced.*

*Rhodes, 1428 August 15*

*AOM 348 fol. 130v-31r (128v-9r), under* prioratus Alamanie, Boemie.

Frater Anthonius etcetera et nos conventus Rhodi domus eiusdem universis et singulis presentes litteras visuris et audituris et presertim bailivis, preceptoribus et fratribus ac subditis nostris quibuscumque per prioratum nostrum Almanie constitutis salutem in Domino sempiternam. Noveritis, quod ad nostram pervenit audienciam, qualiter dissensio seu controversia quedam dampnosa et lamentabilis inter venerabiles et religiosos fratres nostros Hugonem de Monteforti priorem prioratus nostri Alamanie ex una et Iohannem Monreall partibus ex altera occasione domus et camere prioralis Coloniensis exorta sit et iam tempora perplurima – proch dolor! – duravit, ideo et in tantum, ut eciam de dicte camere prioralis et domus perpetua devastacione, nisi celeri succuriatur remedio, formidetur. Unde, cum inibi ex nostri officii debito incumbit talibus inconvenienciis obviare et obstacula adhibere, de maturo nostrorum procerum consilio in finem, ne dicta domus seu prioralis camera Coloniensis durante dicta controversia funditus exterminio et dilapidacione ulteriori subiciatur, eandem domum seu cameram Coloniensem cum omnibus et singulis suis membris, iuribus, redditibus et pertinentiis ad nostras reacceptavimus et revocamus manus ac eciam tenore presencium litterarum nostrarum reacceptamus, revocamus et retenemus neutri partium predictarum in ea ius aliquod relinquendo, donec et quousque controversia huiusmodi iusticia mediante fuerit decisa penitus et terminata. Committentes eciam predictam domum seu cameram Coloniensem predictam dilecto[a] nobis in Christo fratri Karolo de Pingwia arrendatori domus nostre Maguntine tamquam inter predictas partes neutrali et minus suspecto cum omnibus et singulis suis iuribus, fructibus, redditibus et proventibus nomine et loco nostri levandis et percipiendis dictamque cameram et domum tam in capite quam in membris, tam in spiritualibus quam in temporalibus regendam et manutenendam, donec de causa et iure controversie pretacte per venerabilem et religiosum in Christo nobis carissimum fratrem Robertum de Diano priorem Messanensem, visitatorem, reformatorem et commissarium nostrum[b)] cognitum et plene mediante iusticia decisa et terminata fuerit. Precipientes omnibus et singulis dicte domus ac prioratus [131r] camere fratribus, sororibus, donatis, vassallis, reddituariis ac colonis quibuscumque in virtute sancte obediencie, quatenus supradicto fratri Karolo nostro in domo Coloniensi et eius attinentiis hac vice locumtenenti seu eius substituto obediant et pareant sibique de omnibus et singulis iuribus, proventibus, fructibus, redditibus et pertinentiis respondeant et satisfaciant ac sibi tanquam nostro vero locumtenenti tradant et assignent[c)]. Que eciam iura sive reditus, fructus et proventus quascumque sequestramus ac in firmo sequestro apud dictum fratrem Karolum reponi et reservari volumus. In huiusmodi finem, ut divinus cultus, elemosinarum distributio ac status domus prefate secundum bonos et laudabiles usus tam in spiritualibus quam in temporabilibus observentur et quod residuum fructuum sub firmo sequestro, quod apud eundem nostrum locumtenentem maneat usque ad huiusmodi controversie descisionem, parti iusticiam obtinente protunc assignamus. Mandantes insuper presencium tenore vobis fratri Karolo locumtenenti nostro predicto huiusmodi nostre commissioni vobis de domo Coloniensi, ut premittitur, facte sub eadem virtute sancte obediencie firmiter obedire dictamque domum Coloniensem sic, ut premittitur, ad regendam et manutenendam nomine et loco nostro per vos vel alium legalem et fidelem auctoritate nostra vobis substituendum acceptare, cui eciam substituendo per vos vero liceat sub eadem virtute sancte obedientie in hoc casu vobis recalcitrare aut contradicere quovismodo. Vobis eciam venerabilibus et religiosis in Christo nobis carissimis fratribus Hugoni priori ac Iohanni Monreall partibus pretactis in virtute sancte obediencie et sub pena privacionis omnium preceptoriarum ac dignitatum vestrarum districte precipiendo mandamus, quatenus huiusmodi domo seu camera priorali Coloniensi ac omnibus eius iuribus et pertinenciis sic, ut premittitur, ad manus nostras acceptis et retentis desistatis, manus retrahatis neque quovis quesito colore publice vel occulte vos de eadem seu eius iuribus et pertinenciis intromittatis, donec per visitatorem et commissarium nostrum suprascriptum huiusmodi causa diffinita et pronunciata fuerit, quinymo supradicto[d)] fratri Karolo nostro locumtenenti seu eius iuribus substituto de omnibus et singulis iuribus, fructibus, redditibus et pertinenciis pretacte domus seu camere prioralis Coloniensis perceptis et percipiendis tam de anno presenti quam eciam de preteritis huiusmodi controversia durante annis plene et effectualiter et presertim de hiis, que in dicte domus et fratrum ibidem in ea residencium utilitatem et profectum minime conversa sunt, respondeatis, assignatis et computacionem legalem faciatis. Si quis autem vestrum predictorum contra huiusmodi ordinacionem seu disposicionem huiusmodi nostre bulle tenorem in parte vel in toto fecerit aut facere procuraverit seu eciam rebellis fuerit, privacionem suarum preceptoriarum seu dignitatum ac alias nostre religionis penas ipso facto se noverit incursurum. In cuius rei testimonium bulla nostra communis plumbea presentibus est appensa. Dat. Rhodi in nostro conventu anno Domini M° quadringentesimo XX° VIII° mensis Augusti die quinta decima.

*a)* dill *praem. ante corr.* *b)* vestrarum *praem. ante corr.* *c)* assignant *MS* *d)* supradicti *MS*

## 449

*The Master Fr. Antoni de Fluvià and the Convent order the two Bailiffs of Franconia and of the Wetterau to pay to Fr. Gerhard von Werthausen dictus Vuyst, Commander of Duisburg and procurator of the Bailiwicks and Preceptories of Lower* Alamania, *their share of his expenses for travelling to the Convent on Rhodes.*

*Rhodes, 1428 August 15*

*AOM 348 fol. 133r (131r), under* prioratus Alamanie, Boemie.

Frater Anthonius Fluuiani etcetera venerabilibus et religiosis in Christo dilectis fratribus in Franconia ac in der Wederaw balivis domus eiusdem salutem etcetera. Exposuit nobis dilectus nobis in Christo frater Gherardus de Werthusen dictus Vuyst commendator in Duysborgh, procurator balivorum et preceptorum prioratus Almanie inferioris, prout de ipsius procuracionis mandato nobis per instrumentum publice desuper confecti ostensione fidem fecit etcetera, qualiter de premissis sibi expensis faciendi et sallario cum transferendi se nomine vestrorum et per vobis ad conventum Rodi ibique coram nobis conparendi, prout et comparuit etcetera, pro rata seu porcione vos contingente tradere et assignare minime curastis etcetera, vos et cuilibet vestrum iniungimus per presentes, quatenus omni exceptione semota statim[a)] visis presentibus sibi de huiusmodi sumptibus pro rata vestra sub virtute sancte obediencie satisfacere non omittatis, ne nos ad ulteriora contra vos propterea procedere cogamur. Dat. Rodi etcetera M CCCC° XXVIII° die XV mensis Augusti.

*a)* statin *MS*

## 450

*The Master Fr. Antoni de Fluvià and the Convent inform the brethren of the Priory of* Alamania *that the Prior Fr. Hugo von Montfort and Fr. Johann von Monreal have long been quarrelling about the house and prioral chamber of Cologne. To avoid further damages, the Master and Convent sequester the goods and commission Fr. Rembold zum Trübel, Preceptor of Dorlisheim and Rottweil, with their administration until the case is decided. Fr. Rembold may name a sub-administrator. Moreover, he is to pay all necessary expenses for the those who live in the house of Cologne not only from now on but for all the time since the quarrel started.*

*Rhodes, 1428 August 16*

*AOM 348 fol. 131v-2r (129v-30r), under* prioratus Alamanie, Boemie.

Frater Anthonius Fluuian etcetera et nos conventus Rhodi domus eiusdem universis et singulis presentes nostras litteras visuris et audituris et presertim baliviis, preceptoribus, fratribus ac subditis nostris quibuscumque per prioratum nostrum Alamanie constitutis salutem in Domino sempiternam. Ad nostram pervenit audientiam, qualiter dissensio[a] seu controversia quedam dampnosa ac lamentabilis inter venerabiles ac religiosos fratres nostros Hugonem de Monfort priorem prioratus nostri Alamanie ex una ac Iohannem Monreal partibus ex altera occasione domus et camere prioralis Coloniensis exorta sit et iam tempora perplurima – pro dolor! – duravit adeo et in tantum, ut eciam de dicte camere ac domus internitione perpetua ac eius[b] devastacione in temporalibus, nisi celeri succuriatur remedio, formidetur. Unde, cum nobis ex nostri officii debito incumbit talibus obviare inconvenienciis et obstacula adhibere, de maturo nostrorum procerum consilio in fine[m], ne dicta domus seu prioralis camera durante dicta controversia funditus exterminio et delapidacione ulteriori subiciatur, eandem domum seu cameram prioralem Coloniensem cum omnibus [et singulis] suis membris, iuribus, redditibus et pertinentiis ad nostras reacetavimus[!] et retinuimus manus[!] ac eciam presencium nostrarum litterarum tenore reacetamus[!], retinemus ac revocamus manus. Committentes eandem domum sive cameram prioralem Coloniensem dilecto nobis in Christo fratri Rembaldo zum Trubel preceptori in Dorolsoheim et Rotwilere tamquam minus suspecto et inter partes predictas neutrali cum omnibus et singulis suis iuribus, fructibus, proventibus et redditibus loco et nomine nostri levandis et percipiendis dictamque cameram et domum tam in spiritualibus quam in temporalibus regendam et manutenendam, donec et quousque de causa et iure controversie pretacte per venerabilem et religiosum in Christo nobis carissimum fratrem Robertum de Diana priorem Messane, per tota[m] Alamaniam nostrum visitatorem, reformatorem et commissarium cognitum et plene iusticia mediante decissa et determinata fuerit. Precipientes omnibus et singulis dicte domus priori, fratribus, sororibus, donatis, vassallis, reddituariis ac colonis quibuscumque in virtute sancte obediencie ac sub homagii sacramento, quo nobis astricti sunt, quatenus supradicto fratri Remboldo seu omni nostro in dicta Coloniensi domo hac vice[c] locumtenenti obediant et pareant sibique de omnibus et singulis iuribus, proventibus, redditibus et fructibus prefate domus respondeant et eadem[d] sibi tanquam vero nostro locumtenenti assignent. Que iura sive redditus, fructus et proventus sequestramus ac[e] in firmo sequestro apud dictum fratrem Remboldum deponi et reservari volumus in hunc finem, ut dicte domus statui tam in spiritualibus quam in temporabilibus teneat secundum usum et consuetudinem domus eiusdem, et quod residuum fuerit in firmo sequestro teneat usque ad huiusmodi controversie decissionem parti iusticiam obtinenti assignandas. Precipiendo nichilominus vobis Remboldo nostro locumtenenti predicte nostre huiusmodi commissioni sub eadem sancte obedientie virtute firmiter obedire dictamque domum Colloniensem sic, ut premittitur, ad regendam et manutenendam benigne et fideliter per vos vel alium fidelem et neutri partium adherentem auctoritate nostra vobis substituendum absque aliqua excusatione seu exceptione statim visis presentibus dictam domum Colloniensem adire, fructus et proventus eiusdem colligere, partes predictas [132r] nostri nomine requirere et ad obediendum huiusmodi nostre ordinationi compellere et cohercere ac omnia et singula, ut premittitur, sine dolo facere et adimplere, ne mora sive dilactione vestra causantibus domus predicta in aliquo defraudetur. Vobis eciam venerabilibus et religiosis in Christo fratribus Hugoni priori ac Iohanni Monreal partibus predictis in virtute sancte obediencie et sub pena privacionis omnium preceptoriarum ac dignitatum vestrarum districtius precipiendo mandamus, quatenus de huiusmodi domo seu camera priorali Colloniensi ac[f)] omnibus eius[e)] iuribus, pertinenciis et redditibus desistatis, manus retrahatis, ne quovis quesito colore publice vel occulte vos de eadem intromittatis aut prefatum fratrem Remboldum nostrum in hac parte locumtenentem vel eius substituendum quoquomodo usque ad decissionem cause huiusmodi impediatis, quinimo sibi de omnibus et singulis fructibus et proventibus domus pretacte perceptis et percipiendis tam de presenti quam de preteritis huiusmodi controversie annis plene et effectualiter et presertim, que in dicte domus et fratrum ibidem ibidem residencium utilitatem minime conversi sunt, sub penis predictis respondeatis et assignando tradatis. Si quis autem vestrum predictorum contra huiusmodi nostram ordinacionem seu disposicionem fecerit vel ei inobediens fuerit, privacione omnium suarum preceptoriarum ac dignitatum et alias penas nostre religionis contra rebelles et inobedientes fulminandi ipso facto se noverit incursurum. In cuius rei testimonium bulla nostra communis plumbea presentibus est appensa. Dat. Rhodi in nostro conventu die XVI mensis Augusti anno incarnationis Domini M CCCC XXVIII.

*a)* discensio *MS* *b)* ac eius] ad cic *MS* *c)* hac v *praem. ante corr.* *d)* eod *praem. ante corr.* *e) supra lin.* *f) est add. ante corr.*

## 451

*The Master Fr. Antoni [de Fluvià] and the Convent grant for ten years to Fr. Gerhard Vuyst, Commander of Duisburg, the Preceptory or house of Walsum in the Bailiwick of Westphalia (Priory of* Alamania), *which is vacant following the death of Fr. Makarius von Kukelsheim or in some other way.*

*Rhodes, 1428 August 16*

*AOM 348 fol. 132v (130v), under* prioratus Alamanie, Boemie. *Cf. van Winter (1998), 41 no. 31.*

Frater Anthonius etcetera et nos conventus Rhodi domus eiusdem religioso in Christo nobis carissimo fratri Gherardo Vuyst commendatori nostre domus in Duysborgh salutem et sinceram in Domino caritatem. Illos ad honores et regimina domus nostre gratitudine debita evocamus, de quibus accepimus testimonium multipliciter commendandum. Sperantes itaque in commisso vobis regimine favente Domino vos fructus uberiores allaturum, de specialis dono gratie preceptoriam seu domum in Vualscheim in baiulia Westphalie prioratus nostri Almanie per obitum quondam fratris Macharii de Kukelshein vaca[n]tem sive eciam sic, ut premittitur, sive per dimissionem seu liberam resignationem alicuius aut eciam per obitum alterius cuiuscumque seu quocumque alio modo presencialiter vacantem et ad nostram disposicionem propterea racionabiliter devolutam cum omnibus et singulis suis membris, iuribus et pertinentiis ad eam spectantibus et pertinentibus et ad eam spectare et pertinere debentibus quoquomodo habendam, tenendam etcetera invicem deliberato consilio etcetera ad annos decem etcetera. Committentes vobis etcetera. Quocirca universi[s] et singulis etcetera necnon universis etcetera, quinymo eam studea[n]t etcetera. Inhibentes etcetera. Et si, quod absit, etcetera. In cuius rei testimonium bulla nostra communis plumbea presentibus est appensa. Dat. Rhodi in nostro conventu XVI$^{a}$ mensis Augusti anno Domini M° quadringentesimo XX° VIII°.

## 452

*The Master Fr. Antoni de Fluvià and the Convent grant for ten years to Fr. Gerhard Buttermon the house of Wesel (Priory of* Alamania), *which is vacant following its resignation by Fr. Johann Cruze, Bailiff of Westphalia, into the hands of Fr. Hugo von Montfort, Prior of* Alamania.

*Rhodes, 1428 August 16*

*AOM 348 fol. 132v (130v), under* prioratus Alamanie, Boemie. *Cf. van Winter (1998), 41 no. 30.*

Frater Anthonius Fluuian etcetera et nos conventus Rhodi domus eiusdem religioso in Christo nobis carissimo Ghirardo Buttermon domus eiusdem salutem[a)] et sinceram in Domino caritatem. Vite ac morum honestas aliaque laudabilia probitatis et virtutum merita, quibus apud nos fidedignorum testimonio comprobamini, nos inducunt, ut vobis ad gratiam reddamur liberales. De vestra igitur solerti solicitudine, quam in domo Vesaliensi hucusque exercuistis, informati atque de uberiori fructu alaturo per vos sperantes in futurum, speciali dono gratie vos prosequi intendentes, domum sive preceptoriam Vesaliensem baiulie Westfalie ac prioratus nostri Alamanie per liberam resignationem venerabilis et religiosi fratris Iohannis Cruxe balivii Vestfalie sua spontanea et mera voluntate in et ad manus reverendi fratris nostri Hugonis de Montforti prioris nostri prioratus Alamanie factam et per eum acceptatam vacantem presentialiter et ad nostram collationem, provisionem et plenariam dispositionem propterea rationabiliter devolutam sive etiam predicto vel alio quocumque more sive etiam per obitum alicuius vacaverit, eam cum omnibus et singulis suis membris, iuribus et pertinentiis etcetera habendam, tenendam etcetera invicem deliberato consilio de nostra certa scientia et speciali gratia ad annos X continuos et completos a[b)] datis presentium incipiendos etcetera. Committentes vobis fiducialiter etcetera. Quocirca universis et singulis etcetera necnon universis et singulis etcetera ac priori seu presidenti prefato etcetera amoto etiam abinde etcetera. Inhibentes etiam vobis etcetera. In cuius rei testimonium bulla nostra communis plumbea presentibus est appensa. Dat. Rhodi in nostro conventu die XVI mensis Augusti anno[c)] incarnationis Domini M CCCC XXVIII.

*a)* in Domino *add. ante corr.* *b)* ad *corr.* *c)* M CCCC *add. ante corr.*

## 453

*The Master Fr. Antoni de Fluvià and the Convent declare that the Preceptory of Cyprus has suffered serious damages from Saracen raids. With the consent of its Preceptor Fr. Hermann von Ow of the Priory of* Alamania, *who has been in office for a long time, they rent it out to Fr. Angelino Muscetulla and to Fr. Pedro Sarnes who have sent as their plenipotentiary Fr. Brasco Furnari, constituted in an act of the notary public Ludovicus de Sancto Dionysio written at Paphos on 6 May 1428. The two leaseholders receive the preceptory for seven years from 1 September 1428 to 31 August 1435 and with seven annual harvests. (1) They are to maintain the preceptory in good condition, especially the churches and the customary alms. (2) They are to pay 6,000 florins to the preceptory each year. From this sum they are to pay to the preceptor on Rhodes 1,100 florins in two instalments, the first in September and the second in February, and to the Treasury as responsions 4,900 florins, half in February and half in August. (3) They are to spend 500 florins each year for repairs according to the orders of the preceptor or of the visitor whom the Master will send to Cyprus every second year. When the preceptor or the visitor comes to Cyprus, they must provide him with six horses and six servants. (4) After seven years they have to return the preceptory in the state in which they received it. (5) So they have to return 34* mandre *of new sugar cane and 16* mandre *of old sugar cane manured and planted in the* casale *of Kolossi. If they grow more sugar, the preceptor can choose which old sugar and which new sugar he wishes to take, and they may refine their sugar in the factory at Kolossi, provided that the sugar of the preceptor is refined there first. In any case it is the preceptor who has to pay for the people, beasts and instruments necessary for this. The two leaseholders must return the land for the sugar ploughed eight times, 7* mandre *manured and 17* mandre *ploughed eight times. (6) Any unredeemed slaves, animals or other items which exceed the (present) status may be purchased by the preceptor. (7) The two leaseholders are to treat the serfs and subjects of the preceptory in the accustomed way. (8) They are to pay all obligations due. (9) During the seven years they have to pay all officers and servants, (10) but the preceptor has to pay them until 31 August 1428. (11) If there are losses through infertility of the land, fire, war, wind or similar causes, two arbiters or the Master are to decide how much the two leaseholders may deduct from their payments to the preceptor.*

*Rhodes, 1428 August 17*

*AOM 348, fol. 238v-9v (233v-4v) under* partes citramarine. *Ed. Documents concerning Cyprus (2011), 103–6 no. 89.*

Frater Anthonius Fluuian etcetera et nos conventus Rhodi domus eiusdem universis presentibus et futuris nostre religionis fratribus et quibuscumque aliis, ad quos presentes nostre patentes pervenerint littere, salutem in Domino sempiternam. Cum verum sit, quod preceptoria nostra magna regni Cipri iam diu collata fuerit venerabili ac religioso in Christo nobis carissimo fratri Armano de Ovv dicte domus prioratus nostri Alamanie, propter guerrarum tamen tribulationes Saracenorum suis sit viribus et redditibus destituta et, nisi de remedio opportuno celeriter eidem succuramus, posset ad talem pervenire statum et suorum reddituum diminutionem, quod non possemus de remedio salubri ipsi preceptorie imposterum providere. Nos igitur prefatus magister et conventus de consensu nichilominus prefati preceptoris predictam preceptoriam nostram [239r] tradimus, concedimus et arendamus, accensamus et affictamus et ad censum, affictum et arrendamentum tradimus honorabili ac religioso in Christo nobis carissimo fratri Brascho de Fornaris procuratori ac procuratorio nomine religiosorum fratrum Angelini Muscetulla et Petri Carnes dicte domus habenti ad infrascripta sufficiens mandatum, ut de eius mandato constat quodam publico instrumento scripto, confecto[a] Paphi manu Ludouici de Sancto Dionisio notarii publici imperiali auctoritate sub anno subscripto et die Iovis die VI mensis Maii appaltanti nomine et vice dictorum fratrum Angelini et Petri, predictam magnam preceptoriam Cipri cum omnibus et singulis suis membris, caxallibus, villis, edificiis, domibus, silvis, nemoribus, terris[b] aratoriis, cultis et incultis, et cum omnibus assensamentis et successionibus ac omnibus et singulis suis censibus, redditibus, proventibus, obventionibus et emolumentis et cum servis utriusque sexus et cum omnibus et singulis suis serviciis[c] realibus et personalibus et aliis iuribus et pertinentiis quibuscumque, et hoc ad annos septem et recollectas septem recipiendi incoandos a die prima mensis Se[p]tembris presentis anni M CCCC XXVIII et finiendo ultimo die mensis Augusti M CCCC$^{mi}$ XXXV, ad habendum, tenendum, possidendum durantibus dictis septem annis. Et quicquid dictis fratribus Angelino et Petro placuerit faciendum, cum omnibus et singulis, que infra confines rerum dicte preceptorie et membrorum eiusdem ubilibet constitutorum continentur, ac omnibus et singulis ipsi preceptorie et membrorum eiusdem quocumque modo, titulo, occasione seu causa pertinentibus. Que omnia ipsis arrendatoribus pleno iure pertineant et expectant per tempus dictorum septem annorum iure directi dominii ipsi preceptori semper salvo. Et hoc cum pacto, condictionibus et conventionibus infrascriptis:

[I] Primo, quod dicti arrendatores, videlicet fratres[d] Angelinus et Petrus, teneantur et debeant omni contradictione et excusatione cessantibus reparare ecclesias dicte preceptorie et facere eis servire bene et religiose, prout est de bona consuetudine et prout preceptor facere tenetur secundum Deum et suam religionem, necnon largiri et facere elemosinas usitatas ac servire pauperibus melioribus viis, modis et formis, quibus fieri debet de bona consuetudine.

[II] Item quod dicti arrendatores teneantur et debeant pro dicto appalto solvere quolibet anno sex millia florenos, videlicet dicto preceptori hic in Rhodo anno quolibet florenos Rhodi mille centum solvendos in duabus paguis, quarum prima paga erit quolibet mense Se[p]tembris cuiuslibet anni dictorum septem annorum et alia paga quolibet mense Februarii, et de hoc prestare fideiussoriam cautionem bonam et sufficientem dicto preceptori hic in Rhodo. Et insuper teneantur dare et solvere dicti arrendatores anno quolibet dictorum VII annorum communi thesauro Rhodi pro responsionibus ipsius preceptorie florenos Rhodi quatuor millia et VIIII$^{C}$, quorum florenorum IIII$^{M}$ et VIIII$^{C}$ medietatem solvere teneantur et debeant dicto communi thesauro hic in Rhodo de mense Februarii et aliam dimidietatem de mense Augusti cuiuslibet anni dictorum VII annorum.

[III] Insuper quod dicti arrendatores teneantur et debeant anno quolibet exponere et expendere florenos quingentos Rhodi in reparatione et emendatione prefate preceptorie ad ordinationem et dispositionem ipsius preceptoris seu visitatoris, quem nos prefatus magister destinabimus ibidem de duobus annis in duobus annis. Et quod dicti arrendatores teneantur et debeant dare expensas dicto preceptori seu visitatori ipso applicato in Cipro visitatione durante, videlicet dicto preceptori cum VI equis et VI familiaribus seu servitoribus tantummodo.

[IV] Item quod dicti arrendatores teneantur et debeant in fine dictorum VII annorum restituere dicto preceptori, vel cui ius dederit per religionem, statum[e)] dicte preceptorie et suorum pertinentium melioratum et emendatum et non peioratum vel saltim in equali bono statu, in quo ipsam receperunt, excepto statu callamele, quem teneantur dimittere melioratum et statu, quo continebitur inferius in capitulo sequenti.

[V] Propterea, quia dicti arrendatores teneantur et debeant restituere dicto preceptori seu successori suo in prelibata preceptoria dictis septem annis elapsis XXXIIII mandras callamele de muscati et sedecim mandras de callamela antiqua, que erit fimata et plantata ad usum caxallis Collosii. Et in casu, quo dicti arrendatores plantassent ultra dictam summam seu numerum, quod dictus preceptor, seu qui fuerit loco sui, possit eligere meliorem callamelam contiguam tamen, videlicet una sequatur aliam tantum de antiqua quantum de nova, et quod resta callamelarum ipsi arrendatores possint et valeant coquere in coquina Collosii coctis[f)] tamen per prius callamelis ipsius preceptorie. Et ipse preceptor teneatur eis dare magistros, servos, instrumenta, bestialia[g)], carretas et alia neccessaria quecumque cum solutione precii consueti solvere per preceptorem.

Subsequenter quod dicti arrendatores elapsis dictis[h)] VII annis teneantur et debeant dare dicto preceptori, seu qui fuerit loco sui, territorium novum callemelle ruptum [239v] octo vicibus et dare [decem] septem mandras de terrenis fumatis et decem septem mandras terreni rupti octies.

[VI] Etiam si dicti arrendatores dictis VII annis elapsis habuissent seu haberent sclavos, qui non fuerint redempti, ipsius preceptorie seu bestias, frumenta, vina seu alias res, que ascenderunt ultra statum, in quo receperunt, quod sit in potestate preceptoris capere dictas res pro precio illo, quod alius dare voluerit.

[VII] Item quod dicti arrendatores teneantur et debeant tractare[i)] et habere servos et homines ipsius preceptorie modo et forma, quibus sunt consueti tractari per preceptorem dicte preceptorie.

[VIII] Insuper quod dicti arrendatores teneantur et debeant habere dictam preceptoriam cum suo onere et carga quocumque.

[IX] Et quod in fine dictorum VII annorum debeant dimittere dictam preceptoriam libere et expedite dicto preceptori seu suo successori ab omnibus assignationbus et[j)] stipendiis officialium.

[X] Item teneatur dictus preceptor consignare et dare dictis arrendatoribus dictam preceptoriam liberam et francham de et ab omnibus assignationibus et stipendiis officialium, in quibus ipse preceptor fuit et est debitor usque ad primum diem mensis Se[p]tembris proximi futuri.

[XI] Reservatis casibus tam de iure canonico quam civili expressatis capituli 'Propter sterelitatem' Extra 'Locato'[k)] [1)] et legis 'Ex conducto' § 'Si vi[s] tempestatis' ff. eo(dem) ti(tulo),[2)] scilicet incendii, guerrarum, tempestatis et callamelle propter frigi[di]tatem glaciei ac langustarum pestem aliorum malorumque occurrentium ex dispositione planetarum, quibus intellectus humanus non potest providere. Et si in dictis casibus seu aliquo ipsorum ipsa preceptoria[l)] seu ipsi fratres Angelinus et Petrus aliquod dampnum, quod Deus avertat, recipient seu substinere poterunt, quod illud dampnum debeat[m)] dictis fratribus Angelino et Petro defalcari de ipso appaltu ad arbitrium proborum duorum virorum per utramque partem eligendorum seu ad ordinationem nostri magistri hospitalis.

Que omnia et singula promittimus tenere, complere et servare et econtra dictus frater Brascus nominibus quibus supra et contra ea non obicere, dicere vel venire per nos et interpositam personam publice vel secrete, directe vel indirecte de iure vel de facto sub ipotheca et obligatione omnium bonorum nostrorum presentium et futurorum cum omnibus iuris et facti renuntiatione ad hec neccessaria pariter et cautela. In cuius rei testimonium bulla

1) *Extra 3.18.3 De locato et conducto, Propter sterilitatem.*
2) *Dig. 19.2.15 ' 2 Ex conducto, Si vis tempestatis.*

nostra communis plumbea presentibus est appensa. Datum Rhodi in nostro conventu die XVII mensis Augusti anno incarnationis Domini M CCCC XXVIII.

*a) supra lin.* *b)* teriis *MS* *c)* servis *MS* *d)* fratris *MS* *e)* statim *MS* *f)* quotis *MS* *g)* bestilia *praem. ante corr.* *h)* dicti *MS* *i)* dare *praem. ante corr.* *j) supra lin.* *k)* locati *MS* *l)* ipsam preceptoriam *MS* *m)* debeant *ante corr.*

## 454

*Order for Fr. Rembold zum Trübel, Commander of Dorlisheim and Rothenburg, to administer the Preceptory and prioral chamber of Cologne until the Prior of Messina [Fr. Roberto di Diana] as visitor and reformer in the Priory of* Alamania *has decided the lawsuit between Fr. Hugo von Montfort and Fr. Johann von Monreal.*

*Rhodes, [1428] August 18*

*AOM 348 fol. 131r (129r), under* prioratus Alamanie, Boemie.

Fuit factum unum preceptum fratri Rembaldo de Zum Trubel commendatori domorum nostrarum in Toroltzheym et Rotemberg, quatenus preceptoriam sive cameram prioralem Coloniensem debeat in suis manibus retinere et, si ipse illam gubernare non possit, ad illius regimen ponat fratrem religionis honestum et non suspectum, donec venerabilis prior Messane, visitator et reformator dicti prioratus Alamanie de causa vertente inter priorem fratrem Hugonem de Montfor et fratrem Iohannem de Montreal fuerit cognita et determinata. Dat. Rodi XVIII Augusti anno quo supra.

## 455

*Licence to the Fr. Hugo von Montfort, Prior of* Alamania, *to rent out his prioral chambers and preceptories for three years, but only if he travels to the Convent.*

*Rhodes, 1428 October 4*

*AOM 348 fol. 133r (131r), under* prioratus Alamanie, Boemie.

Die[a)] IIII[a] mensis Octobris M° CCCC° XXVIII° fuit data licentia venerabili [et] religioso fratri Hugoni de Monteforti priori[b)] Alamanie arrendandi et affictandi cameras suas priorales et preceptorias, si quas obtinet[c)], usque ad tres anno[s] incipiendos a data dicte arrendacionis vel affictus, ita tamen, quod veniat ad conventum et alius non etcetera ut in forma.

*a)* XXIII *add. ante corr.* *b)* preceptori *praem. ante corr.*, pr *add. ante corr.* *c)* teneat *praem. ante corr.*

## 456

*The Master Fr. Antoni de Fluvià and the Convent grant for ten years to Fr. Gerhard von Werthausen dictus Vuyst the Preceptory (here* baiulia sive preceptoria) *of the house of Steinfurt with its member in the city of Münster (Priory of* Alamania), *which is vacant following its resignation by Fr. Richard von Nordheim into the Master's hands.*

*Rhodes, 1428 October 12*

*AOM 348 fol. 131v (129v), under* prioratus Alamanie, Boemie.

Frater Anthonius Fluuian etcetera et nos conventus Rhodi domus eiusdem religioso in Christo nobis carissimo fratri Girardo de Werthusen dicto Vuyst prioratus nostri Alamanie dicte domus salutem in Domino sempiternam. Commendabilium actuum vestrorum exercitia attendentes, quod in committendis vobis regiminibus in nostro ordine effectus administrationis utilis vos exibebit favente Domino eidem nostri ordini fructuosum nos inducunt, ut vobis ad gratiam reddamur liberales. Hinc est, quod, cum baiulia sive preceptoria domus in Stinfordia[a)] cum membro suo civitatis Monasteriensis sito[b)] in sancto Iohanne in Monte vocato[1)] vacare presentialiter dignoscitur per liberam resignationem religiosi in Christo nobis carissimi fratris Ricardi de Northeym predicte domus et ipsa resignatione in manibus nostri magistri facta et per nos suscepta propterea ad collationem, donationem et dispositionem nostram rationabiliter sit devoluta, cum omnibus et singulis suis membris, iuribus et pertinentiis etcetera habendam, tenendam etcetera invicem deliberato consilio de nostra certa scientia et speciali gratia ad annos X continuos et completos vobis auctoritate presentium conferimus etcetera. Committentes vobis etcetera. Quocirca universis etcetera necnon universis et singulis etcetera. Inhibentes vobis districtius etcetera. Et si, quod absit, in contrarium etcetera. In cuius rei testimonium bulla nostra plumbea presentibus est appensa. Dat. Rhodi in nostro conventu die XII mensis Octobris anne incarnationis Domini M CCCC XXVIII.

*a)* es *add. ante corr.* *b)* scito *MS*

## 457

*Licence for Fr. Gerhard von Werthausen dictus Vuyst, Preceptor of Steinfurt, to leave the Convent and return.*

*[Rhodes], 1428 October 12*

*AOM 348 fol. 133r (131r), under* prioratus Alamanie, Boemie.

1) *The text mentioned the Convent, but the seal was only the Master's bull. The name is missing, and the scribe has left no empty space for it.*

Die XII[a] mensis Octobris M° CCCC° XXVIII° fuit data licentia dicto fratri Gerardo de Werthůsen dicto Vuyst preceptori in Steynfordia recedendi[a)] de conventu et redeundi ut in forma.

*a)* arrend *praem. ante corr.*

## 458

*The Master Fr. Antoni de Fluvià licenses Fr. Gerhard von Werthausen dictus Vuyst, chaplain and familiar of the Master, Preceptor of Steinfurt, Duisburg and Walsum (Priory of* Alamania), *to rent out his preceptories for three years again and again, while he lives. He is also licensed to study the decretals and to receive his doctorate.*

*Rhodes, 1428 November 2*

*AOM 348 fol. 132v (130v), under* prioratus Alamanie, Boemie. *Cf. van Winter (1998), 41 no. 31.*

Frater Anthonius Fluuian Dei gratia sacre domus hospitalis sancti Iohannis Iherosolimitani magister etcetera religioso in Christo nobis carissimo fratri Gherardo de Werthusen dicto Vuyst dicte domus capellano et familiari nostro, preceptori domorum nostrorum Steynfordie, Duysborg ac Walshein prioratus nostri Almanie etcetera. Hinc est, quod vobis harum litterarum tenore de nostra certa scientia et speciali gracia prefatas vestras preceptorias aut aliquas earum, prout vobis videbitur expedire, cum eorum[!] membris, ipsarum redditus, iura et emolumenta etcetera licenciam arrendandi ad tres annos continuos a prima die afficti mandantes etcetera et sic deinceps dictis tribus annis elapsis de tribus annis ad[a)] tres annos, quamdiu vitam duxeritis in humanis etcetera. Item in studio decretorum usque ad gradum doctoratus inclusive ac insignia doctoralia deferre et accipere posse per vos licentiam elargimur et donamus. Dat. Rhodi in nostro conventu anno millesimo CCCC° XXVIII die secunda mensis Novembris.

*a)* in *corr.*

## 459

*Order for Fr. Roberto di Diana, Prior of Messina, to induct Fr. Anton Knoblauch or his procurators into corporal possession of the Preceptory of Regensburg (Priory of* Alamania), *which is vacant following the death of Fr. Peter Salzfaß, despite the protests of Fr. Peter Mersner who claims that Regensburg belongs as a member to one of his preceptories. This claim cannot be substantiated from the Treasury's registers of responsions or other legitimate proofs.*

*Rhodes, 1428 November 3*

*AOM 348 fol. 132r (130r), under* prioratus Alamanie, Boemie.

Fuit factum unum preceptum fratri Roberto de Diana priori Messane, quod cum fratri Anthonio Knobeloch fuit collata preceptoria de Regelspurg prioratus Alamanie, que vacavit per mortem fratris Petri Salzfas, quatenus ipsum fratrem Antonium vel suos legitimos procuratores ponat[a)] in possessionem corporalem dicte preceptorie non obstantibus quibuscumque exceptionibus et cavillationibus fratris Petri Mersner asserentis ipsam preceptoriam de Regelspurg fore membrum unius preceptoriarum suarum, quia ex registris responsionum communis thesauri quam ex aliis legitimis probationibus sint dominus magister et consilium informati[b)], quod dicta preceptoria caput obtinet preceptorio de per se et nullius alterius membrum fuit reputata. Dat. Rhodi die III mensis Novembris anno incarnationis Domini M CCCC XXVIII sub impressione bulle in cera nigra.

*a)* poss *praem. ante corr.* *b)* eciam *add. ante corr.*

## 460

*The Master Fr. Antoni de Fluvià and the Convent inform the brethren in* Alamania *that in the presence of the Master and Convent Fr. Fritz Huber, Commander of Überlingen, has lent 100 florins of the Rhine to Fr. Gerhard von Werthausen dictus Vuyst, Commander of Steinfurt and Duisburg.*

*Rhodes, 1428 November 3*

*AOM 348 fol. 133r (131r), under* prioratus Alamanie, Boemie.

Frater Anthonius Fluuiani Dei gracia etcetera universis et singulis presencia visuris et audituris et presertim[a)] domus nostre fratribus per Almaniam constitutis salutem in Domino sempiternam. Ad vestrorum singulorum noticiam deduci volumus, quod constitutis coram nobis religiosis nostre domus fratribus, videlicet Fritz Huber commendator domus in Vberlinghen ac Gerardo de Werthusen dicto Vůyst commendatore domorum in Steynvorden et in Duysborgh dicte domus, idem frater Gerardus recognovit et in veritate confessus fuit nostra licencia eciam requisita et ad hoc et ad singula infrascripta accedendi se pro suis indigenciis etcetera a dicto fratre Fritzo centum florenos Renenses bonos mutuo etcetera, quas promisit solvere ad suam requisicionem et dampna et expensas, si quas passus fuerit, restituere et obligavit sibi omnia sua bona presencia et futura. In huius testimonium sigillum nostrum etcetera. Dat. Rhodi M CCCC° [b)] XXVIII die 3ª Novembris. – Ego frater Gerardus commendator in Steynfordia et in Duysborg suprascriptus fateor premissa fore vera. In quorum testimonium hic me manu propria subscripsi.

*a)* nostre *add. ante corr.* *b)* die tertia Novembris *add. ante corr.*

## 461

*The Master Fr. Jacques de Milly and the Convent depose the Bailiff Fr. Heinrich von Riedern and, at the suggestion of the Tongue of* Alamania, *grant to Fr. Rudolf von Werdenberg the Bailiwick of Brandenburg with 1,500 florins of responsions, revoking the treaty confirmed by the Master Fr. Juan Fernández de Heredia (no. 115).*

*[Rhodes], 1461 July 9*

*AOM 371 fol. 135r-v (133r-v).* Antea copia ex registris per vicecancellarium fratrem Habele de dato 1633 Februarii 5 (*ut supra no. 115*).

Frater Iacobus de Milly etcetera et nos conventus etcetera nobili ac venerando religioso in Christo nobis precarissimo fratri Rudolffo de Werdenberg ex illustribus comitibus de Werdenberg dicte domus et prioratus nostri Alamanie salutem etcetera. Religionis zelus, morum honestas ac generis claritas, quibus noscimini insignitus, nos merito et racionabiliter inducunt, ut personam vestram ad dicte domus nostre gradus ac dignitates excellentiores tollamus et premiis decoramus, et eo magis, cum ex ipsius promocionis ornatu decus et utilitas religioni nostre provenire censeantur. Itaque humili exposicione[a] venerabilium religiosorum in Christo nobis precarissimorum fratrum venerande lingue Alamanie in hoc nostro conventu Rhodi ad Dei et religionis prelibate obsequia residencium coram nobis nuper facta cerciores effecti de honore, preheminencia, opimo et opulento valore patrie seu baiuliatus nostri de Brandenburg, qui secundum decenciam talis dignitatis et fructuum opulenciam obsequia ac commoda ipsi nostre religioni minime conferre videtur, verum exiguam porcionem respectu tantarum opum, que eciam nonnumquam deperditur, annuatim solvere obligatur. Considerantes igitur huiusmodi baiuliatum per vestram ad ipsum promocionem huius nostre religionis obediencie unire et simplici perpetuis temporibus submitti ac multo maiorem porcionem fructuum, quam hodiernis tribuat temporibus, nostro communi thesauro pro futuro annuatim concedere. Eapropter de consensu, assensu pariter et liberali voluntate ipsorum fratrum lingue antedicte, ad quos presens negocium potissime spectat et pertinet, qui de his coram nobis instantissimam peticionem exhibuerunt et voluerunt huic provisioni nostre licet preter formam stabilimentorum nostrorum ac dicte domus nostre et laudabilium consuetudinum facte in futurum quovismodo per quempiam fratrem vigore huiusmodi stabilimentorum contradici minime posse, verum ipsam in suo robore perpetuo existere. Revocantes, cassantes et annullantes pacta, concordiam et conventiones dudum facta et factas inter preteritos priores et preceptores dicti nostri prioratus Alamanie ac baiulivum et fratres ipsius baiuliatus in et super electione et confirmacione baiulivi et aliis quibusvis eciam litteras confirmatorias postmodum factas de predictis per quondam bone memorie fratrem Iohannem Ferdinandum de Heredia dicte domus olim magistrum, predecessorem nostrum, cum huiusmodi concordia et littere contra honorem et evidentem utilitatem ipsius nostre religionis emenaverint omnes quoque et singulas alias quasvis litteras, provisiones et vocaciones, confirmationes et scripturas factas et concessas quovismodo de dicto baiulliatu et membris eiusdem. Preceptoriam igitur seu baiulliatum prefatum de Brandenburg seu per obitum aut per resignacionem vel per presentes nostras revocaciones sive alias quovismodo vacantem presencialiter et ad nostram ipsorumque fratrum venerabilis lingue Alamanie collacionem, donacionem, ordinacionem et disposicionem pleno iure spectantem et pertinentem cum omnibus et singulis suis preceptoriis, domibus, membris, pertinenciis, fructibus, redditibus, iuribus, honore, onere et emolumentis quibuscunque ad ipsum baiulliatum spectantibus et pertinentibus sive spectare et pertinere debentibus quovismodo habendum, tenendum, possidendum, regendum, gubernandum, augmentandum et meliorandum in spiritualibus et temporalibus tam in capite quam in membris sub annua responsione florenorum auri de Reno mille quingentorum, quos pro responsione ordinaria super ipso baiulliatu per presentes imponimus, ceterisque oneribus impositis aut in futurum quovismodo imponendis in festo nativitatis sancti Iohannis baptiste de mense Iunii nobis et nostro communi thesauro sive deputandis a nobis per vos annis singulis infallibiliter exsolvendis – alias secundum seriem et continenciam statuti etcetera anno sexagesimo sexto celebrato[1] de dicto nostro baiulliatu alteri fratri utili et ydoneo ad eius regimen[b] et gubernacionem[c], qui dictam responsionem et onera solvat et supportet, providere possimus gratia huiusmodi de dicto baiulliatu vobis facta in aliquo non obstante – invicem maturo et deliberato consilio de nostra certa sciencia et speciali gracia vobis prefato fratri Rudolfo, donec vitam duxeritis in humanis, auctoritate presencium conferimus, concedimus et donamus benefaciendo in eadem vosque preceptorem et baiullivum in dicto constituimus baiulliatu harum serie ac eciam ordinamus. Committentes vobis fiducialiter circa curam, regimen et administracionem[d] accomodam dicti baiulliatus bonorumque etcetera. Quocirca etcetera necnon etcetera ne contra presentes nostras litteras revocacionis, cassacionis, annullacionis, imposicionis, collacionis, provisionis, gracie et mandati ac omnia et singula in eis contenta aliquatenus facere etcetera quinymmo iuxta earum mentem et seriem etcetera sic priori etcetera prefati prioratus et cuicunque alteri fratri super hoc primitus requisito, ut vos vel procuratorem etcetera amoto abinde religioso fratre Heinrico de Rideren occupatore dicti baiulliatus et quibusvis aliis ipsius baiulliatus detentoribus, quos nos tenore presencium etcetera. Inhibentes etcetera. Bulla communis plumbea etcetera die nona Iullii M IIII[c] LXI.

Revocatio constitutionis super baiulium[!] Brandenburch *marg.* *a*) exposictione *MS* *b*) regimine *ante corr.* *c*) gubernacioni *MS* *d*) circam curam, regimine et administracioni *MS*

*1) 1367 March 5: Delaville (1913), 161–2.*

## 462

*The Tongue of* Alamania *agrees that Fr. Rudolf von Werdenberg shall have the right to dispose of all preceptories in the Bailiwick of Brandenburg, because it will be difficult for him to obtain the bailiwick at all, but future bailiffs shall dispose of only four preceptories as priors do and a fifth one, whereas the other preceptories shall be disposed of by the Convent and the Tongue of* Alamania.

*[Rhodes, 1461]*

*AOM 371 fol. 137r (135r). Cf. Sarnowsky, Konvent (2001) and Die mittelalterliche Ballei (2001).*

Facta donacione et collacione de baiulliatu de Brandenburg domino fratri Rudolfo de Werdenberg de consensu fratrum venerande lingue Alamanie causis et racionibus in litteris collacionis explicatis fratres huiusmodi lingue predicte fuerunt contenti, quod idem dominus frater Rudolfus consideratis expensis et oneribus, que portabit pro habendo dicto baiulliatu, habeat et possideat ipsum baiulliatum cum suis omnibus preceptoriis, sicuti in bulla continentur, protestantes tamen, quod pro futuro interveniente vacacione ipsius baiulliatus per obitum dicti domini fratris Rudolfi aut alias ille, qui de eo providebitur per conventum seu alias, non teneat et possideat omnes et singulas preceptorias dicti baiulliatus, sed dumtaxat quatuor cameras habeat more reverendorum priorum religionis et unam pro quinta camera sue collacioni spectantem. Cetere autem preceptorie collacioni fratrum ipsius lingue et sacri conventus Rhodi pertineant et spectant et de eis fratres dicte lingue provideantur secundum bonam consuetudinem ordinis. Registrata de mandato reverendissimi domini magistri ad instanciam predictorum fratrum pro futura memoria facti.

Protestatio fratrum venerabilis linguę Alemanniae *marg. (saec. XVII).*

# LIST OF SOURCES

AOM = Archivum Ordinis Melitensis.

Most volumes of the *Libri Bullarum* have a modern pencil folio number. This is today used for ordering copies. The original ink folio numbers are here added in round brackets, because they were used in earlier publications. Where no modern pencil numbers existed when the present book was prepared (AOM 16, 280, 281, 340, 341, 344, 346), the figures – without brackets – indicate the old ink numbers.

Most *Libri Bullarum* cover one or two years. But the Hospitaller chancery on Rhodes commenced its year on the day of the Annunciation, 25 March. For this reason the year 1357 is, for example, hereafter rendered as 1357/8 and so on, because the Hospitallers used the *stilus Annunciationis* according to the *calculus Florentinus*. This meant that their dates given as between 1 January and 24 March 1357 were in fact according to modern style from 1 January to 24 March 1358 and so on, as opposed to the *calculus Pisanus* with dates given as between 25 March and 31 December 1357 being in fact according to modern style from 25 March to 31 December 1356.

AOM 16, originals

10: 2
11: 1
15: 3
34: 5

AOM 280, chapters general

2r-16r: 4
22r-9v: 4
33r-7v: 4
39r-42v: 4
44r-5v: 4
47r-51v: 4

AOM 281, for the Master Fr. Riccardo Caracciolo (obedient to the Roman pope)

1r-9r: 130
26r-7v: 127
29v: 128
33v-4r: 129
40r: 131
56r: 133
56r-v: 134
67r-8r: 149
68r-v: 145
68v-9r: 146
70r-71r: 150
75r: 151
80v: 152
85r: 154
85v-6r: 153
88v: 155
94v: 157
96v: 167

AOM 316 (for 1346/7–58/9)

200v-201r (201v-2r): 16
218r (219r): 14, 15, 17
218v (219v): 18
219r (220r): 20
219r-v (220r-v): 21
219v (220v): 22
219v-20r (220v-21r): 19
220r-v (221r-v): 25
220v (221v): 26
221r (222r): 27
221r-v (222r-v): 28
221v-2r (222v-3r): 29
222r-3r (223r-4r): 30
223r-v (224r-v): 31
223v (224v): 23
223v-4r (224v-5r): 32
224r-v (225r-v): 24
224v (225v): 37
225r (226r): 33, 34
225r-v (226r-v): 35

225v (226v): 36
225v-6r (226v-8r): 38
226r (228r): 39
226r-v (228r-v): 40
226v (228v): 41, 42
227r (229r): 43, 44
227v (229v): 48, 49
227v-8r (229v-30r): 45
228r (230r): 46
228r-v (230r-v): 47
228v (230v): 50, 51, 52, 53
228v-9r (230v-31r): 54
229r-v (231r-v): 55
229v-30r (231v-2r): 56
230v-31r (232v-3r): 57
231r-v (233r-v): 58
231v (233v): 59
232r-v (234r-v): 66
277r (281r): 64
277r-v (281r-v): 13
277v (281v): 65
277v-8r (281v-2r): 60
278r (282r): 61, 67
278r-v (282r-v): 62
278v (282v): 63

AOM 317 (for 1347/8)

100v (88v): 6
152r (140r): 7
152v (140v): 8

AOM 318 (for 1351/5)

150r (142r): 10
150r-v (142r-v): 11
167r-8r (159r-60r): 12
244r (235r): 9

AOM 319 (for 1365/6–66/7)

190r (184r): 70, 71, 72
190v (184v): 69
190v-91r (184v-5r): 68

191r (185r): 76
191v (185v): 75, 78
191v-2r (185v-6r): 73
192r (186r): 74
192v (186v): 77, 80
192v-3r (185v-6r): 79
193r (187r): 81, 82, 83, 84
193v (187v): 86
193v-4r (187v-8r): 87
312r (309r): 85
322r-35v, here 324r (no old fol.): 78

AOM 320 (for 1374/5)

28r-v (19r-v): 88
40r (31r): 90
41r-v (32r-v): 89
54v (45v): 91

AOM 321 (for 1381/2–82/3)

157r (148r): 92, 93, 94
157r-v (148r-v): 95
157v (148v): 96, 100, 101
241r (233r): 99
242r (234r): 97, 98

AOM 322 (for 1382/3–84/5)

18v-19r (9v-10r): 135
145v-6r (140v-41r): 105
203r (195r): 102, 103, 104, 105
203r-v (195r-v): 109
203v (195v): 110, 116, 117
203v-4r (195v-6r): 111
204r (196r): 112, 118
204r-v (196r-v): 113
204r / 207r (196v-7r): 114
207r-v (197r-v): 115
207v (197v): 106, 107
208r (198r): 108, 119, 120, 121, 122
208v (198v): 123, 124
209r (199r): 125, 135
251v-2r (240v-41r): 102

321r (311r): 126
324r (313r$^{bis}$): 132

AOM 323 (for 1385/6–86/7)

153r (145r): 141
153v-4r (145v-6r): 140
154r-5v (146r-7v): 143
155v-6r (147v-8r): 144
156r-v (148r-v): 142
156v (148v): 137, 138
157r (149r): 139, 147, 148
157v (149v): 136
158r (150r): 158
236v (226v): 156

AOM 324 (for 1389/90–90/91)

109r (100r): 160
109r-v (100r-v): 159
109v (100v): 161, 163
110r (101r): 162, 164, 165
110r-11v (101r-2v): 166

AOM 325 (for 1391/2)

134r-v (140r-v): 172
134v (140v): 171
134v-5r (140v-41r): 173
169v (175v): 168, 169
180r-81r (186r-87r): 170

AOM 326 (for 1392/3)

114r (106r): 174

AOM 327 (for 1393/4)

103r (92r): 175, 176
103r-v (92r-v): 177
104r (93r): 178

AOM 328 (for 1394/5)

132r (130r): 179, 180
132v-3r (130v-31r): 181

133r-v (131r-v): 182
133v-4r (131v-2r): 183
134r-v (132r-v): 184
134v (132v): 185

AOM 329 (for 1395/6–96/7)

–

AOM 330 (for 1399/1400–1400/1)

81r (82r): 186, 187
81r-v (82r-v): 188
81v (82v): 189, 190

AOM 331 (for 1401/2)

120r (120r): 191, 192, 194
173v (174v): 193, 198
174r (175r): 195, 197
175r (176r): 196

AOM 332 (for 1402/3–3/4)

120r (120r): 199, 200
120v (120v): 201

AOM 333 (for 1404/5–6/7)

80r (80r): 202
80r-v (80r-v): 203
80v (80v): 204, 205, 206, 207
81r (81r): 208

AOM 334 (for 1407/8–8/9)

113r (112r): 209, 210, 211
113v (112v): 212
114v (113v): 213, 214, 215, 216, 217, 218, 219
115r (114r): 221, 222
115r-v (114r-v): 223
115v (114v): 224
174v (172v): 220

AOM 335 (for 1409/10)

117r (118r): 225, 226
117v-18r (118v-19v): 227
118v (119v): 228
137r-8r (138r-9r): 229
138v (139v): 230
138v-9r (139v-40r): 231

AOM 336 (for 1410/11)

142r (142r): 234
142v (142v): 238
142v-3r (142v-3r): 239
143r-v (143r-v): 240
144v-5r (144v-5r): 242
145r-6v (145r-6v): 243
146v-7v (146v-7v): 235
147v-8v (147v-8v): 236
148v-9r (148v-9r): 237

AOM 337 (for 1409/10–16/17), the Master in the West

26r (77r): 269, 288
35r (86r): 278

AOM 338 (for 1413/14–15/16), the Master in the West

140r (140r): 270, 271
140r-41v (140–41v): 272
141v (141v): 273
141v-2r (141v-2r): 274
142r (142r): 275
142v (142v): 277
142v-3r (142v-3r): 280
143r-v (143r-v): 281
144r-v (144r-v): 282
144ar (144r): 286
144av (144v): 289
144av-5r (144v-5r): 287
145r (145r): 290
145v-6r (145v-6r): 291
146r (146r): 293, 294
146v (146v): 299

147r-v (147r-v): 300
147v-8r (147v-8r): 301
148r-9v (148r-9v): 302
149v (149v): 303
150r (150r): 295, 296, 297, 305
150v (150v): 305
150v-51r (150v-51r): 306
151r (151r): 307, 308
162r-v (162r-v): 292

AOM 339 (for 1409/10–16/17), the Lieutenant and Convent on Rhodes

153v (no old fol.): 310
155r (130r): 249
155r-v (130r-v): 253
155v-6r (130v-31r): 252
156r (132r): 263
156r-v (131r-v): 261
156v-7r (131v-2r): 262
157v (132v): 264
158r (133r): 259
158v (133v): 283
159r (134r): 298, 309
159v (159v): 309
173r-v (148r-v): 246
180r (155r): 260
181v (156v): 254
185r (160r): 268
186r-v (161r-v): 276
192v (no old fol.): 304
203r-v (170r-v): 247
204r (171r): 248
207r-v (174r-v): 255
207v (174v): 256
207v-8r (174v-5r): 257
215r (181r): 265, 266
216v (182v): 267
217r (183r): 279
219r (185r): 284, 285
232v (198v): 232
233r (199r): 233
236r (202r): 245
254r (220r): 243, 244

258r-v (224r-v): 250
260r-v (226r-v): 251
276r (no old fol.): 258

AOM 340 (for 1416/17–17/18), only old fol.

130r: 311, 312
130v: 313
130v-31r: 314
131r-v: 317
131v-4r: 318
134r: 319, 320, 321, 322
134v: 315, 316, 323
135r: 324, 326
137v-8r: 326
138r-v: 327
138v: 326, 328
138v-9r: 329
139r: 331
139v: 332
140r: 333
140v-41r: 334
141r-v: 335
141v: 336, 337
141v-2r: 339
142r-v: 338
143r: 341, 342
143v: 343
143v-4r: 344
144r-v: 346
144v: 349, 351, 352, 353
169v-70r: 348
170v: 352, 353
171r: 354, 355, 356

AOM 341 (for 1416/17–17/18), only old fol.

140r: 312, 325
140v: 330
140v-41r: 340
141r: 345, 347
141v: 350
142r: 357

AOM 342 (for 1418/19–19/20)

17v-18r (17v-18r): 358
141r (141r): 358, 359
141r-v (141r-v): 360
141v (141v): 361, 362, 363
141v-2r (141v-2r): 364
142v (142v): 366, 367, 368
142v-3r (142v-3r): 370
143r-v (143r-v): 371
143v (143v): 372
144r (144r): 373
144r-v (144r-v): 375

AOM 343 (for 1418/19–20/21)

158r (141r): 365, 369

AOM 344 (for 1419/20–20/21), only old fol.

141r: 375
141v: 376

AOM 345 (for 1420/21)

57r-v (57r-v): 399
139r (140r): 377, 378
139r-v (140r-v): 382
139v-40r (140v-41r): 380
140r (141r): 383, 384
140v-41r (141v-2r): 387
141r (142r): 388
141v (142v): 385, 386
141v-2r (142v-3r): 381
142v (143v): 396
142v-3r (143v-4r): 395
143r-v (144r-v): 389
143v (144v): 379, 390
143v-4r (144v-5r): 394
144v (145v): 391, 392, 393, 397, 398
164v-7v (165v-8v): 379
183r (185r): 399
223r (226r): 399

AOM 346 (for 1421/22–22/3), only old fol.

122r: 400
122r-v: 401, 402
122v: 402, 403, 404
122v-3r: 405
123r-4r: 407
123v-4r: 408
124v: 409, 410
125r: 411
125r-v: 412
125v: 414
125v-6r: 413
126r: 415
162r-v: 401

AOM 347 (for 1427/8–28/9)

134r (132r): 416, 417, 418
134v (132v): 420
135v (133v): 422
136r (134r): 419, 421

AOM 348 (for 1428/9)

124r (122r): 424
124r-v (122r-v): 428
124v-5r (122v-3r): 423
125r (123r): 433, 434
125v-6r (123v-4r): 425
126r (124r): 431
126v-8v (124v-6v): 427
127v (125v): 426, 436
128v (126v): 429
129r (127r): 430, 432, 437, 438, 439, 440, 441, 442, 444, 445
129v (127v): 443, 447
130r (128r): 435
130r-v (128r-v): 446
130v-31r (128v-9r): 448
131r (129r): 454
131v (129v): 456
131v-2r (129v-30r): 450
132r (130r): 459
132v (130v): 451, 452, 458

133r (131r): 449, 455, 457, 460
238v-9v (233v-4v): 453

AOM 371 (for 1461/2), here only for Brandenburg

135r-v (133r-v): 461
s137r (135r): 462

# WORKS CITED


Ahn, Sang-Joon, *Die Kölner Johanniterkommende Sankt Johann und Cordula im Spätmittelalter. Geschichte, Besitz, Wirtschaft, Verwaltung und Sozialstruktur*, Kölner Schriften zu Geschichte und Kultur 28 (Cologne, 2006).

*Augenzeuge des Konstanzer Konzils. Die Chronik des Ulrich Richental. Die Konstanzer Handschrift ins Neuhochdeutsche übersetzt von Monika Küble und Henry Gerlach*. Mit einem Nachwort von Jürgen Klöckler (Darmstadt, 2014).

Bonneaud, Pierre, 'La règle de l'*ancianitas* dans l'ordre de l'Hôpital, le prieuré de Catalogne et la *Castellania de Amposta* aux XIVe et XVe siècles', *The Hospitallers, the Mediterranean and Europe* (2007), 221–32.

Borchardt, Karl, *Die geistlichen Institutionen in der Reichsstadt Rothenburg ob der Tauber und dem zugehörigen Landgebiet von den Anfängen bis zur Reformation*, Veröffentlichungen der Gesellschaft für fränkische Geschichte IX/37, 2 parts (Neustadt/Aisch, 1988).

——— 'The Hospitallers in Pomerania: Between the Priories of Bohemia and Alamania', *The Military Orders*, vol. 2: *Welfare and Warfare*, ed. Helen Nicholson (Aldershot, 1998), 295–306.

——— 'The Hospitallers, Bohemia, and the Empire, 1250–1330', *Mendicants, Military Orders and Regionalism in Medieval Europe*, ed. Jürgen Sarnowsky (Aldershot, 1999), 201–31.

——— 'Wirtschaft und Ordensreform im späten Mittelalter: Das Beispiel der Johanniter in Straßburg (mit Ausblick auf Breslau)', *Die Ritterorden in der europäischen Wirtschaft des Mittelalters*, ed. Roman Czaja and Jürgen Sarnowsky, Ordines Militares: Colloquia Torunensia Historica 12 (Toruń, 2003), 35–53.

——— 'Soll-Zahlen zum Personalstand der deutschen Johanniter vom Jahre 1367', *Revue Mabillon* 75 n.s. 14 (2003), 83–113.

——— and Anthony Luttrell, 'Die päpstlichen Enquêten zum Johanniterorden in Lage und Wietersheim (Priorat *Alamania*) vom Jahre 1373', *Deutsches Archiv für Erforschung des Mittelalters* 69 (2013), 615–38.

Bosio, Giacomo, *Dell'Istoria della sacra religione et illustrissima militia di San Giovanni Gierosolimitano*, 3 vols., here vol. 2 (Rome, [2]1629 [[1]1594]).

*Brandenburgisches Klosterbuch. Handbuch der Klöster, Stifte und Kommenden bis zur Mitte des 16. Jahrhunderts*, ed. Heinz-Dieter Heimann, Klaus Neitmann, Winfried Schich, 2 vols., Brandenburgische Historische Studien 14 (Berlin, 2007).

von Bruch, Rudolf, *Die Rittersitze des Fürstentums Osnabrück* (Osnabrück, 1982).

Buchheit, Nicolas, *Les commanderies hospitalières. Réseaux et territoires en Basse-Alsace XIIIe – XIVe siècles*, CTHS Historie 55 (Paris, 2014).

——— 'Strasbourg et les Hospitaliers de Saint-Jean de Jérusalem au XIVe siècle: histoire d'une intégration urbaine', *Les ordres religieux militaires dans la ville médiévale (1100–1350)*, ed. Damien Carraz (Clermont-Ferrand, 2014), 189–204.

Bühler, Hans, *Geschichte der Johanniterkomturei Tobel*, Thurgauische Beiträge zur vaterländischen Geschichte 122 (Frauenfeld, 1985), 5–312.

Burmeister, Karl-Heinz, 'Die Komture des Johanniterhauses zu Feldkirch', *Montfort*, Heft 2 (1969), 185–227.

Büttner, Bengt, *Die Pfarreien der Insel Rügen. Von der Christianisierung bis zur Reformation*, Veröffentlichungen der Historischen Kommission für Pommern 42 (Cologne, 2007).

*Cartulaire générale de l'Ordre des Hospitaliers de S. Jean de Jérusalem 1100–1310*, ed. Joseph Delaville LeRoulx, 4 vols. (Paris, 1894/1906).

*Catalogue of the Records of the Order of St. John of Jerusalem in the Royal* [later: *National*] *Malta Library*, ed. Joseph Mizzi, Antonio Zammit-Gabarretta, Vincent Borg and Francis Azzopardi, vol. 1: Archives 1–72, 2.1: Archives 73–83, 2.2: Archives 84–87, 2.3: Archives 88–90, 2.4: Archives 91–93, 2.5: Archives 94–96, 3.1: Archives 255–260, 3.2: Archives 261–267, 3.3: Archives 268–279, 4: Archives 280–315, 7: Archives 1126–1131, 1135–1138, 1140–1143, 8: Archives 1182–1199, 10: Archives 1649–1712, 11: Archives 1713–1758, 12: Archives 1759–1934b, 13: Archives 1935–2084b (Malta, 1964/90).

*Codex Diplomaticus Maioris Poloniae. Kodeks dyplomatyczny wielkopolski*, ed. Ignacy Zakrzewski, vol. 1: 984–1287 (Poznań, 1877) [= CDMP].

*The Countryside of Hospitaller Rhodes, 1306–1423. Original Texts and English Summaries*, ed. Anthony Luttrell and Gregory O'Malley (London – New York, 2019).

Dauber, Robert L., *Der Johanniter-Malteser Orden in Österreich und Mitteleuropa: 850 Jahre gemeinsamer Geschichte*, vol. 1: Hochmittelalter (12. Jhdt. bis 1291) (Vienna, 1996); vol. 2: Spätmittelalter und frühe Neuzeit (1291 bis 1618) (Vienna, 1998).

Delaville le Roulx, Joseph, *Les Hospitaliers à Rhodes jusqu'à la mort de Philibert de Naillac, 1310–1421* (Paris, 1913, reprint London, 1974).

Dersch, Wilhelm, *Hessisches Klosterbuch. Quellenkunde zur Geschichte der im Regierungsbezirk Kassel, im Kreis Grafschaft Schaumburg, in der Provinz Oberhessen und dem Kreis Biedenkopf gegründeten Stifter, Klöster und Niederlassungen von geistlichen Genossenschaften*, Veröffentlichungen der Historischen Kommission für Hessen und Waldeck 12 (Marburg, [2]1940 [[1]1915]).

Dertsch, Richard, *Die Urkunden des Stadtarchivs Mainz: Regesten*, 4 vols., Beiträge zur Geschichte der Stadt Mainz 20 (Mainz, 1962/67).

*Diplomatarium Danicum*, series 3, ed. Carl Andreas Christensen, vol. 3: 1348–1352 (Copenhagen, 1963).

Dobronić, Lelja, *Posjedi i Sjedišta Templara, Ivanovaca i Sepulkralaca u Horvatskoj* (Zagreb, 1984).

*Documents concerning Cyprus from the Hospital's Rhodian Archives: 1409–1459*, ed. Karl Borchardt, Anthony Luttrell and Ekhard Schöffler, Cyprus Research Centre: Texts and Studies in the History of Cyprus 66 (Nicosia, 2011).

Dörr, Hans, *Mosbach und seine Johanniterkirche: Chronik der Pfarrei Mosbach* (Pfungstadt, 1983).

Engel, Wilhelm, 'Die Krise der Ballei Franken des Johanniterordens zur Mitte des 14. Jahrhunderts', *Zeitschrift für Bayerische Landesgeschichte* 18 (1955), 279–90.

*Estatutos de la Orden de San Juan de Jerusalén: Edición crítica de los manuscritos occitanos (s. XIV)*, ed. Marie-Rose Bonnet and Ricardo Ciérbide Martinena (Bilbao, 2006).

Eubel, Konrad, *Hierarchia catholica medii aevi*, vol. 1: Ab anno 1198 usque ad annum 1431 perducta, ed. Ludwig Schmitz-Kallenberg (Münster/Westfalen, [2]1913 [[1]1898]).

*Europäische Stammtafeln. Neue Folge*, ed. Detlev Schwennicke. Vol. I/3: Die Häuser Oldenburg, Mecklenburg, Schwarzburg, Waldeck, Lippe und Reuß (Marburg, ²2000); Vol. III/1: Herzogs- und Grafenhäuser des Heiligen Römischen Reiches. Andere europäische Fürstenhäuser (Marburg, 1984).

Füßlein, Wilhelm, *Berthold VII., Graf von Henneberg. Ein Beitrag zur Reichsgeschichte des 14. Jahrhunderts. Mit einem Urkundenanhang* (Altenburg, 1905); *Um den bisher unveröffentlichten 2. Teil erweiterter Nachdruck* (Cologne, 1983).

Gahlbeck, Christian, 'Adlige Netzwerke in der mittelalterlichen Ballei Brandenburg des Johanniterordens', *Ordines Militares* 20 (2015), 65–101.

——— 'Strukturreform um der Wirtschaftlichkeit willen? Die Ballei Brandenburg der Johanniter unter Hermann von Warberg nach 1350', *Jahrbuch für die Geschichte Mittel- und Ostdeutschlands* 62 (2016), 97–134.

Gąsiorowski, Antoni, 'Najstarsze dokumenty poznańskiego domu joannitów', *Studia Żródłoznawcz* 8 (1963), 83–95.

*Die geistlichen Ritterorden in Mitteleuropa: Mittelalter*, ed. Karl Borchardt and Libor Jan, Zeme a kultura ve Strední Evrope 20 (Brno, 2011).

von Gierke, Otto, *Das deutsche Genossenschaftsrecht*, vol. 4: Die Staats- und Korporationslehre der Neuzeit durchgeführt bis zur Mitte des siebzehnten, für das Naturrecht bis zum Beginn des neunzehnten Jahrhunderts (Berlin, 1913).

Hartmann, Helmut, 'Die Komture der Mainzer Johanniterkommende', *Mainzer Zeitschrift* 76 (1981), 103–24.

Hatt Olsen, Thomas, *Dacia og Rhodos. En studie over forholdet mellem Johannitterstormesteren på Rhodos og prioratet Dacia i de 14. og 15. århundrede med saerligt henblik på Juan de Carduna's visitation (–1476)* (Copenhagen, 1962).

Hecht, Winfried, *Die Johanniterkommende Rottweil*, Veröffentlichungen des Stadtarchivs Rottweil 2 (Rottweil, 1971).

*Helvetia Sacra 4/7: Die Johanniter, die Templer, der Deutsche Orden, die Lazariter und Lazariterinnen, die Pauliner und die Serviten in der Schweiz*, ed. Petra Zimmer and Patrick Braun, 2 vols. (Basel, 2006).

Hoh, Josef, 'Die Komture der Johanniterkommende Würzburg', *Würzburger Diözesangeschichtsblätter* 11/12 (1950), 113–26.

*The Hospitallers, the Mediterranean and Europe. Festschrift for Anthony Luttrell*, ed. Karl Borchardt, Nikolas Jaspert and Helen J. Nicholson (Aldershot, 2007).

Hubatsch, Walther, 'Der Johanniterorden in Ost- und Westpreußen', *Zeitschrift für Ostforschung* 21 (1972), 1–19.

Hunyadi, Zsolt, *The Hospitallers in the Medieval Kingdom of Hungary, c. 1150–1387*, METEM-Könyvek 70, CEU Medievalia 13 (Budapest, 2010).

Jan, Libor, and Vít Jesenský, 'Hospitaller and Templar Commanderies in Bohemia and Moravia: their Structure and Architectural Forms', *The Military Orders*, vol. 2: *Welfare and Warfare*, ed. Helen Nicholson (Aldershot, 1998), 235–49.

*Jean XXII (1316–1334). Lettres communes analysées d'après les registres dits d'Avignon et du Vatican*, vol. 1, ed. Guillaume Mollat (Paris, 1904).

King, Edwin James, *The Rule, Statutes, and Customs of the Hospitallers, 1099–1310* (London, 1934; reprint New York, 1981).

Klein, Walter Karl, *Die Ausbreitung des Johanniterordens in Oberdeutschland bis zum Jahre 1317*, PhD (Freiburg/Br., 1922) [manuscript].

Koorn, Florence (†) and Johannes A. Mol, 'Netwerken voor het Heilige Land. Jacob van Zuden en de expansie van de johannieters in het bisdom Utrecht', *Jaarboek voor middeleeuwse geschiedenis* 12 (2009), 146–74.

——— 'Jacob van Zuden and the Early Fourteenth-Century Expansion of the Hospitallers in the Bishopric of Utrecht', *Crusades* 14 (2015), 183–207.

Krieger, Albert, *Topographisches Wörterbuch des Großherzogtums Baden*, 2 vols. (Heidelberg, [2]1904/05).

Kürten, Peter, *Das Stift St. Kunibert in Köln von der Gründung bis zum Jahre 1453*. Kölner Schriften zu Geschichte und Kultur 10 (Cologne, 1985).

Lagleder, Gerhard Tonque, *Die Ordensregel der Johanniter/Malteser: Die geistlichen Ritterorden des Johanniter-/Malteserordens, mit einer Edition und Übersetzung der drei ältesten Regelhandschriften* (St. Ottilien, 1983).

Lascurain Bernstorff, Ignacio Garcia, *Die Athleten und der Vikar Christi: Eine Untersuchung zur Semantik der Beziehung zwischen dem Johanniterorden und dem Heiligen Stuhl zwischen Mittelalter und Früher Neuzeit (1393–1503)*, PhD (Munich, 2019) [manuscript].

Lechner, Karl, *Die Kommende Mailberg*, Schriftenreihe des Maltesermuseums Mailberg 3 (Mailberg, 1976).

Legras, Anne-Marie (ed.), *L'enquête pontificale de 1373 sur l'ordre des Hospitaliers de Saint-Jean-de-Jérusalem*. Part 1: L'enquête dans le prieuré de France (Paris, 1987).

Lehmann, Hans, *Das Johanniterhaus Bubikon: Geschichte, Baugeschichte und Kunstdenkmäler*, Mitteilungen der Antiquarischen Gesellschaft in Zürich, 35 Heft 1–3 (Zürich, 1945/7).

Lindenhayn-Fiedorowicz, Agnieszka, 'Johannitisches Patronat und städtische Architektur: die Marienkirche zu Stargard (Stargard Szczecinski) in Pommern', *Regionalität und Transfergeschichte* (2014), 248–70.

Longo, Antonio, *Dell'origine e provenienza in Venezia de' cittadini originari* (Venice, 1817).

Luttrell, Anthony, *The Hospitallers in Cyprus, Rhodes, Greece and the West, 1291–1440* (London, 1978).

——— 'The Later History of the Maussolleion and its Utilization in the Hospitaller Castle at Bodrum', *The Maussolleion at Halikarnassos. Reports of the Danish Archaeological expedition to Bodrum*, vol. 2: The Written Sources and their Archaeological Background, Jutland Archaeological Society Publications 15 (Aarhus, 1986), 114–214.

——— *The Hospitallers of Rhodes and their Mediterranean World* (Aldershot, 1992).

——— *The Hospitaller State on Rhodes and its Western Provinces, 1306–1462* (Aldershot, 1999).

———*The Town of Rhodes, 1306–1356* (Rhodes, 2003).

——— *Studies on the Hospitallers after 1306. Rhodes and the West*, Variorum Collected Studies 874 (Aldershot, 2007).

——— and Elizabeth A. Zachariadou, *Sources for Turkish History in the Hospitallers' Rhodian Archive, 1389–1422* (Athens, 2008).

——— 'The Templars' Archives in Syria and Cyprus', *The Templars and Their Sources* (2017), 38–45.

——— 'Shared Worship at Filerimos on Hospitaller Rhodes 1306–1421', *The Templars, the Hospitallers and the Crusades, Essays in Homage to Alan J. Forey*, ed. Helen J. Nicholson and Jochen Burgtorf (Abingdon – New York, 2020), 116–26.

Mager, Mathis, *Krisenerfahrung und Bewältigungsstrategien des Johanniterordens nach der Eroberung von Rhodos 1522* (Münster/Westfalen, 2014).

Maurer, Bernhard, *Die Johanniter im Breisgau: Aus Geschichte und Gegenwart des Johanniter- und Malteserordens am Oberrhein* (Freiburg/Br., 1978).

Militzer, Klaus, *Die Entstehung der Deutschordensballeien im Deutschen Reich*, Quellen und Studien zur Geschichte des Deutschen Ordens 16 (Bonn, 1970).

——— 'Der Deutsche Orden in seinen Balleien im Deutschen Reich', *Die geistlichen Ritterorden in Mitteleuropa* (2011), 201–14.

Mitáček, Jiři, 'Ziemovit Těšínsky – generální převor řádu johnitů a slezský kníže', *Sborník prací filozofiké fakulty Brnenské univerzity, řada historická* C 46 (1999), 17–40.

——— *Česká provincie řádu sv. Jana Jeruzalémského za vlády Lucemburků (1310–1419)*, PhD (Brno, 2005) [manuscript].

Mol, Johannes Adriaan, 'Die Johanniterklöster im mittelalterlichen Friesland', *Die Johanniterkommende in Bokelesch*, ed. Piotr Piotrowski (Oldenburg, 2005), 9–44.

——— 'The Hospitaller Sisters in Frisia', *Hospitaller Women in the Middle Ages*, ed. Anthony Luttrell and Helen Nicholson (Aldershot, 2006), 179–208.

——— 'Die friesischen Johanniterklöster im Mittelalter', *Zur Geschichte des Johanniterordens im friesischen Küstenraum und anschließenden Binnenland. Beiträge des Johanniter-Symposiums vom 11. bis 12. Mai 2007 in Cloppenburg-Stapelfeld*, ed. Hajo van Lengen (Cloppenburg, 2008), 42–65.

*Monumenta Hohenbergica. Urkundenbuch zur Geschichte der Grafen von Zollern-Hohenberg und ihrer Grafschaft*, ed. Ludwig Schmid (Stuttgart, 1862).

Nisbet, James E., 'Treasury Records of the Knights of St. John in Rhodes', *Melita historica* n. s. 2 (1957), 95–104.

Novotný, Václav (ed.), *Inquisitio domorum hospitalis S. Johannis Hierosolimitani per Pragensem archidioecesim facta anno 1373*, Historický Archiv 19 (Prague, 1900).

Nyberg, Tore, 'Zur Rolle der Johanniter in Skandinavien: Erstes Auftreten und Aufbau der Institutionen', *Die Rolle der Ritterorden in der mittelalterlichen Kultur*, ed. Zenon H. Nowak (Toruń, 1985), 129–44.

Opgenoorth, Ernst, *Die Ballei Brandenburg des Johanniterordens im Zeitalter der Reformation und Gegenreformation*, Beihefte zum Jahrbuch der Albertus-Universität Königsberg/Preußen 14 (Würzburg, 1963).

von Osterhausen, Christian, *Eigentlicher und gründlicher Bericht dessen was zu einer vollkommenen Erkenntnis des hochlöblichen Ritterordens vom hl. Johannes von Jerusalem zu Malta vonnöten* (Augsburg, 1650).

Ożóg, Krzysztof, 'Udział Andrzeja Łaskarzyca w sprawach i sporach polsko-krzyżackich do soboru w Konstancji', *Polska i jej sasiedzi w póznym średniowieczu*, ed. Stanisław Szczur (Kraków, 2000), 159-186.

de Palma, Luigi Michele, *Il consiglio e le costituzioni di fra' Lionardo Bonafedi per le Giovannite di Firenze (14. sec.)* (Bari, 2010).

Paoli, Sebastiano, *Codice diplomatico del sacro militare ordine Gerosolimitano, oggi di Malta*, 2 vols. (Lucca, 1733/37).

von Pflugk-Harttung, Julius, *Der Johanniter- und der Deutsche Orden im Kampfe Ludwigs des Bayern mit der Kurie* (Leipzig, 1900).

*Prier et combattre. Dictionnaire européen des ordres militaires au Moyen Âge*, ed. Nicole Bériou and Philippe Josserand (Paris, 2009).

Prutz, Hans, 'Malteser Studien', *Archivalische Zeitschrift* 8 (1883), 63–105.

Regelmeier, Bernhard, 'Die Johanniterkommende zu Steinfurt', *Zeitschrift für vaterländische Geschichte und Altertumskunde* 69/1 (1911), 367–402.

*Regionalität und Transfergeschichte: Ritterorden-Kommenden der Templer und Johanniter im nordöstlichen Deutschland und in Polen seit dem Mittelalter*, ed. Christian Gahlbeck, Heinz-Dieter Heimann and Dirk Schumann, Studien zur brandenburgischen und vergleichenden Landesgeschichte 9, Schriften der Landesgeschichtlichen Vereinigung für die Mark Brandenburg n.s. 4 (Berlin, 2014).

Reitzel-Nielsen, Erik. *Johanniterordens historie med saerligt henblik på de nordiske land*. Vol. 1: Tiden før Rhodos. Vol. 2: Rhodos og Malta (1309–1798) (Copenhagen, 1984/88).

*Repertorium Germanicum: Verzeichnis der in den päpstlichen Registern und Kameralakten vorkommenden Personen, Kirchen und Orte des Deutschen Reiches, seiner Diözesen und Territorien vom Beginn des Schismas bis zur Reformation*, vol. 2: Urban VI. – Bonifaz IX. – Innozenz VII. – Gregor XII. 1378–1415, ed. Gerd Tellenbach (Berlin, 1933/38; reprint 1961).

Rödel, Walter Gerd, *Das Großpriorat Deutschland des Johanniter-Ordens im Übergang vom Mittelalter zur Reformation anhand der Generalvisitationsberichte von 1494/95 und 1540/41* (Cologne, [2]1972) [Mainz, [1]1966].

———, 'Die Johanniterkommende Heimbach in der Pfalz und ihre Membra: Beiträge zu ihrer Geschichte', *Blätter für pfälzische Kirchengeschichte und religiöse Volkskunde* 40 (1973), 5–55.

Roger, Jean-Marc, *Nouveaux regards sur les monuments des hospitaliers à Rhodes*, II: Les auberges, le baillage du commerce, la maison de F. Hieronimo de Canel (Poitiers, 2010).

Ruppert, Philipp, 'Verzeichnuß aller in Gott ruhenden Personen bei dem Gottshaus S. Johann in Dem Breisgau', *Freiburger Diöcesan-Archiv* 20 (1889), 293–8.

Sarnowsky, Jürgen, *Macht und Herrschaft im Johanniterorden des 15. Jahrhunderts. Verfassung und Verwaltung der Johanniter auf Rhodos (1421–1522)*, Vita regularis 14 (Münster/Westfalen, 2001).

——— 'Konvent, Priorat, Region. Die Johanniter auf Rhodos und die Ballei Brandenburg im Spätmittelalter, 1306–1522', *Jahrbuch für Berlin-Brandenburgische Kirchengeschichte* 63 (2001), 37–50.

——— 'Die mittelalterliche Ballei Brandenburg der Johanniter: Rezeption und Wirklichkeit', *Vergangenheit und Gegenwart der Ritterorden. Die Rezeption der Idee und die Wirklichkeit*, ed. Zenon Hubert Nowak and Roman Czaja, Ordines militares 11 (Toruń, 2001), 165–82.

Sauermann, Franz, *Geschichte der Malteserkommende Glatz [1183–1627], I. Teil: Von der Gründung bis zur Husitenzeit[!]*, Wissenschaftliche Beilage zum Jahresbericht des Königlichen katholischen Gymnasiums zu Glatz, Progr.-No. 261 (Glatz, 1909).

Schmid, Ludwig, *Geschichte der Grafen von Zollern-Hohenberg und ihrer Grafschaft* (Stuttgart, 1862).

Schön, Theodor, *Geschichte der Familie von Ow*, revis. and ed. Hanns Otto von Ow-Wachendorf and Anton von Ow-Felldorf (Munich, 1910).

Schöningh, Enno, *Der Johanniterorden in Ostfriesland*, Abhandlungen und Vorträge zur Geschichte Ostfrieslands 54 (Aurich, 1973).

——— 'Zur Geschichte der Johanniterballei Westfalen', *Osnabrücker Mitteilungen* 81 (1974), 178–85.

Seitz, Johann Karl, 'Die Johanniter-Priester-Komturei Freiburg i. Ü.', *Freiburger Geschichtsblätter* 17 (1910), 1–136.

——— (ed.), 'Regesten der Johanniter-Komturei Freiburg i. Ü.', ibid. 18 (1911), 1–114.

Sgonina, Marc. *Die Johanniterballei Westfalen. Unter besonderer Berücksichtigung der Lebensformen der Zentralkommende Steinfurt und ihrer Membra* (Frankfurt/Main, 2014).

Smoliński, Marek, *Joannici w polityce książąt polskich i pomorskich od połowy pierwszego XII do ćwierćwiecza XIV wieku* (Gdánsk, 2008).

Spufford, Peter, *Handbook of Medieval Exchange*, Guides and Handbooks, Royal Historical Society 13 (London, 1986).

Svátek, Josef, 'Organizace řeholních institucí v českých zemích a péče o jejich archivy, Číslo 2', *Sborník archivních prací* 20 (1970), 505–624.

*Stabilimenta Rhodiorum militum. Die Statuten des Johanniterordens von 1489/93*, ed. Jyri Hasecker and Jürgen Sarnowsky, Nova Mediaevalia. Quellen und Studien zum europäischen Mittelalter 1 (Göttingen, 2007).

Stälin, Paul Friedrich, 'Komthure des Johanniter-Ordens im Gebiet des jetzigen Königreichs Württemberg', *Archivalische Zeitschrift* 8 (1883), 106–11.

Starnawska, Maria, *Między Jerozolimą a Łukowem: Zakony krzyżowe na ziemiach polskich w średniowieczu* (Warsaw, 1999).

——— 'Die Urkunden des Siemowit von Teschen, Komtur in Klein-Oels (ca. 1360–1372) und (Groß)Prior von Böhmen (1372–1390)', *Die geistlichen Ritterorden in Mitteleuropa* (2011), 273–86.

Szczesniak, Boleslaw B., *The Knights Hospitallers in Poland and Lithuania*, Studies in European History 19 (The Hague – Paris, 1969).

*The Templars and Their Sources*, ed. Karl Borchardt, Karoline D. Döring, Philippe Josserand and Helen J. Nicholson, Crusades, Subsidia 10 (London, 2017).

Thomas, Ulrich, *Die Johanniterkomture in Mainfranken: Von den Anfängen bis zum Jahre 1500*, M.A. thesis (Würzburg, 1990) [manuscript].

Tipton, Charles L., 'The 1330 Chapter General of the Knights Hospitallers at Montpellier', *Traditio* 24 (1968), 293–308.

*Die Urkunden der Stadt Neuenburg am Rhein*, 2 parts, ed. Jörg W. Busch and Jürgen Treffeisen (Neuenburg am Rhein, 2019).

Vertôt, René Aubert de, *Historie des Chevaliers hospitaliers de Saint-Jean de Jérusalem, appelés depuis les Chevaliers de Rhodes et aujourd'hui les Chevaliers de Malte*, 5 vols. (Paris 1726). 16th ed. (Lyon, 1959).

Waldstein-Wartenberg, Berthold, *Rechtsgeschichte des Malteserordens* (Vienna – Munich, 1969).

Wienand, Adam (ed.) in association with Carl Wolfgang Graf von Ballestrem and Christoph Freiherr von Imhoff, *Der Johanniter-Orden, Der Malteser-Orden: Der ritterliche Orden des hl. Johannes vom Spital zu Jerusalem, seine Aufgaben, seine Geschichte* (Cologne, [2]1988 [[1]1970]).

van Winter, Johanna Maria, *Sources concerning the Hospitallers of St John in the Netherlands, 14th–18th Centuries*, Studies in the History of Christian Thought 80 (Leiden – Boston – Cologne, 1998).

von Winterfeld, Adolf-Wilhelm Ernst, *Geschichte des ritterlichen Ordens St. Johannis vom Spital zu Jerusalem, mit besonderer Berücksichtigung der Ballei Brandenburg* (Berlin, 1859).

Wunder, Gerd, *Die Schenken von Stauffenberg. Eine Familiengeschichte*, Schriften zur südwestdeutschen Landeskunde 11 (Stuttgart, 1972).

*Württembergische Regesten von 1301 bis 1500: Altwürttemberg*, ed. Württembergisches Hauptstaatsarchiv in Stuttgart, 3 vols. Urkunden und Akten des Württembergischen Staatsarchivs (Stuttgart, 1916/64).

Wyss, Gottlieb, 'Das Basler Ritterordenshaus St. Johann und die Stadt Basel', *Basler Zeitschrift für Geschichte und Altertumskunde* 37 (1938), 169–93.

Zeininger de Borja, Henri-Charles, 'L'Ordre de S. Jean et la Suisse', *Zeitschrift für Schweizer Kirchengeschichte* 40 (1946), 213–34, 269–310.

Ziegler, Peter, *Die Johanniterkomturei Wädenswil 1287–1550* (Wädenswil, 1987).

# INDEX

Note: The index includes persons, places and select offices. Arabic numerals refer to the numbers of the documents, Roman numerals to the pages of the introduction. For the names, English forms are used whenever possible, especially for well-known places and persons. If they are lacking, German forms are used, followed from Czech, Dutch, French, Polish and occasionally other languages. For the alphabetical order the various forms of de, la, le, van, von or z are ignored, e. g. von Montfort is under M. Abbreviations: d. died, n. footnote, r. reigned.

For Product Safety Concerns and Information please contact our EU
representative GPSR@taylorandfrancis.com
Taylor & Francis Verlag GmbH, Kaufingerstraße 24, 80331 München, Germany

www.ingramcontent.com/pod-product-compliance
Ingram Content Group UK Ltd.
Pitfield, Milton Keynes, MK11 3LW, UK
UKHW022006180926
475701UK00003B/217

* 9 7 8 0 3 6 7 6 3 3 7 2 1 *